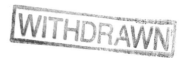
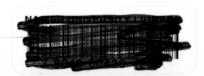

Clinical
Gerontological
Nursing

Clinical
Gerontological
Nursing

A GUIDE TO ADVANCED PRACTICE

Second Edition

Joyce Takano Stone, MS, RNC
Formerly Clinical Nurse Specialist, Gerontology
Department of Veterans Affairs Medical Center
Clinical Professor, Department of Physiological Nursing
School of Nursing
University of California
San Francisco, California

Jean F. Wyman, PhD, RNCS, GNP, FAAN
Professor, Cora Meidl Siehl Chair in Nursing Research
School of Nursing
University of Minnesota
Minneapolis, Minnesota

Sally A. Salisbury, MS, RNCS
Late Coordinator, Hospital Based Home Care
Department of Veterans Affairs Medical Center
Assistant Clinical Professor, Department of Physiological Nursing
School of Nursing
University of California
San Francisco, California

W.B. SAUNDERS COMPANY
A Division of Harcourt Brace & Company
Philadelphia London Toronto Montreal Sydney Tokyo

W.B. SAUNDERS COMPANY
A Division of Harcourt Brace & Company

The Curtis Center
Independence Square West
Philadelphia, Pennsylvania 19106

Library of Congress Cataloging-in-Publication Data

Clinical gerontological nursing: A guide to advanced practice / Joyce Takano Stone,
Jean F. Wyman, Sally A. Salisbury.—2nd ed.

p.   cm.

Rev. ed. of: Clinical gerontological nursing / W. Carole Chenitz, Joyce Takano Stone,
Sally A. Salisbury. 1991.

ISBN 0–7216–5918–7

1. Geriatric nursing.   I. Wyman, Jean Frances.   II. Salisbury, Sally A.
    III. Chenitz, W. Carole—Clinical gerontological nursing.   IV. Title.
    [DNLM: 1. Geriatric Nursing.   WY 152 S878c   1999]

RC954.C457, 1999   610.73'65—dc21

DNLM/DLC   98–12903

CLINICAL GERONTOLOGICAL NURSING:
A Guide to Advanced Practice   ISBN 0–7216–5918–7

Printed in the United States of America.

Last digit is the print number: 9   8   7   6   5   4   3   2   1

To our parents,
Josephine Yetsuko Takano, the late Tsugio Takano, Ruth Julstrom Wyman,
and the late George J. Wyman,
who encouraged and supported all our endeavors;
and to our husbands,
Ronald K. Stone and James W. Begun,
whose sacrifices, understanding, and support enabled us to complete this book.

To our elderly patients
who have shared their life experiences and have taught us about growing old.

To the memory of
W. Carole Chenitz, EdD, RN, and Sally A. Salisbury, MS, RNCS,
our colleagues,
who will never experience the joys and sorrows of old age.

Reviewers

Lynda C. Abusamra, PhD, RNCS
College of Nursing
East Tennessee State University
Johnson City, Tennessee

Sharon L. Carlson, MS, RN
School of Nursing
Otterbein College
Westerville, Ohio

Judith Conway, MS, APRN, CS
Hartford Hospital
Hartford, Connecticut

Karen J. Karner, EdD, RNCS
School of Nursing
East Stroudsburg University
East Stroudsburg, Pennsylvania

Patricia A. O'Neill, MSN, CCRN
School of Nursing
DeAnza College
Cupertino, California

Mary J. Waldo, MS, RN
School of Nursing
Oregon Health Sciences University
Portland, Oregon

Carla Wilhoite, PhD, RN
School of Nursing
Ball State University
Muncie, Indiana

Alice Williams, PhD, RNCS
School of Nursing
Sangamon State University
Springfield, Illinois

Ann Yurick, PhD, RNC
School of Nursing
University of Pittsburgh
Pittsburgh, Pennsylvania

Contributors

Marian L. Baxter, MS, MA, CCRN, RNCS
Rehabilitation Clinical Nurse Specialist, Physical Medicine and Rehabilitation, Hunter Holmes McGuire Department of Veterans Affairs Medical Center, Richmond, Virginia
Ethical Issues

Barbara J. Braden, PhD, RN, FAAN
Dean, Graduate School, Creighton University, Omaha, Nebraska
Pressure Sores

Barbara A. Brant, EdD, RN, CLNC
Consultant and Educator in Aging, Gerontological Nursing, and Long-Term Care; Certified Legal Nurse Consultant, Richmond, Virginia
Sensory Disorders

Kenneth Brummel-Smith, MD
Associate Professor of Family Medicine, Oregon Health Sciences University; Medical Director, Long-Term Care Division, Providence Health System, Portland, Oregon
Impaired Mobility and Deconditioning

Kathleen C. Buckwalter, PhD, RN, FAAN
Associate Provost for Health Sciences, Professor, College of Nursing; Director, Center on Aging, University of Iowa, Iowa City, Iowa
Depression

Virginia Burggraf, DNSc, RNC
Grants Development Associate, American Nurses Foundation, Washington, D.C.
Advanced Practice of Gerontological Nursing

Rebecca Lee Burrage, MSN, FNP-C
Clinical Instructor, College of Nursing, University of Utah; Nurse Practitioner, Department of Veterans Affairs Medical Center, Salt Lake City, Utah
Arthritis

Janet Cuddigan, MSN, RN
PhD Candidate, College of Nursing, University of Nebraska; Nurse Specialist, University of Nebraska Medical Center, Omaha, Nebraska
Pressure Sores

Helen D. Davies, MS, RNCS
Assistant Clinical Professor, Department of Physiological Nursing, School of Nursing, University of California, San Francisco; Psychiatric Clinical Nurse Specialist, Co-Director, Stanford/Veterans Affairs Alzheimer's Center, Veterans Affairs Health Care System, Palo Alto, California
Delirium and Dementia

Glenna A. Dowling, PhD, RN
Associate Adjunct Professor, Department of Physiological Nursing, School of Nursing; Coordinator, Parkinson's Disease Clinic and Research Center, University of California, San Francisco, California
Parkinson's Disease

Sandra J. Engberg, PhD, CRNP
Assistant Professor, School of Nursing, University of Pittsburgh, Pittsburgh, Pennsylvania
Comprehensive Geriatric Assessment

Lois K. Evans, DNSc, RN, FAAN
Professor and Director, Academic Nursing Practices, School of Nursing, University of Pennsylvania, Philadelphia, Pennsylvania
Restraint-Free Care

Kathleen Ryan Fletcher, MSN, RNCS, GNP
Assistant Professor in Patient Care Services, Department of Nursing, University of Virginia Health Sciences Center; Director, Geriatric Services, University of Virginia Health System, Charlottesville, Virginia
Physical and Laboratory Assessment

Terry T. Fulmer, PhD, RN, FAAN
Professor and Director, Center for Nursing Research, New York University; Clinical Associate in Nursing, New York University Medical Center, New York, New York
Elder Mistreatment

Linda A. Gerdner, MA, RN
PhD Candidate, College of Nursing, University of Iowa, Iowa City, Iowa
Managing Problem Behaviors

Geri Richards Hall, PhD Candidate, ARNP, CNS
Adjunct Faculty, College of Nursing, Arizona State University, Tempe; Gerontology Clinical Nurse Specialist, Department of Neurology, Mayo Clinic Scottsdale, Scottsdale, Arizona
Managing Problem Behaviors

Joyce K. Holohan-Bell, MSN, RNCS
Clinical Faculty, School of Nursing, Oregon Health Sciences University; Clinical Nurse Specialist, Gerontology, Department of Veterans Affairs Medical Center, Portland, Oregon
Impaired Mobility and Deconditioning

Mary Ann Johnson, PhD, APRN

Associate Professor Emerita, School of Nursing, University of Utah; Geriatric
Nurse Practitioner/GRECC Investigator, Department of Veterans Affairs
Medical Center/Geriatric Research Education and Clinical Center (GRECC),
Salt Lake City, Utah
  Cardiovascular Conditions

Helen Lamberta, MS, RNCS, ANP

Nurse Practitioner, Department of Orthopedic Surgery, Medical College of
Virginia Hospitals, Richmond, Virginia
  Failure to Thrive

Joan McDowell, PhD, CRNP, FAAN

Associate Professor, Family Nurse Practitioner Program, School of Nursing,
University of Pittsburgh, Pittsburgh, Pennsylvania
  Comprehensive Geriatric Assessment

Christine Miaskowski, PhD, RN, FAAN

Professor and Chair, Department of Physiological Nursing, School of Nursing,
University of California, San Francisco, California
  Pain and Discomfort

Amie Modigh, MSN, RNCS, GNP

Assistant Clinical Professor, Schools of Medicine and Nursing, Virginia
Commonwealth University, Medical College of Virginia Campus; Service Line
Associate Chief, Geriatrics and Extended Care, Hunter Holmes McGuire
Department of Veterans Affairs Medical Center, Richmond, Virginia
  Intimacy and Sexuality

Lynne Morishita, MSN, RNCS, GNP

Clinical Instructor, Department of Family Practice and Community Health,
University of Minnesota; Independent Consultant, Minneapolis, Minnesota
  Practice Models in Gerontological Nursing

Ginette A. Pepper, PhD, RN, CNS, FAAN

Assistant Professor, School of Nursing, University of Colorado Health Sciences
Center, Denver, Colorado
  Drug Use and Misuse

Linda R. Phillips, PhD, RN, FAAN

Professor and Associate Dean for Research, College of Nursing, University of
Arizona, Tucson, Arizona
  Assessment of Social Support

Mary Lynn Scotton Piven, MS, RN

Doctoral Student, College of Nursing, University of Iowa; Advanced Registered
Nurse Practitioner, University of Iowa Hospitals and Clinics, Iowa City, Iowa
  Depression

Sally A. Salisbury, MS, RNCS
Late Coordinator, Hospital Based Home Care, Department of Veterans Affairs
Medical Center; Assistant Clinical Professor, Department of Physiological
Nursing, School of Nursing, University of California, San Francisco, California
Legal Planning Issues
Cognitive Assessment
Alcoholism

Yvonne Browne Sehy, PhD, RNC, FNP/GNP
Assistant Professor, College of Nursing, University of Utah; Nurse Practitioner,
Department of Veterans Affairs Medical Center, Salt Lake City, Utah
Functional Assessment

Catherine Steinbach, MS, RN
Assistant Clinical Professor, Department of Physiological Nursing, School of
Nursing, University of California, San Francisco, California
Iatrogenesis

Joyce Takano Stone, MS, RNC
Formerly Clinical Nurse Specialist, Gerontology, Department of Veterans
Affairs Medical Center; Clinical Professor, Department of Physiological
Nursing, School of Nursing, University of California, San Francisco, California
Constipation, Diarrhea, and Fecal Incontinence
Falls
Iatrogenesis

Neville E. Strumpf, PhD, RNC, FAAN
Associate Professor and Doris Schwartz Term Chair, Director, Gerontological
Nurse Practitioner Program, Director, Center for Gerontologic Nursing Science,
School of Nursing, University of Pennsylvania, Philadelphia, Pennsylvania
Restraint-Free Care

Eileen M. Sullivan-Marx, PhD, RNCS, FAAN
Assistant Professor and Program Director, Adult Nurse Practitioner Program,
School of Nursing, University of Pennsylvania, Philadelphia, Pennsylvania
Restraint-Free Care

Cynthia A. Sutter, MS, ANP-C
Clinical Faculty, College of Nursing, University of Utah; School of Nursing,
Westminster College; Nurse Practitioner, Home-Based Primary Care,
Department of Veterans Affairs Medical Center, Salt Lake City, Utah
Arthritis

Patricia Tobin, JD
Elder Law Attorney, Prensky & Tobin, Mill Valley, California; Director, National
Academy of Elder Law Attorneys, Fellow of Academy
Legal Planning Issues

Marilyn P. Williams, MS, RN
Assistant Clinical Professor, Department of Physiological Nursing, School of
Nursing, University of California; Geriatric Clinical Nurse Specialist, Kaiser
Permanente Medical Center, San Francisco, California
Cognitive Assessment
Functional Assessment

Jean F. Wyman, PhD, RNCS, GNP, FAAN
Professor, Cora Meidl Siehl Chair in Nursing Research, School of Nursing,
University of Minnesota, Minneapolis, Minnesota
Urinary Incontinence
Constipation, Diarrhea, and Fecal Incontinence
Failure to Thrive
Falls

Preface

The purpose of the second edition of *Clinical Gerontological Nursing: A Guide to Advanced Practice* remains the same as that of the first edition: to assist gerontological nurses to fulfill their role in providing healthcare to older adults. This book is written for graduate nursing students specializing in care of the aged and for advanced practice nurses, nurse educators, and generalist nurses who work with the elderly in any healthcare environment. Extensive revisions have been made in this edition to reflect recent changes in healthcare and the current state of advanced practice nursing. Throughout this text, emphasis is placed on research-based clinical practice.

Several theoretical frameworks and practice models are presented in this book. This eclectic approach to theory both reflects the current clinical world and demonstrates the use of theory in practice. The reader does not have to embrace any specific theory or model in order to find this book useful.

There are 5 major sections and 29 chapters in this book. It is designed to be used as a reference. The material is organized so that related chapters can be read together or so the reader can choose to read only selected chapters. Extensive use is made of tables that summarize key aspects of care derived from the research literature. The references listed at the end of each chapter are representative of the research base and can be used by readers to extend their knowledge on the topic.

The second edition contains 12 new chapters. The other 17 chapters have been reorganized and updated. The sections on advanced practice nurses and their management of clinical problems, issues, and concerns have been expanded. The section on settings was deleted and setting-specific information has been integrated throughout the chapters. Twenty-five new contributors have joined us to write the second edition. The contributors are nurses engaged in clinical practice, education, and/or research; they were invited to contribute to this book because of their expertise on a specific topic. Their knowledge and experience have been combined to present this comprehensive, advanced practice textbook on gerontological nursing.

Section I presents an overview of advanced gerontological nursing practice. Trends in healthcare; models for nursing practice; roles and functions of advanced practice nurses; and the impact of financial, social, political, legal, and ethical influences on healthcare and nursing are discussed.

The five chapters in Section II focus on the assessment of the older person. An introductory chapter delineates and discusses the components of a comprehensive geriatric assessment. In the following four chapters, in-depth discussion, guidelines, and instruments for physical, cognitive, social, and functional assessments are presented.

Section III presents nursing management of common clinical problems: urinary incontinence, bowel dysfunction, impaired mobility and deconditioning, pressure sores, failure to thrive, falls, and iatrogenesis. Each chapter addresses what nurses need to know and what nurses can do or are doing about these problems. Theory and research findings relevant to each problem from nursing and other disciplines provide nurses with current information. Guidelines for interventions and protocols are included to assist nurses in the management of these problems.

Section IV consists of seven chapters concerned with nursing management of selected illnesses. Nurses in advanced practice are assuming a greater role in the management of chronic illnesses and selected conditions. To be an effective clinician, the advanced practice nurse must have an understanding of current research in pathophysiology and the treatment of health problems that are prevalent in an elderly population. The chapters in this section are organized to take into account encompassing knowledge of the health problem and the disease process; healthcare factors that impede diagnosis and treatment; and educational, supportive, and clinical nursing interventions across treatment settings. Clinical assessment questionnaires are included to facilitate accurate diagnoses. The health problems included in this section are depression, delirium and dementia, Parkinson's disease, arthritis, cardiovascular conditions, sensory disorders, and alcoholism. This section is not meant to be comprehensive and of necessity includes only selected health problems. Health problems chosen for inclusion in this section are those that may be underdiagnosed and not well understood. Each of these health problems causes functional disability that is primarily managed by the nurse.

Section V examines aspects of care that may be overlooked, inadequately addressed, or poorly managed. These areas of special concern include intimacy and sexuality, restraint-free care for the elderly, drug use and misuse, problem behaviors, pain and discomfort, and elder mistreatment. These subjects are of great importance to both the client and nurse and are presented in depth with a strong theoretical and research base. Each chapter focuses on approaches to intervention.

As stated in the preface of the first edition, knowledge is the key to advancing and changing practice. The ultimate goal of theory development and research in nursing is knowledge development to improve care. Ongoing research in nursing and other disciplines has generated new knowledge. In turn, gerontological nursing practice has continued to change and advance. We hope that the second edition will continue to foster the development of gerontological nursing knowledge and improved healthcare for older adults.

JOYCE TAKANO STONE

JEAN F. WYMAN

Acknowledgments

Many people are responsible for the existence of this book. We are grateful and take this opportunity to give special thanks:

To the staff at W.B. Saunders Company: Terri Wood, Editor; Marie Thomas, Editorial Assistant; Allison Aydelotte, Copy Editor; Jeff Gunning, Production Manager; Ellen Zanolle, Cover Designer; Bill Donnelly, Interior Designer; and Risa Clow, Illustrator, for their unique skills and assistance.

To our contributors, who enthusiastically gave of their time and knowledge to write the manuscripts that became the chapters of this book.

And thanks to our reviewers for their thoughtful critique of the chapters. We made many changes based on their suggestions.

NOTICE

Nursing is an ever-changing field. Standard safety precautions must be followed, but as new research and clinical experience broaden our knowledge, changes in treatment and drug therapy become necessary or appropriate. Readers are advised to check the product information currently provided by the manufacturer of each drug to be administered to verify the recommended dose, the method and duration of administration, and the contraindications. It is the responsibility of the treating physician, relying on experience and knowledge of the patient, to determine dosages and the best treatment for the patient. Neither the publisher nor the editor assumes any responsibility for any injury and/or damage to persons or property.

THE PUBLISHER

Contents

SECTION II
Assessment of the Older Client

SECTION III
Nursing Management of Common Clinical Problems

S E C T I O N I V
Nursing Management of Selected Illnesses

SECTION V
Special Concerns

Overview of Gerontological Nursing

CHAPTER 1

Advanced Practice of Gerontological Nursing

Virginia Burggraf

Each passing year confirms one of the great events of modern times: the triumph of survivorship. It is an event so enormous that we have no handy scale to measure it and its consequences. The increase in the absolute number and relative proportion of people over the age of 65, in our nation and around the world, has been an extraordinary historical phenomenon with fundamental social, economic, cultural, and personal consequences.

ROBERT N. BUTLER, 1981

The dramatic gains in life expectancy and the growing number of people more than 65 years of age are challenging the nursing profession and the healthcare system with an increased need for services. The demographics reveal a changing population; the elderly of tomorrow will be very different from those of today. This chapter discusses the growth of the older population and the projections anticipated into the 21st century and dispels common myths associated with aging. Advanced practice nurses (APNs) with special knowledge and skills in care of the aged will play an increasingly important role in the healthcare delivery system. This chapter also presents the *Scope and Standards of Gerontological Nursing Practice* and the *Scope and Standards of Advanced Practice Registered Nursing*, which were recently published by the American Nurses Association (ANA) and serve as a guide to practice.

THE PRESENT-DAY ELDERLY: SURVIVORS OF THE PAST

The present-day elderly—those more than 65 years of age—were born any time between the late 19th century and 1930. According to present-day standards in the United States, these years were "tough times." Older people living today experienced and survived many events in their lifetime, which may have included wars, emigration, the Great Depression, discrimination, segregation, poverty, and the deaths of children and other family members from what are now preventable diseases. They may have made major sacrifices for their children to receive higher education, often working 12- to 15-hour days, 6 to 7 days a week. Many worked under what are now considered poor or unfair labor practices. Today's older adults ushered in the era of the New Deal, saw the advent of antibiotics and insulin, and engendered in their children (the baby boomers of today) values regarding the importance of country, religion, family, education, and hard work. From these present-day older people—the survivors of the past—younger generations have inherited a tremendous legacy. These older adults have provided many lessons on striving for success, responsibility, coping, and all other aspects associated with succeeding in life.

During the past two to three decades, a new picture of older adults has emerged. We are now witnessing the triumph of survivorship and are facing the social, economic, cultural, and personal consequences referred to by Robert Butler in the opening quotation. The number of people older than 65 years of age has grown tremendously in the United States. In 1900, 4 of every 100 people living in this country made it past their 65th birthday; currently, 13 in 100 people reach this birthday; and in

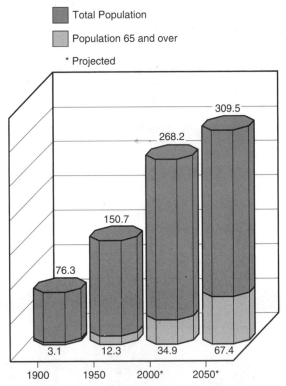

FIGURE 1–1. Growth of the population 65 years and older. The number of people is shown (in millions) for the entire U.S. population and for those older than 65 years. (From U.S. Census Bureau, 1988.)

another 30 years, this number will increase to 1 in every 5 people (Bentley, 1989). Thirteen percent of the population is presently older than the age of 65 years, a statistic that is predicted to increase to 17% (50 million people) by the year 2030. Figure 1–1 depicts the projected growth of the population that is 65 years of age and older from the year 1900 to 2050.

The fastest-growing segment of the population is the octogenarian. The prospect of surviving to 100 years is also real; however, only those older people who enjoy relatively good health and are able to be productive and function independently in the community will welcome this milestone (Baines, 1991). What is not apparent in these demographics is that children who are old themselves will be caring for their very old parents—a reality that is already beginning to occur.

Statistics from the Department of Commerce

(1992) indicate that there are significantly more older women than older men in the United States. There are over 1000 women to 674 men older than the age of 65 years, and at age 75 years, that number increases to 1000 women to 548 men. The preponderance of older women who typically reside alone as widows may increase the importance of family support, as these individuals' health and functional abilities decline.

The *graying* of America also includes fast-growing numbers of older ethnic and racial minorities. Between the years 1970 and 1980 among people 65 years and older, there was a 75% increase in older Hispanics, a 65% increase among older Native Americans, and a 34% increase among older blacks, compared with only a 25% growth in the older white population (American Society on Aging, 1992). Growth in the Pacific Asian elderly population was even more phenomenal, increasing by 400% (Woodruff, 1995).

As providers of healthcare to the elderly, nurses must have more than a statistical picture of the older population. These numbers are important, however, in that they provide a perspective of the growth in the older population, their healthcare needs and problems, and the projected number of gerontological nurses who will be required to provide care.

BABY BOOMERS: THE ELDERLY OF THE FUTURE

With the leading edge of the baby-boomer generation now reaching 50 years of age, their numbers will have a definite impact on the future of healthcare in this country. It is estimated that 20% of the baby boomers will have no children at all and that another 25% will have only one child.

Dychtwald and Flower (1989) claimed that the boomers are not replacing themselves. In 1986 (the latest year for which figures are available) the fertility rate of women was 1%, which is less than half the rate of their mothers, 27% lower than the fertility rate in 1970, and less than one fourth of the rate in 1800. The recent fertility rate is the lowest ever recorded in the United States, revealing a shift from a birthing

nation to an aging nation. This shift is rapidly growing in momentum.

The combined *senior boom* and *birth dearth* is creating a society concerned with the needs and desires of its middle-aged and older citizens (Dychtwald & Flower, 1989). The boomers have dominated U.S. culture since the end of World War II, and their involvement in politics and business is largely responsible for the current "I don't want to grow old" philosophy. They have been and will continue to be a major force in society. As consumers of healthcare, they may demand more services from providers and be more informed about prevention than previous generations. In response, providers will have to become more informed about their consumers, their culture, and their beliefs.

MOVING INTO THE 21ST CENTURY: DISPELLING THE MYTHS ASSOCIATED WITH OLD AGE

What can be expected in the future for the elderly, and what kind of care will be needed? Some of the myths associated with old age (*ageism*) will likely be dispelled (Table 1–1). The misrepresented concepts of old age will need to be replaced to meet the objectives outlined in *Healthy People 2000* (Table 1–2). These objectives serve to guide gerontological nurses

---

TABLE 1-1

New Ideas to Replace Myths Associated with Old Age

Sixty-five is only an arbitrary number for defining old

Old age is not necessarily ill age; preventive and health promotion measures can improve functioning into later decades

Mental ability depends on attitude, motivation, and health—not age

Productivity is possible at ages well over today's retirement age

Sixties are sexually active times for many people

Individual differences among the elderly are as great as at any age

TABLE 1-2

Summary of Objectives for Adults Aged 65 Years and Older: Healthy People 2000

Health Status	Services and Protection

Reduce
  Suicide among white males
  Death by motor vehicle accidents
    (aged 70 years and older)
  Death from falls and fall-related injury
    particularly aged 85 years and older
  Death from residential fires
  Hip fractures
  Number of people who have difficulty
    performing two or more personal care
    activities so as to enhance independence
  Significant visual impairment
  Epidemic-related pneumonia and influenza
    deaths
  Pneumonia-related days of restricted
    activity
Increase
  Years of healthy life to at least 65 among
    Blacks and Hispanics
 	
Risk Reduction
 	
Increase
  Percentage of individuals who regularly
    participate in light to moderate activity
    for at least 30 minutes a day
  Immunization levels for pneumococcal
    influenza among the chronically ill older
    population
  Percentage of older people who receive
    within appropriate intervals screening
    and immunization services and at least
    one counseling service
	Increase
	  Percentage of recipients of home food
	    service
	  Percentage of older adults who have the
	    opportunity to participate yearly in at
	    least one organized health promotion
	    program through senior centers, life care
	    facility, or community-based setting
	    serving the older adults
	  Percentage of states in the United States
	    that have design standards for signs,
	    signals, marking and lighting, and other
	    roadway environmental improvements to
	    enhance visual stimuli and protect the
	    safety of older drivers and pedestrians
	  Proportion of primary care providers who
	    routinely review with their patient
	    prescribed and over-the-counter
	    medications each time a new medication
	    is prescribed
	  Usage of the oral care system
	  Proportion of women aged 40 years and
	    older who receive clinical breast
	    examinations and mammogram
	  Number of women aged 70 years and older
	    with uterine cervix who receive Pap tests
	Extend
	  Long-term institutional facilities, the
	    requirement of oral examinations, and
	    service provided to new admissions no
	    later than 90 days after entering a facility

From U.S. Department of Health and Human Services (1990). *Healthy people 2000: National health promotion and disease prevention objectives* (pp. 23–25). Washington, D.C.: U.S. Government Printing Office.

toward health promotion and disease prevention for older people. Nurses will be caring for a healthier older population. Several myths of old age are briefly discussed here in view of the changes projected for the elderly population in the 21st century.

Myth: Sixty-Five Is Old. The arbitrary designation of 65 years of age as *old* has no scientific merit. It began in Germany in 1889 with Chancellor Bismarck, who chose this as an arbitrary designation for retirement, knowing that most citizens of that day and age did not survive to this age. As a result, he and others in his circle

of leaders would not have to leave office, as they would probably die before that age. As time elapsed, most countries adopted this as the age for retirement.

Sixty-five years may not continue to be the retirement age. Rather, people older than this age may be involved in a new career, work 5 to 10 years in their new "job," and possess a renewed spirit. They may work part time or spend more time in recreation with their family and friends. In response to second or multiple careers, industry may cross-train employees for more than one assignment. Institutions of higher education may design programs specifically for the older returning student.

Myth: Old Age Is Ill Age

Traditional notions about old age and health will have to be rethought. Definitions that have more to do with functional abilities, levels of vigor and vitality, and an individual's own feelings of well-being will become the norm in the years to come. (p. 33)

DYCHTWALD & FLOWER, 1989

Consumers are driven to live longer, healthier lives. Despite the fact that older people are the greatest consumers of healthcare, the later years of life are not destined to be accompanied by declining health (Baines, 1991). In the future, the physical decrements that accompany normal aging may be delayed until the eighth and ninth decades of life. Some individuals may not reach old age because of premature deaths from traumatic injury, the human immunodeficiency virus, and other possible maladies that are presently unknown.

Today, the greatest proportion of chronic illness can be found in the older population. Multiple chronic illnesses tend to coexist, with *longer life* taking on a meaning shrouded in disability and vulnerability to health problems, financial expenses, and increasing care concerns (Lubkin, 1995). Arthritis, hypertension, hearing impairments, heart disease, and cancer remain in the forefront of the chronic conditions affecting the elderly, and thus caregiving for the elderly has become a major burden shared by children, spouses, and significant others.

The challenges of the future are already apparent. The baby boomers are believers in health promotion and disease prevention. As a result, they appear much younger at ages that were previously viewed as old, and they are active in community organizations, setting the agenda and pace for the future. Industry may incorporate health and fitness as part of employee contracts, with nurses providing on-site coordination and responsibility for wellness care. Insurance coverage may include prevention as a key to low copayments. Managed care may become just that—managing the care that

is provided and giving the adult responsibility for his or her own care. The need for sensitivity in dealing with ethnic diversity in this country will have to be more seriously addressed (Yeo, 1996–1997). Gerontological nurses will need to play an advocacy role to ensure that holistic care is provided to all older people.

Myth: Mental Ability Declines with Age. Mental abilities, along with the capacity to learn, do not markedly change with age (Haight, 1991). Attitude, motivation, and health are the key factors that determine one's state of mind. Declines in mental capacity can occur in very late age, however, and are associated with multiple causes such as physiological imbalances, depression, the loss of social supports, and environmental factors. Gerontological nurses should avoid the use of the term *senility.* Senility is not a disease. The alleviation of Alzheimer's disease, a disease feared by many, may become approachable in the 21st century.

Much of what has been attributed to loss of intelligence in older adults is a loss of investment in life as well as a loss of significant others. Many older people retreat from engaging in social activities. If social isolation was a pattern for an individual when he or she was younger, it may be difficult to change.

Caring for older people who experience changes in mental status presents a major challenge for the gerontological nurse. Keen assessments will be necessary to decipher depression from mental decline. Polypharmacy and its inherent drug interactions may cause a blurring of mental acuity. The baby boomers are taking an interest in herbal and other homeopathic remedies, which may be the focus of new research and education.

Myth: Productivity Declines with Age. In all ages, productivity is dependent on a complex interaction of different factors. With the increasing retirement age and the possibility of pursuing a second career in later life, the ideal of a productive older life is becoming a reality.

The myth that productivity declines with age will likely be dispelled by television commercials that depict older people at work as well as by companies increasingly recruiting and hiring the older worker. Older people are reliable employees, and the idea of the seasoned employee is becoming more important. Industry will likely have gerontological nurse practitioners (GNPs) in the work setting to provide care and establish a referral system into the community. Home visitations may become a norm with companies, and homecare may be added to the coverage in health insurance policies, made possible by managed care subcontracting.

Myth: The 60s Are Sexless. Aging is a time for significant reflection, renewal of relationships, and leisure. Old age is an important time to increase one's understanding of sexuality and of people's needs for intimacy and love. The idea of being sexy, sensual, and 60 years of age is becoming increasingly accepted (see Chapter 24). Older people are generally concerned about their liaisons, practice safe sex, and are savvy about their appearance. Baby boomers will age differently than their parents and will likely maintain their health and continue being sexually and socially active well into their 60s and beyond.

Myth: Oldsters Are All the Same. Although gerontology textbooks indicate that the aged are a heterogeneous group, this notion is not universally held by society. "You've seen one, you've seen them all" is a common expression. Yet no two people are alike. Why, then, is there a tendency to believe that older people should think, feel, and act the same way?

The aged should be viewed as a *melting pot* of diversity. Older people are as diverse not only as their ancestries and ethnicities dictate but also as a result of their abilities, education, skills, and individual talents. This melting pot of diversity contains dynamic, unique, wise, well-seasoned individuals.

Future gerontological nursing research will likely delve into this diversity by studying many cultures and their health habits, problems, and environments. Strategies will have to be developed to address the multiple needs of the aged population.

SCOPE AND STANDARDS OF GERONTOLOGICAL NURSING PRACTICE: A MAP INTO THE FUTURE

The ANA's *Scope and Standards of Gerontological Nursing Practice* (1995) is the profession's guide

to gerontological nursing practice and provides the foundation for quality care for older adults. According to the ANA, the scope and standards of gerontological nursing practice are "intended to be used in conjunction with other documents that articulate the values of the nursing profession and the definition and scope of nursing practice" [p. 1] (ANA, 1995). As a resource for assessment tools and plans of care, the standards may be used in peer review and performance appraisal. They apply to all nurses practicing with elderly clients in a variety of settings.

The *Scope and Standards of Gerontological Nursing Practice* describes a competent level of nursing care and delineates basic and advanced practice roles. It is anticipated that these roles will change over time as the specialty of gerontological nursing expands to meet the changing needs and demands of society.

Scope of Gerontological Nursing Practice. The scope of practice is guided by the following beliefs:

- Aging people are a heterogeneous group of unique individuals
- Aging people seek self-fulfillment and are capable of making decisions about matters that affect how they live and die
- Aging is a natural lifelong process; it is not synonymous with disease
- Nursing services should be provided unrestricted by cultural diversity, social or economic status, personal attributes, or the nature of health problems

Gerontological nursing practice involves the same tenets as other areas of practice, such as assessing, planning, and providing appropriate nursing care and other health services as well as evaluating the effectiveness of that care. However, it concentrates more on the assessment of the functional status of aging adults. Emphasis is placed on maximizing functional ability in activities of daily living; promoting, maintaining, and restoring health, including mental health; preventing and minimizing the disabilities of acute and chronic illness; and maintaining life with dignity and comfort.

All professional nurses practicing gerontological nursing should possess the basic knowledge and skills to do the following (ANA, 1995, pp. 8–9):

1. Use the nursing process to develop the aging person's care plan
2. Establish a therapeutic relationship with aging people and their families to facilitate their collaboration with the gerontological nurse in developing a care plan
3. Recognize the age-related changes based on an understanding of physiological, emotional, cultural, social, psychological, economic, and spiritual functioning
4. Collect data to determine health status and functional abilities to plan, implement, and evaluate care
5. Participate as a member of the interdisciplinary team
6. Participate with aging people, families, and other health professionals in ethical decision making that is client centered, empathetic, and humane
7. Serve as an advocate for aging people and their families
8. Teach aging people and families about measures that promote, maintain, and restore health or promote comfort
9. Refer the aging person to other professionals or community resources for assistance as necessary
10. Apply the existing body of knowledge in gerontology to nursing practice and interventions
11. Exercise accountability to the aging person by protecting his or her rights and autonomy
12. Engage in continuing professional development through participation in continuing education, involvement in state and national professional organizations, and certification
13. Use the standards of gerontological nursing practice to increase an aging person's quality of care and quality of life

Standards of Clinical Gerontological Nursing Care. These standards describe a competent level of nursing care as demonstrated by the nursing process. The six standards include assessment, diagnosis, outcome identification, planning, implementation, and evaluation. They form the foundation of all clinical decision making. For each standard, the rationale and measurement criteria are outlined; however, for purposes of this text, only the standards and their rationale are provided (Table 1–3).

Standards of Professional Gerontological Nursing Performance. These standards describe competent levels of behavior in the professional role. The eight standards include activities related to quality of care, performance appraisal, education, collegiality, ethics, collaboration, research, and resource allocation (Table 1–4). The varied professional role activities and expectations of all gerontological nurses are dictated by their educational level, position, and practice setting. Nurses should be self-directed and purposeful in seeking activities such as membership in professional organizations, certification in generalist or advanced specialty practice, participation in continuing education programs, and further academic education.

CHALLENGES WITHIN THE NURSING PROFESSION

The challenges presented to gerontological nurses are significant. Nursing's professional identity will come of age with the graying of America. *Health promotion, cost containment,* and *quality* have become the buzzwords of the 1990s. APNs face the challenge of delineating nursing's contribution in healthcare, measuring patient care outcomes, and providing quality care in the most cost-effective manner. Nurses have the opportunity to advocate for health promotion and disease prevention in the older population. In the future, there may be new, expanding roles in a variety of settings for gerontological nurses; projections for gerontological nursing in the 21st century are presented in Table 1–5.

Advanced Practice Nursing

The APN in gerontological nursing is a clinical nurse specialist (CNS) or nurse practitioner (NP) who holds a master's and/or a doctoral degree in nursing and specializes in the care of

TABLE 1-3

Standards of Clinical Gerontological Nursing Care

Standard I Assessment

The gerontological nurse collects client health data.

Rationale:
   The information obtained from the aging person, significant others, and interdisciplinary team members, in addition to nursing judgment based on knowledge of gerontological nursing, is used to develop the comprehensive plan of care. Interviewing, functional assessment, environmental assessment, physical assessment, and review of health records enhance the nurse's ability to make sound clinical judgments. The assessment is culturally and ethnically relevant.

Standard II Diagnosis

The gerontological nurse analyzes the assessment data in determining diagnosis.

Rationale:
   The gerontological nurse evaluates health assessment data to identify the aging person's state of health and well-being, treatment of and responses to illness, aging, and reduced activity. Each person responds to aging in a unique way. Nursing diagnoses form the basis for nursing interventions.

Standard III Outcome Identification

The gerontological nurse identifies expected outcomes individualized to the client.

Rationale:
   The ultimate goals of providing gerontological nursing care are to influence health outcomes and improve the aging person's health status. Outcomes often focus on maximizing the aging person's state of well-being, functional status, and quality of life.

Standard IV Planning

The gerontological nurse develops a plan of care that prescribes interventions to attain expected outcomes.

Rationale:
   A plan of care is used to structure and guide therapeutic interventions and achieve expected outcomes. It is developed in conjunction with the aging person and appropriate others.

Standard V Implementation

The gerontological nurse implements the interventions identified in the plan of care.

Rationale:
   The gerontological nurse implements a plan of care in collaboration with the aging person, significant others, and the interdisciplinary team. The gerontological nurse provides culturally competent, direct, and indirect care, using concepts of health promotion, illness prevention, health maintenance, rehabilitation, restoration, and palliation. The nurse educates and counsels that aging person and significant others involved in the provision of care to the aging person. In addition, the gerontological nurse supervises and evaluates both formal and informal caregivers to assure that their care is supportive and ethical and demonstrates respect for the aging person's dignity. Gerontological nurses select interventions according to their level of practice.

Standard VI Evaluation

The gerontological nurse evaluates the aging person's progress toward attainment of expected outcomes.

Rationale:
   Nursing practice is a dynamic process. The gerontological nurse continually evaluates the aging person's responses to therapeutic interventions. Collection of new data, revision of the data base, different nursing diagnoses, and modification of plan of care are often required. The effectiveness of nursing care depends on ongoing evaluation.

Adapted from American Nurses Association (1995). *Scope and standards of gerontological nursing practice* (pp. 11–18). Washington, D.C.: American Nurses Publishing.

TABLE 1-4

Standards of Professional Gerontological Nursing Performance

Standard I   Quality of Care

The gerontological nurse systematically evaluates the quality of care and effectiveness of nursing practice.

Rationale:

The dynamic nature of geriatric care and the growing body of gerontological nursing knowledge and research provide both the impetus and the means for gerontological nurses to improve the quality of client care.

Standard II   Performance Appraisal

The gerontological nurse evaluates his/her own nursing practice in relation to professional practice standards and relevant statutes and regulations.

Rationale:

The gerontological nurse is accountable to the public for providing competent clinical care and has an inherent responsibility as a professional gerontological nurse to practice according to standards established by the profession and regulatory bodies.

Standard III   Education

The gerontological nurse acquires and maintains current knowledge in nursing practice.

Rationale:

Scientific, cultural, societal, and political changes require a commitment from the gerontological nurse to the continuing pursuit of knowledge to enhance nursing expertise and advance the profession. Formal education, continuing education, certification, and experiential learning are some of the means for professional growth.

Standard IV   Collegiality

The gerontological nurse contributes to the professional development of peers, colleagues, and others.

Rationale:

The gerontological nurse has the responsibility to share knowledge, research, and clinical information with colleagues and others through formal and informal teaching methods and collaborative educational programs.

Standard V   Ethics

The gerontological nurse's decisions and actions on behalf of clients are determined in an ethical manner.

Rationale:

The gerontological nurse is responsible for providing services and healthcare that are responsive to the public's trust and client's rights. Coworkers and other formal and informal care providers must also be prepared to provide the care needed and desired by the aging person and to render services in an appropriate setting. Special ethical concerns in gerontological nursing care include informed consent, emergency intervention, nutrition and hydration of the terminally ill, pain management, the need for self-determination, treatment termination, quality of life issues, confidentiality, surrogate decision making, nontraditional treatment modalities, fair distribution of scarce resources, and economic decision making.

Standard VI   Collaboration

The gerontological nurse collaborates with the aging person, significant others, and healthcare providers in providing client care.

Rationale:

The complex nature of comprehensive care to aging persons and their significant others requires expertise from a number of different healthcare providers. Collaboration between consumers and providers is optimal for planning, implementation, and evaluation of care. Meetings of the interdisciplinary team provide a forum to evaluate the effectiveness of the care plan and adjust the plan of care.

Standard VII   Research

The gerontological nurse uses research findings in practice.

Rationale:

Gerontological nurses have the responsibility to improve practice and the future healthcare for aging persons by participation in research. At the basic level of practice, the gerontological nurse uses research findings to improve clinical care and identify clinical problems for research study. At the advanced level, the gerontological nurse engages and/or collaborates in the research process.

Standard VIII   Resource Utilization

The gerontological nurse considers factors related to safety, effectiveness, and costs in planning and delivering client care.

Rationale:

The aging person is entitled to healthcare that is safe, effective, and affordable. Treatment decisions must be made in a way to maximize resources and maintain quality of care.

Adapted from American Nurses Association (1995). *Scope and standards of gerontological nursing practice* (pp. 19–26). Washington, D.C.: American Nurses Publishing.

TABLE 1-5

Projections for Gerontological Nursing

Advanced practice nursing will assume a greater role in the provision of healthcare to the elderly; specifically these nurses will become more abundant in nursing homes and in long-term care facilities. These nurses will serve not only as primary care providers but also as case managers assessing clients for discharge and / or placement for rehabilitative services.

There will be more emphasis on health promotion and disease prevention to avoid chronic illness in the "well elderly" and to prevent additional exacerbation of chronic illness both physical and emotional.

Subspecialties will emerge in gerontological nursing, such as geropsychiatric nurse, geriatric nurse care manager, geriatric nurse rehabilitation specialist, and geriatric nurse wellness coordinator.

A changing curriculum will be developed in schools of nursing to meet the increasing need and demand for gerontological nurse specialists.

Caregiving in the "sandwich" generation will be not only discussed but also reimbursed. Gerontological nurses will be leaders in the field, developing policy and drafting legislative language for programs affecting informal caregivers of the elderly.

New gerontological nursing practice models will be developed, such as multidisciplinary practices in the community as well as in industry. Homecare nurse practitioners will make independent house calls to homes and daycare centers. Residential homes and transitional homes for the elderly will proliferate and offer amenities for all group situations and income levels.

Cultural diversity will take on a heightened importance in program planning and the education of gerontological nurses.

Ethics committees incorporated into all institutional as well as community settings will play a major role in healthcare decisions surrounding older people. Gerontological nurses will be placed on these committees as advocates of client rights.

Managed care will employ larger numbers of gerontological nurses as primary care providers. Corporations will contract for advanced practice nursing services.

the elderly. APNs have a "high level of expertise in the assessment, diagnosis, and treatment of the complex responses of individuals, families, or communities to actual or potential health problems, prevention of illness and injury, maintenance of wellness, and provision of comfort" (ANA, 1996). Advanced practice gerontological nurses engage in all activities delineated at the basic level and are guided in their scope of practice by their state's nurse practice acts for advanced practice, which may include prescriptive authority. A major difference in practice from the basic gerontological nurse level is that the APN has a larger knowledge base, with greater ability to synthesize data, particularly in complex situations, and also uses more specialized skills and interventions (ANA, 1996).

Advanced practice roles include practice, case management, education, research, consultation, and administration, all of which require intradisciplinary and interdisciplinary collaboration. Doctorally prepared gerontological nurses are expected to take leadership roles in theory development and in conducting research (ANA, 1995).

Although they do overlap, the roles of the CNS and NP are distinguished in the following descriptions adapted from the *Scope and Standards of Advanced Practice Registered Nurses* (ANA, 1996):

The CNS [clinical nurse specialist] *is an expert clinician and client advocate who provides direct client care, including assessing, diagnosing, planning, and prescribing pharmacologic and nonpharmacologic treatment of health problems, health promotion and preventive care within a specialized area of practice. The sub-roles of the CNS are education, research, and consultation. The CNS is involved in indirect practice activities with the goal of improving the quality of care and serves as a change agent. (p. 3)*

The NP [nurse practitioner] *is a skilled health care provider who utilizes critical judgment in the performance of comprehensive health assessments, differential diagnosis, and the prescribing of pharmacologic and non-pharmacologic treatments in the direct management of acute and chronic illness and disease. NP practice promotes wellness and prevents illness and injury. NPs function in various settings for individuals, families, and communities. This includes working autonomously and in the interdisciplinary teams as resources and consultants. NP sub-roles include research, education, and public policy advocate. (pp. 3–4)*

The new ANA standards of care and professional performance for APNs are summarized in Tables 1–6 and 1–7. Criteria are also defined to measure competent practice.

Credentialing for advanced practice in gerontological nursing is obtained after graduation from an accredited graduate program that provides course work and clinical experiences appropriate for the specialty as well as a national examination offered through the American Nurses Credentialing Center. The appropriate credential depends on the type of educational program completed and may be certification as either a gerontological CNS or a gerontological NP.

Practice Settings

The delivery of healthcare has rapidly changed during the 1990s. Practice settings for APNs in gerontological nursing in the 21st century may evolve in response to the dynamic nature of the healthcare environment. APNs will continue to practice in traditional settings such as hospitals, nursing homes, community or ambulatory settings, and office practices. They will be establishing roles in other settings, such as senior centers, lifecare communities, homecare agencies, adult homes, adult daycare centers, and in multidisciplinary teams for assessing individuals. This will be seen in both rural areas and urban poor areas. There is much to be learned from European colleagues in the field of geriatrics, who carry pagers to be easily accessible to their clients. Nurses will likely do the same here in the near future and may hire

physicians to work in their business practice. In many instances, they will work collaboratively as partners.

Advanced practice gerontological nurses are providing more primary care to older adults who reside in home settings and in nursing homes. In the future, nursing homes may take on a new look and become not only attractive residences within an institutional setting but also places where rehabilitation will take on greater importance. There will be a greater proportion of short-stay residents admitted for rehabilitation only.

The delivery of healthcare services in this century is beginning to come full circle. At the turn of the century, house calls were made and consumers bartered with patients for payment. Few hospitals existed, children were born at home, and people died at home. Healthcare is returning to a similar way of treating illness and promoting health. The paradigm is beginning to shift to a consumer-generated healthcare system that will exist largely in the community.

Creating the Educational Environment: A Vision for a New Curriculum

Current demographic trends will dictate changes in nursing curricula. With increasing numbers of elderly people, every curriculum component will have to integrate gerontological nursing concepts. With the advent of newer roles such as acute care NP, primary care provider, and care manager, faculty may be called on to design programs that address care of the older adult. The diverse health needs of the elderly will require an increased attention to the educational preparation for professional nurses (Timms, 1995).

The challenge for faculty members will be to provide an educational program that prepares nurses to meet the changing needs of the consumer in the community. One potential design for a nursing curriculum would integrate gerontological nursing content and experiences throughout the curriculum; maternal-child nursing courses, for example, would incorporate intergenerational concepts. With the in-

TABLE 1-6
Standards of Care for the Advanced Practice Registered Nurse

Standard I   Assessment

The advanced practice registered nurse collects comprehensive client health data.

Standard II   Diagnosis

The advanced practice registered nurse critically analyzes the assessment data in determining the diagnoses.

Standard III   Outcome Identification

The advanced practice registered nurse identifies expected outcomes derived from the assessment data and diagnoses and individualizes expected outcomes with the client, and with the healthcare team when appropriate.

Standard IV   Planning

The advanced practice registered nurse develops a comprehensive plan of care that includes interventions and treatments to attain expected outcomes.

Standard V   Implementation

The advanced practice registered nurse prescribes, orders, or implements interventions and treatments for the plan of care.

Standard Va   Case Management/Coordination of Care

The advanced practice registered nurse provides comprehensive clinical coordination of care and case management.

Standard Vb   Consultation

The advanced practice registered nurse provides consultation to influence the plan of care for clients, enhance the abilities of others, and effect change in the system.

Standard Vc   Health Promotion, Health Maintenance, and Health Teaching

The advanced practice registered nurse employs complex strategies, interventions, and teaching to promote, maintain, and improve health and prevent illness and injury.

Standard Vd   Prescriptive Authority and Treatment

The advanced practice registered nurse uses prescriptive authority, procedures, and treatments in accordance with state and federal laws and regulations to treat illness and improve functional health status or to provide preventive care.

Standard Ve   Referral

The advanced practice registered nurse identifies the need for additional care and makes referrals as needed.

Adapted from American Nurses Association (1996). *Scope and standards of advanced practice registered nursing* (pp. 11–15). Washington, D.C.: American Nurses Publishing.

creasing numbers of grandparents caring for babies and children, this type of content may be a necessity. Students will be exposed to the *sandwich* generation and the fact that multiple generations exist in one family and significantly affect the health of the whole. Community health, psychiatric mental health, acute care, and critical care may define practice parameters of care for the older client.

An estimated 13.5 million people in the United States have disabled elderly spouses or parents either living at home or in an institution. Because it significantly affects the health of the older adult, the health of caregivers must

TABLE 1-7

Standards of Professional Performance for the Advanced Practice Registered Nurse

Standard I   Quality of Care

The advanced practice registered nurse develops criteria for and evaluates the quality of care and effectiveness of advanced practice registered nursing.

Standard II   Self-Evaluation

The advanced practice registered nurse continuously evaluates his or her own nursing practice in relation to professional practice standards and relevant statutes and regulations and is accountable to the public and to the profession for providing competent clinical care.

Standard III   Education

The advanced practice registered nurse acquires and maintains current knowledge and skills in the area of specialty practice.

Standard IV   Leadership

The advanced practice registered nurse serves as a leader and a role model for the professional development of peers, colleagues, and others.

Standard V   Ethics

The advanced practice registered nurse integrates ethical principles and norms in all areas of practice.

Standard VI   Interdisciplinary Process

The advanced practice registered nurse promotes an interdisciplinary process in providing client care.

Standard VII   Research

The advanced practice registered nurse utilizes research to discover, examine, and evaluate knowledge, theories, and creative approaches to healthcare practice.

Adapted from American Nurses Association (1996). *Scope and standards of advanced practice registered nursing* (pp. 17–20). Washington, D.C.: American Nurses Publishing.

be considered. APNs may dramatically alter the course of life and health events for caregivers. New theories and practice models may emerge in respite and hospice care as well as in occupational health. The shift in delivery of care from the hospital to the community has already resulted in an increased acuity level in the homecare setting (Patton & Patillo, 1995). Clinical settings in senior centers and residential care facilities may become more common. The challenge to faculty members will be to provide clinical experiences that expose students to the myriad settings in which older adults live, work, and play.

As the demands for gerontological nurses become more acute, a new curriculum will evolve. Heine (1993) described varied programs and models currently in existence, including the following:

- Community College–Nursing Home Partnership, through which institutions and community colleges work together to develop positive learning experiences for the associate degree student
- University of Pittsburgh curriculum for undergraduate and graduate students, to include health promotion, clinical experiences in apartment buildings and senior centers, and faculty collaboration with a gerontological CNS who serves as a re-

source person promoting interdisciplinary team planning

- Schools of Nursing partnerships with senior centers for student experiences that focus on health promotion and disease prevention; scientific research on the effectiveness of APNs will be documented
- Elective programs in gerontological nursing offered not only to nursing students but also to practicing nurses for credit to enhance their education and skills
- Treatment of elderly people by rural health nurses through expanding outreach clinics; alternative sites include vans scheduled for certain sites on designated days and school buildings used to treat families; APNs may become "circuit riders" to meet the primary care needs of the rural population

SUMMARY

The future of gerontological nursing is limited only by the visions of today's gerontological nurses. By searching the places where older adults live, work, and recreate and by listening to their concerns and problems, members of the nursing profession can find limitless opportunities for practice and research focused on developing and implementing innovative strategies to prevent and manage chronic illness. Wellness and health promotion are rapidly becoming guiding concepts for nursing curricula, with client education, consumer responsibility, and resource development also being incorporated in nursing education.

In this first chapter, many concepts, visions, and projections for gerontological nursing were discussed. The standards of care to guide practice, information about trends in the field, and opportunities to shape the future of the specialty were presented. Succeeding chapters will discuss (1) current research-based knowledge on comprehensive geriatric assessment, (2) the management of common health problems of the elderly, (3) ethical and legal issues encountered in caring for older adults, and (4) evolving advanced practice models of gerontological nursing.

REFERENCES

American Nurses Association (1996). *Scope and standards of advanced practice registered nursing.* Washington, D.C.: American Nurses Publishing.

American Nurses Association (1995). *Scope and standards of gerontological nursing practice.* Washington, D.C.: American Nurses Publishing.

American Society on Aging (1992). *Serving elders of color: Challenges to providers and the aging network.* San Francisco: American Society on Aging.

Baines, E. M. (1991). *Perspectives in gerontological nursing.* New London: Sage Publications.

Bentley, D. W. (1989). Current challenges and future opportunities. *Infection Control and Hospital Epidemiology, 10,* 481–483.

Butler, R. (1981). Forward. In A. R. Sommers & D. R. Fabian (Eds.), *The geriatric imperative: An introduction to gerontology and clinical geriatrics* (p. iv). New York: Appleton-Century-Crofts.

Department of Commerce (1992). *Statistical abstracts of the United States* (112th ed.). Washington, D.C.: Department of Commerce.

Department of Health and Human Services (1990). *Healthy people 2000: national health promotion and disease prevention objectives* (PHS Publ. No. 91-50212). Washington, D.C.: U.S. Government Printing Office.

Dychtwald, K., & Flower, J. (1989). *Age wave.* Los Angeles: Jeremy P. Torcher, Inc.

Haight, B. (1991). Psychological illness. In E. M. Baines (Ed.), *Perspectives in gerontological nursing* (pp. 296–319). New London: Sage Publications.

Heine, C. (1993). *Determining the future of gerontological nursing education: Partnerships between education and practice.* New York: National League for Nursing Press.

Lubkin, I. M. (Ed.) (1995). *Chronic illness: Impact and interventions* (3rd ed.). Boston: Jones and Bartlett.

Patton, S., & Patillo, M. (1995). Continuing education for nurses in geriatric home care. In C. Heine (Ed.), *Determining the future of gerontological nursing education* (pp. 90–91). New York: National League for Nursing Press.

Timms, J. (1995). Needs assessment: Nursing assessment: Nursing surveys in gerontology. Are we really assessing continuing education needs and priorities. *Journal of Continuing Nursing Education, 26,* 84–88.

Woodruff, L. (1995). Growing diversity in the aging population. *Caring, 12,* 4–10.

Yeo, G. (1996–1997). Ethnogeriatrics. Cross-cultural care of older adults. *Generations, 20*(4), 72–77.

Practice Models in Gerontological Nursing

Lynne Morishita

Practice models in gerontological nursing are evolving with the growing healthcare needs of older adults and the reform of healthcare delivery in the United States. People 80 years of age and older are the fastest-growing segment of our population (Cassel & Brody, 1990). Because of this population growth, a larger proportion of older people will have multiple medical problems and functional deficits, requiring care by teams of professionals from a variety of disciplines and services. By the year 2020, healthcare providers will spend 70% of their time with people older than the age of 70 years (Brand & Gurenlian, 1989). Advances in technology, a growing emphasis on cost containment, and the restructuring of healthcare delivery and payment strategies have given rise to an increased demand for advanced practice nurses (APNs) to provide more cost-effective, quality care for older people (Joel, 1985; Light, 1986). In the future, advanced practice gerontological nurses will have many opportunities for creating innovative roles and practice models for outpatient, home, acute hospital, and community or institutional long-term care settings.

This chapter provides an overall description of existing practice models. These models will be useful for nurses evaluating career opportunities or developing innovative health services, because an established compendium of practice models does not currently exist. (The spe-

17

cific roles and functions of gerontological nurses are covered in Chapter 1.)

A typology of practice models is presented to provide a framework for considering the major factors that affect practice. Interdisciplinary care and case management—two fundamental components of gerontological nursing that must be incorporated into any practice model—are emphasized. Other important subroles of APNs are discussed, including education, administration, and research. Finally, the chapter describes examples of innovative programs designed specifically for older adults that include a critical role for advanced practice gerontological nurses.

It is valuable for nurses to have a framework to review and consider existing practice models, and these models must be clearly defined so that future research can link them with the best client outcomes. In this way, healthcare policy can be established that fosters effective roles for gerontological nurses in providing the highest quality care for older adults.

FACTORS THAT SHAPE GERONTOLOGICAL NURSING PRACTICE

Practice models for gerontological nursing are evolving. The practice situation is determined by many interdependent factors, and changes in any one of these factors can radically alter the practice model. A *shifting sands* metaphor appropriately describes this scenario. All practice models are shaped by five types of factors (Table 2–1).

Client Factors

Older clients can be independent, healthy people who need only preventive care to maintain their health. However, there is a growing population of frail older adults who have multiple problems, including depression, dementia, and urinary incontinence as well as chronic diseases such as congestive heart failure, chronic obstructive pulmonary disease, and osteoarthritis. These clients need assistance with activities of daily living. They require comprehen-

TABLE 2-1

Types of Factors That Shape Practice

Client factors—health problems, functional status, ethnic and cultural diversity, strengths and support

Nurse factors—clinical competency and skill, creativity, communication and leadership skills

Team factors—clinical competency and skill, creativity, communication and leadership skills of others involved in the care of the client

Organizational, payment, and setting factors
  A. Organizational structure—independent, private partnership, employee of private group, employee of institution or managed care organization (e.g., health maintenance organization)
  B. Payment structure—fee-for-service or capitated
  C. Care setting and level of care

Legal factors
  A. Scope of practice
  B. Prescriptive privileges
  C. Third-party reimbursement

sive assessment and management as well as care that is coordinated among providers in nursing, medicine, social work, rehabilitation therapy, and other areas. They also require close follow-up to ensure adherence to treatment plans and continuity of care.

The needs and strengths of the client are factors in determining the practice model. For example, if a client is healthy and independent and needs only preventive care, a nurse in independent solo practice can provide this care in an office or a clinic. If a client has multiple complicated medical problems and psychosocial needs, a collaborative practice with physicians and other healthcare team members will more effectively provide care in the home, outpatient clinic, community or skilled nursing facility, or hospital. Targeting the service to the appropriate client population is critical in attempting to provide appropriate, cost-effective care.

Nurse Factors

Good communication skills and clinical competence contribute to trust and shared decision making, which are critical features of an effective collaborative relationship between a nurse and a physician or other members of the healthcare team. Individual nurses have a wide range of areas of clinical expertise and skills from which to build. For example, if the nurse has expertise in urinary incontinence care and administration, he or she can develop a specialized continence program to complement already existing services. If the nurse has experience with clients with dementia, a program for family caregivers can be established.

Team Factors

Each member of the interdisciplinary team provides services associated with his or her area of clinical expertise; the extent to which the team members enhance and complement each other's skills determines the type of services that can be provided for the client. As with the nurse, the communication skills and clinical competence of physicians and other professionals are key in developing mutual trust and shared decision making, and thus successful, collaborative relationships.

Organizational, Payment, and Setting Factors

The structure of an organization influences how a practice model develops. The nurse can be an independent practitioner in a private corporation, a partner in a group practice that is a privately held corporation, an employee of a group practice, or an employee of a large public or private corporation such as a medical institution or a managed care organization. When the nurse has a private office practice only, the practice may be limited to outpatient care that is provided according to the nurse's scope of practice and standard of care. However, if the nurse is part of a large health maintenance organization (HMO), the nurse may provide care in multiple settings owned by that entity, which may enforce adherence to practice patterns defined by the HMO.

The organizational structure also determines the relationship the nurse has with other professionals involved in the client's care. For example, the nurse partner in a medical group with an office practice who has a client admitted to an acute rehabilitation hospital has only an informal relationship with the therapists in the hospital, whereas the nurse in a large HMO that owns the office practice and acute rehabilitation hospital can continue to work with the client in the rehabilitation facility. As employees of the HMO, the nurse and therapists can all be members of a formal interdisciplinary team working with the client.

The payment structure has a strong influence on the practice model. In a fee-for-service system, the financial incentive to providers is to deliver services that are reimbursed at a high rate by third-party payers. In a prospective payment structure, a set rate per client member is paid to the provider, regardless of the services delivered to the client. The financial incentive in a prospective payment system is to provide the most cost-effective care to the total client population. Medicare was initially established as a fee-for-service payment structure; however, managed care organizations are now also contracting to provide services to Medicare enrollees under a prospective payment structure.

The priority given to preventive services illustrates the impact of the payment system. If third-party payers do not cover preventive care, fee-for-service providers do not have a financial incentive to deliver these services. However, under a prospective payment structure, providing cost-effective preventive health services is encouraged to eliminate the cost of care for clients with preventable disease or declining functional status.

The care setting and level of care influence the type of practice implemented by the nurse. Each setting is licensed to provide a particular level of care, such as acute, outpatient, home, or skilled nursing facility care. Increasingly, healthcare providers are capable of providing a continuum of levels of care. This trend has been accelerated through the development of networks of healthcare organizations to form integrated delivery systems designed to increase efficiency.

If the setting provides outpatient care only, the practice model of course does not include care in the home or a skilled nursing facility.

However, if the setting includes multiple levels of care through an integrated healthcare delivery system, the practice model can ensure continuity with a nurse who provides or coordinates ongoing care in the home, clinic, or acute hospital or any other alternative included in the system of care.

Legal Factors

Three legal factors influence the development of practice models: the scope of practice, prescriptive privileges, and third-party reimbursement.

Legal authority for the scope of practice varies from state to state. In 1997, the Boards of Nursing for 42 states had the sole authority (as opposed to involving nonnursing bodies) over the scope of practice (16 states with requirements for physician collaboration or supervision and 26 without requirements). However, many of the states requiring physician involvement are planning on introducing changes that would eliminate this requirement (Pearson, 1998). Restrictions on the scope of practice also vary among states. Some states require formal practice relationships with physicians, written practice agreements, protocols, collaborative guidelines, and/or physician supervision. (See the January issue of *Nurse Practitioner* for an annual update of legislation affecting advanced nursing practice and prescriptive authority.)

Prescriptive privileges are available in most states, with a varying degree of restrictions. APNs have independent prescriptive authority (in 17 states plus Washington, D.C.), prescriptive authority with the involvement of a physician in 31 states, and no prescriptive privileges in 2 states.

Third-party reimbursement is a major determinant of the viability of any gerontological nurse practice model. Health policy is currently supporting more direct reimbursement for APN services. Historically, the majority of APN services have been reimbursed indirectly, by paying the collaborating physician who billed for APN services. Recent passage of the Balanced Budget Act of 1997 deems that as of January 1998, APN services can be directly reimbursed by Medicare Part B, regardless of geographic area of setting; the amount paid is the lesser of 80% of the actual charge or 85% of the fee schedule amount if provided by a physician. Medicaid pays 70 to 100% of the fee-for-service rates set for physicians by state Medicaid agencies; each state controls its respective rate. APNs are also increasingly gaining admission to provider panels for managed care organizations; in this situation, the payment arrangement is negotiated between the APN and the managed care organization (Balanced Budget Act, 1997).

State legislation is critical to developing practice models. During the past several years, an increasing number of states have allowed the Board of Nursing to authorize the scope of practice and to determine the mechanism for prescriptive privileges and reimbursement (Middelstadt, 1993; Pearson, 1998). There has been a trend in legislation toward less restrictive practice and increasing access to third-party reimbursement, although barriers to practice remain. Nurses can and should play an active role in advocating for legislation that will result in practice models that make effective use of APNs and that make healthcare more accessible to older adults.

KEY PRACTICE COMPONENTS

Interdisciplinary functioning and case management are fundamental components of gerontological nursing and are essential to all practice models of caring for older adults. To address the multiple needs of older adults, interdisciplinary teamwork is vital to the provision of comprehensive care. Case management is necessary to ensure coordination and continuity of care.

Interdisciplinary Functioning

In a traditional healthcare delivery system, care for older adults is frequently fragmented or important health issues are neglected (McCartney & Palmateer, 1985; Siu et al., 1988). Multiple health and social service providers may not coordinate their treatment, resulting in ineffective care of their client. For example, the physical therapist providing stroke rehabilitation may not communicate to the nurse or physician that the client seems oversedated during treatments; under these circumstances, this client will not have the necessary motivation to attain the goal of ambulating independently. Interdisciplinary teams are one solution to the problem of poorly coordinated care, with the aim of achieving the best treatment outcomes.

Frequently, client problems identified by one discipline cannot be managed without treating the whole person with an interdisciplinary care plan. Interdisciplinary teamwork occurs when professionals from different disciplines work interdependently with the client. Each discipline has a representative who performs a separate assessment and exchanges information with the other team members to define treatment goals and collaboratively plan care (Campbell & Cole, 1987; Goldberg et al., 1984). It is important for the interdisciplinary team to define the nursing, medical, social, rehabilitation, and nutritional needs of the older client. Ideally, these professionals should meet to develop an interdisciplinary, team-based plan of care using input from all the providers. *Interdisciplinary collaboration*, a vital element of gerontological nursing, is an American Nurses Association standard of gerontological nursing practice (American Nurses Association, 1995).

Case Management

Case management is a process of coordinating care and services to ensure that client needs are met. Its purpose is to facilitate the early identification of client needs, reduce fragmentation and duplication of services, eliminate delays in receiving services, improve quality of care, and ultimately, to decrease cost.

Case management activities closely approximate the nursing process (assessment, planning, implementation, and evaluation). Key elements of case management are as follows:

- Case finding to identify high-risk, high-cost clients
- Assessment and problem identification

- Care planning
- Procurement of services
- Coordination of the delivery of services
- Monitoring
- Evaluation

When these key elements are implemented, case management can be particularly useful for providing cost-effective care for older adults who are at risk for hospitalization or who generally receive high-cost care (Bower, 1992).

Case management is an important part of the advanced practice gerontological nurse's role (American Nurses Association, 1995). Case management systems may be community or hospital based, or they may provide management across the healthcare continuum. The role of the case manager is defined in different ways, depending on the practice setting. In Carondolet St. Mary's Hospital and Health Center Model in Tucson, Arizona, nurses coordinate care for clients across different health settings. The nurse assesses the client in the hospital and coordinates appropriate care after discharge into the community. This system of case management prevents rehospitalization and decreases the length of hospital stays, thereby decreasing costs (Ethridge & Lamb, 1989).

In the acute hospital of the New England Medical Center Hospitals, nurse case managers monitor patients' progress as well as the resources they have consumed in relation to critical paths developed for a particular admitting medical diagnosis (Zander, 1988). At other hospitals, such as the University of Pennsylvania Hospital, geriatric clinical nurse specialists are used as case managers to implement comprehensive discharge planning protocols. These protocols include a comprehensive patient assessment and discharge plan for posthospital care. Case management has decreased both cost (Naylor et al., 1994; Neidlinger et al., 1987) and readmissions (Naylor et al., 1994) in these systems.

TYPOLOGY OF PRACTICE MODELS

Gerontological nursing practice models are evolving with the restructuring of healthcare

TABLE 2-2

Practice Model Typology: Organizational and Payment Structures

Payment Structure	Type of Practice		
	Independent	Collaborative	Consultant

Fee-For-Service	Solo owner
	Nurse partnership
		Nurse-physician partnership
		Employee
		  Small private organization
		  Large public or private organization
			Solo owner
			Nurse or nurse-physician partnership
			Service provider by contract
			Large public or private organization

Prospective Payment	Service provider by contract Large public or private organization providing managed care	Employee Large public or private organization providing managed care	Service provider by contract Large public or private organization providing managed care

delivery and payment strategies, the growing needs of older adults, and the development of alternative care settings. Although many factors shape practice models into an array of permutations, current practice situations fit conceptually into a typology (Table 2–2). There are three basic practice model types: independent, collaborative, and consultant practice. Each of these practice model types can be implemented through a variety of *organizational structures* listed for each type, depending on the *payment structure* used.

These prototype models can be modified according to the needs of the clients as well as previously discussed factors such as the scope of practice and reimbursement. The concepts of interdisciplinary functioning and case management are universal elements among all practice models in gerontological nursing.

Independent Practice

Increasing numbers of gerontological nurses are establishing independent practices. In this type of practice model, the nurse provides care as an independent practitioner, usually in an outpatient, home, or other community setting. There is a paucity of literature on this subject. As in all practice models, independent practices vary depending on factors such as who

owns the practice and its organizational structure, the scope of practice, third-party reimbursement, prescriptive privileges, and the type of setting. Currently, a major distinguishing feature affecting the practice model is whether the organization has a fee-for-service or a prospective payment structure.

Fee-for-Service Payment Structure. If the nurse is self-employed—that is, the *owner* of a solo practice—he or she can define the practice within legal bounds. There are several examples of independent practices providing primary, preventive, or specialty care (Culbert-Hinthorn et al., 1985; Jimerson, 1986; LaPlante Stein, 1993; Lee & O'Neal, 1994; Levin, 1993; Moll, 1987). Some of these are solo practices, whereas others are *nurse partnerships*. In states with a scope of practice that is unrestricted—not requiring physician supervision or collaboration for providing care or prescribing medications—primary care can be provided by nurses in independent practice. In states that are more restrictive, primary care responsibility that requires prescriptive privileges and a broadly defined scope of practice can only be developed in collaboration with a physician. In these states, nurses have established independent practices that are limited to providing only case management, health education services, or preventive screening and health promotion.

Third-party reimbursement is critical in determining the viability of an independent practice, because most practices serving older adults are financially dependent on Medicare reimbursement and receive only a small proportion of private payment. Where third-party payment is not available, nurses have been creative in obtaining funding for underserved populations through special grants from foundations or local government. Others have contracted to provide health services with a retirement facility or other organization serving older adults, such as the Department of Health or the Department of Aging. The literature includes articles describing independent practices serving populations such as younger women or psychiatric clients who privately pay, as opposed to older adults for whom reimbursement has been a significant barrier. Now that APNs can receive direct Medicare reimbursement, independent practice may become a more viable career option.

Several case examples demonstrate how various factors have shaped some existing gerontological nursing practices. Moll (1987) and a nurse partner are in private practice providing health assessment, health education, and referral to community resources and physicians. They see clients in their office, senior centers, and retirement housing clinics. Unable until recently to receive third-party payment, they have contracts to provide care in these settings supported by the United Way, local churches, and retirement facilities. Harris (M. Harris, personal communication, 1995) works under a broadly defined scope of practice in Oregon, which includes prescriptive privileges and reimbursement by third-party payers. This enables her to assume primary care responsibility for clients. She refers to physicians for consultation when appropriate. Newman (D. K. Newman, personal communication, 1995) has a successful independent practice that provides continence care to clients as outpatients and in their homes. She established a professional nursing corporation and has a medical advisor for consultation and chart review in accordance with the Nurse Practice Act of Pennsylvania. Billing is done directly by the nurses.

Other independent practices have also been developed, such as nurse faculty practices that serve as model teaching centers (Culbert-Hinthorn et al., 1985) or nurse-managed centers in rural areas (Barger, 1991; LaPlante Stein, 1993). The nurse-managed center can assume many forms, such as a community clinic or a mobile unit. It provides rural clients direct access to nursing services, and nurses are directly reimbursed for diagnosing and treating clients. Accountability remains with the nurse, and the overall accountability of the center remains with a nurse executive.

Prospective Payment Structure. As independent practitioners, gerontological nurses can enter into a *contract* with large public or private organizations providing managed care, including preferred provider organizations (PPOs) or HMOs that have capitated prospective payment structures. These nurses are paid by contract with the managed care organization to provide healthcare services. In a Medicare HMO (contracted with the federal government to receive capitated Medicare payment), the capitated amount is paid to the HMO; the HMO then pays a fee to physicians, nurses, and other healthcare professionals for providing services. HMOs often contract with APNs to provide more cost-effective healthcare (Middelstadt, 1993).

These case examples illustrate how nurses have developed creative independent practices. If states legislate less restrictive scope-of-practice definitions, reimbursement from third-party payers, and prescriptive privileges, then more independent practice models will develop and thrive. Although gerontological nurses have successfully established private practices (Henne et al., 1988; Hilderley, 1991; Littell, 1981; Shires & Spector, 1993), most are practicing collaboratively, employed by either physicians, hospitals, or managed care organizations (Moore, 1993).

Collaborative Practice

In simple terms, collaborative practice involves nurses and physicians sharing responsibility and accountability for the care of specific clients. Nurses and physicians provide complementary services and develop their practice patterns to maximize the contribution that each makes to the care of the client. *Collaboration* includes both independent and cooperative decision making, based on the preparation and ability of each practitioner. The need for trust and interdependence as a key to success or failure of the relationship cannot be overemphasized (Shires & Spector, 1993). With the current legal restrictions of many states, collaborative practice is the most commonly used model. In states that require collaboration or supervision by a physician, the term *collaborative practice* is used technically. These states may require mutually agreed-on practice protocols or written guidelines.

As in the independent practice model, the collaborative practice model is shaped by factors including the organizational structure, the scope of practice, reimbursement, prescriptive privileges, and the setting. Again, the payment structure is a distinguishing feature of this practice model.

Fee-for-Service Payment Structure. In this setting, the nurse can be a *partner* (part-owner) of a small partnership or larger group practice or an *employee* of a physician or group practice, a hospital, or a large public or private healthcare organization. The nurse's services are billed either by the physician or directly by the nurse, and the nurse usually receives a salary. In a collaborative practice, nurses can provide primary care or specialty services such as cardiology or oncology.

The collaborative model applies to any setting, outpatient clinic, community, skilled nursing facility, home, acute hospital, or other site providing services for older adults. The collaborative practice model has been used successfully in primary care (Elpern et al., 1983; Kearnes, 1992; Lamper-Linden et al., 1983), specialty care (Burke, 1983; Riegel & Murrell, 1987), skilled nursing facilities (Polich et al., 1990; Rauckhorst, 1989), the home (Zimmer et al., 1985), and acute hospital care (Elpern et al., 1983; Hilderley, 1991; Rimel & Langfitt, 1980; Sawyers, 1993; Walton et al., 1993; Watkins et al., 1992). The nurse functions within the scope of practice for the state and collaborates with the physician according to agreed-on guidelines if required, or when consultation for medical problems is necessary. The collaborative model accommodates restrictions of scope of

practice, lack of prescriptive authority, or inadequate reimbursement; practice guidelines such as prescribing drugs can be developed, and reimbursement is provided to the physician or organization.

At Wilder Senior Clinic in St. Paul, Minnesota, gerontological nurse practitioners collaborate with geriatricians to provide primary care for their caseload of clients who have chronic diseases such as hypertension and recurrent congestive heart failure. The nurse practitioners have prescriptive privileges under written agreement with the geriatricians. Billing is currently done through the geriatricians, although the nurses will be billing directly in the near future.

APNs have been providing clinical consultation, education, and administration in the acute care setting for many years. Nurses have recently begun to provide primary care in the hospital in response to the need to contain costs, prevent complications or detect them earlier, and educate and counsel clients and their families appropriately. These nurses assess, manage, and plan discharge of the acutely ill hospitalized clients. They collaborate with physicians and often work in both the hospital and the outpatient setting to provide continuity of care.

Prospective Payment Structure. Gerontological nurses also work collaboratively with physicians in managed care organizations. In this model, the physician and the nurse are both *employees* of a large public or private organization that provides managed care. They function according to their respective practice acts as they would in private practice. However, the organization receives capitated prospective payments to provide healthcare to its members. Managed care organizations frequently use APNs because they provide a quality, cost-effective alternative to physician care (U.S. Congress Office of Technology Assessment, 1986). Healthcare providers of managed care organizations frequently practice according to guidelines, using critical pathways developed by the organization.

Consultant Practice

A third practice alternative is the consultant model. The consultant model overlaps with the independent and collaborative practice models. The nurse contracts as the *owner* of a solo practice or partnership to provide defined services as an independent practitioner for a fee. These services can be direct client care or indirect care, such as health education. Consultant work can be done with a private or managed care organization. The nurse consultant may also contract with an HMO to participate in a collaborative practice model for providing care; the nurse is a consultant but working clinically in a collaborative relationship with a physician. The roles and functions can be similar to those of nurses working in independent or collaborative practice models, but the nurse is not an owner or employee of the organization and thus is *outside* the organizational structure, with a financial arrangement by contract.

ADVANCED PRACTICE NURSING SUBROLES

The practice models that have been discussed relate to clinical practice. However, additional subroles of administration, education, and research may be assumed by the APN. Administrative functions include activities such as developing and directing gerontological programs (the Geriatric Day Hospital [GDH] and EverCare programs discussed later were started by gerontological nurse practitioners), establishing standards of practice, participating in strategic planning of gerontological programs, and reviewing institutional policies and procedures. The nurse may educate clients, their families, nursing students, or other health professionals. Research activities may include identifying researchable clinical problems, evaluating the impact of clinical programs or interventions on client care, or participating with an institutional research committee.

Another role the APN can develop is that of the entrepreneur. Some nurses use their skills to begin a business. Clark and Quinn (1988), for example, described Lifewise, a private business that assists the elderly to stay as independent as possible or helps adult children cope with caring for their elderly parents. Chicken Soup Plus is a nursing practice and home health agency that is owned and operated by

a family nurse practitioner (Baker & Pulcini, 1990).

INNOVATIVE MODELS FOR THE FUTURE

This section presents three examples of innovative programs that serve older clients with multisystem disease, physical disabilities, and psychosocial problems and also incorporate the concepts of interdisciplinary teamwork and case management. Each program has a nurse practitioner as the primary care provider. The programs are as follows: (1) GDH, a fee-for-service model of outpatient care for frail older adults; (2) On Lok Senior Health Services, a managed care program that provides community-based long-term care for frail older adults; and (3) EverCare, a managed care program that provides institutional long term care.

The Geriatric Day Hospital, Los Angeles, California. The GDH is an outpatient service that goes beyond a clinic or office by providing subacute or acute medical, nursing, social, and rehabilitative services at any time of the day, with return visits as necessary. The GDH provides comprehensive geriatric assessment by an interdisciplinary team including a gerontological nurse practitioner, a social worker, and a geriatrician; these team members attend to problems such as memory loss, depression, urinary incontinence, and inappropriate medications. Physical, occupational, and speech therapists; dietitians; and medical subspecialists participate when needed. Multiple diagnostic tests that may be too debilitating to perform in frail elderly patients in a typical outpatient setting, such as barium enema exams and biopsies, are performed with careful monitoring. Acutely ill clients who do not require overnight hospital stay, such as those with dehydration who need intravenous fluids, receive acute nursing care during the day. Intensive coordinated rehabilitation services as well as case management are provided to ensure continuity of care. These functions fill gaps between traditional levels of care, thereby enabling the team to provide complex care on an outpatient basis. Without such a service, physicians would often use the hospital or nursing home as an alternative (Morishita et al., 1989).

The GDH is a fee-for-service, hospital-based outpatient setting with gerontological nurse practitioners as primary care providers and key members of the interdisciplinary team. The hospital employs the nurses, and the nurses have a collaborative relationship with the geriatricians, using agreed-on standardized procedure guidelines.

On Lok Senior Health Services, San Francisco, California. On Lok Senior Health Services is a successful managed care model of community-based long-term care for older adults who are eligible for nursing home services. It employs nurse practitioners as primary care providers who work collaboratively with physicians, social workers, and other healthcare professionals who are also employees of On Lok (Morishita & Hansen, 1986). Nurses and physicians are part of an interdisciplinary team that authorizes and offers comprehensive medical, nursing, and social services to the On Lok participants. These services cover the continuum of healthcare needs, including acute care, homecare, skilled nursing level care, social services, personal care, homemaker and chore services, daycare, meals, transportation, and case management. The program's foundation is the adult day health center, where meals and outpatient health, social, rehabilitation, and recreational therapy services are provided. On Lok is a consolidated model of case management that provides all services under a capitated reimbursement structure. It has demonstrated that close oversight of participants enables the staff to prevent costly, unnecessary hospitalizations, thereby containing costs. The On Lok model is being replicated throughout the country as the Program of All-inclusive Care of the Elderly (PACE) (Zawadski & Eng, 1988).

EverCare, Minneapolis, Minnesota. EverCare was developed by two APNs to provide healthcare services to nursing home residents who are members of a managed care organization. The nurse practitioner plays a key role in this program as both primary care provider and case manager for a caseload of residents. The nurse practitioners and physicians either are EverCare employees or have an independent contractual arrangement. The nurse prac-

---

TABLE 2-3

Questions for Considering Practice Options

1. What are the needs of the older client served?
2. What other professional consultation is available from other disciplines? What would your relationship be?
3. How are clinical decisions made?
4. What is the organizational structure?
5. Who owns the practice?
6. What is the payment structure?
7. What is the healthcare setting?
8. How are you going to manage your client throughout a continuum of care? Is there an integrated delivery system?
9. What is the scope of practice in the state?
10. What third-party reimbursement or other funding is available?
11. What prescriptive privileges are available?

---

titioner works collaboratively with physicians and ensures coordination and communication with the nursing home staff. Preventive care is emphasized. Financial incentives encourage the nurse practitioner and physician to make more frequent visits to the nursing home and also deter the unnecessary use of hospital admissions or emergency room visits. The increased oversight of the client—beyond that allowed by a traditional care system—minimizes hospitalizations and therefore costs (Polich et al., 1990).

Developing New Practice Models. These three innovative programs use advanced practice gerontological nurses in key roles and also incorporate the concepts of case management and interdisciplinary team care to meet the healthcare needs of frail older adults. They provide examples for how an advanced nursing practice model can be developed. Table 2–3 includes questions that should be addressed in developing or evaluating one's own practice. The answers to these questions will indicate potential practice options as well as how to most effectively develop a practice. As a practice evolves, the nurse should answer these questions periodically to reevaluate his or her own practice.

SUMMARY

Practice models in gerontological nursing are evolving with the growing need for specialized healthcare of older adults in this country, along with the changes in healthcare delivery and payment structures that have been developed to contain costs. Independent, collaborative, and consultant practice models are shaped by client, nurse, team, organizational, third-party reimbursement, and legal factors that affect the actual practice that is developed. These factors are interdependent; a change in any factor can have an impact on the practice model. As changes occur, gerontological nurses must anticipate how these changes affect their practice options and position themselves for expanded practice roles in the care of older adults.

Gerontological nurses will have opportunities to develop practice models that respond to trends such as the dramatic increase in managed care, expansion of community-based services, and an increasing need to address health issues of older women and a more culturally diverse older population.

It is important to define practice models and to conduct critically needed research that links models of practice with client outcomes and cost-effectiveness measures. This work will be important in formulating future healthcare policy that leads to the effective use of advanced practice gerontological nurses and establishment of practice models that provide accessible, high quality care for older people.

Acknowledgments

The author thanks Mary Cadogan, PhD, RN, CS, and Ryu Kanemoto, MN, RN, CS, for their review and helpful suggestions.

REFERENCES

American Nurses Association (1995). *Scope and standards of gerontological nursing practice.* Washington, DC: American Nurses Publishing.

Baker, M. M., & Pulcini, J. A. (1990). Innovation: Nurse practitioners as entrepreneurs. *Nurse Practitioner Forum, 1*(3), 169–174.

Balanced Budget Act of 1997. Pub. L. No. 105-33 (5 August 1997).

Barger, S. E. (1991). The nursing center: A model for rural nursing practice. *Nursing and Health Care, 12*, 290–294.

Bower, K. A. (1992). *Case management by nurses.* Kansas City, MO: American Nurses Publishing.

Brand, M. K., & Gurenlian, J. K. (1989). Extending access to care: Preparing allied health practitioners for non-traditional settings. *Journal of Allied Health, 18(3),* 261–270.

Burke, L. E. (1983). The clinical nurse specialist in collaborative practice. *Momentum, 1,* 3–5.

Campbell, L. J., & Cole, K. D. (1987). Geriatric assessment teams. *Clinics in Geriatric Medicine, 3,* 99–110.

Cassel, C. K., & Brody, J. A. (1990). Demography, epidemiology, and aging (pp. 16–27). In C. K. Cassel, D. E. Riesenberg, L. B. Sorenson & J. R. Walsh (Eds.), *Geriatric medicine* (2nd ed.). New York: Springer-Verlag.

Clark, L., & Quinn, J. (1988). The new entrepreneurs. *Nursing and Health Care, 9*(1), 7–15.

Culbert-Hinthorn, P., Fiscella, K. D., & Shortridge, L. M. (1985). A nurse-managed clinical practice unit: Part I—The positives. *Nursing & Health Care, 6*(2), 97–100.

Elpern, E. H., Rodts, M. F., DeWald, R. C., & West, J. W. (1983). Associated practice: A case for professional collaboration. *Journal of Nursing Administration, 13*(11), 27–35.

Ethridge, P. H., & Lamb, G. S. (1989). Professional nursing case management improves quality, access and costs. *Nursing Management, 20,* 30–35.

Goldberg, R. J., Tull, R., Sullivan, N., & Wool, M. (1984). Defining discipline roles in consultation psychiatry: The multidisciplinary team approach to psychosocial oncology. *General Hospital Psychiatry, 6,* 17–23.

Henne, S. J., Warner, N. E., & Frank, K. J. (1988). Ambulatory care centers: A unique opportunity for nurse practitioners. *Nurse Practitioner, 13,* 45–55.

Hilderley, L. J. (1991). Nurse-physician collaborative practice: The clinical nurse specialist in a radiation oncology private practice. *Oncology Nursing Forum, 18,* 585–591.

Jimerson, S. S. (1986). Expanded practice in psychiatric nursing. *Nursing Clinics of North America, 21,* 527–535.

Joel, L. (1985). Economics of health care: Trends and problems. In The American Academy of Nursing (Ed.), *The economics of health care and nursing* (pp. 7–18). Kansas City, MO: American Nurses Publishing.

Kearnes, D. R. (1992). A productivity tool to evaluate NP practice: Monitoring clinical time spent in reimbursable, patient-related activities. *Nurse Practitioner, 17,* 50–55.

Lamper-Linden, C., Goetz-Kulas, J., & Lake, R. (1983). Developing ambulatory care clinics: Nurse practitioners as primary providers. *Journal of Nursing Administration, 13*(12), 11–18.

LaPlante Stein, L. M. (1993). Health care delivery to farmworkers in the southwest: An innovative nursing clinic. *Journal of the American Academy of Nurse Practitioners, 5,* 119–124.

Lee, E. J., & O'Neal, S. (1994). A mobile clinic experience: Nurse practitioners providing care to a rural population. *Journal of Pediatric Health Care, 8,* 12–17.

Levin, T. E. (1993). The solo nurse practitioner: A private practice model. *Nurse Practitioner Forum, 4,* 158–165.

Light, D. (1986). Surplus versus cost containment: The changing context for health providers (pp. 519–542). In L. Aiken & D. Mechanic (Eds.), *Applications of social science to clinical medicine and policy.* New Brunswick, NJ: Rutgers University Press.

Littell, S. C. (1981). The clinical nurse specialist in a private medical practice. *Nursing Administration Quarterly, 6*(1), 77–85.

McCartney, J. R., & Palmateer, I. M. (1985). Assessment of cognitive deficit in geriatric patients. *Journal of the American Geriatrics Society, 33*, 467–471.

Middelstadt, P. C. (1993). Federal reimbursement of advanced practice nurses' services empowers the profession. *Nurse Practitioner, 18*, 43–49.

Moll, J. A. (1987). Private practice for older adults: Models for long-term care. *National League for Nursing Publications, 20-2188*, 15–21.

Moore, S. (1993). Promoting advanced practice nursing. *American Association of Critical-Care Nurses, Clinical Issues in Critical-Care Nursing, 4*(4), 603–608.

Morishita, L., & Hansen, J. C. (1986). GNP and the long-term care team. *Journal of Gerontological Nursing, 12*(6), 15–20.

Morishita, L., Siu, A. L., Wang, R. T., et al. (1989). Comprehensive geriatric care in a day hospital: A demonstration of the British model in the United States. *Gerontologist, 29*, 336–340.

Naylor, M., Brooten, D., Jones, R., et al. (1994). Comprehensive discharge planning for the hospitalized elderly. *Annals of Internal Medicine, 120*(12), 999–1006.

Neidlinger, S. H., Scroggins, K., & Kennedy, L. M. (1987). Cost evaluation of discharge planning for hospitalized elderly. *Nursing Economics, 5*(5), 225–230.

Pearson, L. J. (1998). Annual update of how each state stands on legislative issues affecting advanced nursing practice. *Nurse Practitioner, 23*(1), 14–66.

Polich, C. L., Bayard, J., Jacobson, R. A., & Parker, M. (1990). A nurse-run business to improve health care for nursing home residents. *Nursing Economics, 8*, 96–101.

Rauckhorst, L. M. (1989). Impact of a physician/nurse practitioner team primary care delivery model on selected geriatric long-term care outcomes. *Journal of Nursing Quality Assurance, 4*, 62–72.

Riegel, B., & Murrell, T. (1987). Clinical nurse specialists in collaborative practice. *Clinical Nurse Specialist, 1*, 63–69.

Rimel, R. W., & Langfitt, T. W. (1980). The evolving role of the nurse practitioner in neurosurgery. *Journal of Neurosurgery, 53*, 802–807.

Sawyers, J. E. (1993). Defining your role in ambulatory care: Clinical nurse specialist or nurse practitioner? *Clinical Nurse Specialist, 7*, 4–7.

Shires, B. W., & Spector, P. M. (1993). The clinical nurse specialist and psychiatrist in joint practice. *Perspectives in Psychiatric Care, 29*, 21–24.

Siu, A. L., Leake, B., & Brook, R. K. (1988). The quality of care received by older patients in 15 university-based ambulatory practices. *Journal of Medical Education, 63*, 155–161.

U.S. Congress Office of Technology Assessment, HCS 37 (1986). *Nurse practitioners, physician assistants, and certified nurse-midwives: A policy analysis.* Washington, D.C. Congress of the United States, Office of Technology Assessment.

Walton, M. K., Jokobowski, D. S., & Barnsteiner, J. H. (1993). A collaborative practice model for the clinical nurse specialist. *Journal of Nursing Administration, 23*(2), 55–59.

Watkins, S., Kirchhoff, K. T., Hartigan, E. G., & Karp, T. (1992). Development of a program for neonatal intensive care units managed by neonatal nurse practitioners. *Nursing Clinics of North America, 27*, 87–96.

Zander, K. (1988). Nursing case management: Strategic management of cost and quality outcomes. *Journal of Nursing Administration, 18*(5), 23–30.

Zawadski, R. T., & Eng, C. (1988). Case management in capitated long-term care. *Health Care Financing Review, (suppl.)*, 75–81.

Zimmer, J. G., Groth-Jucker, A., & McCusker, J. (1985). A randomized controlled study of a home health care team. *American Journal of Public Health, 75*(2), 134–141.

APPENDIX 2-1

Resources

National Association of Professional Geriatric
Care Managers
1604 N. Country Club Road
Tucson, AZ 85716
Phone: (602) 881-8008

Individual Case Management Association
11830 Westline Industrial Drive
St. Louis, MO 63146
Phone: (800) 664-2620

National Gerontological Nursing Association
7250 Parkway Drive, Suite 510
Hanover, MD 21706

National Conference of Gerontological Nurse
Practitioners
P.O. Box 270101
Fort Collins, CO 80527-0101
Phone: (970) 493-7793

Legal Planning Issues

Patricia Tobin
Sally A. Salisbury

The issues involved in healthcare for the elderly are far reaching, complex, and often protracted. When a patient requires long-term healthcare or personal care, numerous decisions must be made beyond those that pertain to healthcare treatment: selecting a caregiver or care setting; paying for services; applying for aid (if any is available); obtaining access to records; resolving problems of insurance coverage; and settling conflicting opinions of family members.

This chapter discusses the legal problems encountered by patients and their families when faced with chronic, debilitating, or de-menting conditions. It is designed to inform the advanced practice nurse of the options and resources available to patients and their families so that informed, timely, and appropriate referrals can be made.

THE LAWYER AS A MEMBER OF THE HEALTHCARE TEAM

Legal consultations can be provided by attorneys experienced in estate and financial matters, conservatorships, powers of attorney, and eligibility for government programs and other benefits (Family Caregiver Alliance, 1993). Although elderly people as well as spouses or children who care for the chronically ill elderly need information about legal planning, these individuals and healthcare professionals seldom consider attorneys their allies. Yet if elderly people and their families planned and were better prepared to meet the multiple and fluctuating needs created by illness, healthcare providers would be better able to make treatment decisions and discharge plans.

PHASES OF LEGAL PLANNING

The legal planning process involves several phases: consideration, choice, identification of legal steps and tools, expression, and formalities. This process starts when an individual begins to *consider* future health and financial needs, such as controlling healthcare decision making and finances; facing the possibility of declining health, disability, or mental incapacity; and considering one's own death and the *choices* to be made about the disposition of property to survivors after death.

The individual then educates himself or herself or consults an attorney for guidance in legal planning to *identify the legal steps or tools* available for implementing a plan. The individual *expresses* choices and makes plans through informal discussion with family members, consultation with physicians, written informal letters or instructions to family members, or formal legal documents. Some of the written documents can be private, meaning they are disclosed only after the individual dies. Usually directions are written in a format that includes the necessary legal *formalities* to ensure legal force and effect when the need arises.

The creation of a will provides an example of all the phases of legal planning. In the simplest context, this process is initiated when a *planner* (the individual who initiates the legal process) acknowledges, "I think, at my age, it is time for me to write a will" [*consideration*]. For example, a woman making a will (known as a *testator*) may implicitly choose to leave all her property to her family and explicitly choose her eldest daughter to implement her plan [*choice*]. The person who is selected in the will

to manage the estate is known as the *executor*. The planner selects a lawyer and discusses the plan with him or her. Ideally, the lawyer outlines the legal ramifications of each choice and the options, advantages, and disadvantages of the plan [*identification of legal steps and tools*]. After learning the person's wishes, the lawyer drafts an appropriate document to be signed by the person [*expression*]. If the document is signed with the appropriate formalities, it is treated as binding. This process is known as executing the document [*formalities*]. On the death of the planner, the designated family member becomes responsible for carrying out the terms of the will.

Legal planning can also involve much more sophisticated and considered plans. A more comprehensive plan might include planning for financial and healthcare issues during the life of the planner as well as specific concerns such as tax avoidance, charitable intentions, anatomical gifts, and funeral arrangements.

The legal planning process requires the involvement of a motivated planner who can on some level—no matter how superficial—formulate a plan, understand the choices to be made, and express the plan by discussing it with others and/or writing the plan down. Further, the planner must have the mental capacity—again, at least at some level—to understand the options and express a preference. (The most common legal planning tools are listed in Table 3–1.)

In a crisis situation, such as when a parent is ill, family caregivers often see the value of planning and, with good intentions, try to orchestrate the creation of a legal plan on the parent's behalf. One often hears caregivers say, "we need to get Mom a durable power of

---

TABLE 3-1

The Most Common Legal Planning Tools

Durable power of attorney for health care (DPAHC)
Living will
Declaration to physicians
Durable power of attorney for finances (DPA)
Living trust (intervivos trust, revocable trust, private will)
Will

attorney" or "here, Dad, sign this" or "you wouldn't want to be kept alive on machines, would you, Aunt May?" Although family members can assist a planner, caregivers and professionals sometimes hold the misconception that concerned friends or family members can complete the legal planning on behalf of the planner.

By understanding the phases of legal planning and the appropriate responses at each phase, the advanced practice nurse can avoid misdirecting families and patients and can make better referrals for services needed by families and patients.

COMPETENCE AND CAPACITY

This brief discussion focuses on competence and capacity related to long-term planning and decision making (see also Chapter 4). *Capacity,* for the purposes of this chapter, is defined as the functional ability to understand, appreciate, and either take or direct certain actions. *Competence* is best defined as a legal term of art in which the individual's actions are given effect in various legal contexts.

The central idea of competence is that it is not a static entity but one that fluctuates over time, in periods of health and illness. Elderly people may hesitate to formalize the delegation of authority because they feel it is not yet needed, or they may wish to avoid thinking of themselves as incapacitated. However, any person suddenly very ill has diminished capacity: All thought and energy are absorbed in dealing with pain, fear of the unknown, and the work of recovery. Someone else needs to handle daily living matters such as paying bills, arranging for aftercare, and tending the home. In other words, life outside of the illness event will proceed more smoothly if someone is empowered to assist on the patient's behalf. This is not to imply that the patient is rendered powerless; rather, his or her energy can be better directed toward dealing with immediate treatment concerns and making those immediate decisions that affect the treatment given and the responses to treatment. One study found that mildly demented, chronically ill inpatients did not differ from nondemented co-

horts in their ability to communicate their desires and adjust treatment decisions using prognostic information; further, both groups were consistent in their choices regarding treatment (Gerety et al., 1993).

In legal usage, competence may simply be determined by age. For example, a healthy, functioning adult who witnessed an event is typically termed competent to testify as a witness in a trial. However, a 4-year-old child who witnessed the same event may be deemed incompetent to testify. The child is legally disqualified as a witness and is considered an inherently unreliable witness because a child of this age lacks the judgment and experience to correctly report on past events. This finding of incompetence for a specific legal purpose in no way means the child is disabled, nonfunctional, or otherwise impaired.

In other legal contexts, such as a protective proceeding known in various states as a *guardianship* or *conservatorship proceeding*, an elderly person may be adjudged incompetent. This would likely mean that after some (at times, cursory) review of the situation, a judge has imposed a legal disability on the elderly person that disqualifies the elderly person from participation in managing his or her normal affairs. Although it varies among states, a finding of incompetence could legally disqualify an elderly person from voting, driving, marrying, signing a contract, consenting to medical treatment, writing a will, buying or selling property, using credit, or choosing a place of residence. This *legal disability* can prevent the incompetent elderly person from effectively engaging in any transaction with legal ramifications as well as other specific transactions. The characterization of incompetence is designed to protect an individual from the consequences of his or her own actions or the undue or harmful influence of others. During the proceeding, someone else is usually appointed to make judgments on behalf of the incompetent person.

For example, a person who is deemed incompetent by a court in a guardianship or conservatorship matter may have the apparent ability to sign a contract under which his or her home is sold for a fraction of its value. Thus, this legal disability (i.e., the finding of incompetence) cannot in itself physically prevent an otherwise unconfined individual from engaging in any business that he or she can initiate. However, when the buyer tries to enforce the sale (by taking money from the incompetent "seller" and publicly recording the deed), the previous characterization of incompetence may be used by the incompetent individual or his or her *surrogate* (conservator or guardian) to invalidate the sale and shield the individual from the consequences of his or her own actions. Further, if a surrogate decision maker has been appointed in the competency procedure, that person—and not the person judged incompetent—would have the legal authority to enter into a contract and sell the house for a fair value on behalf of the incompetent individual.

In various states, the court review of competency and the appointment of a substitute decision maker may be called a conservatorship, a protective procedure, an adult guardianship proceeding, or another title. The protected person may be known as a conservatee, a ward, or a committee. The surrogate decision maker may be termed a surrogate, a conservator, or a guardian.

These kinds of proceedings have recently begun to focus more on identifying the functional abilities of the protected person. The court system has begun to move away from a global characterization of an individual as incompetent and toward identifying specific transactions in which the protected person is incapable of participating or dysfunctional disabilities that render a person—of any age—incapable of carrying out certain transactions (Hurme, 1991). Similarly, the trend is to move toward a review of functional capacities and functional disabilities and to limit protection and intrusion only to those functional disabilities. For this reason, planning issues discuss incapacity rather than incompetence. It is essential that a person who creates a legal plan has capacity.

ELEMENTS OF A LEGAL PLAN FOR OLDER ADULTS

There are three primary elements in a legal plan for older adults:

- Estate planning for property
- Estate planning for personal or healthcare issues
- Planning for access to care and resources

Estate Planning for Property

Estate planning describes the process of using legal tools to plan for the preservation, appreciation, or control of property. In this context, estate planning does not include any steps concerning healthcare management.

The legal steps available for estate planning are typically the creation of legal documents and the application of principles contained in laws, regulations, and court cases. Patients may also concurrently employ the tools of other estate planning disciplines, which can include financial, investment, and tax planning. These three areas can and should be integrated; however, patients often focus on legal estate planning, rather than investment or tax planning, because these legal tools are often the key to implementing any other investment or tax strategy.

Common Legal Documents. The most common legal documents that patients consider or create are the following:

- *Durable Power of Attorney (DPA) for Property.* The patient (the *principal*) appoints someone else (the *agent* or *attorney in fact*) to manage his or her financial affairs. The DPA can become effective when the patient no longer wants the responsibility of managing his or her own affairs or becomes mentally incapacitated. It is considered durable because it endures even in the event of mental incapacity; however, it is not effective after death.
- *Living Trust.* This is a special framework for one's own property. The person who creates the trust is called a settlor, trustor, grantor, or creator. This framework is established by a written and signed document (like an agreement). However, the trust is not effective unless arrangements are made to ensure that the existence of the trust is reflected in the ownership of the creator's property. (Just signing documents is usually not enough to make an

effective trust.) The instructions contained in the trust direct how the trust will operate. When property is held in this trust, another person—the *trustee*—manages the property for the creator's benefit when the creator becomes unable to do so. The trustee can be a friend, a family member, or a professional worker such as a bank officer. When the creator dies, the trustee can distribute the property in the trust without going through the court process (known as probate). On the death of a client, a trust can substitute for a will.

- *Will.* A will appoints an executor and directs the executor in distributing the property to friends and family after death. The person making the will is referred to as the testator. A will gives *no* authority over property until the testator dies. During the life of the testator, the executor has no right to manage the testator's property if he or she is unable to manage or make healthcare decisions for someone who is ill. When the testator dies, a court supervises the executor in carrying out the directions in the will. This court supervision process is known as a probate administration. Certain types or small amounts of property can be passed to heirs without probate.

Estate Planning for Personal or Healthcare Issues

Although they are dependent in many instances on finances, personal or healthcare planning issues are best viewed as a separate component of an estate plan. Much has been written about advance directives and their effect on end-of-life treatment. *Advance directives* are legal documents used to indicate individuals' wishes concerning medical care and treatment when the individuals are no longer able to express their wishes themselves (Hague & Moody, 1993).

Common Types of Advance Directives. There are three common advance medical directive documents used to express personal or healthcare preferences:

- *Durable Power of Attorney for Health Care*

(DPAHC). A patient may appoint someone (known as an agent [used in this chapter], proxy, surrogate, or attorney in fact) to consent to (or refuse) healthcare treatment for the patient. This can include consent to invasive tests, the release of medical records, and even the withdrawal of life-sustaining treatment. This power is effective only if the patient is (temporarily or permanently) mentally unable to make decisions. If the patient has the capacity to make healthcare decisions, the patient's choice—not the choice of the agent—governs. The Uniform DPA Act has been adopted in 22 states, and all 50 states have enacted some version of a DPAHC (Regan & Gilfix, 1993).

- *Living Will.* This is a formal written statement of a patient's wishes concerning the use or discontinuance of life-sustaining treatments; it is not necessarily binding in all states.

- *Declaration to Physician.* A type of living will, this document is a written, enforceable statement that is signed in the presence of independent witnesses. It states the declarant's wishes for future medical treatment to be withdrawn if the declarant is ever permanently unconscious or suffers from an incurable, irreversible terminal condition.

Hospitals, nursing facilities, homecare agencies, and health maintenance organizations receiving Medicare and Medicaid reimbursement are now required to adhere to the regulations of the Patient Self-Determination Act (PSDA) and inform all their patients over the age of 18 years of their right to plan for their future care (PSDA, 1990). Providers must give patients the agency's written policy concerning this right and take steps to educate their staff about these provisions (Holly, 1993). The new legislation has done much to bring issues of advance planning to the attention of healthcare providers and consumers of healthcare, but it has not clarified the misconceptions held by consumers, their families, or healthcare providers.

Four common misconceptions are the following:

1. *Myth*: When a patient has a DPAHC and

is admitted to a hospital, the healthcare agent decides what treatment is given.

Fact: The agent has no greater rights than the patient to demand any particular treatment. Typically, the treatment providers propose certain treatments (often with input from insurance representatives or the utilization review team). The patient has a complete right to accept or refuse the treatment. The agent has input *only* when the patient is unable to express his or her wishes concerning the treatment or lacks the capacity to give informed consent.

2. *Myth*: Family members should obtain a form so they can make a decision for the patient.

   Fact: A DPA can be *executed* (i.e., signed with specific legal formalities) only by the patient when the patient has capacity and chooses to sign.

3. *Myth*: When the patient goes to a hospital, he or she must have a DPA for healthcare.

   Fact: The PSDA requires only that the hospital give notice to the patient of his or her right to execute a DPA for healthcare. The provider cannot require a patient to complete any form.

4. *Myth*: A DPA for healthcare tells the hospital when to "pull the plug."

   Fact: The discontinuance of life support is first a medical recommendation and then a decision for the patient. If the patient cannot express a preference, the agent must review and follow the preferences expressed in the document. If the preferences are not clear, the agent must use his or her judgment to act in the best interest of the patient, which could mean either continuing or discontinuing life support. A DPA for healthcare can express a preference to use all medically feasible treatment to maintain life; such a document need not specify only the withdrawal of treatment.

Researchers have examined several problems in the use of advance medical directives. Although patients may have heard of living wills or powers of attorney for healthcare, many do not fully understand them or the conditions under which they may be implemented; still fewer patients have executed one. Jacobson and associates (1994) found that some patients who have completed the legal formalities to create power of attorney for healthcare do not fully understand what it means. Therefore, although more patients are aware of advance planning and discuss this with their surrogates and physicians, the PSDA has not caused a significant change in the number of patients who formalize their choices through legal documents (Emanuel et al., 1993).

To competently fulfill their role as advocates for patients, advanced practice nurses need a working knowledge of the types of formal decisions available to patients and the circumstances under which they may be invoked. However, nurses often have not been prepared adequately and feel uncomfortable talking to patients and their families about these issues and the process of estate planning (Barta & Neighbors, 1993).

Planning for Access to Public Resources

For several reasons, patients who would ordinarily consider themselves self-sufficient and not needing help from the government should consider the availability of public services such as Medicaid. First, functionally dependent older patients and their families are likely to need healthcare or personal care services and respite for months or even years. The costs of healthcare have made most long-term care services unaffordable, even to the middle class. Second, the somewhat arbitrary categories of private healthcare insurance coverage (most critically, the limits on home services and custodial long-term care) render some patients ineligible for coverage of necessary services. Managed care can be expected to sharply curtail the services available through both private and public healthcare payers. Third, many patients may be excluded from purchasing private healthcare insurance coverage because of preexisting health problems.

Entitlement Versus Welfare. Several factors can influence an inpatient's decision to use or reject social services and public resources. Elderly people may reject the intrusiveness of government bureaucracies that provide services, or they may hold cultural values that conflict with the use of such services. They may reject or deny that they are an appropriate beneficiary of services. Many elderly people do not wish to be identified as a user of "senior services," or they may view public resources as charity. Advanced practice nurses can expect to find among their patients a variety of opinions on this issue.

The United States currently has two main systems of care for the elderly: Social Security, which pays income to individuals who worked and contributed to the system; and Medicare, a universal health insurance system for certain people who have disabilities and/or who are over 65 years of age. However, there are no constitutional guarantees that these systems will remain viable. As early as 1983, the Reagan administration declared that as part of the Medicaid program, states could legally require children to contribute to the support of their elderly parents (Callahan, 1987). As the cost of care escalates and reimbursement and coverage dwindle, however, a justifiable concern is that families will have to bear an increasing share of the cost of care. In the future, the decision of whether to view cure and care services for the elderly as an entitlement or as welfare may influence methods of payment for these services as well as the steps families must take to ensure that such care is received when needed. Planning for illness will become increasingly critical.

Callahan (1987) defined three concepts as possible moral and social foundations for care: need, veteranship, and intergenerational reciprocity. The *need* and vulnerability of the sick elderly generate a corresponding obligation to have those needs met, and family members may perceive this as a moral imperative to respond—but for how long and at what cost? Is it appropriate for society to expect that caregivers sacrifice their own health to provide care or that adult children deprive their children financially to meet the needs of sick, elderly parents?

Veteranship defines the past of the elderly in terms of their work, parenting, investing, soldiering, and building. Old age is therefore viewed as a compensation and an earned status (Callahan, 1987). From this cognitive set, programs such as Social Security and Medicare are viewed as entitlements, not giveaway programs, and the elderly regard a comfortable and secure life in old age as a right purchased with a life of labor. This view is widely held by the present cohort of elderly patients and their families. Moreover, veteranship views the contribution of the elderly as embracing not only the nuclear family but also society and the country as a whole. It follows, then, that the elderly look to society and government to provide for their needs. However, the need for elderly people to impoverish themselves to qualify for care under Medicaid creates a forced dependency on government, deprives them of dignity, and is inconsistent with the concept of veteranship. (A more detailed description of Medicaid rules is given later.)

Reciprocity between generations implies that all generations are interdependent and have an interest in social policies and intergenerational transfers that meet people's needs throughout life (Kingson et al., 1986). Thus, although young people today may be paying an inordinate share of the taxes to provide services and care for the elderly, they can expect to reap the same benefits when they become old. This idea operates within families as well. Senior family members who have inherited and built on property or wealth—no matter how meager it may seem—often feel a moral imperative to pass this on to the next generation. For this reason, there is often bitter resentment at the idea of "spending down" to reach Medicaid limits to qualify for long-term care services. There is also concern on the part of young people who are now heavily taxed to support the elderly that future policy changes may deprive them of needed care when they are old.

In summary, most elderly and their families view care for the elderly as an entitlement. When care is framed as welfare, they may balk at accepting it—not because they feel it is undeserved, but because they feel unfairly stigmatized by having care equated with welfare.

The advanced practice nurse's decision over whether to encourage patients to use government services should rest on many factors: the availability, suitability, and quality of local services; the needs and values of patient and family members; and the nature of the healthcare enterprise in which the nurse practices. To ensure informed decision making by patients, the facility should at a minimum inform the family of these potential resources.

Types of Public Benefits. The following is a list of the public benefits most relevant to elderly patients (Table 3–2):

- *Social Security.* This benefit of a check is available to retired workers, disabled workers, or certain dependents of those workers. Payment is usually received on the third day of the month; for new beneficiaries (after April 1997), this date may vary. The Old-Age Survivors and Disability Insurance and Social Security Disability Insurance programs are *not* based on financial need. Divorced spouses at 62 years of age can qualify on the earnings records of former spouses or as caregivers to the former spouse's child(ren). Children of disabled workers and disabled adult children of retired or disabled wage earners can also qualify (Table 3–3).
- *Supplemental Security Income.* This check from the Social Security Administration is normally received on the first day of the month. The supplemental security income program *is* based on financial need. An applicant must be a citizen or lawful resident of the United States and must have disabilities and/or be over 65 years of age. Single people must have countable assets of less than $2000 as well as low income. Certain assets, such as a home, can be treated as exempt.
- *Medicaid.* Medicaid benefits are based on

TABLE 3-2

Types of Public Benefits

Social Security
Supplemental security income (SSI)
Medicaid
Medicare
Care services at home, also known as in-home support
  services (IHSS) or personal care option (PCO)
Veteran's benefits

TABLE 3-3

Social Security Benefits

The following people can qualify on the work record of a **disabled** or **retired** wage earner:

- Spouse at 62
- Spouse of any age if caring for wage earner's child under 16 or for disabled child
- Ex-spouse at age 62 if marriage lasted over 10 years
- Unmarried child under 18 (up to 19 if full time high school student)
- Unmarried disabled child of any age—if disability began before 22

The following people qualify on the work record of a **deceased** wage earner:

- Widow(er) at age 60
- Disabled widow(er) at age 50 (with certain limits)
- Widow(er) at any age if caring for a child under 16 or a disabled child
- Unmarried ex-spouse over 60 if marriage lasted 10 or more years
- Remarried ex-spouse if marriage lasted 10 years and remarriage occurred after age 60
- Unmarried ex-spouse over 50, if disabled and marriage lasted over 10 years
- Remarried disabled ex-spouse if marriage lasted over 10 years and remarriage occurred after age 50
- Ex-spouse of any age if caring for wage earner's eligible child

Actual benefits depend on contributions. If a beneficiary is eligible on his/her own record or in more than one category, only one benefit is paid. Status as natural, adopted, foster, step or illegitimate child or status as putative or common-law wife may require case-by-case review. Payments to beneficiaries will be affected by earnings. Wage earners or their dependents who receive workers' compensation benefits, government pensions, or retirement pensions from local or state government will be subject to "offsets" which will reduce their Social Security benefits.

financial need. People who receive care through Medicaid are given a plastic or other card or a form with evidence of eligibility or a "share of cost." Clients use the card like a membership card when they see their physician or care provider during each month of eligibility. The provider then bills the state Medicaid program for services. Clients do not receive cash from Medicaid; however, Medicaid can be used as health insurance to cover the costs of physicians, hospitals, prescriptions, and skilled nursing facility care. Although eligibility requirements vary from state to state, a single person can currently have no more than $2000 in assets. In 1998, married couples could keep $3000 to $82,760 in assets, depending on the type of care needed and the state rules. The most generous levels are applicable only when one spouse is in a nursing facility and the other remains at home. Currently, a recipient must be disabled or over 65 years of age and a citizen or lawful U.S. resident; however, these program requirements and the financial standards are likely to change.

- *Medicare.* This benefit is available only to people who receive Social Security retirement or disability benefits. It is not usually available to people who receive Social Security as dependents or survivors; however, children of wage earners who receive benefits on their parents' work record can receive Medicare linked to their Social Security disability insurance if they were disabled prior to 22 years of age. Their Medicare benefits begin 2 years after they start receiving checks. Medicare is a completely different program from Medicaid and is *not* based on financial need. People with Medicare coverage receive only a small paper card that states the person's health insurance claim number. It indicates whether the person is qualified for Part A (hospitalization) and/or Part B (medical) insurance. This card does not usually cover prescriptions or the costs of long-term care in a skilled nursing facility.

- *Care Services at Home (also known as In-Home Support Services or Medicaid Personal Care Option).* This program pays for *chore workers* or aides to provide personal care services to aged or disabled people in their own homes. It varies widely among states and is not always available. It is provided only to financially needy people. In-home support services can provide homemaker services to people with disabilities to enable them to remain in their homes and avoid institutionalization. Benefits are almost never available for 24-hour-a-day care, but depending on the availability of services, current budget funding, and the disability of the individual, significant homecare services may be provided.

- *Veteran's Benefits.* Veterans may be eligible for cash benefits or homecare services known as *aid and attendant* services. These benefits are one type of cash grant available to low-income, disabled, or aged veterans. The other major veteran's cash benefit—veteran's compensation—is available to veterans of any age who have a "service-connected" injury. Access to veterans hospitals is granted on a priority system, and those veterans without such injuries often cannot qualify for inpatient care.

GUIDING FAMILIES THROUGH THE LEGAL MAZE

Stages of Legal Planning

Legal planning can be viewed in three stages—planning, crisis, and postcrisis stages—distinguished by the type of legal issues that can arise:

- *Planning Stage.* During this stage, the planner, who can be of any age or health condition, must have adequate capacity to understand and make choices. This individual can use any of the legal tools described earlier in the chapter and make decisions about his or her finances and their use, investment and/or conservation. The planner may also make decisions concerning the disposition of property after death. During this stage, issues of personal care and healthcare planning are identified, and many choices are often available. Options for access to government resources are typically wide open at this point.

- *Crisis Stage.* During a crisis, the patient experiences a reduction or loss of functioning and may already be incapacitated. Planning options are now severely curtailed; some may be precluded owing to a reduction in mental capacity, or court proceedings may be needed to designate a substitute decision maker for the protected person. When the financial realities have been identified, it may become clear that the patient is unable to afford the costs of his or her own healthcare, and the availability of government resources may need to be considered.

- *Postcrisis Stage.* The situation of the principal person is settled during this stage and is likely to be predictable, if not stable. There may be sufficient recovery that capacity is restored, and the planner may consider all viable options. Unfortunately, in many cases, the principal person clearly no longer has or will regain capacity to make decisions about his or her own healthcare, personal care, or finances. It may be necessary to liquidate funds to pay for medical care, annuitize pensions to begin to provide a steady source of income, or plan for the disposition of the estate after death. Decisions regarding personal care and healthcare may require plans for placement, withdrawal or withholding of certain treatment modalities, or the use of psychiatric care. However, if the planner lacks capacity, a substitute decision maker must handle the planning and postcrisis management and ongoing care management. To have authority as a substitute decision maker, previously created estate or personal care plans may be implemented or a surrogate may be appointed by the court.

Barriers to Advance Planning and the Implementation of the Selected Plan

Most people live to old age and also face a period of incapacitation or diminished capacity before they die. Why, then, do so few families take steps to ensure the orderly flow of responsibility and authority within the family? The reasons can be roughly categorized under avoidance and assumptions. Shawler and colleagues (1992) found that although many hospitalized elderly people were seriously ill, they did not expect to suffer from decisional incapacity and often procrastinated regarding issues of legal planning. Many people interviewed hoped to be able to make their own decisions throughout their lives.

Another study found that among hospitalized patients who stated that they planned to execute a power of attorney for healthcare, few had done so (Cohen-Mansfield et al., 1991). More than half had not discussed their wishes with potential surrogate decision makers or with their physicians. Some stated that it was too early to execute a power of attorney, suggesting that they may have been denying both their age and their illness (Cohen-Mansfield et al., 1991).

Families likewise avoid bringing up what is perceived as an unpleasant topic. When the elderly family members are doing well, other family concerns usually take precedence. When the elderly person becomes ill, families hesitate to broach a topic that implies that recovery may not occur. Avoidance and denial on the part of the spouse or adult children of a failing elderly person often prevent those closest to the patient from seeing how impaired the elderly person has become. Many spouses of patients with Alzheimer's disease later disclose how they ignored subtle signs of deterioration early in the disease. Similarly, children, even those who visit their parents regularly, typically do not assess function in a meaningful way and miss or deny subtle signs of loss of function. In other instances, decline may be so gradual that children slowly take on more and more instrumental tasks, such as shopping, cleaning, or gardening, without considering the ramifications of the parent's diminished ability to perform these tasks.

The elderly and their families often operate on false assumptions regarding care for their needs if they become ill. Many are shocked to learn that Medicare often does not provide sufficient long-term care in an institution or at home. Some veterans mistakenly assume that they will be provided for in veterans hospitals or homes. Others simply underestimate the expense of private in-home care services. When the very old think of approaching death, few contemplate a long period of dwindling strength and ability.

Other assumptions concern the process within the family itself. Historically, children and families have been the first to care for the dependent elderly person; in many countries and cultures, this is still largely true. Even in the United States, with its mobile population and two-worker or single-parent households, most elderly people live near at least one child whom they see regularly.

The elderly often assert that they have spent most of their lives providing a good life for their children and they expect their children to love and be concerned about them during old age (Pillari, 1986). When they were younger, many elderly people sacrificed and postponed their own gratification to provide their children with a better chance in life. Even in families whose children and parents are not close, elderly people often assume that the children will take on responsibility for their care, should they need it (Pillari, 1986).

Parents often assume that legal documents and advance planning are not needed because the child or children selected as the caregiver(s) know their wishes, even if these matters have never been discussed (Shawler et al., 1992). Adult children, if they consider these matters at all, may also hold mistaken assumptions. They may assume that their parents have been more diligent in planning for old age and illness than they actually have.

Practitioners often hear children express dismay when they assume caretaking for an incapacitated elderly person and learn that financial and other affairs are hopelessly muddled or incomplete. Even functional, normally coping families tend to avoid potentially painful issues. It is not surprising, therefore, that adult children often avoid asking their parent or parents questions about preparations for catastrophic or long-term illness, fearing that they will hurt or anger their parents.

Family Decision Making

Every family has its own style of relating and assigning tasks and responsibilities. Early in the family history, family members are assigned roles that persist into old age and illness, even though they may not work well during times of crisis. When the elderly first begin to demonstrate dependency and the

need for care, a filial crisis is precipitated—even in very functional families. Old ways of relating do not always facilitate problem solving and decision making. In some families, the passing of authority to succeeding generations occurs by tacit agreement among members, usually based on formal or informal prior role assignment. Men usually defer to their spouses, but women tend to select an adult child, usually the oldest female, to assume responsibility (Cohen-Mansfield et al., 1991).

Unfortunately, this process does not always occur. Faced with a major change in the family that precipitates a crisis, family members may struggle with loyalties, fear, guilt, and doubts. These disabling conflicts may cause family members to seek absolution from familiar authority figures, rather than use deliberation and reflection to find answers (Smyer et al., 1988).

One of the worst-case scenarios occurs when a matriarch or patriarch who holds the decision-making power and authority within the family becomes disabled. Other family members are often too paralyzed by old family rules to challenge the identified patient, who may make very irrational choices. Healthcare providers often struggle—sometimes without success—to educate and support someone else in the family so he or she will intervene. In other instances, old sibling rivalries and conflicts may be acted out around the decision-making process concerning treatment, with siblings undermining each other's authority and giving conflicting instructions to physicians and nurses (Molloy et al., 1991).

Family communication often lacks clarity. The message sent is often not the message received, and members of the same family may mistakenly think they understand each other. Studies of end-of-life treatment decisions have shown that in simulated situations surrogate decision makers tend to make choices in accordance with the patients' wishes; however, their choices did not always concur with what the patients chose (Seckler et al., 1991). Another study showed that prior discussion between surrogate decision makers and patients regarding treatment and care options increased agreement on the simulated test (Sulmasy et al., 1994). Still another study showed that even when siblings share the same culture and religion and think that they know the elderly person's wishes, they do not all make the same choices if asked separately (Sonnenblick et al., 1993).

Religious beliefs, values, and ethical and cultural factors all influence how the elderly person and family members view options and express preferences (Meyer, 1993). For many elderly people, religion is the lens through which their situation is viewed. Religious experience is inherently subjective but nevertheless defines reality; it may also provide a context for decision making that contrasts with the objective medical data that frame the decision for the healthcare professional (O'Connell, 1994). Deliberation about healthcare decisions often requires a careful examination of conscience and perhaps consultation with clergy. However, waiting for a health crisis to make such decisions precludes this type of careful consideration.

In times of illness or decline, family decision making takes place within the unfamiliar arena of a healthcare setting. Physicians, nurses, and social workers become a part of the decision making, further complicating the process. Even when every possible action has been taken to meet the elderly person's wishes, the emotional intensity of the healthcare crisis may undermine former plans. If families are not clear and informed about what legal steps have been taken to ensure autonomy, and if they are not in agreement and accepting of these legal decisions, they are in a position to sabotage former plans.

Two studies using simulated situations showed that if physicians were pressured by families to insert a feeding tube in a nonresponding patient, they would overrule the provisions of a living will that specifies nonaggressive means of sustaining life (Ely et al., 1992; Watts, 1992). Family misunderstanding and conflict, the family history of communicating and deciding, the influence of culture and religion, and the emotional intensity that surround a health crisis in an elderly patient all potentially undermine the patient's autonomy. New treatment options continually offer more choices, and financial constraints are becoming

more burdensome; therefore, it is increasingly critical for advanced practice nurses to refer family members for legal counsel that will assist them in choosing and formulating plans before care is actually needed.

SUMMARY

The advanced practice nurse can assist older people and their families in addressing the many legal issues that arise with declining health, disability, mental incapacity, and death. Knowledge of sources for legal information and assistance enable the advanced practice nurse to properly direct older people to the appropriate services.

This chapter presented the phases of legal planning, described legal documents for estate planning, identified the types of public benefits available to the elderly, and described how the advanced practice nurse can guide families through the legal maze.

REFERENCES

Barta, K., & Neighbors, M. (1993). Nurses' knowledge of—and role in—patients' end-of-life decision making. *Trends in Health Care, Law & Ethics, 8*(4), 50–52.

Callahan, D. (1987). *Setting limits: Medical goals in an aging society.* New York: Simon & Schuster.

Cohen-Mansfield, J., Droge, J. A., & Billig, N. (1991). The utilization of the Durable Power of Attorney for Health Care among hospitalized elderly patients. *Journal of the American Geriatrics Society, 39,* 1174–1178.

Ely, J. W., Peters, P. G., Jr., Zweig, S., et al. (1992). The physician's decision to use tube feedings: The role of the family, the living will, and the Cruzan decision. *Journal of the American Geriatrics Society, 40,* 471–475.

Emanuel, E. J., Weinberg, D. S., Gonin, R., et al. (1993). How well is the Patient Self-Determination Act working: An early assessment. *American Journal of Medicine, 95,* 619–628.

Family Caregiver Alliance (1993). *Taking good care.* San Francisco: Family Caregiver Alliance.

Gerety, M. B., Chiodo, L. K., Kanten, D. N., et al. (1993). Medical treatment preferences of nursing home residents: Relationship to function and concordance with surrogate decision-makers. *Journal of the American Geriatrics Society, 41,* 953–960.

Hague, S. B., & Moody, L. E. (1993). A study of the public's knowledge regarding advance directives. *Nursing Economics, 11,* 303–307, 323.

Holly, C. M. (1993). Advance directives: A program design for home health care. *Home Health Care Nurse, 11*(5), 34–38.

Hurme, S. B. (1991). *Steps to enhance guardianship monitoring*. Washington, D.C.: American Bar Association.

Jacobson, J. A., White, B. E., Battin, M. P., et al. (1994). Patient's understanding and use of advance directives. *Western Journal of Medicine, 160*, 232–236.

Kingson, E. R., Hirshorn, B. A., & Cornman, J. M. (1986). *Ties that bind: The interdependence of generations*. Cabin John, MD: Locks Press.

Meyer, C. (1993). 'End-of-life' care: Patient's choices, nurses' challenges. *American Journal of Nursing, 93*(2), 40–47.

Molloy, D. W., Guyatt, G. H., Alemayehu, E., et al. (1991). Factors affecting physicians' decisions on caring for an incompetent elderly patient: An international study. *Canadian Medical Association Journal, 145*, 947–952.

O'Connell, L. J. (1994). The role of religion in health-related decision making for elderly patients. *Generations, 18*(4), 27–30.

Patient Self-Determination Act (PSDA) of 1990, Omnibus Budget Reconciliation Act of 1990; P.L. 101–508, Sections 4206 and 4751, November 5, 1990 (effective December 1, 1991).

Pillari, V. (1986). *Pathways to family myths*. New York: Brunner/Mazel.

Regan, J. J., & Gilfix, M. (1993). *Tax, estate, and financial planning for the elderly: Forms and practice*. New York: Matthew Bender & Co.

Seckler, A. B., Meier, D. E., Mulvihill, M., & Cammer, B. E. (1991). Substituted judgment: How accurate are proxy predictions? *Annals of Internal Medicine, 115*, 92–98.

Shawler, C., High, D. M., Moore, K. K., & Velotta, C. (1992). Clinical considerations. Surrogate decision making for hospitalized elders. *Journal of Gerontological Nursing, 18*(6), 5–11.

Smyer, M. A., McHale, S. M., Birkel, R. C., & Madle, R. A. (1988). Impairments, handicapping environments, and disability: A life-span perspective. In V. B. Van Hasselt, P. S. Strain & M. Hersen (Eds.), *Handbook of developmental and physical disabilities, vol. 148* (pp. 9–20). Oxford, England: Pergamon Press.

Sonnenblick, M., Friedlander, Y., & Steinberg, A. (1993). Dissociation between the wishes of terminally ill parents and decisions by their offspring. *Journal of the American Geriatrics Society, 41*, 599–604.

Sulmasy, D. P., Haller, K., & Terry, P. B. (1994). More talk, less paper: Predicting the accuracy of substituted judgments. *American Journal of Medicine, 96*, 432–438.

Watts, D. T. (1992). The family's will or the living will: Patient self-determination in doubt. *Journal of the American Geriatrics Society, 40*, 533–534.

Resources

Several organizations and agencies are available to provide older adults, their families, and the advanced practice nurse with information and assistance on legal issues, concerns, and problems.

National Academy of Elder Law Attorneys, 1604 North Country Club Road, Tucson, AZ, 85716, (520) 881-4005. An organization of attorneys who focus on legal problems of the elderly and their families. They can provide the names of local law attorneys for the elderly as well as information on law topics pertaining to the elderly.

National Association of Private Geriatric Care Managers, 655 North Alvernon Way, Suite 108, Tucson, AZ, 85711, (520) 881-8008. An organization of private care managers, usually nurses or social workers who provide private (usually paid) care management services for the elderly and their families. They can provide the names of local care managers.

Eldercare Locator, (800) 677-1116. A national telephone line for long-distance caregivers (i.e., friends or family members who take responsibility for the well-being of but are not physically located near the elderly person) that provides referrals to services for the elderly nationwide.

National Citizens' Coalition for Nursing Home Reform, 1424 16th St., NW, Suite L-2, Washington, D.C., 20036-2211, (202) 797-0657. National organization that provides information on rights of nursing home patients and referrals to state or local agencies that can give assistance.

Area Agency of Aging. Federally funded agency that can provide information and referrals to state, regional, or local providers of nutritional, transportation, and legal services.

Other. Information on government programs may be obtained through the Social Security Administration and the U.S. Department of Health and Human Services, Health Care Financing Administration.

Ethical Issues

Marian L. Baxter

Nurses frequently find themselves in patient care situations that require ethical thinking and decision making—often when they lack training in such matters. Nurses may wonder how to best approach an ethical problem and the resources to use when doing so; one cannot always rely on common sense or intuition to resolve a troubling circumstance. Advanced practice nurses (APNs) may be called on by other members of the clinical team, patients, and families to serve as a resource in helping resolve ethical dilemmas. This chapter orients the APN on ethical issues that may arise in the care of geriatric patients and also offers guidance in ethical decision making.

DEFINING ETHICAL DILEMMAS

Morals, ethics, integrity, and *laws* are words frequently used in conjunction with each other.

Morals can be thought of as what is "right" or "good." They are learned from families, social and religious communities, schools, peers, and other sources. Ethics is the study of morality, or the study of what is right or good. Professionals may interchange the terms *ethics* and *integrity*; for example, a person is considered ethical if he or she has professional integrity, and vice versa. *Webster's dictionary* (1983) defines integrity as "the quality or state of being of sound moral principle; uprightness, honesty, and sincerity" (p. 953). Nursing has moral principles, or parameters, that distinguish it as a profession (Table 4–1). Thus, a nurse has integrity or is ethical if he or she follows these parameters of the profession.

Adding laws to the moral parameters increases the complexity of these concepts. When determining the right thing to do in a particu-

TABLE 4-1

Moral Rules or Parameters of the Nursing Profession

American Nurses Association's Code for Nursing
American Nurses Association's Standards of Practice
Nightingale Pledge
Institutional policies and procedures
Laws

TABLE 4-3

American Nurses Association's Code for Nurses

1. The nurse provides services with respect for human dignity and the uniqueness of the client, unrestricted by considerations of social or economic status, personal attributes, or the nature of health problems.
2. The nurse safeguards the client's right to privacy by judiciously protecting information of a confidential nature.
3. The nurse acts to safeguard the client and the public when healthcare and safety are affected by the incompetent, unethical, or illegal practice of any person.
4. The nurse assumes responsibility and accountability for individual nursing judgments and actions.
5. The nurse maintains competence in nursing.
6. The nurse exercises informed judgment and uses individual competence and qualifications as criteria in seeking consultation, accepting responsibilities, and delegating nursing activities to others.
7. The nurse participates in activities that contribute to the ongoing development of the profession's body of knowledge.
8. The nurse participates in the profession's efforts to implement and improve standards of nursing.
9. The nurse participates in the profession's efforts to establish and maintain conditions of employment conducive to high-quality nursing care.
10. The nurse participates in the profession's effort to protect the public from misinformation and misrepresentation and to maintain the integrity of nursing.
11. The nurse collaborates with members of the health professions and other citizens in promoting community and national efforts to meet the healthcare needs of the public.

Adapted from American Nurses Association (1985). *Code for nurses with interpretive statements.* Kansas City, MO: American Nurses Association.

lar situation, people often consult the law for factual information. Laws are an incomplete source of information, however. For example, using a legal loophole when filing one's taxes may indeed be legal but not always ethical. In addition, because not every act is covered by a particular law, it may be difficult if not impossible to find a law that speaks to every potential situation. A decision made, therefore, can be legal without being ethical or ethical without being legal. This situation may increase the level of anxiety of those who turn only to the law for ethical decision making.

An ethical dilemma may be described as a conflict between two equally difficult choices. It may involve conflicts between two or more values, principles, moral duties, or obligations. The conflicts may be *intrapersonal* (within one person) or *interpersonal* (between two or more people). Ethics in the patient care setting is referred to as *clinical ethics* and applies to the institutions that provide patient care as well as the individuals involved in that care. For gerontological nurses, these settings may in-

TABLE 4-2

Conditions in the Clinical Setting in Which Ethical Dilemmas May Arise

Communication
Privacy and confidentiality
Truthtelling and disclosure
Informed consent
Determining capacity
Refusal of treatment
Foregoing life-sustaining treatments
Death and dying
Access to healthcare and rationing

clude hospitals, long-term care facilities, offices, clinics, and community settings. The goal of clinical ethics is to identify, analyze, and resolve the ethical dilemmas that arise in the delivery of patient care. When ethical dilemmas arise, it is natural and logical to turn to the parameters of the profession for guidance in seeking resolution. For most of the ethical situations faced by clinicians today, however, these parameters often fall short. Table 4–2 lists those conditions of the clinical setting in which ethical dilemmas may arise; excluding the issue of access to healthcare and rationing, gerontological nurses face problems related to these areas on almost a daily basis.

The American Nurses Association's *Code for nurses with interpretive statements* (1985) (Table 4–3) advises nurses to respect and maintain privacy and confidentiality. This task can be complicated, however, when care is delivered to a patient with dementia, for example, for whom the situation necessitates disclosing information to others. Although having a diagnosis of dementia does not necessarily preclude a patient from being involved in decision making, the gerontological nurse must ensure that a patient does indeed have the capacity to understand and make decisions. Answers to specific situations cannot generally be found in codes and standards, which do not provide a "cookbook" approach for the right or best thing to do. Matters become even grayer because what might be right for one person in one situation might be considered very wrong for another. The United States is a pluralistic society, composed of many different cultures, communities, values, and beliefs, and individuals learn what is right or good from many sources. Each patient holds a unique set of beliefs and values, as does each clinician who cares for that patient. It is no wonder that conflicts arise when so many different values can potentially collide.

APPLYING PRINCIPLES TO ETHICAL PROBLEMS

A principles approach is a common means of resolving ethical dilemmas. Principles used in clinical practice are listed in Table 4–4.

Autonomy means to have self-rule or self-governance, and respect for autonomy means respect for another person's right to self-governance. Translated in the clinical setting, then, respect for autonomy means respect for anoth-er's right to self-determination (Beauchamp & Childress, 1994). Autonomy is an important concept in the United States, as evidenced by the enactment of the Patient Self-Determination Act in 1991. This act mandated that healthcare institutions receiving federal monies inform patients of their right to be involved in decisions about their own care. One of the ways patients can ensure their own involvement, even when unable to speak on their own behalf, is to execute an advance directive (see Chapter 3).

Beneficence, the principle of doing good, also includes preventing harm. Sometimes in trying to do good and prevent harm, clinicians mistakenly ignore respect for autonomy and decide what they think is best for the patient. In contrast, it is appropriate to assess what is medically indicated and to share that information with the patient. Patients need this information to make informed decisions. According to the *rule of veracity*, patients expect clinicians to communicate with them and to be truthful with them. To decide what is best for a patient is a paternalistic approach that was common practice prior to the civil rights movement. Before the 1960s, respect for autonomy was not an issue. A physician would assess a situation, decide what was the best thing to do, and inform the family of this decision. In *A theory of medical ethics* (1981), Veatch warned against the practice of paternalism, as it places beneficence in conflict with autonomy and can erode the trust between the clinician and the patient.

Nonmaleficence is the principle of doing no harm. It goes beyond beneficence and preventing harm to an obligation to not intentionally inflict harm, a principle found within the Hippocratic tradition of the 5th century B.C. (Veatch, 1981). Included in the teachings of Hippocrates was the practice of not giving patients bad news, which is now termed benevolent deception. It was thought that relaying bad news might impair healing and take away hope, thus causing more harm than good. The use of benevolent deception became standard practice and was not formally addressed until 1980, by the American Medical Association (AMA) (1981). The use of deception in caring for the elderly is often more common than the exception. For example, well-intentioned

TABLE 4–4
Ethical Principles in Healthcare

Autonomy	Nonmaleficence
Beneficence	Justice

family members may instruct nursing staff members to not inform an elderly patient or nursing home resident of the death of a loved one, for fear of "upsetting" them. Clinicians may find several principles in conflict and not know how to best proceed. It can be difficult to discern whether one's actions are benevolent or malevolent. In other words, will this action do good or cause harm? Similarly, actions to adequately control pain may hasten death, as may foregoing life-sustaining treatments.

Justice, as described by Beauchamp and Childress (1994), involves fairness and equity—getting what one is due. Issues of access and allocation must be considered in the provision of healthcare. Until recently, healthcare professionals were not encouraged to consider inadequacies in the distribution of services. Many thought that there were ample resources that could be accessed by those who needed them. However, these misinformed opinions are now beginning to give way to a realization that not everyone who needs medical care has access to it—often through no fault of his or her own.

Since the late 1980s and early 1990s, much public and political debate has revolved around the issue of healthcare reform. Thirty-seven to 40 million Americans lack basic healthcare, and reports indicate that healthcare costs continue to skyrocket. The United States spent almost $1 trillion on healthcare during 1994, an amount that has more than tripled since 1981. As the cost of healthcare has increased, so has the percentage of the gross national product (GNP) spent on healthcare, nearly doubling from 7.6% in 1980 to 14% in 1993 (Gaylin, 1993). Considering the rate of this recent growth, questions have been raised about how profits in this industry will be distributed. If healthcare expenditures (measured as the percentage of the GNP) continue on their current course, other services may have to be decreased as a result. Possible solutions include cost containment and rationing.

Cost containment is a concept with which many people can agree, as long as it pertains to other individuals rather than to the individual who is in need of a particular service. In Beauchamp and Childress's discussion (1994), the principles of autonomy, beneficence, non-

maleficence, and justice clearly exist in a balance; no single principle reigns supreme over the other three principles. Within the past 20 years, however, situations have occurred in which honoring one patient's autonomy has paralyzed the entire medical community. Treatments of questionable benefit are provided for indefinite periods of time, because patients or their families demand them or because clinicians feel better doing something rather than nothing. Situations such as these are frequently considered futile and are receiving attention within the medical community as well as in the media. Some argue that society cannot continue to bear the financial burden for this type of care, and others argue that providing these treatments is a disservice to humanity that only perpetuates suffering and prolongs the dying process. Still others argue that an individual should have the right to request continued treatments, no matter how others view that quality of life. Finding satisfactory answers to these and other difficult questions continues to be a slow and sometimes painful process.

Whereas cost containment is a relatively new idea in healthcare, *rationing* is not. Critical care nurses are familiar, for example, with the practice of moving a less critical patient out of an intensive care unit to allow a patient in a more critical condition to use that bed. Transplant organs are also rationed, because there is simply a greater demand than supply. It is not uncommon for age to be considered when allocating resources, as shown by the practice of denying dialysis to the elderly in the United Kingdom. Veatch (1981) argued that societal accord could only be achieved through an acceptance of the practice of rationing. Consensus has yet to be reached on whether access to basic healthcare is a right to which all people are entitled; other issues under debate are the amount of healthcare that should be provided and the specific circumstances under which it should be offered or terminated. There is general agreement on the need to respect autonomy regarding the wishes of an individual. What is now being questioned at a national level, however, is whether the autonomous decisions of some to receive healthcare justify others doing without.

EXAMINING THE CAPACITY TO MAKE DECISIONS

A key feature of the principle of autonomy is the capacity to make decisions. *Capacity* is different from *competence*, although the two terms are often used to mean the same thing. *Competence* is a legal term used by the courts rather than by healthcare professionals. A patient may have been determined legally incompetent to handle his or her financial affairs and yet may still have the capacity to be involved in medical decision making.

Deciding whether an individual has capacity can be one of the most challenging components of caring for the elderly population. The capacity for decision making may be altered by many factors, including an acute process such as an infection, the side effects of medications, or the effects of more chronic influences such as a dementing illness. The prevalence of dementia in the elderly and its effects on capacity are well known to gerontological clinicians. Further, capacity may not always be present in an individual, thus increasing the complexity of the situation. It is often difficult to know whether a patient truly has capacity. Clinicians need to know how to increase patient participation in decision making in light of the difficulties involved and the resources available to assist in the process. A case discussion may help illustrate the point.

Case Study

M, a woman in her early 80s, was admitted to the nursing home. She was Jewish by birth and faith and had survived the Holocaust, forced to witness the murder of her husband and children. She had experienced what might be considered a schizophrenic break. Eventually, M immigrated to the United States and lived alone in New York until she became increasingly unable to care for herself. A guardian was appointed to handle her affairs. Her adjustment to nursing home life was slow; the high, wooden privacy fence brought back memories of the concentration camp.

One day her usually cheerful demeanor was replaced by a furrowed brow and silence; something was wrong. M finally admitted that she had been experiencing chest pain. When the electrocardiogram machine was brought to her room, she expressed an emphatic "no!" She did not want to be "electrocuted." The next strategy was to discern whether the symptoms were cardiac or gastrointestinal. An antacid and nitroglycerine were offered, to which M again expressed a resounding "no." She announced that she was not going to be "poisoned." The staff was in a dilemma, wanting to respect her autonomy and yet unsure about her capacity to refuse treatment.

Capacity includes but is not limited to the ability to form a decision and to make a choice that is consistent over time. Consistency over time is important to ensure that the decision is indeed what the patient—and not someone else—desires. Individuals may make a decision based on how it will affect not only them but also their relationship with a family member or their physician. As previously mentioned, capacity may wax and wane, depending on the health status of that person. Decision making should be attempted during the patient's "best" times, when participation is enhanced, just as therapeutic modalities should be attempted when the patient is more rested and responsive.

Capacity also involves understanding the consequences of a particular choice. This was the element that posed the dilemma for the staff in the case of M. Did M understand what refusal of an evaluation and then treatment might mean? Because the staff was unsure about her ability to fully understand, the home's consulting psychiatrist was called.

Case Study *(Continued)*

Dr. E conducted an evaluation of M's capacity and found her capable of making this decision. M had lived more than 80 years and had lost everyone in her family. She did not want to endure any procedures or take any medications, no matter how easy and pain free they were. She understood that refusing any evaluations and treatments might mean that she would die. She informed Dr. E that if this was her time to die, she was ready.

Continued on following page

M returned to the home without medical evaluation or treatment and died 3 weeks later. Her death brought sorrow and a sense of failure to many staff members; they saw her death as needless when "simple" medical interventions could have extended her life, which was felt to be of high quality. What helped mitigate their feeling of medical failure was the realization that M's autonomy had been respected.

M had been declared legally incompetent and had been appointed a guardian who could have made the decision to force treatments on M. M's condition might have improved, and she might have forgiven those who forced treatments on her; conversely, she might not have forgiven. The issue also had to be considered in terms of other nursing home residents' perceptions: If M were forced to undergo medical treatments, would they become afraid that their wishes would be ignored as well? The actions and behaviors of healthcare professionals in their delivery of care to one patient can affect the perceptions of care delivery by the community and society at large.

SURROGATE DECISION MAKING

When surrogates are called on to make decisions for patients, healthcare professionals must be careful not to place the entire burden on them. Those acting on behalf of a patient need information regarding the medical appropriateness of a treatment or procedure. Questions by practitioners such as "Well, Mrs. Y, what do you want us to do?" can change the focus of the surrogate's responsibility. Mrs. Y most likely does not want to lose her loved one, so asking her what she wants may cause her to request that "everything" be done. In addition, posing the question in terms of what she wants may imply to her that doing everything is appropriate and will result in restoring her husband to his premorbid state. If Mrs. Y requests that everything be done, the clinicians may feel frustrated because they know that, medically, this will result in a situation quite the opposite from what she anticipates.

In general, if doing everything is not medically appropriate, it should not be considered an option. Information should be offered regarding what options are appropriate. When Mrs. Y is asked to assist in decision making for her husband, it may help to pose the question in reference to what her husband would have wanted, or to ask her, based on what she knows about her husband and his values, what her husband might say if he could speak to them at that time. Using this approach changes the burden from Mrs. Y to one that is shared with the clinical team; it may also help relieve any guilt over feeling that one has not done everything, whatever that may entail.

INFORMED CONSENT

Informed consent is a process of educating and sharing information that promotes informed decisions. It includes the information itself as well as the way in which that information is presented. Within the shared information are the elements of prognosis, risks and benefits of treatment options, expected outcomes, probable recovery time, limits of medical treatment, and recommendations to withdraw or withhold treatments. Clinicians may unconsciously or consciously bring their own biases into the discussion. Biases are different from data that help provide a realistic picture about prognosis; rather, they give a subjective slant regarding what the clinician feels should happen and also include the clinician's own values and beliefs, which may be entirely different from the patient's. The amount of information given is also important. Does the patient have enough information to make a truly informed decision based on his or her own value system, or is it only enough information for the patient to choose what the clinician wants for the patient?

How the information is delivered is as important as the information itself. Is the information shared in language the patient understands, or is it full of medical jargon that may be misconstrued? Is the discussion unhurried, or is the presenter standing, posed at the door, ready to exit? Time needs to be allowed for questions, both during the initial discussion and after the patient has had time to digest the original information shared. What does the patient understand; more important, does the patient have the capacity to understand?

It is not uncommon for clinicians to sidestep the issue of capacity as long as the patient is making choices that are in agreement with those of the clinician. Often it is only when the patient's choice differs that capacity is called into question. As long as the patient says "yes" (or at least does not say "no"), the patient is viewed as cooperative and rational. In a *Hastings center report* (1989), Brody cautioned practitioners to take a closer look at the process of informed consent. The decisions that patients make have far-reaching consequences that each patient has to live with after he or she leaves the hospital. Clinicians generally see outcomes and consequences limited to the time the patient is under that clinician's care. The American Hospital Association's *A patient's bill of rights* (1992) affirms the patient's right to information and informed consent (Appendix 4–1).

REFUSAL OF TREATMENT: WITHHOLDING VERSUS WITHDRAWING

People have the right to make their own decisions, even if these decisions are painful for the people who render care or if they are not the decisions that the clinician desires for a patient. Some of the most troubling situations for clinicians involve cases in which patients forego life-sustaining treatments. Individual philosophies on the meaning of life and death enter into the responses offered. Does an individual believe in a right to death? Conversely, does he or she believe that as long as there is life there is hope, and as long as there is breath there is life? The latter would necessitate continuing treatments at all cost. Clinicians must examine their own beliefs on this subject, realizing that their values can influence behavior and practice.

In geriatric practice, a common example of conflict regarding the withholding and withdrawing of a treatment concerns feeding tubes. If a feeding tube is withdrawn and the patient dies, does this constitute mercy killing (euthanasia)? Does the withdrawal of a life-sustaining treatment constitute euthanasia or phy-

sician-assisted suicide, or does it merely allow the patient to die? Perhaps the feeding tube should never have been offered, thus preventing the current dilemma of whether to withdraw the tube. Morally, the withholding and withdrawing of treatments can be considered equal, since it should be equally difficult to not start a treatment that may offer some benefit as it should be to stop a treatment that is not providing the intended benefit.

These alternatives may be considered morally equivalent, but emotionally, they appear to be different, especially when the situation involves a feeding tube. Families and clinicians may view the removal of a feeding tube as actively ending that person's life. It is not uncommon to hear that the patient is being "starved to death." In contrast, although it is accepted practice to withdraw ventilators when the burdens for a patient are seen to outweigh the benefits, it is uncommon to hear accusations of "suffocating the patient to death" when the ventilator is removed. One reason for this discrepancy is the symbolic nature of food. Food denotes caring and nurturing and is usually present at family events in American culture, be they happy or sad in nature. Eating is equated with regaining one's strength. The issue at hand, however, is not one of eating but rather of artificial feeding. Feeding tubes are an artificial means of supplying nutrition, just as respirators are an artificial means of supplying respiration. Feeding tubes are medical interventions that patients, or surrogates, may refuse.

Refusing medical treatments can include refusing the continuation of treatment after it has been started. In 1973, the AMA provided a statement that distinguished between killing and allowing a patient to die (Beauchamp & Childress, 1994). Allowing a patient to die by removing treatments is permissible and is referred to as *passive euthanasia*. However, this differs from killing a patient, which is known as *active euthanasia*. The AMA strictly prohibits active euthanasia.

RESOURCES FOR INSTITUTIONAL ETHICS

Refusing, withholding, and withdrawing treatments are but a few of the ethical dilemmas encountered by clinicians. Finding resolution can seem overwhelming. Resources are available both within and outside most healthcare institutions. Institutions may have an ethics committee, or they may employ an ethicist full time or contract for services as needed. An ethicist usually has a doctoral degree in philosophy and/or religious studies including advanced education in ethics. Physicians, nurses, and social workers who have studied ethics at an advanced educational level may also consider themselves to be ethicists, although consensus certainly has not been reached on this matter. In contrast to ethicists, ethics committees are more interdisciplinary and are typically composed of individuals from different disciplines.

The functions of ethics committees may include policy development, education, case consultation or review, research, or providing a forum for ethical discussions. In a study of 1278 long-term care facilities, Glasser and colleagues (1988) found education, case review, and policies and procedures to be the main functions of those committees. Ethical issues most commonly addressed included (1) orders to not resuscitate a patient; (2) patient refusal of treatments; (3) starting, continuing, or stopping treatments; and (4) patient competence and capacity for decision making. Clinicians may want to investigate the existence of an ethics program within their facility and what services it provides. A newly forming committee may be limited to committee education and a retrospective review of cases. More seasoned committees, however, may be experienced and capable in all the previously mentioned functions.

Styles and approaches to resolving ethical problems vary widely. La Puma and Schiedermayer (1991) advocated a medical model of consultation that provides expert opinion and may also include managing or directing a patient's plan of care. In contrast, Fletcher (1991) supported an interdisciplinary approach that offers education about existing options and provides an approach similar to mediation to facilitate communication. Limitations of the medical, or expert, model include being perceived as judge and jury over the outcome of the situation. Committee work, which concen-

trates on education and mediation rather than on giving the answer, may be more welcomed by clinicians than the expert model but is frequently criticized for having a slower response to requests for help.

Ethics committees may find that they are called to assist with a situation after it has escalated to crisis proportions. A request may also be made when communication between parties has come to a standstill. Requesting assistance sooner, in a more proactive manner, can prevent ethical dilemmas from becoming unmanageable.

USING A CASE METHOD APPROACH TO ETHICAL PROBLEMS

Ethical dilemmas may be grouped by subject, such as *issues at the end of life* or *refusal of treatments*. Each dilemma, however, occurs differently in each patient situation. Once a dilemma has been identified, the challenge then becomes how to best approach the situation. It may be tempting to look for a rule that directs the individuals involved on how to proceed. However, applying rules about what should or should not be done before the situation has been examined—that is, using a cookbook approach—precludes the use of moral reasoning. The subtleties and uniqueness of the situation may be missed. Fletcher (1979) referred to this approach as *rule ethics*, stating that "the rule decides, and you, the moral agent, have no part to play" (p. 3). Using a rule, commandment, or principle to choose an action without regard for the consequences of that action falls within a deontological approach. Fletcher instead advocated a *situation ethics* approach, in which the situation and the consequences of the situation must be considered and decisions are made only after the consequences are known. Fletcher (1979) stated that "in act or situation ethics the moral agent, the decision maker, judges what is best in the circumstances and in view of the foreseeable consequences" (p. 3). This approach is also known as *consequentialism*.

The most common example of consequentialism is *utilitarianism*, in which an action is considered right or good if it produces the desired outcomes; in other words, the end justifies the means. Questions may arise within a consequentialist approach regarding (1) who the moral agent or decision maker is, (2) how a particular decision was derived, (3) what if any motives there may be, (4) how *moral agent* is defined, or (5) what makes a moral agent. These questions are not easy to answer. No matter how objective one tries to be, subjectivity may enter into the decision making. Each person brings his or her own set of beliefs and values, which may include biases that affect the decision making. To limit subjectivity, Fletcher (1991) encouraged the use of shared decision making in addressing ethical dilemmas, which flowed from a similar recommendation by the President's Commission for the Study of Ethical Problems in Medicine and Biomedical and Behavioral Research (1982).

Jonsen and colleagues (1992) identified four "topics" for clinicians to consider in the analysis of every case:

- Indications for medical interventions
- Preferences of patients
- Quality of life
- Socioeconomic factors

Fletcher and Miller (1994) built from a similar approach and established a four-step approach to case analysis (Table 4–5). Both groups of ethicists placed the patient's medical condition, as diagnosed by medical personnel, first among the topics to be discussed. Using these approaches, patient values are not disclosed until after medical information has been presented. Encouraging the presentation of medical information before information about the patient may give the impression that medical information is more important than the patient as a person. A discussion of the patient's preferences must include the patient's values and beliefs as a whole.

Historically, patient-clinician relationships developed gradually over time, and medical situations that allowed for discussions about sensitive issues were common. Today, patients interact with practitioners of many disciplines, such as physicians, nurses, social workers, dieticians, and others who help plan and direct care. Health maintenance organizations and di-

---

TABLE 4-5
Four-Step Approach to Case Analysis

I. Assessment

    A. What are the relevant contextual factors?
    B. What are the patient's medical condition and indications for treatment?
    C. Is the patient capable of decision making?
    D. What are the patient's preferences?
    E. What are the preferences of the family or surrogate decision makers?
    F. What are the needs of the patient as a person?
    G. Are there interests other than, and potentially competing with, those of the patient that need to be considered?
    H. Are there institutional or legal factors contributing to the ethical problem?

II. Identification of Ethical Problems

    A. What are the ethical problems in the case? (Rank the problems by magnitude.)
    B. What ethical considerations are most relevant? (What is ethically at stake?)
    C. What are the most analogous cases?
    D. What are the most relevant guidelines for clinicians regarding the problem(s)?

III. Decision Making and Implementation

    A. What are the ethically acceptable options?
    B. What justification can be given for the preferred resolution of the case?
    C. How is a satisfactory resolution of the case to be accomplished?
    D. Is ethics consultation necessary or desirable?
    E. Is judicial review necessary or desirable?

IV. Evaluation

    A. Current: Is the plan working? If not, why not?
    B. Retrospective: What might have been done to improve the care of the patient? Would changes in institutional policy or education help prevent or better resolve ethical problems posed by similar cases?

Adapted from Fletcher, J., & Miller F. (1994). A case method in planning for the care of patients. In J. Fletcher, C. Hite, P. Lombardo & M. Marshall (Eds.), *Introduction to clinical ethics* (pp. 27–58). Charlottesville, VA: University of Virginia Center for Biomedical Ethics.

---

agnostic-related groups dictate time constraints in an effort to contain healthcare costs. As a result, the patient can end up in a system that offers a fragmented delivery of care. Even when a patient's care is overseen by a primary care physician, third-party payers—who are often guided by manuals and people who will never meet the individual whose care is being deliberated—may dictate limitations that cause care to be delivered in segments. An approach that emphasizes quantity rather than quality prevents discussions that were once commonplace and a normal part of care. Patients appear for care with their entire life history generally unknown to the healthcare team that is providing care. Bits and pieces of the patient's story are told, but usually only as they relate to the presenting illness. Rarely do clinicians have the time to get to know their patients as they once did. This is especially true of patients who cannot speak for themselves.

NARRATIVE IN ETHICAL DECISIONS

Stories or narrative may be useful in resolving ethical dilemmas. Storytelling is as old as humankind. It is the method used for informing generations about family traditions and cultures as well as the way history continues to be communicated. Hauerwas and Jones (1989) offered narrative ". . . to explain human action, to articulate the structures of human consciousness, to depict the identity of agents, . . . to justify a view of the importance of 'story-telling,' . . . and to develop a means for imposing order on what is otherwise chaos" (p. 2). Narrative can be applied to ethical decision making in clinical situations by providing a method for argument and depicting personal identity and convictions. In shared decision making, clinicians try to understand the patient's values and preferences. At times, clinicians may also attempt to predict what a patient may choose for himself or herself. MacIntyre (1989) referred to this as *epistemology*, the study of being able to predict what one might do or desire based on what one did or the choices one has made in the past. Epistemology is used in ethical situations as a means of attempting to discover the truth. However, clinicians may try to second guess what a particular patient or family might choose, only to find that their predictions are in error. Choosing options that are within the norm is usually not questioned; a person's mental state and his or her choices are questioned only when choices fall outside the norm. The realization of unsuspected truth that

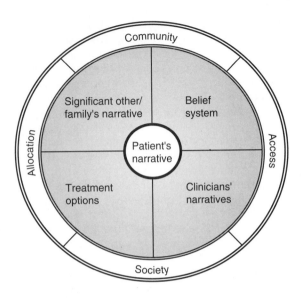

FIGURE 4–1. Conceptualization of narratives.

becomes evident through patients' choices reinforces the necessity of shared decision making.

Figure 4–1 provides a diagram conceptualizing the use of narrative in ethical decision making. At the center of this model is the patient's narrative, which is the patient's own account of present events as they relate to his or her life story. At the second level, the patient's narrative interacts with and occurs within the context of other narratives. The patient's family members and/or significant others bring their own narratives to their relationship and interactions with the patient and caregivers. Similarly, the narratives or stories of family members and clinicians may also influence the patient's system of values and beliefs, which in turn have an effect on the patient's narrative. Patients are also presented with treatment options that they must examine within the contexts of their own narrative and value system and the narratives of those individuals who are closely involved with the patient (i.e., the clinicians and significant others). The third and outermost layer of this model is composed of the larger forces of community and society. The narratives of the patient, the clinicians, and family members interact within a community that has its own story and then within the larger society. Issues of access and allocation interact with and affect the narratives of society and community. Treatment options may also be affected. No story exists in isolation; rather, all exist within larger circles of community and society.

The patient's story forms the center of all these interactions, and it is told first. Conducting the narrative with a patient who has decision-making capacity may be as simple as asking a few questions, such as "How are you?," "What is your understanding of your condition?," and "What are your thoughts about how things have gone thus far as well as how things are going now?" When the diagnosis is the focus, however, patients must make decisions about their illness as though it were separate from themselves. Instead, allowing the patient to be heard—before others have been heard— places the focus on the patient rather than on the patient's condition or diagnosis. Treatment becomes not a matter of what to do about a heart condition or a cancer but rather how to treat a person who has this condition.

The narratives of patients who lack capacity must be told by others. Clinicians can pose open-ended questions in the form of statements to help the storyteller know where and how to start. Clinicians might state, "Tell us about your husband. We have only known him since his illness. What was he like as a husband, a father, a man? What are some of the things you remember that make him who he is? Tell us about his sense of humor." Statements that acknowledge the short time the clinical team has interacted with the patient reinforce to the family that the clinicians do not know him as well as the family and that the family has an important role to play.

ROLE OF THE ADVANCED PRACTICE NURSE

Advanced practice gerontological nurses may find themselves in many different settings, working wherever there are aging people in need of healthcare. Delivering care to the elderly presents challenges and opportunities that are complex and multidimensional. Because the potential for ethical problems is so great, APNs must take a proactive approach.

First, APNs need to be informed about the relevant ethical issues common to the population served. Clinicians should be familiar with institutional policies on the subject as well as laws that govern the locality where practice occurs. Topics that particularly affect practice within the geriatric population include, but are not limited to, capacity and decision making; stopping, starting, or refusing treatments; and issues surrounding the end of life.

Second, education must occur for both staff members who provide hands-on care and patients and their surrogates. Patients should be educated about directing surrogates to speak on their behalf when they are no longer able, and surrogates need information regarding their responsibilities when speaking on behalf of another person. Education should also address the limits of available medical technology and the options of withholding treatments or withdrawing treatments once they have been started. By using the term *medical treatment* instead of *care*, nurses can convey to patients and family members that when treatments are withdrawn, care will still be provided. Information is needed for staff members and patients about the differences between *care* and *cure*—that is, when cure is no longer possible, care will remain. Nurses must speak to the issue of the care that is needed by a patient. Care may include adequate and aggressive pain control, not only for terminal pain but also for chronic and debilitating pain. It is certainly not suggested that each APN be an expert in ethics, but he or she should be informed about the issues to be addressed and the resources that can assist with this process.

Third, APNs can and should become comfortable with discussions about what may seem to be sensitive topics. Discussions need to occur over time, as the nurse-patient relationship develops, but also before an ethical crisis arises. Discussions must be incorporated into the nursing process as part of a thorough assessment and the development, implementation, and evaluation of a plan of care. Often the discomfort surrounding death and dying lies with the nurse and not with the patient. Table 4–6 presents the American Nurses Association's statement on nursing and the Patient Self-Determination Act.

TABLE 4-6
American Nurses Association's Position Statement on Nursing and the Patient Self-Determination Act

Summary: The American Nurses' Association (ANA) believes that nurses should play a primary role in implementation of the Patient Self-Determination Act, passed as part of the Omnibus Budget Reconciliation Act of 1990. It is the responsibility of nurses to facilitate informed decision making for patients making choices about end-of-life care. The nurse's role in education, research, patient care and advocacy is critical to implementation of the Patient Self-Determination Act within all healthcare settings.

The Patient Self-Determination Act became effective December 1, 1991. This federal law applies to all healthcare institutions receiving Medicaid funds and requires that all individuals receiving medical care be given written information about their rights under state law to make decisions about medical care, including the right to accept or refuse medical or surgical treatment. Individuals must also be given information about their rights to formulate advance directives such as living wills and durable powers of attorney for healthcare. Patients must be made aware of the rights to make decisions about these issues on admission (to hospitals or skilled nursing facilities), enrollment (in health maintenance organizations), on first receipt of care (in the case of hospices), or before the patient comes under an agency's care (in the case of home health personal care agencies).

The ANA supports the patient's right to self-determination and believes that nurses will and must play a primary role in implementation of the law. Ideally, decisions about advance directives should be made by the patient with the family and the primary care provider prior to admission. The formation of advance directives is an important decision that will inevitably involve nurses, who are the most omnipresent professionals in healthcare facilities. It is imperative that nurses facilitate the decision making that will fall to patients and their families as they make choices about end-of-life care.

- Each nurse should know the laws of the state in which he or she is practicing that pertain to advance directives and should be familiar with the strengths and limitations of the various forms of advance directive.
- The nurse is one of several healthcare professionals who has a responsibility for ensuring that the advance care directives initiated by the patient are current and reflective of the patient's choices. Facilitating the self-determination of patients with respect to end-of-life decisions is a process that includes evaluating changes in the patient's perspective and health state.
- The nurse has a responsibility to facilitate informed decision making, including but not limited to advance directives.
- The ANA recommends that the following questions about advance directives be part of the nursing admission assessment: Do you have basic information about advance care directives, including living wills and durable power of attorney? Do you wish to initiate an advance care directive? If you have already prepared an advance care directive, can you provide it now? Have you discussed your end-of-life choices with your family and/or designated a surrogate and a healthcare team worker?
- The role of the nurse is critical in implementing the Patient Self-Determination Act. It includes public education, research, patient care, advocacy, education of the profession, and inservice education of other healthcare providers.

Adapted from American Nurses Association. (1992). *Code for nurses with interpretive statements.* Kansas City, MO: American Nurses Association.

Fourth, APNs need to be familiar with and able to access the resources for ethics in healthcare. As part of the Joint Commission on Accreditation of Healthcare Organization's standards for institutional ethics (1993), programs are being established that address how patients, families, and staff members can learn their institution's program for resolving ethical dilemmas. By becoming familiar with a facility's program, the advanced practitioner can assist with this process of resolving ethical issues. If a committee exists, the advanced practitioner may want to petition the committee for membership. In the absence of an ethics program, the advanced practitioner may want to begin the process of developing such a program. Until a program is in place, the APN can lead nursing focus groups to review cases retrospectively, whereby ethical problems are identified and discussion is fostered. A process of this kind can be informal and can help nurses work through unresolved issues that can affect the delivery of future care.

SUMMARY

Gerontological APNs serve individuals whose beliefs and values may be very different from their own. They need to first understand their own story to be able to hear what the patient is trying to say, both verbally and nonverbally, about his or her own goals and desires.

APNs must become aggressive with comfort care and understand pain control. At the same time, they must become aware of their own attitudes about life and death and the differences between suffering and survival. Shared decision making must be fostered and encouraged, along with discussions of prognosis and the option of providing no treatment. Gerontological APNs must realize that decisions are not made in isolation but within the context of an individual within a community. Resources are available to assist with challenging ethical situations.

REFERENCES

American Hospital Association (1992). *A patient's bill of rights*. Chicago: American Hospital Association.

American Medical Association (1981). *Current opinions of the judicial council of the American Medical Association*. Chicago: American Medical Association.

American Nurses Association (1985). *Code for nurses with interpretive statements*. Kansas City, MO: American Nurses Association.

Beauchamp, T., & Childress, J. (1994). *Principles of biomedical ethics* (4th ed.). New York: Oxford University Press.

Brody, H. (1989). Transparency: Informed consent in primary care. *Hastings Center Report, 19*(5), 5–9.

Fletcher, J. (1979). *Humanhood: Essays in biomedical ethics*. Buffalo, NY: Prometheus Books.

Fletcher, J. (1991). Ethics consultation: A service of clinical ethics. *Newsletter of the Society for Bioethics Consultation, Spring*, 1.

Fletcher J., & Miller, F. (1994). A case method in planning for the care of patients. In J. Fletcher, C. Hite, P. Lombardo & M. Marshall (Eds.), *Introduction to clinical ethics* (pp. 27–58). Charlottesville, VA: University of Virginia Center for Biomedical Ethics.

Gaylin, W. (1993). Faulty diagnosis. *Harper's Magazine*, October. 57–64.

Glasser, G., Zweibel, N., & Cassel, C. (1988). The ethics committee in the nursing home. *Journal of the American Geriatrics Society, 36*, 150–156.

Hauerwas, S., & Jones, L. (1989). *Why narrative? Readings in narrative theology*. Grand Rapids, MI: William B. Eerdmans Publishing Company.

Joint Commission on Accreditation of Healthcare Organizations (1993). Patients rights. *Accreditation manual for hospitals, 1993* (pp. 9–10). Oakbrook Terrace, IL: Joint Commission on Accreditation of Healthcare Organizations, Department of Publication.

Jonsen, A., Siegler, M., & Winslade, W. (1992). *Clinical ethics*. New York: Macmillan Publishing Company.

La Puma, J., & Schiedermayer, D. (1991). Ethics consultation: Skills, roles, and training. *Annals of Internal Medicine, 114*, 155–160.

MacIntyre, A. (1989). Epistemological crises, narrative, and philosophy of science. In S. Hauerwas & L. Jones (Eds.), *Why narrative?* (pp. 138–147). Grand Rapids, MI: William B. Eerdmans Publishing Company.

President's Commission for the Study of Ethical Problems in Medicine and Biomedical and Behavioral Research (1982). *Making health care decisions, vol. 1*. Washington, D.C.: U.S. Government Printing Office.

Veatch, R. (1981). *A theory of medical ethics*. New York: Basic Books, Inc.

Webster's new universal unabridged dictionary (2nd ed.). (1983). New York: Simon & Schuster.

American Hospital Association: A Patient's Bill of Rights

1. The patient has the right to considerate and respectful care.
2. The patient has the right to and is encouraged to obtain from physicians and other direct caregivers relevant, current, and understandable information concerning diagnosis, treatment, and prognosis.

   Except in emergencies when the patient lacks decision-making capacity and the need for treatment is urgent, the patient is entitled to the opportunity to discuss and request information related to the specific procedures and/or treatments, the risks involved, the possible length of recuperation, and the medically reasonable alternatives and their accompanying risks and benefits.

   Patients have the right to know the identity of physicians, nurses, and others involved in their care, as well as when those involved are students, residents, or other trainees. The patient also has the right to know the immediate and long-term financial implications of treatment choices, insofar as they are known.
3. The patient has the right to make decisions about the plan of care prior to and during the course of treatment and to refuse a recommended treatment or plan of care to the extent permitted by law and hospital policy and to be informed of the medical consequences of this action. In case of such refusal, the patient is entitled to other appropriate care and services that the hospital provides or transfer to another hospital. The hospital should notify patients of any policy that might affect patient choice within the institution.
4. The patient has the right to have an advance directive (such as a living will, healthcare proxy, or durable power of attorney for healthcare) concerning treatment or designating a surrogate decision maker with the expectation that the hospital will honor the intent of that directive to the extent permitted by law and hospital policy.

   Healthcare institutions must advise patients of their rights under state law and hospital policy to make informed medical choices, ask if the patient has an advance directive, and include that information in patient records. The patient has the right to timely information about hospital policy that may limit its ability to implement fully a legally valid advance directive.
5. The patient has the right to every consideration of privacy. Case discussion, consultation, examination, and treatment should be conducted so as to protect each patient's privacy.
6. The patient has the right to expect that all communications and records pertaining to his or her care will be treated as confidential by the hospital, except in cases such as suspected abuse and public health hazards when reporting is permitted or required by law. The patient has the right to expect that the hospital will emphasize the confidentiality of this information when it releases it to any other parties entitled to review information in these records.

Adapted from American Hospital Association. *A patient's bill of rights*. Chicago: American Hospital Association. Reprinted with permission of the American Hospital Association, copyright 1992.

7. The patient has the right to review the records pertaining to his or her medical care and to have the information explained or interpreted as necessary, except when restricted by law.

8. The patient has the right to expect that, within its capacity and policies, a hospital will make reasonable response to the request of a patient for appropriate and medically indicated care and services. The hospital must provide evaluation, service, and/or referral as indicated by the urgency of the case. When medically appropriate and legally permissible, or when a patient has so requested, a patient may be transferred to another facility. The institution to which the patient is to be transferred must first have accepted the patient for transfer. The patient must also have the benefit of complete information and explanation concerning the need for, risks, benefits, and alternatives to such a transfer.

9. The patient has the right to ask about and be informed of the existence of business relationships among the hospital, educational institutions, other healthcare providers, or payers that may influence the patient's treatment and care.

10. The patient has the right to consent to or decline to participate in proposed research studies or human experimentation affecting care and treatment or requiring direct patient involvement, and to have those studies fully explained prior to consent. A patient who declines to participate in research or experimentation is entitled to the most effective care that the hospital can otherwise provide.

11. The patient has the right to expect reasonable continuity of care when appropriate and to be informed by physicians and other caregivers of available and realistic patient care options when hospital care is no longer appropriate.

12. The patient has the right to be informed of hospital policies and practices that relate to patient care, treatment, and responsibilities. The patient has the right to be informed of available resources for resolving disputes, grievances, and conflicts, such as ethics committees, patient representatives, or other mechanisms available in the institution. The patient has the right to be informed of the hospital's charges for services and available payment methods.

These rights can be exercised on the patient's behalf by a designated surrogate or proxy decision maker if the patient lacks decision-making capacity, is legally incompetent, or is a minor.

Assessment of the Older Client

Comprehensive Geriatric Assessment

Sandra J. Engberg
Joan McDowell

One of the major challenges facing the healthcare system in our society is the provision of quality care for the rapidly expanding population of older adults. At the beginning of this century, only 1 in 25 people was 65 years of age or older. By the middle of the next century, it is estimated that 1 in 5 people will be of this age (Windom, 1988). Of even greater concern is the aging of the elderly population itself, which is reflected in the categories used for these individuals: *young old*, those people 65 to 74 years of age; *middle old*, 75 to 84 years of age; and *old old*, 85 years of age and older (Brody, 1980). The old old age group is the most rapidly increasing population in this country (Randall, 1993). Unfortunately, these individuals are much more likely to have significant functional deficits and frequent contact with the healthcare system.

Although older adults constitute only 12% of the population, they account for a much higher proportion of the people receiving healthcare services. In primary care settings, over one third of the patients receiving care

are 65 years of age or older (Kane et al., 1994), and older adults constitute a disproportionately large percentage of the patients in acute care settings (Abrams et al., 1995). In 1992, the hospital discharge rate per 1000 people was 336.5 for individuals age 65 years and older, compared with 131 and 96 for people 45 to 64 years of age and 15 to 44 years of age, respectively (Graves, 1994). Older adults constitute 74% of the people who receive home healthcare (Straham, 1994), and the vast majority of long-term care patients are 65 years of age or older. Thus, nurses working in a variety of care settings, including homecare, must possess the skills required for assessment of the elderly.

UNIQUENESS OF OLDER ADULTS

Assessment provides the basis for planning and implementing care, and the quality of subsequent care is often contingent on nurses' abilities to adequately assess older adults. The evaluation of older patients is a challenge to nurses' assessment skills. Just as children should not be considered "miniature adults," one should not consider the aged as simply "old adults." Providing healthcare for elderly people requires special approaches and an understanding of the physiological, psychosocial, and pathological impacts of aging. Older adults are the most diverse of all the age groups. The combined effects of genetic factors and lifelong exposure to health habits, medical problems, lifestyles, environmental factors, and sociocultural influences intensify the differences between individuals, making it difficult to absolutely predict the effects of "normal aging." In addition, there is tremendous variability within each person's body systems. Chronological age is thus a convenient marker but not necessarily a good predictor of biological age.

SPECIAL PROBLEMS AFFECTING ASSESSMENT

Several factors complicate the assessment of older patients. These include differentiating the effects of aging from those caused by disease, the coexistence of multiple diseases, the underreporting of symptoms by patients, atypical and nonspecific presentations of illnesses, and increased iatrogenic illnesses.

When assessing older adults, it is often difficult to differentiate the effects of aging from those of disease. Physiologically, normal aging involves the steady erosion of organ reserves and homeostatic mechanisms. Lifestyle factors, however, have a much more profound effect on biological functioning (Williams, 1994). Researchers are just beginning to be able to differentiate the effects of aging from those of pathology. A lack of awareness of the normal effects of aging can lead to overdiagnosing or underdiagnosing diseases in the older patient. For example, glucose tolerance decreases with age and results in an increase in the blood glucose following a glucose load. Thus, postprandial glucose levels are normally higher in older patients. An unawareness of this effect of aging can result in an overdiagnosis of diabetes (see Appendix 6–1 for the changes associated with normal aging). More common than overdiagnosis, however, is underdiagnosis—attributing pathological conditions to normal aging rather than to disease. Examples of pathological processes that may be inappropriately attributed to aging include urinary incontinence, fatigue, depressive symptoms, and decreased cognitive functioning.

The presence of multiple chronic diseases complicates the assessment of older patients. Four out of five older adults have at least one chronic disease (Fowles, 1991), and community-dwelling and hospitalized older adults each have an average of three and a half and six pathological conditions, respectively (Rowe, 1985). Symptoms of one condition can exacerbate or mask those of another, thus complicating clinical evaluation. The patient with degenerative joint disease of the knees or hips, for example, may severely limit his or her physical activity, thereby masking the symptoms of coronary artery disease.

Many older adults tend to underreport symptoms, further complicating assessment (Williams, 1994). This tendency may be affected by the individual's cultural or educational background, ageism, fear, depression, and cognitive dysfunction. Older adults may believe that morbidity and disability are a nor-

TABLE 5-1

Nonspecific Symptoms

Symptom	Examples of Possible Causes
Sudden confusion	Infections (urinary tract infection, pneumonia) Congestive heart failure Myocardial infarction Adverse drug reactions Stroke Metabolic disorders (hyperglycemia or hypoglycemia, azotemia, electrolyte imbalances) Fecal impaction Transfer to unfamiliar surroundings (particularly if sensory input is compromised)
Failure to thrive	Cancer Endocrine disorders (diabetes, hypothyroidism) Infections Congestive heart failure Depression Dementia Parkinson's disease Isolation Neglect Dental problems
Fatigue	Depression Congestive heart failure Anemia Hypothyroidism
Insomnia	Age-related changes in sleep patterns Anxiety Congestive heart failure with orthopnea Urinary frequency with nocturia
New urinary incontinence	Uncontrolled diabetes Adverse drug reactions Delirium Fecal impaction Immobility

Data from Kane et al. (1994) and Verdery (1994).

mal consequence of aging and therefore dismiss symptoms as age related.

Another factor confounding assessment is that illness may present with atypical and nonspecific symptoms such as confusion, weakness, and functional decline. For this reason, the patient history may be less useful in ruling out health problems (Table 5–1).

Iatrogenic illnesses are common in the elderly and can also complicate assessment (see Chapter 16). Drugs can have paradoxical and bizarre side effects in the elderly. One should always suspect that medications may be the cause of a patient's illness. Because symptoms of adverse drug reactions can be nonspecific or can mimic those of other illnesses, these reactions may be ignored or unrecognized.

MULTIDISCIPLINARY ASSESSMENT

The complex healthcare needs of many older adults, particularly the frail elderly, can often best be met through a multidisciplinary approach to assessment and management (Allen et al., 1986; Katz et al., 1985; Lichtenstein & Winograd, 1985; Rubenstein et al., 1987). The composition of multidisciplinary teams varies widely, but the core team commonly consists of medical, nursing, and mental health professionals. Successful multidisciplinary assessments can lead to improved diagnostic accuracy, more appropriate placements, improved functional status, improved affect or cognition, fewer prescribed medications, decreased use of nursing homes, increased use of home health services, fewer acute care admissions, reduced healthcare costs, and prolonged survival (Rubenstein et al., 1987).

COMPREHENSIVE GERIATRIC ASSESSMENT

Functional ability rather than disease should be the focus of geriatric assessment and care (Kane et al., 1994; Rubenstein, 1995; Rubinstein et al., 1989; Williams, 1994). Many of the healthcare problems of older adults are chronic, with little or no potential for cure. Although it is important to identify potentially reversible illnesses, the goal of healthcare for older adults shifts from curing underlying problems to maximizing functional ability and well-being.

Comprehensive assessment of the older adult should address biological, psychological, and social functioning. (Table 5–2 outlines the components of a comprehensive gerontological assessment.) Completing such an assessment is time consuming and can be particularly tiring for the frail older adult. It is often best accomplished in multiple sessions. If the patient seems tired or overwhelmed, consider scheduling another visit to complete the assessment. Subsequent chapters focus on the physical examination (Chapter 6), the assessment of cognitive status (Chapter 7) and affective status (Chapter 17), mobility assessment (Chapter 12), and activities of daily living (Chapter 9). The remainder of this chapter is devoted to the health history, the assessment of health risks and preventive health practices, and developmental and environmental assessment.

TABLE 5-2

Components of a Comprehensive Gerontological Assessment

1. Health history
2. Health risk appraisal and preventive health practices
3. Developmental assessment
4. Environmental assessment
   Physical environment
   Social environment
5. Physical examination
6. Functional assessment
   Cognitive function
   Affective function
   Mobility
   Activities of daily living

HEALTH HISTORY

The assessment of all patients, regardless of age, should begin with the health history. This history provides the basis for interpreting subsequent assessment data and suggesting a plan of care.

Effective Interviewing Skills

The ability to obtain a complete health history requires learning and practice. An effective clinical interview is characterized by objectivity, precision, sensitivity, and specificity. *Objectivity* refers to the removal of one's beliefs, biases, and preconceptions from the interview process (Coulehan & Block, 1992). To achieve objectivity during the interview, one should focus on listening to what the patient is saying, provide effective feedback on what is heard, and avoid jumping to premature conclusions about the nature of the patient's problem. One should avoid being influenced by the patient's interpretation of his or her own symptoms. For example, when a patient says he has the flu or heart problems, the nurse should ask what symptoms the patient is experiencing.

Ageism is a bias that often interferes with effectively interviewing older adults. A nurse may believe, for example, that a functional disability is an inevitable consequence of aging, rather than pursue the problem to identify a potentially correctable cause. Ageism may also be a patient bias. Older adults often inappropriately attribute potentially correctable health problems such as urinary incontinence to normal aging, and they frequently fail to report symptoms.

Effective interviewing also requires *precision*, the ability to understand as completely as possible what the patient is experiencing. What exactly does Mrs. Smith mean when she says she doesn't sleep well? Precision requires obtaining as much detail as possible about the patient's complaint.

In relation to the health history, *sensitivity* and *specificity* refer to the ability of a symptom or complex of symptoms to accurately identify a particular health problem. Individual symptoms vary widely in their sensitivities (ability to identify actual problems) and specificities (ability to rule out other problems), and thus symptom complexes are often critical in diag-

nosing health problems. An objective and precise interview allows the nurse to accurately identify symptom complexes. In younger adults, these complexes are typically sensitive and specific for particular health problems. Unfortunately, health problems often present atypically or nonspecifically in the frail older patient, decreasing the sensitivity and specificity of the health history (see Tables 5–1 and 5–3).

Interviewer qualities that enhance communication with the patient are respect, genuineness, and empathy (Coulehan & Block, 1992). *Respect* refers to the clinician's ability to value the patient's beliefs and to view the patient's responses as valid adaptations to his or her illness or life circumstances. Clinicians need to separate their personal feelings about the patient's beliefs or behaviors from their concerns about helping the patient. The following are simple behaviors clinicians can use to dem-

TABLE 5-3
Common Atypical Disease Presentations

Illness	Atypical Presentations
Hyperthyroidism	Apathetic (lethargy and intellectual blunting) rather than hyperkinetic symptoms Nonspecific presentation with failure to thrive, anorexia, change in alertness Suspect hyperthyroidism in unexplained heart failure or tachyrhythmia, a new onset psychiatric disorder, or profound myopathy
Hypothyroidism	Apathy, depression, mental and physical slowness, or nonspecific deterioration in health
Pneumonia	Confusion, anorexia, weakness, lethargy, unsteadiness, and slight dyspnea
Congestive heart failure	Urinary incontinence Confusion
Myocardial infarction	Dyspnea, syncope, weakness, vomiting, or confusion instead of chest pain
Urinary tract infection	Urinary tract infection Confusion
Depression	Constitutional (physical) symptoms or failure to thrive
Adverse drug reaction	Confusion Many medications can cause paradoxical or bizarre side effects in older patients and should always be considered when new symptoms occur

Data from Beers & Besdine (1987), Hodkinson (1973), Kane et al. (1994), and Starer & Libow (1995).

onstrate respect for the patient (Coulehan & Block, 1992):

- Introducing themselves before beginning the interview and explaining their role in the patient's care
- Using the patient's last name when addressing him or her
- Making sure that the patient is comfortable before starting the interview
- Sitting at the patient's level during the interview
- Telling the patient what they are going to do
- Responding in a way that lets the patient know they have heard what the patient said

Genuineness means not pretending to be someone or something that you are not and being oneself both as a person and as a professional. *Empathy* means showing understanding. In a clinical interview, it involves the clinician listening to the patient's total communication—words, emotions, and gestures—and providing feedback to indicate that he or she hears what the patient is saying.

Asking Questions

The quality of the information obtained during the health history is strongly influenced by the way questions are asked. When conducting a clinical interview, the clinician should begin each area of inquiry with an open-ended question; for example, "what is the pain like?" Once the patient has been given an opportunity to talk, follow with more directed questions to clarify and amplify information as needed. When the patient is having difficulty finding the words to describe certain characteristics, such as the nature of the pain, it may be helpful to provide a list of possible descriptions to choose from; for example, "would you describe the pain as sharp, dull, achy, burning, or pressure?" Avoid the use of leading questions as well as compound questions. Examples of poor questions include "it hurts in your right lower abdomen, doesn't it?" (a leading question) and "do you have any pain in your abdomen and are your bowels moving regularly?" (a compound question).

Interviewing the Older Adult

Various difficulties can be encountered when obtaining a medical history from an older person. Vision and hearing impairments are prevalent and can interfere with effective communication (see Chapter 22). Several techniques may be useful when interviewing the patient with sensory impairment: (1) make sure the room is well lit but do not sit or stand in front of a strong light or window, since older people are often sensitive to glare; (2) eliminate as much background noise as possible; (3) face the patient and sit comfortably close to him or her (many older patients with a hearing impairment read lips and use body language as cues to enhance communication); and (4) speak slowly and clearly, amplify the volume of the voice only slightly (being careful not increase the pitch), and do not shout; if the patient has a hearing aid, make sure it is turned on, that the volume is high enough, and that the batteries work. When interviewing patients who are very hard of hearing, a pocket sound amplifier may be helpful; with these devices, the patient wears Walkman-like earphones, and the clinician speaks into the amplifier.

Cognitive problems are also common in older adults, especially among the old old. The patient with significant cognitive impairment cannot provide a reliable history, and thus the nurse will need to use secondary sources to obtain information about the patient's health history. Unfortunately, the older adult with excellent social skills may be able to mask mild and even moderate cognitive deficits. If there is any question about the reliability of information a patient is providing, it may help to evaluate the patient's cognitive function early in the encounter (see Chapter 7). This will help the clinician judge the reliability of subsequent data provided by the patient. At the very least, the health history provides the basis for subsequent evaluation of the patient. In some situations, however, the clinical diagnosis and subsequent management may be based entirely on the history. Thus, it is critical to establish the reliability of the data being collected. When documenting the health history, it is important to include a notation about the reliability of the information.

Many older patients have lengthy histories with multiple health complaints. The clinician should keep in mind, however, that multiple somatic complaints can sometimes be a manifestation of depression in the older patient (Kane et al., 1994). In general, more time is required to obtain a health history from an older adult than from a younger person.

Components of the Complete Health History

The components of a health history are listed in Table 5–4. The format of taking a health history is similar to that for younger adults; however, emphases on certain components of the history as well as the information collected during parts of the history differ somewhat for the older adult.

TABLE 5-4
Complete Health History

Chief complaint
Patient profile
Present illnesses
  Characterization of the present complaint
  Known illnesses
  Self-rated health
  Medications
Past medical history
  Serious childhood illnesses
  Other illnesses
  Hospitalizations/surgical procedures/injuries
  Allergies
  Other drug reactions
  Alcohol and tobacco use
Health promotion and preventive practices
  Use of health services
  Screening practices
  Nutrition
  Exercise
  Sleep patterns
  Safety
  Immunizations
Family history
Review of systems

TABLE 5-5
Patient Profile Data

Marital status
  If widowed
    How long widowed
    Adjustment to being widowed
  If spouse is living
    Health of spouse
    Relationship with spouse
Children
  Relationships with children
  Frequency of contact with children
  Telephone numbers
Living arrangements
Support systems
  Family/friends
  Community services
Recent losses, including pets
Education/occupation/retirement
Adequacy of finances and health insurance
Transportation, particularly access to healthcare
Hobbies
Social/organizational activities
Typical day

Chief Complaint. The health history begins with the chief complaint—the reason for the patient encounter. Because many older adults have multiple health problems, however, there may not be a single chief complaint. When the patient presents with multiple health problems or complaints, the clinician may need to help the patient identify which is of greatest concern to him or her and focus on that complaint; this is particularly important when there is limited time for the assessment. When a chief complaint does exist in the elderly, the nonspecific and atypical presentations of disease make it less sensitive and specific in identifying health problems than in younger adults.

Patient Profile. The patient profile provides an opportunity to learn more about the patient as a person and to identify potential risk factors for health problems. Table 5–5 summarizes the information typically included in a patient profile. Questions address marital status, relationships, living arrangements, support systems, losses, education, occupation, access to healthcare, and activities.

Present Illnesses. This component of the health history focuses in greater detail on the presenting complaint as well as known illnesses. If there is a presenting complaint, start with open-ended questions about the complaint. For example, "Tell me about your knee pain." Once the patient has been given an opportunity to talk about the problem, ask additional questions as necessary to characterize it. As needed, ask about the symptom's onset and progression, location, character, severity, factors that aggravate or lessen it, and associated symptoms.

When inquiring about the onset and progression of a symptom, ask when the symptom started, what the patient was doing when it started, and how it has changed since its onset ("Has it stayed the same, increased, or decreased in severity?"). If the symptom is intermittent, ask how often it occurs; what precipitates an episode; how long episodes last; if the patient can identify anything that alleviates the episode; and how, if at all, episodes have changed over time.

For symptoms such as pain, ask about the location and any radiation. To determine the location of symptoms, ask the patient to point to where it hurts. Ask if the location of the pain has changed since its onset and if it radiates to any other area.

Do not accept symptoms at face value. Ask the patient to describe the symptom—what it is like; for example, "Could you describe the pain?," "Could you describe how you feel when you get dizzy?," "What do you mean when you say that you are constipated?," or "You said that you're tired; could you describe how you feel?" Start by trying to get the patient to describe the symptom in his or her own words. If the patient is unable to describe the symptom, provide a list of possible descriptors and have the patient select the one that most closely describes what he or she is experiencing.

Try to establish the severity of the symptoms. For symptoms such as vomiting, diarrhea, or constipation, questions should focus on the frequency and severity of symptoms. For symptoms such as pain, it may be helpful to ask the patient to rate the severity of the pain by comparing it to the most severe pain he or she has ever experienced; for example, "on a scale from 0 to 10, with 10 being the most severe pain you have ever experienced, how would you rate this pain?" Asking the patient about the impact of the symptom on activities of daily living and sleep may also help in quantifying its severity.

Ask the patient about factors that alleviate or aggravate the symptom (e.g., "Is there anything that makes the symptom worse?"). Depending on the nature of the symptom, the clinician may want to ask about specific aggravating factors such as activity, movement, food, and stress. Ask if the patient has tried or noticed anything that lessens the symptom. Again, the clinician may want to follow this general question with more directed questions about specific factors known to alleviate the symptom in select illnesses.

Finally, ask about associated symptoms. Start with an open-ended question such as "Are you experiencing any other problems in addition to the pain?" Follow this with questions about specific symptoms known to be associated with select illnesses.

In addition to collecting data on the presenting complaint, ask the patient about other current illnesses, their onset and progression, and any complications. Ask how the problem has been and is being treated. Question the patient about compliance as well as side effects related to treatment. Finally, inquire about the functional impact of each problem. To what extent does this problem interfere with the patient's ability to do things he or she needs or wants to do?

Self-Rated Health. It is useful to ask the older adult to rate his or her current health. Older patients tend to see themselves as healthier than clinicians see them. Despite increasing numbers of medical problems, most rate their health as good, as long as they can perform activities related to maintaining independence and social roles (Mezey et al., 1993).

Past Medical History. Older adults often have fairly involved past medical histories, and they may have had multiple illnesses and surgeries. The past medical history can help put current problems in perspective and may even offer diagnostic clues about the cause of current problems. Ask the patient specifically about illnesses he or she reports having had in the past; never simply accept a diagnosis. After asking an open-ended question about past illnesses, ask specifically about major or common illnesses such as diabetes, hypertension, heart problems, tuberculosis, cancer, and depression. Inquire about past hospitalizations and their reasons, previous surgical procedures, and past injuries. During the physical examination, ask about any scars observed. This may help the patient recall procedures he or she may have forgotten to mention during the history. Childhood illnesses are less important in older patients. It is generally adequate to ask only about unusual or serious childhood illnesses (e.g., those causing them to miss a lot of school) (Coulehan & Block, 1992; Fields, 1991).

Ask the patient about past blood transfusions. When acquired immune deficiency syndrome and hepatitis occur in older adults, they are most often secondary to blood transfusions (Starer & Libow, 1995).

The medication history is extremely important in the elderly because of the high risk for adverse drug reactions (ADRs) (see Chapter 26). Chronic and multiple illnesses are often associated with polypharmacy in the elderly, and older adults take an average of four and a half medications at any one time (Beers & Ouslander, 1989). The pharmacokinetic and pharmacodynamic changes that occur with aging and polypharmacy increase the risk of ADRs (Schwartz, 1994). It is important to review all medications the patient is taking or supposed to be taking. The best approach is to ask the patient or family to bring in all medications the patient has—both prescription (including topical medications) and nonprescription. Go through each medication and ask the patient if he or she is currently taking it and how. Do not assume that the medication is being taken according to the label instructions. By asking the patient why he or she is taking each medication, the nurse can evaluate the patient's knowledge of the medication and uncover health problems previously unidentified in the history.

Patients frequently do not mention over-the-counter medications unless asked about them specifically. Ask about the use of vitamins, mineral supplements, pain medications, laxatives, nonprescription sleep aids, and cold and allergy medications. These medications can have significant negative health effects. For example, over-the-counter cold medications can cause urinary retention or confusion in some older adults.

The medication history provides an excellent opportunity for assessing the patient's understanding of the medications he or she is taking and for providing patient education. It is also a good opportunity to assess the patient's ability to open the medication containers and read the labels. Patients with mobility impairments or arthritis in their hands, for example, may have considerable difficulty opening the containers. Those with visual impairments often cannot read medication labels unless the print is large.

Query the patient about allergies, particularly to medications. If the patient reports being allergic to a medication, ask about the nature of the reaction. Patients may misinterpret a medication side effect as an allergic reaction. Also ask about other adverse reactions to medications.

Finally, question the patient about current and past use of tobacco and caffeine. Although it is a serious problem in the elderly, alcoholism is often not recognized (see Chapter 23). Structured instruments such as the Michigan Alcoholism Screening Test (MAST) may be useful in screening for alcoholism (Selzer, 1971; Willenbring et al., 1987). Willenbring and colleagues (1987) examined the validity of the original 25-item MAST and two short versions of the questionnaire, the Brief MAST and the Short MAST, in groups of elderly people with and without alcoholism and found that although the MAST showed excellent sensitivity and specificity, the shorter versions were less sensitive and/or specific.

All older adults who smoke should be advised to stop. Caffeine intake may be an important area of inquiry, particularly for those with urinary incontinence, palpitations, nervousness, or difficulty sleeping.

Health Promotion and Prevention Practices. The health history provides an excellent opportunity to screen for health promotion and disease prevention practices. Table 5–6 summarizes health promotion and screening recommendations of the U.S. Preventive Services

TABLE 5-6

Health Promotion and Disease Prevention
Recommendations for Older Adults

Activity	Recommendations
Physical examination	Annual, based on clinical judgment
Blood pressure	Every 2 years if the diastolic pressure is less than 85 mm Hg and the systolic less than 140 mm Hg, or annually if last diastolic pressure is 85–89 mm Hg
Dental examination	Every 1 to 2 years
Vision examination	Routine visual acuity screening; with Snellen chart; interval based on clinical judgment
Hearing examination	Periodic evaluation by patient inquiry; frequency not specified
Serum cholesterol	Every 5 years (based on expert opinion rather than scientific data); there are few data to recommend or not recommend routine screening of asymptomatic older adults over 65 years of age, but screening may be considered for high-risk individuals
Height and weight	Periodic assessment; interval not specified
Breast cancer screening	
Self breast examination	No specific recommendations
Clinical breast examination	Every 1 to 2 years
Mammography	Every 1 to 2 years; can be discontinued after age 75 years if no pathology detected; the American Cancer Society recommends continued screening as long as the patient's life expectancy exceeds 5 years
Colon cancer	
Digital rectal examination	Routine screening if at high risk for colon cancer (e.g., first-degree relative with colorectal cancer; positive personal history of endometrial, ovarian, or breast cancer; previous diagnosis of inflammatory bowel disease, adenomatous polyps, or colorectal cancer); otherwise, based on clinical judgment
Fecal occult blood test	Annual
Sigmoidoscopy	Routine screening; interval not specified
	The American Cancer Society recommends digital rectal exam and stools for occult blood annually; sigmoidoscopy is recommended every 3 to 5 years for persons over age 50 years, and periodic colonoscopy is recommended for high-risk patients
Cervical cancer	
Papanicolaou smear	Every 1 to 3 years; can discontinue screening at age 65 years if there has been documented regular negative screening
Prostate cancer	
Digital rectal examination	Based on clinical judgment; the American Cancer Association recommends annual screening
Prostate-specific antigen	Not recommended
Oral cancer	Routine screening for high-risk patients only
Lung, skin, ovarian, and pancreatic cancer	Routine screening not recommended
Osteoporosis screening	All postmenopausal women should be counseled about prevention measures; selective screening for high-risk women considering hormone prophylaxis
Immunizations	
Influenza	Annual
Tetanus-diphtheria	Every 10 years
Pneumovac	At least once; revaccination may be appropriate for high-risk people who have not been vaccinated in 6 or more years and for those who received the older 14-valent vaccine

Recommendations of the U.S. Preventive Services Task Force (1996). *Guide to clinical preventive services* (2nd ed.). Baltimore: Williams & Wilkins.

Task Force and, where they differ, of the American Cancer Society.

Use of Health Services and Screening Practices. Ask the patient about his or her use of health services, including the frequency of routine medical care, dental examinations, eye examinations, and hearing tests. Inquire about health screening activities, including screening for colorectal cancer (stool for occult blood, sigmoidoscopy, and colonoscopy) and high cholesterol. Women should be asked about their last pelvic examination and Papanicolaou (Pap) smear, self-breast examinations, their last clinical breast examination, and their last mammogram. Men should be asked about clinical examinations of the prostate and being tested for prostate specific antigen (PSA).

The U.S. Preventive Services Task Force (1996) does not recommend routine screening for dementia for asymptomatic older adults. It does, however, recommend that the clinician periodically inquire about the older adult's functioning at work or home. Some geriatric experts recommend routine screening for cognitive impairment, particularly in the frail elderly and the middle old and old old (Murphy & Jones, 1993; Siu et al., 1994).

The older adult should also be asked about immunizations. (Table 5–6 summarizes the U.S. Preventive Services Task Force recommendations regarding immunizations for older adults.) Unless the patient has a serious egg allergy, influenza vaccine is recommended yearly, and pneumococcal vaccine should be given at least once to everyone 65 years of age and older. There is some evidence that pneumococcal antibody levels decrease over time in some elderly patients and that revaccination (6 years after the initial pneumococcal vaccine) helps ensure that high-risk patients have adequate levels of pneumococcal antibodies (Davidson et al., 1994). A tetanus-diphtheria booster (Td) should be given at least once every 10 years. Some older adults will have not received the primary Td series; they should be advised that it is recommended for all older adults.

Nutrition. Older adults may be at increased risk for nutritional problems owing to the effects of chronic illnesses, immobility, sensory deficits, difficulty chewing or swallowing, limited incomes, limited access to food stores, and eating alone. Thus, a nutritional history should be included as part of the comprehensive geriatric assessment. The purpose of this assessment is twofold: (1) to determine if food intake is adequate and appropriate and (2) to identify those at risk for malnutrition. Symptoms that place the older adult at increased risk for malnutrition include anorexia, weight loss, early satiety, difficulty chewing or swallowing, dental problems, nausea and vomiting, a change in bowel habits, fatigue, apathy, depression, and cognitive impairment. Illnesses that are associated with malnutrition include chronic alcoholism, cognitive disorders, chronic myocardial disorders, chronic pulmonary disease, renal insufficiency, and malabsorption syndromes (Lipschitz, 1994). Polypharmacy also increases the risk of malnutrition. Patients should be asked specifically about these problems during the health history.

The Nutritional Screening Initiative, a national consortium of health professionals, developed a self-administered nutritional health checklist (Fig. 5–1) to help individuals assess their risk for nutritional problems (Lipschitz, 1994). A questionnaire such as this can be included as part of the nutritional assessment.

When doing a complete health history on older adults, it is important to assess dietary intake. One approach is to ask the patient what he or she ate during the last 24 hours, asking first about each meal and then about snacks. The clinician should then ask if this is typical of what the patient eats. When evaluating the adequacy and appropriateness of the patient's diet, determine the following:

Is the representation of each food group adequate?
Is the fat content within the recommended limits?
Is fiber intake adequate?
Is sodium intake excessive?
Is the patient on a special diet? If so, is it prescribed or self-defined and are there problems with compliance?

Exercise. Ask the patient about regular exercise. How often and how long does he or she exercise? What type of physical activity? Most older adults are sedentary; only 30% report

The warning signs of poor nutrition are often overlooked. Use this checklist to find out if you or someone you know is at nutritional risk.

Read the statements below. Circle the numbers in the "yes" column for those that apply to you or someone you know. Total your nutritional score.

	Yes
I have an illness or condition that made me change the kind and/or amount of food I eat	2
I eat fewer than two meals per day	3
I eat few fruits, vegetables or milk products	2
I have three or more drinks of beer, liquor or wine almost every day	2
I have tooth or mouth problems that make it hard for me to eat	2
I don't always have the money to buy the food I need	4
I eat alone most of the time	1
I take three or more different prescribed or over-the-counter drugs a day	1
Without wanting to, I have lost or gained 10 pounds in the last six months	2
I am not always physically able to shop, cook and/or feed myself	2

Total your nutritional score   ⎯⎯

If it's:

0–2	Good! Recheck your nutritional score in six months.
3–5	You are at moderate nutritional risk. See what can be done to improve your eating habits and lifestyle. Your office on aging, senior nutrition program, senior citizens center or health department can help. Recheck your nutritional score in six months.
6 or more	You are at high nutritional risk. Bring this checklist the next time you see your doctor, dietitian or other qualified health or social service professional. Talk with them about any problems you have. Ask for help to improve your nutritional health.

FIGURE 5–1. Checklist to Determine Your Nutritional Health. (From Lipschitz, D. A., Ham, R. J., & White, J. V. [1992]. An approach to nutrition screening for older Americans. *American Family Physician, 45,* 603. Reprinted with permission from American Family Physician, published by the American Academy of Family Physicians.)

regular exercise (U.S. Department of Health and Human Services, 1996). Lack of physical activity is a risk factor for coronary artery disease, hypertension, hypercholesterolemia, obesity, glucose intolerance, breast and colon cancer, and increased rates of bone loss (U.S. Department of Health and Human Services, 1996).

Sleep Patterns. Sleep disturbances are among the most common age-related complaints (Haponik, 1994). Aging has varied effects on sleep, including increased sleep latency (taking longer to fall asleep), more frequent and longer arousals, and decreased sleep efficiency. The following changes related to sleep structure are frequently observed in sleep laboratories: (1) increased nonrapid eye movement stage 1 sleep (the transition time from drowsiness to sleep), (2) decreased stages 3 and 4 (deep) sleep, and (3) decreased and early-onset rapid eye movement sleep (Haponik, 1994).

These changes result in common sleep-related complaints such as (1) difficulty falling asleep, (2) awakening more often, (3) being tired during the day, and (4) increased difficulty adjusting to changes in sleep routine. During the assessment of older adults, the nurse should evaluate the characteristics of sleep by asking what time the patient normally goes to bed and gets up, how long it takes him or her to fall asleep, how often he or she awakens during the night and for how long, if he or she feels rested and refreshed in the morning, and if he or she feels sleepy or naps during the day. If the patient presents with a sleep-related complaint, also inquire about snoring, periodic breathing, or abnormal motor activity during the night (Haponik, 1994). The assessment should include questions about exercise patterns, alcohol and caffeine intake, and eating habits.

Safety. Injuries are a significant cause of morbidity among older adults, and the time required for recovery is often prolonged. Older patients should be questioned about safety practices. (Safety practices related to the home are discussed in the section on environmental assessment.) Ask patients about the use of seat belts and when they last took a driving test. Sensory and cognitive changes can have an adverse affect on driving ability, and older adults are involved in proportionately more motor vehicle accidents than are younger people (Stamatiadis & Deacon, 1995).

Family History. The major purpose for collecting the family history is to help clinicians develop a patient's health risk profile. In the middle old adult (75 to 84 years of age) and old old adult (older than 85 years), this becomes less of an issue. With the possible exception of Alzheimer's disease, familial diseases generally express themselves before the person reaches old age (Coulehan & Block, 1992; Fields, 1991).

Review of Systems. This section of the history gives the nurse an opportunity to ask about a variety of symptoms, with the goal of detecting any previously missed problems. The information collected is similar to that for younger individuals except that the nurse should be careful to inquire specifically about symptoms that are commonly seen in older adults. Table 5–7 summarizes those symptoms that should receive special attention and that are associated with illnesses commonly encountered in older patients.

DEVELOPMENTAL ASSESSMENT

Developmental Tasks

A variety of theories address development in later life. The theories of Erikson and colleagues (1986) and Peck (1968) are briefly reviewed here as they relate to the older adult. Erikson and colleagues described eight stages

TABLE 5-7

Important Symptoms in the Review of Systems

System	Symptoms
Head, eyes, ears, nose, throat	Visual impairment Hearing impairment Problems with dentition Decreased sense of smell Altered sense of taste Dry mouth
Cardiovascular	Dyspnea Orthopnea Chest pain Edema Dizziness or syncope Decrease in energy level
Gastrointestinal	Anorexia Frequency of bowel movements Change in bowel habits Difficulty swallowing Heartburn Abdominal pain
Genitourinary	Nocturia Urgency Frequency Hesitancy Difficulty emptying bladder Incontinence Hematuria Dysuria Women: vaginal bleeding or discharge Men: impotence
Musculoskeletal	Joint pain Limitation of range of motion Difficulty walking or using assistive devices Difficulty getting out of chair or bed Balance problems Falls
Neurological	Tremors Numbness or tingling Weakness Paralysis Decreased sensory perception
Psychological	Problems with sleep Depression Problems with memory
Skin	Dryness Pruritus Rashes or lesions Open areas

in the development of a healthy personality over one's life span. The last stage—which has the greatest significance for older adults—is that of integrity versus despair, during which earlier life experiences are integrated. The outcome can be either integrity (acceptance of one's life and life changes) or despair (Erikson et al., 1986).

Peck (1968) identified three developmental tasks of old age:

1. Ego differentiation versus role-work preoccupation—the successful substitution of other roles and activities for those lost through retirement and changes in parental responsibilities
2. Body transcendence versus ego preoccupation—acceptance of and adjustment to the physical changes and discomforts that occur with aging
3. Ego transcendence versus ego preoccupation—acceptance of one's life rather than preoccupation with the prospect of dying

Based on these developmental theories of aging, Mezey and colleagues (1993) further identified the developmental tasks of old age (p. 8):

• Maintaining independence
• Relinquishing power
• Coping with losses
• Initiating a life review process
• Developing a philosophical perspective on life

The comprehensive health history allows nurses to assess the older adult's achievement of the developmental tasks of this stage of life. To what extent has the person accepted the aging process? How has he or she adjusted to the physical and role changes that have occurred with aging? The nurse might ask, "How do you feel about being retired?" or "How do you feel about not being able to get out as much as you could in the past?" Assess how well the patient has integrated and accepted his or her life experiences. During the interview, patients often mention things that have happened to them during their lives; by exploring with the patient how he or she feels about the event, the nurse can better evaluate

how well the patient has accepted and integrated the experience.

Spirituality

Although religion can be considered an aspect of spirituality, *spirituality* is broader than just religion and encompasses one's personal interpretation of life and inner resources. Heriot (1992) described the needs of the spirit as "the development of a sense of meaning and purpose of life, including finding meaning in suffering; a means of forgiveness; a source of love and relatedness, including the ability to both give and receive love; a sense of transcendence; a sense of awe or wonder about life; and a deep experience of trustful relatedness to God, a Supreme Being, or a universal power or force" (p. 23). Traditionally, nurses have limited their spiritual assessment to inquiries about the patient's religious affiliation. Heriot suggested that the spiritual history should also include questions to elicit patients' ideas about the meaning of life, how they express love for others, if they feel loved, what gives them a sense of wonderment about life, and what their sources of forgiveness are. Stoll (1979) developed a spiritual history guide to help nurses assess spirituality; suggested questions for use are presented in Figure 5–2.

ENVIRONMENTAL ASSESSMENT

The physiological changes that occur as a result of aging and the illnesses that commonly accompany it increase the importance of environment for older adults. For them, the environment can either facilitate or be a barrier to independence. Thus, the assessment of the physical and social environment is a critical aspect of comprehensive geriatric assessment.

Physical Environment

The physical environment can be critical to effective functioning, particularly for the frail elderly. Although the nurse can gain some insight into the patient's physical environment

1. Concept of God or deity
   • Is religion or God significant to you? If yes, can you describe how?
   • Is prayer helpful to you? What happens when you pray?
   • Does God or a deity function in your personal life? If yes, can you describe how?
   • How would you describe your God or what you worship?

2. Sources of hope and strength
   • Who is the most important person to you?
   • To whom do you turn when you need help? Are they available?
   • In what ways do they help?
   • What is your source of hope and strength?
   • What helps you the most when you feel afraid or need special help?

3. Religious practices
   • Do you feel your faith (or religion) is helpful to you? If yes, would you tell me how?
   • Are there any religious practices that are important to you?
   • Has being sick made any difference in your practice of praying? Your religious practices?
   • What religious books or symbols are helpful to you?

4. Relation between spiritual beliefs and health
   • What has bothered you the most about being sick (or about what has happened to you)?
   • What do you think is going to happen to you?
   • Has being sick (or what has happened to you) made any difference in your feelings about God or the practicing of your faith?
   • Is there anything especially frightful or meaningful to you now?

FIGURE 5–2. Spiritual Assessment Guide (From Stoll, R. I. [1979]. Guidelines for spiritual assessment. *American Journal of Nursing, 79,* 1574–1577.)

by asking questions during the health history, a home visit is the most effective way to assess the patient's physical environment. An in-home assessment is strongly recommended for older patients with significant functional deficits and a history of falls and for whom the history suggests some concern about the physical environment.

During the environmental assessment, the nurse should assess the safety of the patient's environment and environmental barriers to effective functioning. If the assessment is conducted in the patient's home, the nurse can also observe the patient's ability to perform the physical and instrumental activities of daily living that are necessary for independent functioning (see Chapter 9).

The safety of the older adult's environment is important particularly because of the risk of falls. Approximately 30% of community-dwelling older adults fall each year (Sattin, 1992). Most of these falls occur in the home and are the result of both intrinsic factors affecting the person's stability and extrinsic factors such as environmental hazards (see Chapter 15). Environmental safety can be assessed by asking the patient about potential hazards; having the patient or family complete a questionnaire about safety practices such as the Home Safety Checklist developed by the National Safety Council (Appendix 5–1); or ideally, by directly observing the patient's environment.

The following are key areas to assess in the older patient's physical environment:

1. Check that the lighting is adequate. Are light switches within easy access? Are stairways well lit? Is the pathway to the bathroom well lit? Are there problems with glare?
2. Check that the flooring is safe. Throw rugs, loose or frayed carpeting, and slippery floors are potential safety hazards. Look for objects that the older adult could trip over, such as cords going across the floor, small objects on the floor, or furniture obstructing the pathway across or in and out of a room.
3. Check that the stairways are safe. Is there adequate lighting, are there securely fastened handrails, and are the stairs and their covering in good condition?

4. Examine the bathroom for potential safety hazards. Are there grab-bars to help the person get in and out of the tub or shower and on and off the toilet? Is the height of the toilet appropriate? If the individual needs an assistive device for walking, does it fit in the bathroom? If there are rugs, are they nonskid? Is there a nonskid surface or mat in the tub?

5. In the kitchen, check that items used on a regular basis are within easy access.

6. Consider other safety hazards. Does the home or apartment have smoke or fire alarms? Is there excessive environmental clutter? Are there other fire hazards such as frayed electrical cords and space heaters? Is there spoiled food in the refrigerator or cupboards? Are medications properly labeled? Is there alcohol in the house? Are there firearms in the house that the older adult could use to harm himself or herself or others? Is the yard cluttered or is the ground uneven? Is there adequate lighting if the patient goes out at night? Is the neighborhood safe? Are sidewalks in good repair? Are there street lights?

7. Detect barriers to optimal functioning. Does the patient with incontinence or urinary frequency have to go up and down the steps to reach the bathroom? Is the bathroom a long distance from where the person sleeps? Can the person easily get out of the chair he or she usually sits in? Can he or she get out of bed easily?

Social Environment

In addition to looking at the physical environment, the nurse should assess the social environment (see Chapter 8). Does the older adult live with anyone else? If so, what is their relationship? If there is another person (or people) living in the home, is that person able to help the older adult or is he or she dependent on the older adult for care?

If the older adult has a caregiver, it is important to include him or her in the assessment. Is he or she physically able to provide the care that the older adult needs? How often is he or she available to provide care? Nearly half of the caregivers in this country are also in the work force, and up to one third of these individuals report conflicts between their work and caregiving responsibilities (American Association of Retired Persons and the Travelers Companies Foundation, 1989). Is the caregiver emotionally able to provide the care the patient needs? Caregiver burden is an important factor in the decision to admit frail older adults to long-care services (Brown et al., 1990; Zarit et al., 1986). Nurses can use a variety of scales to measure caregiver burden (Kosberg & Cairl, 1986; Lawton et al., 1989; Zarit et al., 1986). Is the caregiver aware of community services such as daycare, respite care, and support groups? If the caregiver is stressed, the nurse needs to be alert to the risk of elder abuse (Chapter 29). Additional information on social assessment is provided in Chapter 8.

SUMMARY

The purpose of comprehensive geriatric assessment is to identify actual and potential problems that can compromise the functional status of the older adult so that interventions can be planned and initiated to reverse or compensate for these problems. A major goal of the advanced practice nurse should be to maximize functional status and quality of life for older patients. This process begins with the health history.

REFERENCES

Abrams, W. B., Beers, M. H., & Berkow, R. (1995). *The Merck manual of geriatrics* (2nd ed.). Whitehouse Station, NJ: Merck & Co., Inc.

Allen, C. M., Becker, P. M., McVey, L. J., et al. (1986). A randomized controlled clinical trial of a geriatric consultation team: Compliance with recommendations. *Journal of the American Medical Association, 255*, 2617–2621.

American Association of Retired Persons and the Travelers Companies Foundations (1989). *A national survey of caregivers: Working caregivers report.* Washington, D.C.: American Association of Retired Persons.

Beers, M., & Besdine, R. (1987). Medical assessment of the elderly patient. *Clinics in Geriatric Medicine, 3*(1), 17–27.

Beers, M. H., & Ouslander, J. G. (1989). Risk factors in geriatric drug prescribing: A practical guide to avoiding problems. *Drugs, 37*, 105–112.

Brody, S. J. (1980). The graying of America. *Hospitals, 54*(10), 63–66, 123.

Brown, L. J., Potter, J. F., & Foster, B. G. (1990). Caregiver burden should be evaluated during geriatric assessment. *Journal of the American Geriatrics Society, 38,* 455–460.

Coulehan, J. L., & Block, M. R. (1992). *The medical interview: A primer for students of the art* (2nd ed.). Philadelphia: F. A. Davis Company.

Davidson, M., Bulkow, L. R., Grabman, J., et al. (1994). Immunogenicity of pneumococcal revaccination in patients with chronic disease. *Archives of Internal Medicine, 154,* 2209–2214.

Erikson, E. H., Erikson, J. M., & Kivnick, H. Q. (1986). *Vital involvement in old age.* New York: W. W. Norton & Company.

Fields, S. D. (1991). History-taking in the elderly: Obtaining useful information. *Geriatrics, 46*(8), 26–44.

Fowles, D. G. (1991). *A profile of older Americans.* Washington, D.C.: American Association of Retired Persons, Administration on Aging.

Graves, E. J. (1994). 1992 summary: National hospital discharge survey. *Advance data from vital and health statistics* (Report No. 249). Hyattsville, MD: National Center for Health Statistics.

Haponik, E. F. (1994). Sleep problems. In W. R. Hazzard, E. L. Bierman, J. P. Blass, et al. (Eds.), *Principles of geriatric medicine and gerontology* (3rd ed., pp. 1213–1228). New York: McGraw-Hill, Inc.

Heriot, C. S. (1992). Spirituality and aging. *Holistic Nursing Practice, 7*(1), 22–31.

Hodkinson, H. M. (1973). Non-specific presentation of illness. *British Medical Journal, 4,* 94–96.

Kane, R. L., Ouslander, J. G., & Abrass, I. B. (1994). *Essentials of clinical geriatrics* (3rd ed.). New York: McGraw-Hill, Inc.

Katz, P. R., Dube, D. H., & Calkins, E. (1985). Use of a structured functional assessment format in a geriatric consultation service. *Journal of the American Geriatrics Society, 33,* 681–686.

Kosberg, J. I., & Cairl, R. E. (1986). The cost of care index: A case management tool for screening informal carers. *Gerontologist, 26,* 273–278.

Lawton, M. P., Kleban, M. H., Moss, M., et al. (1989). Measuring caregiving appraisal. *Journal of Gerontology, 44*(3), P61–P71.

Lichtenstein, H., & Winograd, C. H. (1985). Geriatric consultation: A functional approach. *Journal of the American Geriatrics Society, 33,* 422–428.

Lipschitz, D. A. (1994). Screening for nutritional status in the elderly. *Primary Care, 21*(1), 55–67.

Mezey, M. D., Rauckhorst, L. H., & Stokes, S. A. (1993). *Health assessment of the older individual* (2nd ed.). New York: Springer.

Murphy, J. B., & Jones, T. F. (1993). Screening for older persons. *Rhode Island Medicine, 76,* 47–53.

Peck, R. C. (1968). Psychological developments in the second half of life. In B. L. Neugarten (Ed.), *Middle age and aging* (pp. 88–92). Chicago: University of Chicago Press.

Randall, T. (1993). Demographers ponder the aging of the aged and await unprecedented looming elder boom. *Journal of the American Medical Association, 269,* 2331–2333.

Rowe, J. W. (1985). Health care of the elderly. *New England Journal of Medicine, 312,* 827–835.

Rubenstein, L. Z. (1995). Comprehensive geriatric assessment. In W. B. Abrams, M. H. Beers & R. Berkow (Eds.), *The Merck manual of geriatrics* (2nd ed., pp. 224–235). Whitehouse Station, NJ: Merck & Co., Inc.

Rubenstein, L. Z., Calkins, D. R., Greenfield, S., et al. (1989). Health assessment for elderly patients: Report of the Society of General Internal Medicine Task Force on Health Assessment. *Journal of the American Geriatrics Society, 37,* 562–569.

Rubenstein, L. Z., Josephson, K. R, Wieland, G. D., et al. (1987). Geriatric assessment in a subacute hospital ward. *Clinics in Geriatric Medicine, 3,* 131–143.

Sattin, R. W. (1992). Falls among older persons: A public health perspective. *Annual Review of Public Health, 13,* 489–508.

Schwartz, J. B. (1994). Clinical pharmacology. In W. R. Hazzard, E. L. Bierman, J. P. Blass, et al. (Eds.), *Principles of geriatric medicine and gerontology* (3rd ed., pp. 259–276). New York: McGraw-Hill, Inc.

Selzer, M. L. (1971). The Michigan Alcoholism Screening Test: The quest for a new diagnostic instrument. *American Journal of Psychiatry, 127,* 1653–1658.

Siu, A. L., Reuben, D. B., & Moore, A. L. (1994). Comprehensive geriatric assessment. In W. R. Hazzard, E. L. Bierman, J. P. Blass, et al. (Eds.), *Principles of geriatric medicine and gerontology* (3rd ed., pp. 203–212). New York: McGraw-Hill, Inc.

Stamatiadis, N., & Deacon, J. A. (1995). Trends in highway safety: Effects of an aging population on accident propensity. *Accident Analysis and Prevention, 27,* 443–459.

Starer, P. J., & Libow, L. S. (1995). History and physical examination. In W. B. Abrams, M. H. Beers & R. Berkow (Eds.), *The Merck manual of geriatrics* (2nd ed., pp. 205–224). Whitehouse Station, NJ: Merck & Co., Inc.

Stoll, R. I. (1979). Guidelines for spiritual assessment. *American Journal of Nursing, 79,* 1574–1577.

Strahan G. W. (1994). An overview of home health and hospice care patients: Preliminary data from the 1993 National Home and Hospice Care Survey. *Advance data from vital and health statistics, No. 256.* Hyattsville, MD: National Center for Health Statistics.

U.S. Department of Health and Human Services (1996). *Physical activity and health: A report of the Surgeon General.* Atlanta, GA: U.S. Department of Health and Human Services, Centers for Disease Control and Prevention, National Center for Chronic Disease and Health Promotion.

U.S. Preventive Services Task Force (1996). *Guide to clinical preventive services* (2nd ed.). Baltimore: Williams & Wilkins.

Verdery, R. B. (1994). Failure to thrive. In W. R. Hazzard, E. L. Bierman, J. P. Blass, et al. (Eds.), *Principles of geriatric medicine and gerontology* (3rd ed, pp. 1205–1211). New York: McGraw-Hill, Inc.

Willenbring, M. L., Christensen, K. J., Spring, W. D., & Rasmussen, R. (1987). Alcoholism screening in the elderly. *Journal of the American Geriatrics Society, 35,* 864–869.

Williams, M. E. (1994). Clinical management of the elderly patient. In W. R. Hazzard, E. L. Bierman, J. P. Blass, et al. (Eds.), *Principles of geriatric medicine and gerontology* (3rd ed., pp. 195–202). New York: McGraw-Hill, Inc.

Windom, R. E. (1988). An aging nation presents new challenges to the health care system. *Public Health Reports*, 103(1), 1–2.

Zarit, S. H., Todd, P. A., & Zarit, J. M. (1986). Subjective burden of husbands and wives as caregivers: A longitudinal study. *Gerontologist*, 26, 260–266.

Home Safety Checklist

	YES	NO

HOUSEKEEPING

1. Do you clean up spills as soon as they occur?

2. Do you keep floors and stairways clean and free of clutter?

3. Do you put away books, magazines, sewing supplies, and other objects as soon as you're through with them and never leave them on floors or stairways?

4. Do you store frequently used items on shelves that are within easy reach?

FLOORS

5. Do you keep everyone from walking on freshly waxed floors before they're dry?

6. If you wax floors, do you apply two thin coats and buff each thoroughly or else use self-polishing, nonskid wax?

7. Do all small rugs have nonskid backing?

8. Have you eliminated small rugs at the tops and bottoms of stairways?

9. Are all carpet edges tacked down?

10. Are rugs and carpets free of curled edges, worn spots and rips?

11. Have you chosen rugs and carpets with short, dense pile?

12. Are rugs and carpets installed over good-quality, medium-thick pads?

BATHROOM

13. Do you use a rubber mat or nonslip decals in the tub or shower?

14. Do you have grab bars securely anchored over the tub or on the shower wall?

15. Do you have a nonskid rug on the bathroom floor?

16. Do you keep soap in an easy-to-reach receptacle?

TRAFFIC LANES

17. Can you walk across every room in your home, and from one room to another, without detouring around furniture?

18. Is the traffic lane from your bedroom to the bathroom free of obstacles? _____ _____

19. Are telephone and appliance cords kept away from areas where people walk? _____ _____

LIGHTING

20. Do you have light switches near every doorway? _____ _____

21. Do you have enough good lighting to eliminate shadowy areas? _____ _____

22. Do you have a lamp or light switch within easy reach from your bed? _____ _____

23. Do you have night lights in your bathroom and in the hallway leading from your bedroom to the bathroom? _____ _____

24. Are all stairways well lighted? _____ _____

25. Do you have light switches at both the tops and bottoms of stairways? _____ _____

STAIRWAYS

26. Do securely fastened handrails extend the full length of the stairs on each side of stairways? _____ _____

27. Do rails stand out from the walls so you can get a good grip? _____ _____

28. Are rails distinctly shaped so you're alerted when you reach the end of a stairway? _____ _____

29. Are all stairways in good condition, with no broken, sagging, or sloping edges? _____ _____

30. Are all stairway carpeting and metal edges securely fastened and in good condition? _____ _____

31. Have you replaced any single-level steps with gradually rising ramps or made sure such steps are well lighted? _____ _____

LADDERS AND STEP STOOLS

32. Do you have a sturdy step stool that you use to reach high cupboards and closet shelves? _____ _____

33. Are all ladders and step stools in good condition? _____ _____

34. Do you always use a step stool or ladder that is tall enough for the job? _____ _____

35. Do you always set up your ladder or step stool on a firm, level base that is free of clutter? _____ _____

36. Before you climb a ladder or step stool, do you always make sure it is fully open and that the stepladder spreads are locked? _____ _____

37. When you use a ladder or step stool, do you face the steps and keep your body between the side rails? _____ _____

38. Do you avoid standing on top of a step stool or climbing beyond the second step from the top on a stepladder? _____ _____

OUTDOOR AREAS

39. Are walks and driveways in your yard and other areas free of breaks? _____ _____

40. Are lawns and gardens free of holes? _____ _____

41. Do you put garden tools and hoses away when they're not in use? _____ _____

42. Are outdoor areas kept free of rocks, loose boards, and other tripping hazards? _____ _____

43. Do you keep outdoor walkways, steps, and porches free of wet leaves and snow? _____ _____

44. Do you sprinkle icy outdoor areas with deicers as soon as possible after a snowfall or freeze? _____ _____

45. Do you have mats at the doorway for people to wipe their feet on? _____ _____

46. Do you know the safest way of walking when you can't avoid walking on a slippery surface? _____ _____

FOOTWEAR

47. Do your shoes have soles and heels that provide good traction? _____ _____

48. Do you wear house slippers that fit well and don't fall off? _____ _____

49. Do you avoid walking in stocking feet? _____ _____

50. Do you wear low-heeled oxfords, loafers, or good-quality sneakers when you work in your house or yard? _____ _____

51. Do you replace boots or galoshes when their soles or heels are worn too smooth to keep you from slipping on wet or icy surfaces? _____ _____

PERSONAL PRECAUTIONS

52. Are you always alert for unexpected hazards, such as out-of-place furniture? _____ _____

53. If young grandchildren visit, are you alert for children playing on the floor and toys left in your path? _____ _____

54. If you have pets, are you alert for sudden movements across your path and pets getting underfoot? _____ _____

55. When you carry bulky packages, do you make sure they don't obstruct your vision? _____ _____

56. Do you divide large loads into smaller loads whenever possible? _____ _____

57. When you reach or bend, do you hold onto a firm support and avoid throwing your head back or turning it too far? _____ _____

58. Do you use a ladder or step stool to reach high places and never stand on a chair? _____ _____

59. Do you always move deliberately and avoid rushing to answer the phone or doorbell? _____ _____

60. Do you take time to get your balance when you change position from lying down to sitting and sitting to standing?   _____   _____

61. Do you hold onto grab bars when you change position in the tub or shower?   _____   _____

62. Do you keep yourself in good condition with moderate exercise, good diet, adequate rest, and regular medical checkups?   _____   _____

63. If you wear glasses, is your prescription up to date?   _____   _____

64. Do you know how to reduce injury in a fall?   _____   _____

65. If you live alone, do you have daily contact with a friend or neighbor?   _____   _____

This checklist is used to identify fall hazards in the home. After identification, hazards should be eliminated or reduced. One point is allowed for every *no* answer. A score of 1 to 7 is excellent, 8 to 14 is good, 15 or higher is hazardous. (Developed by the National Safety Council in cooperation with the National Retired Teachers Association and the American Association of Retired Persons. Reprinted with permission from the National Safety Council, 444 North Michigan Avenue, Chicago, IL 60611.)

Physical and Laboratory Assessment

Kathleen Ryan Fletcher

Subjective Assessment: Evaluation of the Symptoms of Disease and Illness
Symptom and Sign Differentiation
Complete and Episodic History
Dimensions of Symptomatology

Objective Assessment: Evaluation of the Signs of Disease and Illness

Systems Assessment*
Integumentary System
Respiratory System

Cardiovascular System
Neurological System
Musculoskeletal System
Gastrointestinal System
Genitourinary and Reproductive Systems
Hematological System
Endocrine System
Immune System

Summary

Physical assessment of the older adult is challenging in light of the multiple, complex, and often interrelated problems experienced by this rapidly growing age group. The elderly population today is vastly diverse and may include individuals nearly twice as old as others considered to be within the same cohort. The assessment of a healthy 55-year-old is quite different from the assessment of a frail 110-year-old. Even the most skilled and experienced advanced practice nurse may feel intimi-

dated in evaluating an older adult who has a chronic disease superimposed with an acute illness and who is taking multiple medications, is nutritionally compromised, and is severely limited in function. The assessment process becomes a forensic endeavor as one attempts to distinguish what is normal; what defies the expected process of health and disease; what is acute and what is chronic; what one might repair or alleviate; and what must be accepted or tolerated. When equipped with advanced physical assessment skills, nurses are better able to identify, assess, refer, treat, and teach self-management so that less illness is tolerated and more illness is alleviated.

*Includes physiological changes, assessment parameters, laboratory tests, and symptoms and signs. The sensory system is presented in Appendices 6–1 and 6–2 and discussed in Chapter 22.

SUBJECTIVE ASSESSMENT: EVALUATION OF THE SYMPTOMS OF DISEASE AND ILLNESS

The patient really knows the diagnosis, you just have to ask the right questions.

SIR WILLIAM OSLER

Symptom and Sign Differentiation

The two major goals in problem identification are to recognize the disease and to describe the impact that the disease has on the individual patient. The process of collecting data involves both subjective and objective assessment. *Symptoms* are defined as sensations or changes in body function that the patient regards as abnormal, and *signs* are abnormal findings on physical examination. Both are essential components of the database, and each builds on the other. The symptom of pruritus, for example, leads one to look for signs of rash. The respiratory finding of crackles generates questions about dyspnea and changes in respiratory function. Discrepancies between what is reported in the history and what is found on the physical examination should lead to further exploration about possible hidden problems such as falls and physical abuse.

The patient history guides the clinician in selecting an approach and method for conducting the physical examination. Varying levels of assessment can be used, including (1) a screening examination, often chosen when the purpose is early case finding (e.g., breast examination); (2) a comprehensive examination, selected when determining general health level or care requirements (e.g., Minimum Data Set for Long-Term Care); and (3) a problem-focused examination, conducted when the patient is experiencing a new sign or symptom of a disease or illness.

Complete and Episodic History

When evaluating a complaint, it is helpful to place this complaint in the context of the pa-tient's previous health and illness experiences. However, detailed patient health histories are available only under the best of circumstances (see Chapter 5). The chief complaint is typically the patient's main reason for requesting the visit. Unfortunately, in geriatric patients there is not usually a single complaint or symptom, but rather a constellation of symptoms that gives the clinician cues to the diagnosis. It may be helpful to ask the patient to bring a list of concerns to his or her appointment, preferably listed in order of importance.

Older adults, particularly those with several chronic diseases, may present with multiple complaints. Clustering the symptomatology around a known existing chronic illness may be revealing. Prioritizing the assessment and the treatment of symptoms is usually best accomplished by considering first what is life threatening or potentially life threatening, and then what is most bothersome to the patient. Another differential used to diagnose the patient with multiple symptoms is depression.

The complaints of older adults may be nonspecific, vague, and atypical. When the subjective data are less clear, a more methodical and detailed physical examination should be conducted. Emphasis on functional assessment may prove enlightening in this situation (see Chapter 9). Functional assessment may be best accomplished prior to the visit using a self-report checklist.

Attention to and accommodation of sensory and communication impairments are necessary during the evaluation process. The preparative ritual for physical assessment should include a minimization of environmental distractors and the use of aids to maximally compensate for deficits. For cognitively impaired people, a mental status evaluation performed early in the assessment process might facilitate recognition of the patient as an unreliable historian. Unfortunately, this does have a serious drawback, in that prematurity in mental status testing might threaten a trusting relationship and serve to restrict valuable information that the cognitively impaired patient might offer. Clinicians should avoid the trap of low expectation by first eliciting details of the symptom from the patient and then supplementing the information with contributions from caregiver informants. If an impaired patient is unable to report an abnormal sensation such as pain, depression, or anxiety, it may be helpful to question the patient's caregiver about any behavioral or functional changes that he or she has noticed, even if the caregiver is unaware of their potential significance.

Dimensions of Symptomatology

Once the symptoms have been identified and prioritized, the episodic history is guided by the seven dimensions of symptomatology (Wasson et al., 1984). These dimensions (Table 6–1) may be applied to any symptom, with occasional emphasis on selected components. For example, if a patient reports abdominal pain as the chief symptom, the clinician should have the patient locate a specific quadrant or region and describe the depth of the experience (superficial is somatic; deep is more visceral) and trace the radiation with his or her finger. The pain experience can be quantified using a scale in various ways (see Chapter 28). A more modest scale of 0 to 4 (rather than 0–10) might be less overwhelming to the patient. Researchers have noted that older adults prefer verbally descriptive scales (Herr & Mobily, 1993).

Quality refers to a specific descriptor of the experience. Patients typically have the most difficulty expressing symptom quality and often use analogies (e.g., "my chest pain is like an elephant sitting on my chest" or "dizziness like whirling on a merry-go-round"). At times, an adjective list may facilitate the narrative (e.g., "is the pain sharp, dull, aching, boring,

burning, stabbing, or cramping?"). Because of the leading nature of this approach, it must be used judiciously and selectively.

Eliciting the chronological evolution of the symptom (i.e., when and how the symptom began and the circumstances at that time) might reveal physical as well as psychosocial contributions to the patient's present experience. There may have been considerable delay between the symptom's or sign's first appearance and the current presentation and finding. After determining the onset of a symptom, it may be useful to ask about its variability; most symptoms are not constant, and a pattern might be discerned in this way.

What makes the symptom worse and what makes it better? Aggravating and relieving factors for abdominal pain may include food intake or a lack of it; certain foods may be problematic, others therapeutic. The pain may be associated with or relieved by certain movements, in which case the clinician should consider the patient's environment (i.e., whether it occurs in certain circumstances, locations, or with certain individuals). It is rare for a patient to have a single symptom; most disease processes are identified by a constellation of symptoms. Recording the absence of associated symptoms and signs is as important as recording their presence. In the previous example of abdominal pain, the examiner should ask about nausea, vomiting, changes in bowel habits, fever, chills, flatus, and belching. Charting by exception is not advisable when taking a geriatric history, owing to the more common atypical presentations. Additional documentation of the absence of symptoms and signs should support the clinical decision made and the judgment used to make it.

The examiner should determine what the patient has tried so far and what has been effective by eliciting from the patient all attempts at alleviation, including self-management strategies (i.e., medication, home remedies, or other therapeutic measures). Gathering explicit details of all medication usage is critical, because these details may be a contributing factor to the presentation, if not the precipitant of it. The narrative of an episodic history should also include the patient's relevant past history and previous history of similar symp-

---

TABLE 6–1

Seven Dimensions of the Symptom

1. Location and depth
2. Quality or character
3. Quantity or severity
4. Timing or chronology (onset, duration, frequency, course)
5. Setting in which symptoms present
6. Aggravating or alleviating factors
7. Associated manifestations (including significant negatives)

tomatology, the evaluation and outcome, and any significant family history.

The greatest problem in communication is the illusion that it's been accomplished.

GEORGE BERNARD SHAW

After completing a geriatric symptom assessment, the clinician should summarize the narrative details for the patient. This process allows the patient to embellish, clarify, or refute the clinician's interpretation. A conclusion to the subjective data collection process might be accomplished by asking the patient if he or she would like to make any final points. This is the opportune time for the patient to reveal any hidden agenda; occasionally the chief complaint is not the real reason for the presentation, and after a relationship has been established the patient may be open about more pressing concerns.

OBJECTIVE ASSESSMENT: EVALUATION OF THE SIGNS OF DISEASE AND ILLNESS

Uncommon presentation of common conditions is more common than common presentation of uncommon conditions.

SLOAN, 1991

Because older adults frequently present with vague, nonspecific, and atypical symptoms, the physical examination and functional assessment are pivotal in identifying the problem. To place the physical findings in a proper context, the examiner must be familiar with the expected changes that accompany aging (Appendix 6–1). The appropriate extent and detail of a physical assessment are controversial. Primary care professionals have recognized the need to perform a focused physical examination rather than an exhaustive, time- and resource-consuming version of the complete examination that is taught in schools (Frank et al., 1992). The physical assessment of a symptomatic patient is guided by the symptom(s).

Appendix 6–2 presents an overview of the most common presentations of disease in older adults, including the most common signs and symptoms, contributing factors, and potential causes. Laboratory values in older adults can be found in Appendix 6–3.

For the asymptomatic patient, screening criteria specifically for patients older than 65 years of age are summarized in the *Guide to clinical preventive services* by the U.S. Preventive Services Task Force (1996) (see also Chapter 5). When deciding whether to abbreviate the physical assessment, the examiner should consider that the examination often accomplishes more than problem identification. Particularly for geriatric patients, the therapeutic value of the examiner's touch and the opportunity taken to teach the patient self-assessment and self-care (e.g., a breast or testicular examination) may have even greater value than the diagnosis of illness or disease.

When conducting a physical assessment, it is often necessary to modify the examination procedure or equipment for more functionally dependent patients. A specially equipped examination chair or table with hydraulic features can facilitate access to the patient and allow a greater degree of comfort.

SYSTEMS ASSESSMENT

Integumentary System

PHYSIOLOGICAL CHANGES

A multitude of factors influence the aging of the skin, including hereditary factors, nutrition, and exercise; however, the most damaging factor is usually the environmental influence of the sun (Lober & Fenske, 1990). More is being learned about the distinctions between intrinsic aging and actinic skin aging (Yaar & Gilchrest, 1990). An overview of the expected changes that occur with the aging process is presented in Appendix 6–1. Specific reference is given here to those changes that create the most risk for vulnerable patients. For example, the fact that the dermis and epidermis thin and subcutaneous fat is lost with age has great significance in evaluating a patient who is bedbound with his or her head elevated. The patient may continue to slide down (producing a shearing force) and may thus require pulling and sometimes dragging (producing a friction force) to achieve a more comfortable and acceptable position. In the older patient with trauma, just a few hours on a backboard in the emergency room may initiate ulcer formation for the individual at risk.

Atrophy of the sweat glands, if considered in a positive light, results in a decreased body odor and need for bathing. However, evaluation of the older adult with a history of heart failure who is maintained on diuretic therapy may reveal dehydration during the summer months, which may necessitate seasonal adjustment of the therapeutic regimen. The loss of skin vascularity and elasticity places functionally limited patients at a higher risk for skin tears and contributes to delayed healing once the skin is no longer intact. Postoperative older patients generally require a longer time for wound healing.

ASSESSMENT PARAMETERS

Subjective assessment of the skin should be guided by a review of the entire system. If positive symptomatology is present, the seven dimensions of the symptom should be reviewed. Although the chronological evolution of a symptom is often overlooked, it can provide invaluable information because lesion characteristics may change over time. A significant component of the patient history is the patient's medication profile. Drug-related skin eruptions generally occur within a short time (1–10 days) after the initiation of therapy and disappear within 14 days after the drug has been discontinued (Gilchrest, 1995). Highly medicated older adults are less likely to present with a drug-induced adverse reaction than are their younger counterparts (Williams, 1993). Significant information also includes the patient's history of atopy or allergy, environmental history of exposure (including solar), and work history. With the presence of any skin complaint, a general review of systems should be completed, owing to the plethora of systemic causes in geriatric patients that reveal themselves through the integumentary system.

The general physical examination should incorporate a skin assessment with the evaluation of each more specific system. The entire body surface of a patient with a skin complaint or an identifiable lesion should be examined, including the hair, nails, and mucous membranes; the assessment is incomplete unless the more hidden skinfold areas are also inspected. Lesions are characterized according to type (primary, secondary, or vascular); distribution (flexor, extensor, dermatomal, or intertriginous); and configuration or shape. Palpation of the skin should include a determination of the temperature, texture, mobility, thickness, and turgor. In geriatric patients, the non–sun-exposed surfaces of the abdomen or inner thigh are the best areas to check skin turgor and resiliency.

LABORATORY TESTS

Skin evaluation is enhanced through simple magnification and good lighting. In a pruritic patient, for example, the burrows of a mite could be conclusive for pediculosis. Vascular lesions can be blanched using microscopic slide compression. Direct microscopy of skin scrapings under a Wood's light with potassium hydroxide can identify the hyphae characteristic of a fungal lesion. Culturing draining lesions for common bacteria is nearly always advantageous and is inexpensive. The differentiation of pathological and nonpathological lesions is being performed more often in office settings through punch biopsy.

Skin testing may be a method for detecting a person's hypersensitivity to toxic products, determining the susceptibility or resistance to infection, checking for past or present exposure to an infectious agent (tuberculosis skin testing), or evaluating impaired cellular immunity.

COMMON SYMPTOMS AND SIGNS

Nearly half of all older adults suffer from a skin disorder that causes them to seek treatment. Pruritus is the most common skin complaint, the cause of which is typically dry skin (xerosis). Overlooking a systemic process causing this symptom, such as iron deficiency anemia or hypoglycemia, is ill afforded in older adults because they often present atypically.

Skin lesions may be characterized as benign, premalignant, malignant, inflammatory, or infectious (Table 6–2); all types of lesions are

TABLE 6-2

Common Skin Lesions in the Elderly

Classification	Lesion	Description
Benign	Acrochodon (skin tag)	Small flesh-colored pediunculated papules, usually on neck or trunk
	Lentigines (liver spot)	Hyperpigmented patches on sun-exposed surfaces
	Seborrheic keratosis	Waxy, verrucous, often appearing stuck on papules or patches
	Cherry angiomas	Very small red papules usually on trunk; blanch with pressure
	Senile purpura	Ecchymotic areas that appear after minor injury, usually to hand and forearm, and may last several weeks
	Telangiectasis	Dilated and tortuous superficial capillaries on the face
	Venous lakes	Purplish macules or plaques, especially on lower lips and ears
Premalignant	Actinic keratosis	Erythematous scaly areas of cellular dysplasia
	Leukoplakia	White areas of cellular dysplasia, seen often in oral or vaginal membranes
Malignant	Squamous cell	Erythematous, often indurated; may be scaly or hyperkeratotic ulcerated areas arising in sun-exposed or chronically inflamed areas
	Basal cell	Pearly papular or plaquelike lesion that may be ulcerated; generally found on head and neck
	Malignant melanoma	Pigmented macular or nodular lesions with irregular borders; predominating on sun-exposed surfaces
Infectious	Fungal	*Feet:* scaly, maceration, in interdigital spaces *Nails:* grossly thickened *Groin or vaginal areas:* maceration, scaly, erythematous, may be edematous; vaginal discharge may be present
	Bacterial (*Staphylococcus* and *Streptococcus* common)	Vesicles or pustules, sometimes bullous lesions; swelling & erythema may be present; constitutional symptoms might include fever, malaise, lymphadenopathy
	Herpes zoster (shingles)	Acute eruption of vesicular lesions in dermatological distribution; prodromal symptoms may include pain, paresthesias in defined area
	Parasites	*Scabies:* excoriated burrow (linear ridge with vesicle at one end); found in interdigital webs, flexor areas of wrist, umbilicus, nipple or genital areas *Lice:* eczematous areas in scalp or pubic areas; small grey white nits
Inflammatory	Seborrheic dermatitis	Scaly and erythematous eruptions (often appearing greasy) affecting central face and hair areas
	Contact dermatitis	Inflamed erythematous areas; scaly or vesicular lesions appearing at a source of contact
	Stasis dermatitis	Erythematous inflammatory areas of the dependent lower extremities, generally coexisting with edema
	Psoriasis	Erythematous plaques often with a silvery scale appearance usually on the extensor surfaces, scalp, and buttocks; nails may be pitted, discolored, and thickened

Data from Gilchrest (1995); and Lober & Fenske (1990).

more commonly experienced by older adults than by younger people. Although the majority of skin lesions are benign, the type of skin lesion may need to be differentiated more conclusively, thus requiring a biopsy. Even benign lesions (e.g., skin tags, seborrheic keratosis) may warrant removal for cosmetic reasons or because they are an irritant. The removal and biopsy of lesions is performed by practitioners who have received the necessary education.

Premalignant types of lesions include actinic keratosis, which may evolve into a squamous cell lesion and should therefore be treated. Fortunately, there is a long latency period with this type of lesion, which increases the likelihood of identification. Distinguishing among the various malignant types (i.e., basal and squamous cell, malignant melanoma) is achieved only through biopsy. The people at highest risk for malignant skin disease are fair-skinned individuals with a low melanin level. The course of treatment should be determined according to histological confirmation, the size and depth of invasion of the lesion, and the patient's history. The general location of malignant skin lesions is on sun-exposed skin; however, even malignant melanoma lesions may appear on non–sun-exposed surfaces. The prognosis for this type of lesion is determined by the depth of the lesion rather than the type.

Skin infections are most commonly caused by a chronic fungal process or *Staphylococcus* or *Streptococcus* bacteria. The incidence of herpes zoster peaks in people 50 to 70 years of age, and the incidence of herpetic neuralgia is almost 40% in people older than 60 years of age (Gilchrest, 1995). Patients may present with a burning type of prodromal symptom prior to the appearance of the vesicular lesions; if a viral process is not considered at this time, the clinician may miss the window period of effective treatment with acyclovir (Zovirax). Parasitic infections are frequently transmitted by skin-to-skin contact, and the presentation is usually intense pruritus with excoriations.

The superficial inflammation of dermatitis is often due to irritant exposure, allergic sensitization, or idiopathic factors. The most characteristic symptoms of dermatitis are pruritus, erythema, edema, vesiculization, and oozing or crusting of the skin. In very chronic cases, the skin becomes thickened or lichenified with linear excoriations frequently seen from repeated scratching.

Drug-related skin eruptions most often present as maculopapular-type lesions. Although over-the-counter drugs might cause a skin reaction, the medications most frequently implicated include the penicillins, sulfonamides, gold, phenylbutazone, and gentamycin (Gilchrest, 1995).

Skin ulcers and tears are most often seen in the very debilitated elderly. Pressure ulcers are discussed in Chapter 13.

Respiratory System

PHYSIOLOGICAL CHANGES

Age-related physiological changes in the respiratory system (see Appendix 6–1) have little functional impact on resting ventilation. The aging process appears to cause metabolic demand and pulmonary reserve to decline in parallel, a change that is notable when effort is expended at higher altitudes or in the heat (Johnson et al., 1994). The reduced elasticity and recoil of the lung tissue can result in a diminished maximal breathing capacity and an early collapse of poorly supported peripheral airways. Calcification of the thoracic wall and a visible barrel-chested appearance may have some impact on the chest wall compliance in patients who are supine. The thickened chest wall may be most significant to the examiner, who finds the lung sounds more distant and therefore less discernable. Cilial atrophy has a negative impact on older adults' abilities to handle secretions during a debilitated or dehydrated state. The people at highest risk are smokers, because nicotine further compromises ciliary movement (Lareau, 1993).

ASSESSMENT PARAMETERS

When collecting the subjective details of respiratory assessment, the clinician should remember that older adults may not present with respiratory symptomatology until late in the course of disease. The dyspnea of left-sided heart failure, for example, may not be evident in a patient who only minimally exerts himself or herself. Dyspnea is subjective, and the patient's experience may provide little objective evidence. The onset of a respiratory symptom can often guide clinicians in making a differential diagnosis. In patients with pulmonary embolus, the onset is quite rapid, whereas the dyspnea of most forms of obstructive disease is insidious. The dyspnea of congestive heart failure tends to be in an interim range. Significant past medical history information includes smoking, heart disease, cardiac risk factors, and environmental and work exposures.

The physical examination of the lung includes all the parameters of inspection, palpation, percussion, and auscultation. Assessment must be conducted with an exposed chest wall to include inspection for the barrel chest; the use of accessory muscles; and the rate, rhythm, and pattern of respiration. Palpation for tenderness in patients with a respiratory complaint may give evidence of musculoskeletal injury. Percussion is used to assess for the dullness of a possible lesion, in which resonance percussed over an inflated lung is the expected finding. Auscultation for adventitious sounds is accomplished by checking for crackles (fluid signs) and wheezes (constricted airway sign) and the less frequent rubs of an inflamed pleura (Fig. 6–1). A pediatric diaphragm may be helpful in older adults with predominant ribs, allowing a more firm application of the stethoscope between the interspaces. A func-

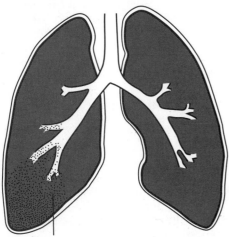

Consolidation
(crackles)

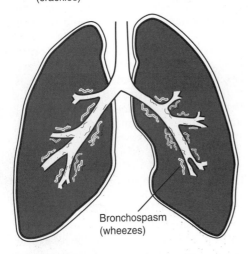

Bronchospasm
(wheezes)

FIGURE 6–1. Abnormal lung sounds. (From Jarvis, C. [1996]. *Physical examination and health assessment* [2nd ed., pp. 505–507]. Philadelphia: W. B. Saunders.)

TABLE 6-3
Breathlessness Scale

Grade	Degree	Characteristics
0	None	Not troubled with breathlessness except with strenuous exercise
1	Slight	Troubled by shortness of breath when hurrying on the level or walking up a slight hill
2	Moderate	Walks slower than people of the same age on the level because of breathlessness or has to stop for breath when walking at own pace on the level
3	Severe	Stops for breath after walking about 100 yards or after a few minutes on the level
4	Very severe	Too breathless to leave the house; breathless when dressing or undressing

Data from Ferris (1978).

tional assessment (e.g., the Breathlessness Scale) may be helpful in evaluating the effect of exertion on ventilatory effort (Table 6–3).

LABORATORY TESTS

Chest x-rays are more frequently ordered in the elderly than in other populations, owing to the high incidence of pulmonary infections, which are the fourth leading cause of death in older adults (Neiderman, 1991). In the elderly, the recognizable signs of an infectious process (e.g., elevation in white blood count, fever, and tachycardia) occur with declining frequency. Findings from the chest x-ray are reviewed in light of the clinical picture; for example, the patient may have normal findings with significant pulmonary compromise. Interstitial changes are often age related.

Pulmonary function studies are not indicated in a routine screening. The clinician may use spirometry to get a general sense of the patient's breathing capacity or may use pulse oximetry to determine oxygenation status. Pulmonary function studies done on healthy older individuals have demonstrated an increase in the residual volume (RV) and a decline in the total lung capacity (TLC) (Tockman, 1995). The actual declines in forced vital capacity (FVC) and maximum expiratory flow rates are attributed more to changes in body weight and strength rather than to changes in the pulmonary tissue. Arterial blood gas also reflects a functional decline in lung tissue with age, as the arterial $PaCO_2$ rises and the PaO_2 falls. Lower diffusion capacity results from a thickening of the alveolar-capillary membrane and a reduced ability of gas to combine with elements in the blood (Tockman, 1995). Gradual decline in the PaO_2 is attributed to a loss of elastic recoil and a subsequent reduction in airway caliber, early airway closure, and a maldistribution of ventilation. This is further affected by a significant (50%) drop in the ventilatory response to hypoxia and a more modest (40%) drop related to hypercapnia (Tockman, 1995). Maximal O_2 consumption with exercise has been shown to decline with age. However, with regular endurance training, even previously sedentary older adults are able to breathe the same percentage of maximal voluntary ventilation as athletes (Johnson et al., 1994).

Expectorated specimens are often unreliable because of pharyngeal colonization; however, if a gram stain of the specimen can be made, it may provide information to guide the therapeutic decision (McClure, 1992).

COMMON SYMPTOMS AND SIGNS

The most common pulmonary complaint in older adults is dyspnea. With aging, breathing becomes more of a conscious effort, particularly in deconditioned patients who exert themselves. The cause of dyspnea may be cardiac, pulmonary, metabolic, mechanical, or hematological, and the presence of this symptom therefore requires an assessment of these various systems. Anemia is underdiagnosed, whereas congestive heart failure is overdiagnosed.

Crackles are the most common physical finding, with contributing factors including atelectasis and age-related fibrotic changes in the lungs. The crackle is always an abnormal finding because the areas filled with fluid are not adequately exchanging air and are a potential source of infection. The wheeze is characteristic of airflow obstruction, which may indicate airway disease but may also be a side effect of a beta-blocker. A chronic cough may be a side effect of an angiotensin-converting enzyme inhibitor.

Cardiovascular System

PHYSIOLOGICAL CHANGES

It is difficult to determine what constitutes expected cardiac function in a group with such a high prevalence of disease. Approximately half of all people older than 60 years may have severe narrowing of the coronary artery, which increases myocardial demand; yet only 50% of these individuals exhibit clinical signs and symptoms of this process (Lakatta, 1995). The size of the heart remains unchanged over the years, with only a slight hypertrophy of the left ventricle that is not statistically significant. Muscle fibers that line the endocardium atrophy, and increased deposits of collagenous and fibrous tissue form in the lining of the heart chambers. Peripherally, the vessels become atherosclerotic and arteriosclerotic. This in part accounts for the increase in systolic blood pressure seen with aging. As the left ventricle becomes less compliant, the rate of ventricular relaxation decreases, subsequently causing more emphasis on atrial contraction so a fourth heart sound is commonly heard.

Over time, fat deposits form along the sinoatrial node and the number of pacemaker cells decreases. These changes may cause an irregular pulse and predispose the heart to arteriovenous block and arrhythmias. Baroreceptors become less sensitive with age, and the effectiveness of compensatory mechanisms to hypertensive and hypotensive stimuli is therefore decreased. Because of the blunted baroreceptor response, the Valsalva maneuver may cause a sudden uncompensated drop in blood pressure, and with postural hypotension the patient is more likely to fall.

At rest, these changes have little functional impact, but with exercise or postural stress the aging heart is less able to increase and sustain an increase in cardiac output. Compensatory cardiac dilatation and increased stroke volume in part compensate for a diminished heart rate during exercise (Gawlinski & Jensen, 1991). More recent studies have shown that lifestyle and peripheral vascular disease have a greater impact on cardiac exercise tolerance than does age alone (Lakatta, 1995).

ASSESSMENT PARAMETERS

The techniques of cardiac assessment are the same for both young and old adults; however, auscultation is more of a challenge with barrel-chested patients. Inspection may not reveal the pulsating point of maximal impulse of a left ventricle because it is obscured by a thickened chest wall. Jugular venous distension should be assessed in people with cardiac disease. Peripheral vascular inspection should note the presence of vascular markings, edema, or loss of hair in distal extremities.

The valvular areas should be palpated to determine the presence of a palpable murmur (the *thrill*). The palpable point of maximal impulse may be displaced to the left anterior or mid-axillary line in patients with left ventricular hypertrophy. The pulses should be checked throughout for rate, rhythm, volume, and symmetry. A portable Doppler may facilitate recognition of an otherwise imperceptible pulsation. Asymmetrical findings may indicate an occlusion of a vessel branch. If edema is present, it should be palpated, as the fingertips are more sensitive than the eyes. The presence of a pitting or nonpitting edema should be recorded. Circumferential measurements should be made using a tape measure, which is preferred over the less objective rating scale of +1 through +4. For repeated measurements, a skin marking pencil can ensure reliability. Capillary refill should be checked, although hyperkeratotic toenails make this procedure less reliable in the lower extremities of certain older adults. Clubbing should be noted, and a review of possible causes should be considered.

Auscultation should be performed with a diaphragm, using a bell at the valvular areas to detect murmurs and at the carotids to detect bruits. Asymptomatic carotid bruit is a major risk factor for stroke and should be a part of the routine cardiac examination. All detectable carotid bruits should be further evaluated, as studies have shown that the vessel is occluded over 50% by the time turbulence is audible. Although the fourth heart sound is common because of the changes of normal aging, a third heart sound warrants a search for other signs of congestive heart failure. Prolonged extra heart sounds (murmurs) are quite common, particularly systolic murmurs. Systolic ejection murmurs occur in as many as 55% of adults older than 70 years and frequently indicate aortic valve disease (Fleg, 1995). Diastolic murmurs are less frequent and are always pathological.

Blood pressure should be measured in both arms to check for stenosis and should be checked positionally because of the prevalence of orthostatic hypotension. Two positions are usually adequate, and the clinician should wait at least 2 minutes after changing a position to recheck the pressure, thereby permitting the baroreceptors to compensate. A drop of 20 mm Hg in the systolic is significant; however, in symptomatic patients a drop of 10 mm Hg should be pursued. The lack of a compensatory pulse elevation with position change suggests autonomic insufficiency, sinus node dysfunction, or drug effect (Fleg, 1995).

LABORATORY TESTS

The electrocardiogram (ECG) of a normal aging person may show a decrease in precordial QRS voltage and ST segment and T-wave changes (Kane et al., 1994). The most common ECG abnormality is nonspecific changes in ST segments and/or T waves due to medications such as digoxin, diuretics, antiarrythmias, and psychotropics (Fleg, 1995). The prognostic evidence of ectopic beats on ECG is less clear, although dysrhythmias rise in incidence with age (Wajngarten et al., 1990). Ventricular and supraventricular ectopic beats are extremely common, particularly in men (Manolio et al., 1994). Premature ventricular contractions (PVCs) and atrial fibrillation may occur in asymptomatic older adults. Sick sinus syndrome is also fairly common. The recognition and treatment of dysrhythmias is important in preventing syncopal events.

As measured by the VO_2 max, the overall

decline in cardiovascular function with age is 13% per decade; however, it is less than half that (5%) for adults who exercise regularly (Kasch et al., 1993).

The chest x-ray may reveal calcification around the area of the aortic knobs without pathology; however, any intracardiac findings are pathological. Echocardiography may further detect thickened valve leaflets or a calcified mitral annulus. This testing may be inadequate in patients with chest wall abnormalities or pulmonary inflation.

Total cholesterol values are increased in patients 60 to 90 years of age, with increases greater in women than in men. In the very old, however, cholesterol values decrease (Tietz et al., 1992) but still remain higher than those of young adults. Low-density lipoprotein (LDL) cholesterol levels have similar changes, whereas high-density lipoprotein (HDL) levels remain constant in later years (Stulnig et al., 1993). Triglyceride levels are increased in older adults 60 to 90 years of age but then decrease in very old adults (Tietz et al., 1992).

COMMON SYMPTOMS AND SIGNS

Chest pain is an early sign of aortic valvular disease, and in patients with occlusive coronary artery disease it reflects increased myocardial demand. Chest pain is not always present, even in patients with severe myocardial ischemia, and myocardial infarctions often present silently in older adults.

Syncope (the sudden loss of consciousness) or *presyncope* (a transient alteration in consciousness) results from diminished cerebral metabolism. When cardiac pathology is the cause, it often results from a rhythm disturbance, valvular disease, or hypertrophic cardiomyopathy (Gawlinski & Jensen, 1991). The most common form is the simple faint (*vasodepressor syncope*), with the principal mechanism being peripheral arterial vasodilation. Hypertension is present in over 50% of people older than 65 years of age, with many cases involving isolated systolic hypertension (>160 mm Hg). Because the risk of a cardiovascular event rises as blood pressure rises, more consideration is now being given to better blood pressure control. Clinicians are advised to take the elevated pressure on several occasions, taking two measurements each time (Roben, 1993).

Claudication is pain, tightness, or weakness in an exercising muscle that is promptly relieved by rest. Indicated by diminished pedal pulses, it is the cardinal and only specific symptom of peripheral arterial disease. Ankle systolic pressures 50 mm Hg or less or toe pressures 30 mm Hg or less are diagnostic (Thompson et al., 1993). The major correlates for symptomatic arterial disease are current smoking and elevation in systolic blood pressure (Vogt et al., 1993).

Edema is a commonly recognized sign of right-sided heart failure; however, it is less specific to this cause in the older population. Other known causes include protein calorie malnutrition, peripheral vascular disease, venous varicosities, and lymphatic obstruction (Ciocon et al., 1993).

Neurological System

PHYSIOLOGICAL CHANGES

Aging is manifest in the nervous system by a decrease in the number of neurons and an increase in the size and number of neuroglial cells (Boss, 1991). Because there are few significant neurological changes with aging, most neurological decline is evidence of a disease process. The most common disorders involve degenerative and cerebrovascular processes. Aging can cause a decline in nerves and nerve fibers and a slower conduction of fibers across the synapses. Neurofibrillary plaques and tangles that are characteristic of Alzheimer's disease are also seen with normal aging, leading to the speculation that the *location* of these plaques (rather than their presence) is more predictive of cognitive loss. Atrophy of the brain occurs with aging, with maximal loss occurring in the frontal and temporal associative cortex (Morris & McManus, 1991). There is a modest decline in short-term memory, with benign loss restricted to more trivial events. Psychomotor movements such as gait are slower. Gait pattern is often wide based, shorter stepped, and flexed forward.

ASSESSMENT PARAMETERS

Changes in mental status may be overlooked unless a mental status evaluation (Table 6–4) is specifically conducted. This evaluation might be included with the history-taking process. Cognitive function can be assessed using a variety of mental status instruments (see Chapter 7). The Folstein Mini-Mental State Examination is one of the most widely used screening tools; a score of 23 or below out of 30 is considered abnormal (Folstein et al., 1975); however, the total score is of less use to the clinician than is the identification of specific areas of deficit. Successful use of such an instrument is contingent on a certain level of education, literacy ability, and communication competency. Other parameters in mental status testing include tests of memory and judgment. Both of these require an ability to validate the patient's report and an appreciation of cultural and ethnic differences. A brief screening instrument for depression should be considered (see Chapter 17).

Cranial nerve testing has limited clinical utility in a screening evaluation but is useful in evaluating specific neurological deficits. An evaluation of the facial nerve is indicated, for example, when there appears to be some asymmetry of facial movements. When asymmetry is present, the possibility of a stroke (due to an upper-motor or supranuclear lesion) or Bell's palsy (the facial paresis of lower motor neuron origin) must be considered. The only specific age-related changes in cranial nerve function are pupils reacting more slowly and a progressive limitation of upward gaze in some patients (Morris & McManus, 1991).

Sensory testing is crucial in older adults. Screening should include the most distal upper and lower extremities and a comparative evaluation of both sides of the body. Checking sensations of both light touch and pain is important, because these sensations are transmitted by different nerve endings. Cutaneous sensory dysfunction may also be demonstrated by a diminished vibratory sense in the distal lower extremities, which can be assessed by placing the vibrating tuning fork over a bony prominence and testing for residual vibration after the patient reports the vibration has ceased. This somesthetic change is present in approximately one third of the elderly (Morris & McManus, 1991). For patients at risk for neuropathy (i.e., with diabetes, alcoholism, or pernicious anemia), this screening for vibratory sense may detect a decline before it is detected by other forms of sensory testing.

Cerebellar function can be tested using the Romberg test, checking for nystagmus, and evaluating finger-to-nose and heel-to-shin movements. Deficiencies should be followed as they would be in younger patients, while recognizing that the ability to balance and approximate might be influenced by musculoskeletal changes. A gait evaluation is essential for most aged individuals. A variation on the Get Up & Go test (Mathias et al., 1986) is a quick way to assess gait. The patient is asked to get up from a chair quickly without using the arms of the chair, if possible. Once stabilized, the patient is asked to walk 10 feet, turn, and then return to the chair. The examiner notes gait fluidity and balance during the stance and swing phases of the gait. If a patient requires arm support to rise from the chair or has to shift weight, this may indicate some lower muscle weakness (Fleming et al., 1991). A shuffling gait (the inability to elevate the feet during walking) and turning abnormalities (marked reduction in the speed of walking during the turn) are also important observations (Odenheimer et al., 1994). Elderly individuals tend to abduct their upper limbs more abruptly when rapidly changing direction (Lassau-Wray & Parker, 1993). Gait abnormali-

---

TABLE 6-4

Elements of the Mental Status Evaluation

State of consciousness
General appearance and behavior
Orientation
Memory (immediate, recent, remote)
Language
Perception
Insight
Judgment
Thought process
Mood and affect

ties common to aged individuals are presented in Figure 6–2.

Deep tendon reflex evaluation is a useful part of the screening examination, using a scale of 0 to 4 (0 = no response, 1 = sluggish or diminished, 2 = active or expected, 3 = more brisk than expected, 4 = brisk or hyperactive). As in younger adults, hyperactive and hypoactive responses are significant. All stretch reflex responses (except perhaps the Achilles result) are expected to fall in the +2 range. With normal aging, the distal Achilles reflex may be diminished (Morris & McManus, 1991). Reflexes are also considered abnormal if they are not bilaterally symmetrical, indicated by two or more reflexes in a limb consistently decreased or increased compared with those of the opposite limb (Odenheimer et al., 1994). This assessment is complicated by a fear of failure on the part of the client; thus, it may be helpful to use distractors to achieve greater validity of response (e.g., having the patient interlock the fingers of both hands and pull so that the upper limbs are isometrically contracted while the lower limbs are being tested).

LABORATORY TESTS

In older adults, electroencephalogram results typically show reduced slow-wave amplitude and more interrupted rapid eye movement episodes during sleep (Morris & McManus, 1991). Depressed elderly patients have shown significantly higher than normal absolute alpha amplitude and lower than normal beta values (Roemer et al., 1992), whereas patients with Alzheimer's disease exhibit highly significant increases in delta and theta activity as well as lower beta values (Elmstahl et al., 1994).

Cerebral white matter lesions are a common finding from magnetic resonance imaging in elderly people with cerebrovascular risk factors (Breteler et al., 1994). Cross-sectional magnetic resonance imaging and computed tomography

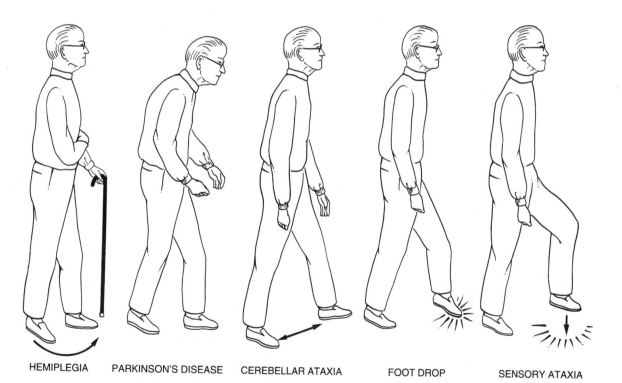

HEMIPLEGIA   PARKINSON'S DISEASE   CEREBELLAR ATAXIA   FOOT DROP   SENSORY ATAXIA

FIGURE 6–2. Common types of gait abnormalities. (From Swartz, M. H. [1997]. *Textbook of physical diagnosis* [3rd ed., p. 543]. Philadelphia: W. B. Saunders.)

studies have shown that ventricular dilatation, brain atrophy, and an increased variability of brain size are all associated with normal aging (Morris & McManus, 1991). Among elderly patients with acute neurological defect, computed tomography is most useful in those patients presenting with signs of atypical stroke and unexplained confusion (Brown et al., 1993).

COMMON SYMPTOMS AND SIGNS

Neurological disorders such as a stroke, Alzheimer's disease, and Parkinson's disease are the most common causes of disability in the elderly, accounting for almost half of recognized functional incapacity (Morris & McManus, 1991).

Dizziness is a complex symptom involving integration of the visual, proprioceptive, somatosensory, and vestibular pathways. Evaluation of this complaint requires a complete examination, as it may be caused or exacerbated by a broad spectrum of disorders of the eye, ear, cardiac, musculoskeletal, and neurological systems. In older adults, dizziness and disequilibrium may represent *presbystasis*, a general problem involving many systems rather than a local lesion in any one area (Baloh, 1992). It is important to address the symptom because these individuals experience a higher rate of falls.

Tremors are not a normal finding and should be evaluated if present. The essential or familial tremor is considered to be genetically predetermined and may be responsive to treatment with propranolol or primidone (Koller et al., 1994). Other potential causes include Parkinson's disease, choreiformic movements, and dyskinesia. To facilitate the clinical assessment, a clinical rating scale has been proposed that measures the severity of the postural and resting tremor (Bain et al., 1993).

Assessment for mental status changes and memory decline is indicated in this age group. Chapter 7 discusses the evaluation of cognitive status in greater detail.

Musculoskeletal System

PHYSIOLOGICAL CHANGES

The muscles, joints, and bones undergo significant changes with aging, and the decline is often first noticed in the middle years. There is a loss of muscle mass secondary to a reduction in muscle cells, connective tissue, and muscle tissue fluid as well as a 12 to 15% loss in muscle strength between the ages of 30 and 70 years (Blocker, 1992). Arthritis is one of the most prevalent chronic diseases in the older adult population (see Chapter 20), and the majority of individuals experience some osteoarthritic pain by the age of 60 years (Matteson, 1997). Women begin to lose cortical bone density at a rate of 10 to 20% per decade postmenopausally, and men experience bone loss of 3 to 5% per decade (Zorowitz et al., 1990). Physical signs of bone loss include kyphosis, reduced lumbar lordosis, and decreased body height. The patient at highest risk for osteoporosis is the thin postmenopausal female with reduced calcium and vitamin D intake. Other patients at high risk for bone loss include those with alcoholism or metastatic disease or who are taking steroid replacements.

Muscle response time is 10% slower in older adults than in their younger counterparts. This change has been attributed to a slowing of the central processes involving stimulus identification and registration rather than to decreases in neurotransmitter supply and reduced nerve conduction velocity (Lassau-Wray & Parker, 1993). The rehabilitative time for older adults is considerably longer, owing in part to these changes.

Older adults at highest risk for musculoskeletal decline are immobile patients. Tendons begin to shrink and muscle weakens within a day of immobility, with actual decline in the range of motion apparent within 48 hours. A daily loss of 1.3 to 3.0% of muscle strength results in a significant loss within a very short period (Hoenig & Rubenstein, 1991). Additional information on immobility is described in Chapter 12.

ASSESSMENT PARAMETERS

Although the most valuable screening assessment of the musculoskeletal system is conducted during the functional assessment, a working familiarity with the bones, joints, and muscles and the normal range of motion for each joint is required while conducting the episodic examination. A regional approach to the assessment is limited, as it is difficult to isolate the movements of a specific joint or muscle. The body moves in an integrated fashion, with loss in one area generally compensated for by another. The muscles should be inspected for signs of atrophy, and the bones for any deformities. Asymmetrical findings are the most significant. Muscle tone is measured by passive movement. Increased tone is present when there is marked sustained resistance, rigidity, or spasms; and decreased tone is present when there is no or minimal resistance to passive motion.

Palpation is used to check for any tenderness, bony enlargement, soft tissue swelling, or crepitation. The joints should all be evaluated for range of motion using a *goniometer*, a simple protractor with movable arms. After evaluating the fullness of the range of joint movement, each muscle group should be evaluated for strength using a scale of 0 to 5 (0 = no movement; 1 = barely detectable flicker; 2 = active movement without gravity; 3 = active movement against gravity; 4 = active movement against some resistance; and 5 = active movement against full resistance without fatigue [normal strength]).

LABORATORY TESTS

Bone loss, as measured by a roentgenogram, is not observed until nearly 30% loss has occurred. Earlier loss can be detected with more sophisticated and expensive bone densitometry techniques, which measure the decrease in bone mineral density that occurs with osteoporosis and osteomalacia. Several prospective studies now support the measurement of bone mineral density at several skeletal sites to permit stratification of fracture risk (Mitlak & Nussbaum, 1993).

There is no definitive testing for musculoskeletal disease. The *rheumatoid factor* is a macroglobulin type of antibody that is found in many individuals with rheumatoid arthritis. It is not limited to blood from patients with rheumatoid arthritis but may sometimes be found in the serum of patients with other inflammatory or infectious diseases. The level of rheumatoid factor in an individual rises with age,

and the specificity of testing in a geriatric population is lower than in a younger population (Wernick, 1989). Antinuclear antibody (ANA) testing used to evaluate patients with systemic lupus erythematosus is highly sensitive but has low specificity; positive results of this test have been seen in healthy elderly patients (Duthie & Abbas, 1991).

The erythrocyte sedimentation rate has been shown to change significantly with normal aging, with mild elevations (10–20 mm) assumed to be age related (Kane et al., 1994). Because the sedimentation rate represents complex changes in fibrinogens, globulins, and albumin and is also influenced by the hematocrit, it is not a very specific test. Despite these limitations, the sedimentation rate is helpful in identifying conditions such as malignancy, infection, and connective tissue disorders.

Serum albumin shows a steady decline with age throughout adult life. The reasons for this change are not fully understood. Possible causes include a decrease in liver size, blood flow, enzyme production, and protein intake.

Increases in osteoblastic and osteoclastic activity cause a rise in bone alkaline phosphatase. A rise to more than 20% above the normal range may be an indicator of disease (Melillo, 1993a). This test is useful in identifying treatable bone disease that may otherwise go undetected. Mildly elevated levels have been noted with healing fractures, Paget's disease, osteomalacia, fracture, or cancerous diseases. Modest elevations have been noted with myocardial infarctions (representing hepatic congestion associated with congestive heart failure) and pulmonary infarction. Other valuable tests for bone disease include serum osteocalcin concentration, which reflects the rate of bone turnover as a predictor of bone loss, and urinary hydroxyproline as a standard for determining bone resorption (Mitlak & Nussbaum, 1993).

Mean creatine kinase isoenzyme values typically decline in adults older than 70 years of age (Tietz et al., 1992). This change is caused by a decrease in total muscle mass as well as a decrease in creatine kinase activity in the muscle tissue itself.

COMMON SYMPTOMS AND SIGNS

Pain and stiffness are the most prevalent musculoskeletal complaints of older adults. Osteoporosis is generally asymptomatic, although some patients experience the first symptom as pain from a resultant fracture. Discomfort from osteoarthritis occurs with weight bearing and motion and usually worsens by the end of the day. In contrast, the pain and stiffness of rheumatoid arthritis are most pronounced in the morning after several hours of inactivity. Additional findings in patients with rheumatoid arthritis include swelling and joint deformities. Although the onset of rheumatoid disease usually occurs earlier in life, the first presenting symptoms may be revealed in later years. See Chapter 20 for a discussion of the various degenerative joint diseases.

A loss of joint mobility is generally caused by disuse in those patients who are unable to move without considerable discomfort or who are cognitively unaware of the need to stretch the muscles or tendons. In some instances, the first sign of a fracture is the loss or limitation of joint mobility.

Muscle weakness can result from disuse or may be a focal sign evident in the neurological evaluation. The major contributors to decline in muscle function include senescent changes in the neuromuscular tissue, chronic diseases, medications, the atrophy of disuse, and malnutrition (Fiatarone et al., 1993).

Gastrointestinal System

PHYSIOLOGICAL CHANGES

With age, dental enamel wears and gums recede, thereby exposing more of the teeth and increasing the likelihood of decay. In the past, there was little concern over dental disease, as most older adults had their teeth removed during middle age. However, with fluoride in the water system and better dental hygiene, people are now keeping their teeth longer and periodontal disease has become more common. The prevalence of coronal caries has decreased in children and young adults, but dentate elderly people appear to remain at risk for both coronal and root caries (Dolan et al., 1990). Atrophy and fibrosis of the salivary glands make the breakdown of protein and starches more difficult, and patients with dry oral membranes (a condition termed *xerostomia*) often have trouble eating. Xerostomia is no longer accepted as a normal consequence of aging but is instead related to salivary gland pathology or dysfunction resulting from radiation therapy, drugs, or systemic disease (Dolan et al., 1990). Xerostomia causes a diminished sensation of taste, which frequently causes alterations in nutrition.

Aging is associated with a decrease in the level of negative pressure that is created when the esophageal sphincter opens and fails to completely relax between swallows (Dejaeger et al., 1994). Swallowing disorders are common; most people older than 70 years of age have some functional abnormality of the oral, pharyngeal, or esophageal stage of swallowing (Ekberg & Fernberg, 1991).

Gastrointestinal muscular tension changes with age. A decrease in gastric pH may result in an altered effect of drugs. The size of the liver decreases over time, which also has a significant effect on drug metabolism. Although constipation is a frequent complaint in the aged population, there is no physiological decline in colonic motility. The sluggish colon is often indicative of functional changes related to a lack of fiber, fluid intake, and exercise (Harari et al., 1993).

ASSESSMENT PARAMETERS

One of the most overlooked systems of assessment in the geriatric patient is the mouth. An oral examination is more important in the elderly than in younger patients because they have higher rates of cancerous and precancerous lesions and a greater risk of periodontal disease. Inspecting the mucosa includes checking the teeth and gums, the base of the tongue, and the posterior pharyngeal wall for lesions and evaluating the moisture content of the oral cavity. For edentulous patients, the dentures must be removed and the palate and alveolar ridges checked for irritation and proper fit. During palpation, attention should be paid to the base of the tongue, where lesions may be less obvious.

Abdominal assessment in geriatric patients should follow the same process as that used in younger adults. Inspection is done for a pulsating abdominal aorta and for the visible peristalsis indicative of early intestinal obstruction. The contour of the abdomen should be checked from the side, noting any distension of the abdominal wall. At this time the patient can be asked to lift his or her head up off the table to check for hernia protrusion. Auscultation always precedes palpation so that the examiner does not influence bowel sounds or risk palpating a potential leaking abdominal aortic aneurysm. The frequency of bowel sounds per quadrant and the presence or absence of abdominal bruit should be recorded. Aortic aneurysms are more common in older adults and are often misdiagnosed in elderly men experiencing abdominal or back pain (Marston et al., 1992).

Tenderness is assessed through palpation. Tortuosity or aneurysm of the abdominal aorta may be felt as a pulsatile mass in the abdomen. Aneurysms are usually wider than 3 cm and often have an associated bruit (Fields, 1991). The abdomen should also be palpated for masses and organ enlargement. When a mass in the area of the distal colon is found, the examiner should ask about the frequency of bowel movements.

A digital rectal examination should be performed with the patient in the left lateral decubitus position to check for the presence of stool and masses. Approximately 15% of colorectal cancers are detectable, although the majority of cancerous lesions are too high to palpate. A check for occult blood in the stool might be done at this time; however, a positive test in the patient who has not been properly prepared should be repeated after restrictive dietary measures have been taken.

LABORATORY TESTS

The American Cancer Society recommends an annual digital rectal examination for all people older than 40 years of age, an annual stool occult blood test for people older than 50 years of age, and a sigmoidoscopy every 3 to 5 years in people older than 50 years of age if two consecutive examinations have been negative. The U.S. Preventive Services Task Force (1996) noted that there is insufficient evidence to recommend for or against such screening in asymptomatic individuals and that it may be clinically prudent to offer screening to people who have a positive family history or other risk factors.

Liver function tests do not typically change with aging. Such tests include aspartate aminotransferase (aspartate transaminase [AST] or serum glutamic-oxaloacetic transaminase [SGOT]), alanine aminotransferase (ALAT) or serum glutamate pyruvate transaminase (SGPT), gamma-glutamyltransferase (GGTP), and serum bilirubin (Cavalieri et al., 1992). The alkaline phosphatase level discussed earlier *does* increase, although this is thought to be more an influence of extrahepatic sources.

COMMON SYMPTOMS AND SIGNS

Constipation, experienced as either infrequent or difficult elimination and/or straining, is a frequent symptom of older adults. True clinical constipation reveals a large amount of stool by digital examination and/or fecal loading of the colon or rectum detected with abdominal film. This phenomenon has been attributed to chronic illness, medications, a decrease in water content and dietary bulk, and a decrease in the motor complexes normally stimulated by bulk. Studies have also revealed colorectal dysmotility, increased colorectal diameter, and sometimes impaired rectal sensation in patients with constipation (Harari et al., 1993). Chronic laxative use is common in this population and thus complicates measurements of the true prevalence of this symptom among the elderly.

Swallowing dysfunction or dysphagia may be caused by a variety of defects that affect the oropharyngeal or esophageal phases of deglutition (Castell, 1990). Oropharyngeal defects (i.e., neuromuscular disease, tumors, vertebral osteophytes, and thyroid disease) can result in an inability to initiate the act of swallowing. Esophageal causes result from motility or mechanical disorders (e.g., spasm or stricture, displaced aorta, and medication-induced disorders) and produce difficulty in transporting material down the esophagus.

Gastroesophageal reflux disease (GERD) commonly affects all age groups but is more pronounced in the elderly. An estimated 60% of reflux episodes can be attributed to a mechanically defective lower esophageal sphincter (Morton & Fomkes, 1993). Heartburn is the most common symptom and is often described as a retrosternal burning sensation associated with meals, position, sleep, or exercise (Morton & Fomkes, 1993). Additional symptoms include hypersalivation (the body's attempt to dilute to a more alkaline saliva). Chest pain can be a common presenting symptom of this disorder.

Abdominal pain is a challenging complaint in any age group but particularly in the elderly. Causes include gall bladder disease, small bowel obstruction, appendicitis, pancreatic disease, mesenteric infarction, and any form of abdominal cancer. Diverticulitis is perhaps the most common cause of abdominal pain in the elderly; its hallmark is abdominal pain in the presence of an inflammatory process (Deckman & Cheskin, 1993). Diverticula (lesions without inflammation) cause a typically asymptomatic diverticulosis.

Genitourinary and Reproductive Systems

PHYSIOLOGICAL CHANGES

Of all the aging changes in body systems, the most influential may be the decline in kidney function resulting from the loss of glomeruli and reduced renal mass. Older adults at highest risk include those who are (1) taking multiple medications that compete for excretion receptor sites, (2) taking the more toxic medications or receiving contrast material for diagnostic procedures, (3) experiencing some degree of renal impairment, or (4) having a water balance disorder.

Women experience changes that include decreased (1) elasticity and tone of the pelvic ligaments, (2) connective tissue strength, and (3) estrogen level. The loss of estrogen contributes to dry, friable, vaginal mucosa and an increased frequency of dyspareunia. In addition, there is the loss of estrogen's protective effect on bones and the cardiac system. These factors should be considered when assessing the risk and benefits of estrogen replacement therapy (McKeon, 1994).

In men there is a decrease in (1) testosterone level, (2) sperm production, (3) muscle tone of the scrotum, and (4) size and firmness of the testicles. The relationship of these physiological changes to the increased complaint of impotence and sexual dysfunction is unclear. The prostate enlarges significantly over time, with one in four males older than 80 years of age requiring prostatic surgery when it creates obstructive symptoms (Roberts, 1994).

In both sexes there is a reduction in bladder muscle tone, resulting in decreased bladder capacity and increased residual volume in some individuals. Voiding patterns tend to change with the aging process (see Chapter 10).

ASSESSMENT PARAMETERS

Direct physical assessment of the urinary system is limited to palpation over the kidneys and an evaluation for costovertebral tenderness in patients with urinary symptoms. The examiner should check the prostate while conducting the digital rectal examination. Although the gland may be enlarged, it should feel soft and smooth. Tumors often occur in portions of the prostate (medial and anterior) that are not accessible to the examiner's finger. Patients with any suspicious findings should be referred for further evaluation (Fields, 1991). A symptom assessment for evaluating benign prostatic hyperplasia is recommended (Roberts, 1994).

A breast examination is important in aged women, who are at a higher risk for breast cancer. An annual breast examination provides the clinician an opportunity to teach patients how to perform the examination, which may be more difficult when arthritis also prevails. The breasts become more pendulous over time owing to a loss of hormonal stimulation and the atrophying of the mammary and glandular tissue of the breast. In older women, any mass palpated may be a malignant lesion.

A modified position for the pelvic examination may be necessary because of the prevalence of hip osteoarthritis in older women. The left lateral position with the hips slightly flexed may allow the examiner to perform a gynecological examination. External genitalia should be checked for dryness and atrophic changes. The patient can be asked to cough at this time so the examiner can check for the presence of stress incontinence. The assessment should also include an examination for cystocele, rectocele, or a prolapsed uterus. Normal gynecological findings include a smaller uterus and unpalpable ovaries. Because hormonal stimulation decreases with age, any vaginal discharge is suspect.

LABORATORY TESTS

Although the frequency of Papanicolaou (Pap) smear screening varies, most clinicians recommend one test every 3 years for sexually active women who have had normal examinations in the past. Pap smear screening can be discontinued after 65 years of age if all tests have been normal (U.S. Preventive Services Task Force, 1996). Mammography every 1 to 2 years continues to be recommended for older women but may be discontinued at 75 years of age if pathology has not been previously detected (Fields, 1991).

Protein levels in the urine rise slightly with age, reflecting changes in the kidney basement membrane. Proteinuria may also signify renal pathology or subclinical urinary tract infection. Thus, although trace or +1 protein may be clinically insignificant for kidney disease, a differential diagnosis of urinary tract infection should be considered. Urine specific gravity declines with age, owing to the loss of nephrons, which impair the kidneys' ability to concentrate urine.

A loss of one third to one half of functioning glomeruli occurs by the age of 70 years, reducing the glomerular filtration rate. As a result, blood urea nitrogen steadily rises beginning in middle life and continuing into old age. A similar increase occurs with serum creatinine, although it is less striking because the reduction in muscle mass caused by aging leads to a lower production of creatinine from the breakdown of cells. Thus, the creatinine clearance test is the most sensitive indicator of renal function for older patients (Melillo, 1993b). The creatinine clearance level does decline with age and is thus an important consideration in preventing toxicity from medications, particularly those that are excreted unchanged by the kidney (e.g., digoxin, aminoglycosides). The fol-

lowing formula is useful in obtaining a more accurate estimate of how the kidneys may handle drugs or toxins:

$$\text{Creatinine clearance (mL/min)} = \frac{(140 - \text{age}) \times \text{lean body weight (kg)}}{72 \times \text{serum creatinine (mg/dL)}}$$

Similar antagonistic effects account for the relative stability of reference ranges for serum uric acid, which remain stable throughout middle age and begin to rise in later years (Tietz et al., 1992). An important factor in interpreting geriatric renal values is that high normal values of blood urea nitrogen (BUN) and creatinine can indicate substantially reduced function.

COMMON SYMPTOMS AND SIGNS

Incontinence is a hidden and distressful symptom in older adults. The assessment and management of urinary incontinence are covered in Chapter 10.

Benign prostatic disease in men presents initially with obstructive or irritative symptoms (e.g., hesitancy, straining to void, intermittency, urgency, frequency, nocturia). The prostate begins to enlarge in men 50 or more years of age, and enlargement is nearly universal in men who reach 80 years of age. Prostate hyperplasia is most common in the central zone when it is benign and in the peripheral zone if prostatic cancer is present (Roberts, 1994). Because of its lack of specificity, the prostatic surface antigen (PSA) has not yet been recommended for annual screening. However, serum creatinine should be screened, and if it is abnormal, the use of imaging studies such as intravenous urography (IVU) may be more conclusive.

Hematological System

PHYSIOLOGICAL CHANGES

The percentage of bone marrow space occupied by the hematopoietic tissue varies throughout life, declining progressively in individuals older than 70 years of age. With aging, the hematopoietic tissue is replaced with fat and connective tissue. Thus, an ineffective erythropoiesis results in an impaired incorporation of iron into the tissues (Freedman, 1995). Patients at risk for problems are those who lose blood, who have an adverse hematological effect of medication, or who have multisystem chronic disease.

ASSESSMENT PARAMETERS

Assessment of the hematological system is typically confined to laboratory analysis, although the physical examination may give clues to an underlying hematological disorder. The skin, for example, may demonstrate petechiae or purpura, or the conjunctivae or buccal mucosa may give evidence of the pallor of anemia. A hematological disorder may be best detected with a careful review of general well-being that assesses fatigue, weakness, or any decrease in exercise tolerance.

LABORATORY TESTS

Hemoglobin and hematocrit levels show a modest decline with age, although normal elderly people still remain within the limits typical of younger adults. Misattributing an abnormal value to normal aging can lead to a failure to assess and correct an underlying anemia. The hematocrit, although it does not change appreciably with the aging process, is influenced dramatically by the level of hydration, which can vary considerably in older people. Mean corpuscular volume (MCV) increases slightly with age, although red blood cells do not change significantly (Freedman, 1995). Reports differ regarding normal age-related changes in the white blood cell count and differential levels. The total leukocyte count in older adults is usually lower than in younger adults; this difference is attributed primarily to a decline in total lymphocytes caused by a decrease in the T-cell lymphocytes (Cavalieri et al., 1992). All changes in lymphocytes and granulocytes may be reflective of alterations in the immune status and antimicrobial activity in the elderly. There is no appreciable change in the platelet level (Duthie & Abbas, 1991), although survival may be shortened because of the change in bone marrow. There may also be a reduced ability to regenerate platelets after

a severe loss. Age-related changes in the erythrocyte sedimentation rate were discussed previously in the musculoskeletal section. Coagulation studies reveal no change in the prothrombin time (PT) and the partial thromboplastin time (PTT) in healthy older adults (Davis, 1993).

Reports differ on whether there is an age-related decline in serum levels of vitamin B_{12}. However, most studies report that vitamin B_{12}, serum iron, transferrin, total iron binding capacity, and serum folate levels do not change with age. Changes in these values are more likely to be associated with malnutrition or drug-nutrient interactions (Cavalieri et al., 1992).

Many hematological tests are used in the assessment of older adults. The complete blood count (CBC) includes a measure of hemoglobin, hematocrit, total leukocyte count, and red blood cell indices. It may be useful to conduct an initial screening in all elderly patients and to subsequently test specific components in patients at risk. The differential leukocyte count (DLC) estimates the percentages of leukocytes that are mature polymorphonuclear neutrophils, lymphocytes, eosinophils, basophils, monocytes, and band neutrophils. Indications for testing include patients with newly suspected infection, those suspected of having hematological malignancies, and those at risk for leukopenia due to chemotherapy or bone marrow disease (Duthie & Abbas, 1991). The reticulocyte count estimates the numbers of young, immature, and nonnucleated red blood cells that are formed in the bone marrow. It is helpful in differentiating anemias caused by bone marrow failure from those caused by hemorrhage or hemolysis and also in reevaluating the effectiveness of therapy and the recovery of bone marrow function. Coagulation studies are indicated only in those patients who have a coagulative disorder and are receiving anticoagulant therapy or who are preparing for procedures that will interfere with hemostasis.

COMMON SYMPTOMS AND SIGNS

Anemia is common in the elderly, occurring in over 33% of geriatric outpatients (Freedman, 1995). This symptom is a manifestation of underlying disease processes and, if suspected, should be further examined with diagnostic efforts aimed at detecting its cause. The typical signs of mild anemia are fatigue and a decreased level of activity. The two most prevalent types of anemia are associated with iron deficiency and chronic disease (Joosten et al., 1992). Iron deficiency anemia is more frequently caused by blood loss than by dietary deficiency or malabsorption (Scott, 1993). The anemia of chronic disease is associated with chronic infections, inflammations, or malignancies. *Anemia of chronic disease* is a bit of a misnomer, as it can also accompany acute inflammation, trauma, or protein energy malnutrition (Lipschitz, 1990). The presentation here is more subtle, and in many patients the clinical symptoms reflect the underlying disease rather than the anemia itself.

Hematopoietic malignancies are becoming more prevalent as the population ages. Chronic lymphocytic leukemia (CLL) is sometimes associated clinically with a mild symmetrical lymphadenopathy and splenomegaly. It is further confirmed if the lymphocyte count is elevated significantly and the smaller lymphocytes are affected (Scott, 1993). During the past decades, the incidence of acute myeloid leukemia (AML) has decreased in the younger population and significantly increased in the elderly population (Heinemann & Jehn, 1991). AML is a heterogeneous disease, and there is speculation that the increase in incidence with age may be caused by an accumulation of mutagenic events over time that frequently occurs in patients with antecedent hematological disorders.

Endocrine System

PHYSIOLOGICAL CHANGES

Aging is marked by an overall decline in hormone secretion. More significant, however, is the diminished tissue sensitivity to secreted hormones. The thyroid gland undergoes fibrosis and increases in nodularity with age but overall is able to produce a normal amount of hormone during later years (Levy, 1991). As people age, deposits of amyloid form in the pancreatic islets of Langerhans. There is also a change in glucose tolerance, with postprandial levels jumping by 6 to 13 mg/dL (Deakins, 1994). The change in glucose tolerance is attributed primarily to a decrease in tissue sensitivity to insulin, which results from a postreceptor defect and an overall decrease in the number of insulin receptors. There is also an inability to adequately inhibit glucose output from the liver, which results in a prolonged glycemic response to a meal (Davidson, 1995). As a result of these changes, endocrine diseases are most common in later years; diabetes mellitus affects as many as one in two people older than 80 years, and thyroid disease affects one in four people in this age group. The presentation of these disorders may markedly differ among older adults, often delaying diagnosis and risking a more adverse outcome.

Basal metabolic rate declines with age. Age-related changes in the thermoregulatory response increase the risk of hyperthermia and hypothermia for people residing in environments with more extreme climates. Along with changes in body composition (increased body fat and decreased lean body mass), changes in food preferences, and diminished physical activity, these factors increase the likelihood of being overweight or obese.

Because carbohydrate metabolism affects and is affected by changes in fluid and electrolyte balance, the metabolic systems of the body are related to the endocrine system. Although there are no known changes in calcium, sodium, or regulatory potassium with aging itself, disorders are common, owing to multisystem disease, the adverse effects of medication, and a diminished reserve capacity. Plasma renin levels and aldosterone concentrations decline with age (Solomon, 1995). Patients at risk for disorders of the renin-angiotensin-aldosterone system are those with diabetes and renal insufficiency.

ASSESSMENT PARAMETERS

Routine screening for diabetes or thyroid disease has yet to be consistently recommended except for those individuals considered at risk (i.e., those who are markedly obese or have a family history of disease, and women with history of gestational diabetes) (U.S. Preventive Services Task Force, 1996). Because of the frequency of these diseases, clinicians are advised to conduct a review of systems as part of the screening assessment. History-taking questions for thyroid disease include questions on confusion, memory loss, apathy, dyspnea, constipation, dry skin, gait disturbance, arthralgias, weakness, tremors, and anorexia. A patient history for diabetes should cover the metabolic and vascular systems. The classic symptomatologies of polyuria, polydipsia, and polyphagia are good screening criteria for older adults; however, these symptoms may be attributed to other commonly known geriatric problems. Polyuria, for example, can be mimicked by the use of diuretics and the presence of prostatic hypertrophy. Polyphagia is often hard to quantify in the elderly; in fact, they are more likely to present with anorexia. Older adults with an impaired thirst response do not respond to the increase in osmolarity caused by drinking fluids. Atypical presentations include altered mentation, behavioral changes, sleep disturbances, incontinence, weight loss, anorexia, and falls.

Earlier warning signs of diabetes include shin spots and recurrent skin infections. Because the complications of diabetes occasionally develop before the diabetes itself is apparent, neuropathy, nephropathy, and vascular changes should be assessed. Early warning signs include eye changes, kidney dysfunction, numbness and tingling in the feet or legs, vascular disease, and hardening of the arteries. The thyroid should be checked for enlargement or swelling. Any changes in eye appearance or heart rate should warrant a more thorough evaluation for thyroid disorder.

Measuring body composition is frequently overlooked in favor of simply weighing a patient. The latter method, however, is a better indicator of fluid status in the geriatric patient than it is of muscle mass stores and body fat accumulation. Anthropometric measurements including skinfold thickness and body frame size should be evaluated in patients known to have or be at risk for nutritional compromise.

LABORATORY TESTS

With aging, fasting glucose levels increase slightly, and glucose levels more dramatically increase after a glucose load. Blood glucose testing has become a simple, readily available method for screening and monitoring patients. Glycosylated hemoglobin (HbAlc) and fructosamine assays give a better view of long-term glucose control and are good supplementary methods for monitoring the effectiveness of therapy (Duthie & Abbas, 1991).

There is a possible decrease in thyroxine (T_4) and triiodothyronine (T_3) production with age as well as a slight increase in thyroid-stimulating hormone (TSH) levels (Cavalieri et al., 1992). Thyroid hormone concentration is generally well maintained as thyroid hormone degradation or disposal is increased (Levy, 1991).

Calcium balance is maintained by the endocrine system in concert with intestinal absorption, bone exchange, and renal excretions. Hypocalcemia is rare in both the young and the old and is more often seen in patients with hypoalbuminemia, hypoparathyroidism, renal insufficiency, acute pancreatitis, and calcitonin-producing tumors (Miller & Gold, 1994). The predominant acute symptom of hypocalcemia is increased neuromuscular excitability, which may proceed to tetany. Long-term manifestations include lens opacities, abnormalities of the nails, and dry skin. The most frequent causes for hypercalcemia in elderly patients are malignant disease and primary hyperparathyroidism. Vitamin D helps metabolize calcium and is a common deficiency in the housebound or institutionalized population.

Although sodium is not known to change with aging, the elderly are predisposed to overhydration and dehydration. As part of normal aging, there is decreased activity in the renin-angiotensin-aldosterone system, increased activity of the atrial natriuretic hormones, and increased antidiuretic hormone excretion, all of which can increase the risk of hyponatremia (Miller & Gold, 1994). Hyponatremia (less than 136 mEq/L) can result from the syndrome of inappropriate antidiuretic hormone. This type of water retention can occur secondarily to sulfonylureas (e.g., chlorpropamide), thiazide diuretics, carbamazepine (Tegretol), thioridazine hydrochloride (Mellaril), cytotoxics (e.g., vincristine, vinblastine), and tricyclic antidepressants. It can also occur with renal disorders, pulmonary disease, central nervous system disorders, vomiting, and diarrhea. Symptoms and signs typically involve the central nervous system (e.g., depressed sensorium, decreased deep tendon reflexes, seizures, muscle cramps, nausea). Hypernatremia usually occurs because of excessive water loss with inadequate intake. The usual initial thirst response may be blunted in the aged; thus, initial symptoms are mild. Other symptoms often follow, including altered mental status with drowsiness.

Potassium balance disturbances are important. The range for the normal potassium levels is narrow and easily fluctuates between hypokalemia and hyperkalemia. Hypokalemia is often associated with diuretic use, diarrhea, laxative use, vomiting, malnutrition, and diabetic acidosis. With moderate loss there are no symptoms, but with larger losses neuromuscular symptoms can develop, including weakness, myalgias, cramps, and sometimes neuropsychiatric symptoms (e.g., depression). Cardiac changes may include ST-segment depression, T-wave flattening, and prominent U waves. Severe depletion can lead to disturbances in atrioventricular conduction.

The risk for hyperkalemia may be associated with age-related decreases in renin and aldosterone; at normal levels, these hormones facilitate potassium excretion. Hyperkalemia is most common in those patients with renal disease. Several drugs may antagonize potassium excretion; these include digitalis, nonsteroidal antiinflammatory agents, beta-blockers, and angiotensin-converting enzyme (ACE) inhibitors. The symptoms of hyperkalemia are nonspecific and include anxiety, restlessness, apprehension, weakness, stupor, hyporeflexia, paresis, and fasciculation.

COMMON SYMPTOMS AND SIGNS

The signs and symptoms of endocrine disturbances are vague and nonspecific. Thus, clinicians should consider the possibility of an endocrine disturbance given the relative frequency with which they appear.

Immune System

PHYSIOLOGICAL CHANGES

Age-associated decline in immune function includes both spontaneous (e.g., serum isoagglu-

tinins) and induced (e.g., antibody response to the influenza vaccine) immunity and reflects a generalized decline in the immune system response to foreign antigens (Ben-Yehuda & Weksler, 1992). There is a decline in both T-cell and B-cell functions, with a dramatic effect on cell-mediated immunity. An important example of this defect in cell mediation is the inability of many elderly people to mount a delayed cutaneous hypersensitivity response. The decline in B-cell function may be indirectly related to a decline in T-cell function (Plewa, 1990). The decreased numbers of B cells secreting immunoglobulin (Ig) G result in a generally poor humoral immune response (Burns et al., 1993). With aging, the thymus gland involutes and there is a decrease in the thymic hormone level; the number of autoantibodies also increases (Fraser, 1993).

Patients at risk for disease associated with impaired immune function are those who are nutritionally compromised or immunosuppressed. Chronic disease, debility, and institutional living increase the risk of an infectious process. Protein energy malnutrition impairs (1) further cell-mediated immunity, (2) the ability of phagocytes to kill ingested bacteria and fungi, (3) several components of the complement system, (4) mucosal secretory IgA antibodies, and (5) the affinity of antibodies (Chandra, 1990). In addition to alterations in the immune system, organ-specific host resistance decreases; for example, cilial atrophy and detrusor muscle weakness both increase the risk of an infectious process.

ASSESSMENT PARAMETERS

When an older adult presents with symptoms or signs of an immune system process (e.g., infection, autoimmune disease) the physical assessment may give evidence of an underlying pathology. The usual symptoms of infection—fever, chills, leukocytosis, or even tachycardia—may be absent or sometimes blunted in the elderly, and changes in function may be an indication of immune system alteration. Confusion or incontinence, for example, may be the only presenting symptoms of respiratory or urinary tract infections. Pneumonia and influenza constitute the leading infectious causes of death in the elderly and the fourth most common cause of death overall (Musgrave & Verghese, 1990). The other most common infections include urinary tract and skin infections. It is important to pay particular attention to these high-risk areas. Infections can occur anywhere, and overlooked sites often include the lining of the heart, the teeth, the feet, and the gastrointestinal tract.

Cancer is the second most common cause of mortality in the elderly, increasing with age and leveling off in individuals by approximately 84 years of age (Guralnik & Havik, 1995). Leukemia and cancers of the digestive system, breast, prostate, and urinary tract increase with age. Symptoms may be generalized or organ specific, and the clinician must be vigilant.

LABORATORY TESTS

Hematological tests of white blood count and other indices often provide clues of the immunological responses that accompany excess or impaired function. Anergy and lymphopenia are grave prognostic indicators; they have a 28% survival rate 3 years posttesting in asymptomatic, apparently healthy elderly people (Chandra, 1990). Although the absolute number of peripheral blood polymorphonuclear leukocytes remains unchanged with age, the functional capacity of these is less clear (Plewa, 1990). A significant decrease in the number and functional capability of both T lymphocytes and B lymphocytes has been shown to be a component of the altered immune status of the elderly (Kelso, 1990). Neutrophil adherence is a critical component of host defense against infection. In many elderly people, neutrophil plasma adherence is depressed (Damtew et al., 1990), resulting in impaired phagocytosis.

The immunoglobulins demonstrate some change with aging. The mean and median values for IgA and IgG are higher than those of the younger population (Tietz et al., 1992). IgM values for people older than 90 years are lower, and IgE levels appear to be unchanged.

COMMON SYMPTOMS AND SIGNS

Decreases in both immune competency and the sensitivities of several homeostatic mecha-

nisms contribute to the risk of infection and also reduce the probability that infection will present with classic signs and symptoms. The most common atypical symptoms and signs of infection include failure to thrive and changes in mental status, activity, appetite, or weight. Infection should be suspected any time an older patient presents with a decline in well-being or with nonspecific symptoms such as falls, dizziness, confusion, anorexia, or weakness (McClure, 1992). The sudden development of urinary frequency or incontinence may be the hallmark of a urinary tract infection.

When assessing a patient, the examiner should review the seven warning signals of cancer: (1) a change in bowel or bladder habits, (2) a sore that does not heal, (3) unusual bleeding or discharge, (4) a thickening or lump in the breast or elsewhere, (5) indigestion or difficulty swallowing, (6) obvious change in a wart or mole, and (7) a nagging cough or hoarseness. These warning signs are not exclusive signals of malignancy in the aged and may be attributed to the aging process or other chronic illness.

SUMMARY

It is more important to know the patient who has the disease than it is to know the disease the patient has.

SIR WILLIAM OSLER

The techniques and parameters of physical examination form the cornerstone of assessment by the advanced practice nurse. Being familiar with the physiological changes of aging, knowing the classic and atypical disease presentations, and appreciating the value of laboratory assessment are all important components of providing quality care to older adults.

REFERENCES

Bain, P. S., Findley, L., Atchison, P., et al. (1993). Assessing tremor severity. *Journal of Neurology, Neurosurgery and Psychiatry, 56*(8), 868–873.
Baloh, R. W. (1992). Dizziness in older people. *Journal of the American Geriatrics Society, 40*(7), 713–721.

Ben-Yehuda, A., & Weksler, M. (1992). Host resistance and the immune system. *Clinics in Geriatric Medicine, 8*(4), 701–711.

Blocker, W. (1992). Maintaining functional independence by mobilizing the aged. *Geriatrics, 47*(1), 28–50.

Boss, B. (1991). Normal aging in the nervous system. Implications for SCI nurses. *Spinal Cord Injury Nursing, 8*(2), 42–47.

Breteler, M., Van Swieten, J., & Bots, M. (1994). Cerebral white matter lesions, vascular risk factors and cognitive function in a population-based study: The Rotterdam Study. *Neurology, 44*(7), 1246–1252.

Brown, G., Warren, M., Williams, J., et al. (1993). Cranial computed tomography of elderly patients: An evaluation of its use in acute neurological presentations. *Age and Ageing, 22*(4), 240–243.

Burns, E., Lum, L., L'Hommedieu, G., & Goodwin, J. S. (1993). Specific humoral immunity in the elderly: In vivo and in vitro response to vaccination. *Journal of Gerontology, 48*(6), 231–236.

Castell, D. (1990). Esophageal disorders in the elderly. *Gastroenterology Clinics of North America, 19*(2), 235–254.

Cavalieri, T., Chopra, A., & Bryman, P. (1992). When outside the norm is normal: Interpreting lab data in the aged. *Geriatrics, 47*(5), 66–70.

Chandra, R. (1990). The relation between immunology, nutrition and disease in elderly people. *Age and Ageing, 19*, 25–31.

Ciocon, J., Fernandez, B., & Ciocon, D. (1993). Leg edema clinical cues to the differential diagnosis. *Geriatrics, 48*(5), 34–40.

Damtew, B., Spagnuolo, P., Goldsmith, G., & Marino, J. A. (1990). Neutrophil adhesion in the elderly: Inhibitory effects of plasma from elderly patients. *Clinical Immunology and Immunopathology, 54*(2), 247–255.

Davidson, M. (1995). Diabetes mellitus and other disorders of carbohydrate metabolism. In W. Abrams, M. H. Beers, R. Berkow & A. J. Fletcher (Eds.), *The Merck manual of geriatrics* (2nd ed., pp. 997–1023). Whitehouse Station, NJ: Merck & Co., Inc.

Davis, C. (1993). Laboratory values for the elderly. In D. L. Carnevali & M. Patrick (Eds.), *Nursing management for the elderly* (3rd ed., pp. 141–170). Philadelphia: J. B. Lippincott.

Deakins, D. (1994). Teaching elderly patients about diabetes. *American Journal of Nursing, 4*, 38–42.

Deckman, R., & Cheskin, L. (1993). Diverticular disease in the elderly. *Journal of the American Geriatrics Society, 41*(9), 986–993.

Dejaeger, E., Pelemans, W., Bibau, G., & Ponette, E. (1994). Manofluorographic analysis of swallowing in the elderly. *Dysphagia, 9*(3), 156–161.

Dolan, T., Monopoli, M., Kaurich, M., & Rubenstein, L. S. (1990). Geriatric grand rounds: Oral diseases in older adults. *Journal of the American Geriatrics Society, 38*(11), 1239–1250.

Duthie, E., & Abbas, A. (1991). Laboratory testing: Current recommendations for older adults. *Geriatrics, 46*(10), 41–50.

Ekberg, O., & Fernberg, M. (1991). Altered swallowing function in patients without dysphagia. *American Journal of Roentgenology, 156*(6), 1181–1184.

Elmstahl, S., Rosen, I., & Gullberg, B. (1994). Quantitative EEG in elderly patients with Alzheimer's disease and healthy controls. *Dementia, 5*(2), 119–124.

Ferris, B. (1978). Epidemiology standardization project: Recommended respiratory disease questionnaire for use with adults and children in epidemiological research. *American Review of Respiratory Diseases, 118*, 6.

Fiatarone, M., O'Neill, E., Doyle, N., et al. (1993). The Boston FICSIT Study: The effects of resistance training and nutritional supplementation on physical frailty in the oldest old. *Journal of the American Geriatrics Society, 41*(3), 333–337.

Fields, S. (1991). Special considerations in the physical exam of older patients. *Geriatrics, 46*(8), 39–44.

Fleg, J. (1995). Cardiovascular disorders: Diagnostic evaluation. In W. Abrams, M. H. Beers, R. Berkow & A. J. Fletcher (Eds.), *The Merck manual of geriatrics* (2nd ed., pp. 441–445). Whitehouse Station, NJ: Merck & Co., Inc.

Fleming, B. E., Wilson, D. R., & Pendergast, D. R. (1991). A portable, easily performed muscle power test and its association with falls by elderly persons. *Archives of Physical Medicine and Rehabilitation, 72*, 886–882.

Folstein, M. F., Folstein, S., & McHugh, P. R. (1975). Mini-Mental State: A practical method for grading the cognitive state of patients for the clinician. *Journal of Psychiatric Research, 12*, 189–198.

Frank, S., Stange, K., Moore, P., & Smith, C. K. (1992). The focused physical examination: Should checkups be tailor-made? *Postgraduate Medicine, 92*(2), 171–186.

Fraser, D. (1993). Patient assessment: Infection in the elderly. *Journal of Gerontological Nursing, 19*(7), 5–11.

Freedman, L. (1995). Age-related hematologic changes and anemias. In W. Abrams, M. H. Beers, R. Berkow & A. J. Fletcher (Eds.), *The Merck manual of geriatrics* (2nd ed., pp. 847–861). Whitehouse Station, NJ: Merck & Co., Inc.

Garner, B. C. (1989). Guide to changing lab values in elders. *Geriatric Nursing, 10*(3), 144–149.

Gawlinski, A., & Jensen, G. (1991). The complications of cardiovascular aging. *American Journal of Nursing, 11*, 26–32.

Gilchrest, B. (1995). Skin changes and disorders. In W. Abrams, M. H. Beers, R. Berkow & A. J. Fletcher (Eds.), *The Merck manual of geriatrics* (2nd ed., pp. 1255–1286). Whitehouse Station, NJ: Merck & Co., Inc.

Guralnik, J. M., & Havik, R. J. (1995). Epidemiology and demographics. In W. Abrams, M. H. Beers, R. Berkow & A. J. Fletcher (Eds.), *The Merck manual of geriatrics* (2nd ed., pp. 1351–1365). Whitehouse Station, NJ: Merck & Co., Inc.

Harari, D., Gurwitz, J., & Minaker, K. (1993). Constipation in the elderly. *Journal of the American Geriatrics Society, 41*(10), 1130–1140.

Heinemann, V., & Jehn, V. (1991). Acute myeloid leukemia in the elderly: Biological features and search for adequate treatment. *Annals of Hematology, 63*(4), 179–188.

Herr, K., & Mobily, P. (1993). Comparison of selected pain assessment tools for use with the elderly. *Applied Nursing Research, 6*(1), 39–46.

Hoenig, H., & Rubenstein, L. (1991). Hospital associated deconditioning and dysfunction. *Journal of the American Geriatrics Society, 39*(2), 220–222.

Johnson, B. D., Badr, M. S., & Dempsey, J. A. (1994). Impact of the aging pulmonary system on the response to exercise. *Clinics in Chest Medicine, 15*(2), 229–245.

Joosten, E., Pelemans, W., Hiele, M., et al. (1992). Prevalence and causes of anaemia in a geriatric hospitalized population. *Journal of Gerontology, 38*(1–2), 111–117.

Kane, R., Ouslander, J., & Abrass, I. (Eds.). (1994). *Essentials of clinical geriatrics* (3rd ed.). New York: McGraw-Hill.

Kasch, F., Boyer, J. L., Van Camp, S. P., et al. (1993). Effects of exercise on cardiovascular aging. *Age and Ageing, 22,* 5–10.

Kelso, T. (1990). Laboratory values in the elderly: Are they different? *Emergency Medical Clinics of North America, 8*(2), 241–254.

Koller, W. C., Busenbark, K., & Miner, K. (1994). The relationship of essential tremor to other movement disorders. Report on 678 patients in the essential tremor group. *Annals of Neurology, 35*(6), 717–723.

Lakatta, E. (1995). Normal changes of aging. In W. Abrams, M. H. Beers, R. Berkow & A. J. Fletcher (Eds.), *The Merck manual of geriatrics* (2nd ed., pp. 625–657). Whitehouse Station, NJ: Merck & Co., Inc.

Lareau, S. C. (1993). Respiratory problems. In D. L. Carnevali & M. Patrick (Eds.), *Nursing management for the elderly* (3rd ed., pp. 625–657). Philadelphia: J. B. Lippincott.

Lassau-Wray, E. R., & Parker, A. W. (1993). Neuromuscular responses of elderly women to tasks of increasing complexity imposed during walking. *European Journal of Applied Physiology and Occupational Physiology, 67,* 476–480.

Levy, E. (1991). Thyroid disease in the elderly. *Medical Clinics of North America, 75*(1), 151–167.

Lipschitz, D. A. (1990). The anemia of chronic disease. *Journal of the American Geriatrics Society, 38*(11), 1258–1267.

Lober, C., & Fenske, N. (1990). Photoaging and the skin: Differentiation and clinical response. *Geriatrics, 45*(4), 36–42.

Manolio, T. A., Furger, C., Rautaharja, P., et al. (1994). Cardiac arrhythmias on 24-hour ambulatory electrocardiology in older women and men: The Cardiovascular Health Study. *Journal of the American College of Cardiology, 23*(4), 916–925.

Marston, W., Ahlquist, R., Johnson, G., & Meyer, A. A. (1992). Misdiagnosis of ruptured abdominal aortic aneurysms. *Journal of Vascular Surgery, 16*(1), 17–22.

Mathias, S., Nayak, U., & Issacs, I. (1986). Balance in elderly patients: The "get up and go test." *Archives of Physical Medicine and Rehabilitation, 67,* 387–389.

Matteson, M. A. (1997). Age-related changes in the musculoskeletal system. In M. A. Matteson, E. S. McConnell & A. D. Linton (Eds.), *Gerontological nursing: concepts and practice* (2nd ed., pp. 196–221). Philadelphia: W. B. Saunders.

McClure, C. (1992). Common infections in the elderly. *American Family Physician, 45*(6), 2691–2696.

McKeon, V. A. (1994). Hormone replacement therapy: Evaluating the risks and benefits. *Journal of Obstetric, Gynecologic and Neonatal Nursing, 23*(8), 647–657.

Melillo, K. D. (1993a). Interpretation of abnormal laboratory values in older adults: Part I. *Journal of Gerontological Nursing, 19*(1), 39–45.

Melillo, K. D. (1993b). Interpretation of abnormal laboratory values in older adults: Part 11. *Journal of Gerontological Nursing, 19*(2), 35–40.

Melillo, K. D. (1993c). Interpretation of laboratory values in older adults. *Nurse Practitioner, 18*(7), 59–67.

Miller, M., & Gold, G. (1994). Acute endocrine emergencies. *Clinics in Geriatric Medicine, 10*(1), 161–183.

Mitlak, B. H., & Nussbaum, S. R. (1993). Diagnosis and treatment of osteoporosis. *Annual Review of Medicine, 44,* 265–277.

Morris, J., & McManus, D. (1991). The neurology of aging: Normal versus pathologic change. *Geriatrics, 46*(8), 47–54.

Morton, L., & Fomkes, J. (1993). Gastroesophageal reflux disease: Diagnosis and medical therapy. *Geriatrics, 48*(3), 60–66.

Musgrave, T., & Verghese, A. (1990). Clinical features of pneumonia in the elderly. *Seminars in Respiratory Infection, 5*(4), 269–275.

Neiderman, M. (Ed.). (1991). Community acquired pneumonia in the elderly. *Respiratory infections in the elderly.* New York: Raven Press.

Odenheimer, G., Funkenstein, H., Beckett, L., et al. (1994). Comparison of neurological changes in "successfully aging" persons vs. the total aging population. *Archives of Neurology, 51,* 573–580.

Plewa, M. (1990). Altered host response and special infections in the elderly. *Emergency Medical Clinics of North America, 8*(2), 193–206.

Roben, N. (1993). Hypertension. In D. Carnevali & M. Patrick (Eds.), *Nursing management for the elderly* (3rd ed., pp. 529–542). Philadelphia: J. B. Lippincott.

Roberts, R. (1994). BPH: New guidelines based on symptoms and patient preference. *Geriatrics, 49*(7), 24–31.

Roemer, R., Shagass, C., Dubin, W., et al. (1992). Quantitative EEG in elderly depressives. *Brain Topography, 4*(4), 285–290.

Scott, R. B. (1993). Common blood disorders: A primary care approach. *Geriatrics, 48*(4), 72–76.

Sloan, J. P. (1996). *Protocols in primary care geriatrics* (2nd ed.). New York: Springer-Verlag.

Solomon, D. M. (1995). Age-related endocrine and metabolic changes. In W. Abrams, M. H. Beers, R. Berkow & A. J. Fletcher (Eds.), *The Merck manual of geriatrics* (2nd ed., pp. 981–984). Whitehouse Station, NJ: Merck & Co., Inc.

Stulnig, T., Mair, A., & Jarosch, E. (1993). Estimation of reference intervals from a senieur protocol compatible age population for immunologerontological studies. *Mechanisms of Aging and Development, 68,* 112.

Thompson, M., Sayers, R. D., Varty, K., & Reid, A. (1993). Chronic critical leg ischaemia must be redefined. *European Journal of Vascular Surgery, 7*(4), 420–426.

Tietz, N., Shuey, D., & Wekstein, D. (1992). Laboratory values in fit aging individuals—sexagenarians through centenarians. *Clinical Chemistry, 38*(6), 1167–1185.

Tockman, M. (1995). The effects of age on the lung. In W. Abrams, M. H. Beers, R. Berkow & A. J. Fletcher (Eds.), *The Merck manual of geriatrics* (2nd ed., pp. 569–574). Whitehouse Station, NJ: Merck & Co., Inc.

U.S. Preventive Services Task Force (1996). *Guide to clinical preventive services* (2nd ed.). Baltimore: Williams & Wilkins.

Vogt, M., Cauley, J., Kuller, L., & Hulley, S. B. (1993). Prevalence and correlates of lower extremity arterial disease in elderly women. *American Journal of Epidemiology, 137*(5), 559–568.

Wajngarten, M., Grupi, C., DaLuz, P., et al. (1990). Frequency and significance of cardiac rhythm disturbances in healthy elderly individuals. *Journal of Electrocardiology, 23*(2), 171–176.

Wasson, J., Walsh, B., Tompkins, R., et al. (1984). *The common symptom guide* (2nd ed.). New York: McGraw-Hill.

Wernick, R. (1989). Avoiding laboratory test misinterpretation in geriatric rheumatology. *Geriatrics, 44*(2), 61–63, 67–68, 73–78.

Williams, B. (1993). Prescribing for older patients. *Practitioner, 237*(3), 260–262.

Yaar, M., & Gilchrest, B. (1990). Cellular and molecular mechanisms of cutaneous aging. *Journal of Dermatologic Surgery and Oncology, 16*(10), 915–922.

Zorowitz, R. A., Luckey, M. M., & Meier, D. E. (1995). Metabolic bone disease. In W. Abrams, M. H. Beers, R. Berkow & A. J. Fletcher (Eds.), *The Merck manual of geriatrics* (2nd ed., pp. 897–917). Whitehouse Station, NJ: Merck & Co., Inc.

Physiological Influences of the Aging Process

AGE-RELATED CHANGE	APPEARANCE OR FUNCTIONAL CHANGE	IMPLICATION
Integumentary System		
Loss of dermal and epidermal thickness Flattening of papillae	Paper-thin skin Shearing and friction force more readily peels off the epidermis Diminished cell-mediated immunity in the skin	Prone to skin breakdown and injury
Atrophy of the sweat glands Decreased vascularity	Decreased sweating Slower recruitment of sweat glands by thermal stimulation Decreased body odor Decreased heat loss Dryness	Frequent pruritus Alteration in thermoregularity response Fluid requirements may change seasonally Loss of skin water Increased risk of heat stroke
Collagen cross-linking Elastin regression Loss of subcutaneous fat Decreased elasticity Loss of subcutaneous tissue	Increased wrinkling Laxity of skin Intraosseous atrophy, especially to back of hands and face Purpuric patches after minor surgery	Potential effect on one's morale and feeling of self-worth Loss of fat tissue on soles of feet—trauma of walking increases foot problems Reduced insulation against cold temperatures; *prone to hypothermia* Check why injury is occurring; be alert—potential abuse or falls
Decreased number of melanocytes	Loss of pigment Pigment plaque appears	Teach importance of using sun block creams; refer to dermatologist as needed
Decline in fibroblast proliferation	Decreased epidermal growth rate Slower reepithelialization Decreased vitamin D production and synthesis	Decreased tissue repair response

AGE-RELATED CHANGE	APPEARANCE OR FUNCTIONAL CHANGE	IMPLICATION
Decreased hair follicle density	Loss of body hair	
Decreased growth phase of individual fibers	Thin, short villus hairs predominate Slower hair growth	
Loss of melanocytes from the hair bulb	Graying of the hair	Potential effect on self-esteem
Alternating hyperplasia and hypoplasia of nail matrix	Longitudinal ridges Thinner nails of the fingers Thickened, curled toenails	Nails prone to splitting Advise patient to wear gloves, keep nails short, avoid nail polish remover (causes dryness); refer to podiatrist May cause discomfort

Respiratory System

Decreased lung tissue elasticity	Decreased vital capacity Increased residual volume Decreased maximum breath capacity	Reduced overall efficiency of ventilatory exchange
Thoracic wall calcification	Increased anteroposterior diameter of chest	Obscuration of heart and lung sounds Displacement of apical impulse
Cilia atrophy Decreased respiratory muscle strength	Change in mucociliary transport Reduced ability to handle secretions and reduced effectiveness against noxious foreign particles Partial inflation of lungs at rest	Increased susceptibility to infection Prone to atelectasis

Cardiovascular System

Heart valves fibrose and thicken	Reduced stroke volume, cardiac output may be altered Slight left ventricular hypertrophy	Decreased responsiveness to stress Increased incidence of murmurs, *particularly aortic stenosis and mitral regurgitation*
Mucoid degeneration of mitral valve	S4 commonly heard Valve less dense; mitral leaflet stretches with intrathoracic pressure	
Fibroelastic thickening of the sinoatrial (SA) node; decreased number of pacemaker cells	Slower heart rate Irregular heart rate	Increased prevalence of arrhythmias

Appendix continued on following page

AGE-RELATED CHANGE	APPEARANCE OR FUNCTIONAL CHANGE	IMPLICATION
Increased subpericardial fat		
Collagen accumulation around heart muscle		
Elongation of tortuosity and calcification of arteries	Increased rigidity of arterial wall Increased peripheral vascular resistance	Aneurysms may form Decreased blood flow to body organs Altered distribution of blood flow
Elastin and collagen cause progressive thickening and loss of arterial wall resiliency		Increased systolic blood pressure, contributing to coronary artery disease
Loss of elasticity of the aorta dilation		
Increased lipid content in artery wall	Lipid deposits form	Increased incidence of atherosclerotic events, such as *angina pectoris*, stroke, gangrene
Decreased baroreceptor sensitivity (stretch receptors)	Decreased sensitivity to change in blood pressure Decreased baroreceptor mediation to straining	Prone to loss of balance—potential for falls Valsalva maneuver may cause sudden drop in blood pressure

Gastrointestinal System

AGE-RELATED CHANGE	APPEARANCE OR FUNCTIONAL CHANGE	IMPLICATION
Liver becomes smaller	Decreased storage capacity	
Less efficient cholesterol stabilization absorption	Increased evidence of gall stones	
Dental enamel thins	Staining of tooth surface occurs	Tooth and gum decay; tooth loss
Gums recede	Teeth deprived of nutrients	
Fibrosis and atrophy of salivary glands	Prone to dry mucous membranes Decreased salivary ptyalin	Shift to mouth breathing is common Membrane more susceptible to injury and infection May interfere with breakdown of starches
Atrophy and decrease in number of taste buds	Decreased taste sensation	Altered ability to taste sweet, sour, and bitter Change in nutritional intake Excessive seasoning of foods
Delay in esophageal emptying	Decline in esophageal peristalsis Esophagus slightly dilated	Occasional discomfort as food stays in esophagus longer
Decreased hydrochloric acid secretion	Reduction in amount of iron and vitamin B_{12} that can be absorbed	Possible delay in vitamin and drug absorption, *especially calcium and iron*
Decrease in gastric acid secretion		Altered drug effect Fewer cases of gastric ulcers

AGE-RELATED CHANGE	APPEARANCE OR FUNCTIONAL CHANGE	IMPLICATION
Decreased muscle tone Atrophy of mucosal lining	Altered motility Decreased colonic peristalsis Decreased hunger sensations and emptying time	Prone to constipation, functional bowel syndrome, esophageal spasm, diverticular disease
Decreased proportion of dietary calcium absorbed	Altered bone formation, muscle contractility, hormone activity, enzyme activation, clotting time, immune response	Symptoms more marked in women than in men
Decreased basal metabolic rate (rate at which fuel is converted into energy)		May need fewer calories Possible effect on life span

Genitourinary and Reproductive Systems

Reduced renal mass Loss of glomeruli	Decreased sodium conserving ability Decreased glomerular filtration rate Decreased creatinine clearance Increased blood urea nitrogen concentration	Administration and dosage of drugs may need to be modified
Histological changes in small vessel walls Sclerosis of supportive circulatory system	Decreased renal blood flow	
Decline in number of functioning nephrons	Decreased ability to dilute urine concentrate	Altered response to reduced fluid load or increased fluid volume
Reduced bladder muscular tone	Decreased bladder capacity or increased residual urine	Sensation of urge to urinate may not occur until bladder is full Urination at night may increase
Atrophy and fibrosis of cervical and uterine walls Reduced number and viability of oocytes in the aging ovary	Menopause; decline in fertility Narrowing of cervical canal	
Decreased vaginal wall elasticity	Vaginal lining thin, pale, friable Narrowing of vaginal canal	Potential for discomfort in sexual intercourse
Decreased levels of circulating hormones	Reduced lubrication during arousal state	Increased frequency of sexual dysfunction
Degeneration of seminiferous tubules	Decreased seminal fluid volume Decreased force of ejaculation Reduced elevation of testes	

Appendix continued on following page

AGE-RELATED CHANGE	APPEARANCE OR FUNCTIONAL CHANGE	IMPLICATION
Proliferation of stromal and glandular tissue	Prostatic hypertrophy	Potentially compromised genitourinary function; *urinary frequency, and increased risk of malignancy*
Involution of mammary gland tissue	Connective tissue replaced by adipose tissue	Easier to assess breast lesions

Neuromuscular System

AGE-RELATED CHANGE	APPEARANCE OR FUNCTIONAL CHANGE	IMPLICATION
Decreased muscle mass	Decreased muscle strength Tendons shrink and sclerose	Decreased tendon jerks Increased muscle cramping
Decreased myosin adenosine triphosphatase (ADT) activity	Prolonged contraction time, latency period, relaxation period	Decreased motor function and overall strength
Deterioration of joint cartilage	Bone makes contact with bone	Potential for pain, crepitation, and limitation of movement
Loss of water from the cartilage	Narrowing of joint spaces	Loss of height
Decreased bone mass Decreased osteoblastic activity Osteoclasts resorb bone	Decreased bone formation and increased bone resorption, leading to osteoporosis Hormonal changes	More rapid and earlier changes in women Greater risk of fractures Gait and posture accommodate to changes
Increased proportion of body fat Regional changes in fat distribution	Centripetal distribution of fat and invasion of fat in large muscle groups	Anthropometric measurements required Increased relative adiposity
Thickened leptomeninges in spinal cord Accumulation of lipofuscin	Loss of anterior horn cells in the lumbosacral area Altered RNA function and resultant cell death	Leg weakness may be correlated
Loss of neurons and nerve fibers	Decreased processing speed and vibration sense Altered pain response Decreased deep tendon, Achilles tendon	Increased time to perform and learn Possible postural hypotension Safety hazard
Decreased conduction of nerve fibers	Decreased psychomotor performance	Alteration in pain response
Few neuritic plaques Neurofibrillary tangles in hippocampal neurons		Possible cognitive and memory changes Heavy tangle formation and neuritic plaques in cortex of those with Alzheimer's

AGE-RELATED CHANGE	APPEARANCE OR FUNCTIONAL CHANGE	IMPLICATION
Changes in sleep-wake cycle	Decreased stage 4, stage 3, and rapid eye movement phases Deterioration of circadian organization	Increased or decreased time spent sleeping Increased nighttime awakenings Changed hormonal activity
Slower stimulus identification and registration	Delayed reaction time	Prone to falls
Decreased brain weight and volume		May be present in absence of mental impairments

Sensory System

AGE-RELATED CHANGE	APPEARANCE OR FUNCTIONAL CHANGE	IMPLICATION
Morphological changes in choroid, epithelium, retina	Decreased visual acuity Visual field narrows	Corrective lenses required Increased possibility of disorientation and social isolation
Decreased rod and cone function		Slower light and dark adaptation
Pigment accumulation		
Decreased speed of eye movements	Difficulty in gazing upward and maintaining convergence	
Sclerosis of pupil sphincter	Difficulty in adapting to lighting changes Increased threshold for light perception	Glare may pose an environmental hazard Dark rooms may be hazardous
Increased intraocular pressure		Increased incidence of glaucoma
Distorted depth perception		Incorrect assessment of height of curbs and steps; potential for falls
Ciliary muscle atrophy	Altered refractive powers	Corrective lenses often required
Nuclear sclerosis (lens) Reduced accommodation Increased lens size Accumulation of lens fibers	Presbyopia Hyperopia Myopia	Near work and reading may become difficult
Lens yellows	Color vision may be impaired	Less able to differentiate lower color tones: blues, greens, violets
Diminished tear secretion	Dullness and dryness of the eyes	Irritation and discomfort may result Intactness of corneal surface jeopardized

Appendix continued on following page

AGE-RELATED CHANGE	APPEARANCE OR FUNCTIONAL CHANGE	IMPLICATION
Loss of auditory neurons	Decreased tone discrimination and voice localization High frequency sounds lost first	Suspiciousness may be increased because of paranoid dimensions secondary to hearing loss Social isolation
Angiosclerosis calcification of inner ear membrane	Progressive hearing loss, especially at high frequency Presbycusis	Difficulty hearing, particularly under certain conditions such as *background noise, rapid speech, poor acoustics*
Decreased number of olfactory nerve fibers	Decreased sensitivity to odors	May not detect harmful odors Potential safety hazard
Alteration in taste sensation		Possible changes in food preferences and eating patterns
Reduced tactile sensation	Decreased ability to sense pressure, pain, temperature	Misperceptions of environment and safety risk

Endocrine System

AGE-RELATED CHANGE	APPEARANCE OR FUNCTIONAL CHANGE	IMPLICATION
Decline in secretion of testosterone, growth hormone, insulin, adrenal androgens, aldosterone, thyroid hormone	Decreased hormone clearance rates	Increased mortality associated with certain stresses (burns, surgery)
Defects in thermoregulation Reduction of febrile responses	Shivering less intense Poor perceptions of changes in ambient temperature Reduced sweating; increased threshold for the onset of sweating Fever not always present with infectious process	Susceptibility to temperature extremes (*hypothermia/ hyperthermia*) Unrecognized infectious process operative
Alteration in tissue sensitivity to hormones	Decreased insulin response, glucose tolerance, and sensitivity of renal tubules to antidiuretic hormone (ADH)	
Enhanced sympathetic responsivity		
Increased nodularity and fibrosis of thyroid		Increased frequency of thyroid disease
Decreased basal metabolic rate	Alteration in carbohydrate tolerance	Increased incidence of obesity

AGE-RELATED CHANGE	APPEARANCE OR FUNCTIONAL CHANGE	IMPLICATION
Hematological System		
Decreased percentage of marrow space occupied by hematopoietic tissue	Ineffective erythropoiesis	Risky for patient who loses blood
Immune System		
Thymic involution and decreased serum thymic hormone activity Decreased T-cell function Appearance of autoantibodies	Decreased number of T cells Production of antiself reactive T cells Impairment in cell-mediated immune responses Decreased cyclic adenosine monophosphate (AMP) and glucose monophosphate (GMP) Decreased ability to reject foreign tissue Increased laboratory autoimmune parameters	Less vigorous and/or delayed hypersensitivity reactions Increased risk mortality Increased incidence of infection Reactivation of latent infectious diseases Increased prevalence of autoimmune disorders
Redistribution of lymphocytes	Impaired immune reactivity	
Changes in serum immunoglobulin	Increased immunoglobulin A (IgA) levels Decreased immunoglobulin G (IgG) levels	Increased prevalence of infection

6 - 2

Common Presentations in the Older Adult

COMMON SYMPTOMS OR SIGNS	CONTRIBUTING FACTORS	POTENTIAL SIGNIFICANCE
Integumentary System		
Pruritus	Changes in central nervous system perception Low relative humidity Cool air Excessive bathing Harsh detergents or cleansing agents	Dry skin (xerosis) Hyperthyroidism Renal disease Iron deficiency anemia Drug allergy Diabetes Lymphomas Parasitic infections Liver disease
Decreased skin turgor	Atrophy of skin tissues	Dehydration or volume depletion
Discoloration	Increased vascular fragility	Peripheral vascular disease Senile purpura Vitamin C deficiency Bruising Physical abuse
Loss of body hair	Decrease in hair follicle density	Abdominal, pubic, or axillary hair loss may suggest hormonal imbalance Localized loss seen with peripheral vascular disease Diffuse alopecia may be caused by iron deficiency, hypothyroidism, hypoproteinemia, skin inflammatory diseases
Surface-type pain parasthesias		Nerve involvement
Lesions	Sun exposure Excoriation from scratching	Actinic keratosis Basal cell carcinoma Squamous cell carcinoma Inflammation Skin tags (acrochordons)

COMMON SYMPTOMS OR SIGNS	CONTRIBUTING FACTORS	POTENTIAL SIGNIFICANCE
Lesions (Continued)		Drug reactions
		Infection (e.g., herpes zoster)
		Vascular lesions (e.g., venous lakes, senile angiomas, telangiectasia)
Scaliness	Scratching	Dermatitis
	Wool clothing	Psoriasis
	Strong soaps	
	Excessive bathing	
	Edema	Vascular insufficiency
	Heat	Fungal infections
	Moisture	

Respiratory System

COMMON SYMPTOMS OR SIGNS	CONTRIBUTING FACTORS	POTENTIAL SIGNIFICANCE
Diminished breath sounds	Kyphosis, scoliosis	Pleural effusion
	Pleural thickening	Pneumothorax
	Emphysema	Pneumonia
		Atelectasis
		Chronic obstructive pulmonary disease
Increased breath sounds	Thin chest wall	Pulmonary fibrosis
Crackles	Deconditioning, age-related fibrotic changes	Congestive heart failure
		Pulmonary edema
		Pneumonia
Wheezes	Bronchospasm	Airway obstruction
	Side effect of beta-blocker	Airway occlusion or narrowing
	Environmental pollutants	Cardiac asthma
Dyspnea	Bedrest	Atelectasis
	Cigarette smoking	Pulmonary embolism
	Deconditioning	Chronic obstructive pulmonary disease
	Obesity	Congestive heart failure
	Abdominal mass	Pneumonia
	Organomegaly	Obesity
		Poor physical condition
		Systemic acidosis
		Renal failure
		Presence of foreign body
		Anemia
Cough		Congested mucous membrane
		Acute bronchitis
		Chronic bronchitis
		Bronchogenic cancer
		Tuberculosis
		Angiotensin-converting enzyme inhibitor side effect

Appendix continued on following page

COMMON SYMPTOMS OR SIGNS	CONTRIBUTING FACTORS	POTENTIAL SIGNIFICANCE
Loss of an effective cough	Sedative use Reduced consciousness Neurological disease	Increased risk of aspiration
Fatigue	Excessive energy demand Deconditioning Nutritional deficiency Drug therapies	Emphysema Anemia Cardiac disease
Barrel chest	Kyphosis	Emphysema

Cardiovascular System

COMMON SYMPTOMS OR SIGNS	CONTRIBUTING FACTORS	POTENTIAL SIGNIFICANCE
Elevated blood pressure	Associated risk factors (e.g., smoking, family history, obesity)	Hypertensive heart disease Hyperthyroidism Anemia Hyperparathyroidism Stroke
Wide pulse pressure	Increased vascular resistance (increased systolic) Decreased catecholamine response (decreased diastolic)	Shock difficult to recognize
Systolic murmurs	Common; most often benign	Rheumatic fever Chronic obstructive pulmonary disease Aortic stenosis Aortic sclerosis Mitral regurgitation Idiopathic hypertrophic subaortic stenosis
Irregular pulse or palpitations	Alcohol Caffeine	Arrhythmia (e.g., atrial fibrillation, premature ventricular complexes [PVCs], sick sinus syndrome) Isolated premature beats
Diminished distal pulses		Embolism
Edema	Excess sodium intake Dependent position Lack of exercise	Venous insufficiency Decreased serum albumin Congestive heart failure Unilateral edema-proximal obstruction Claudication Decreased perfusion
Postural hypotension	Decreased baroreceptor sensitivity Deconditioning Drug treatment (e.g., vasodilators, antihypertensives, diuretics, psychotropics)	Volume depletion (dehydration, blood loss)

COMMON SYMPTOMS OR SIGNS	CONTRIBUTING FACTORS	POTENTIAL SIGNIFICANCE
Sustained apical pulse Point of maximal impulse displacement	Increased anterior-posterior diameter	Left ventricular hypertrophy Atherosclerotic occlusive disease
Vascular bruits		Hypertension Ventricular dysfunction (R or L) Stenosis
Claudication	Inadequate collateral circulation Peripheral vascular disease Exercise	Debilitating pain, which limits function Loss of limb
Extra heart sounds		S4 arterial kick May mean congestive heart failure
Syncope	Diminished cerebral metabolism	Hyperventilation, hypoglycemia Seizure disorder Cardiovascular disorder Neurological disorder

Gastrointestinal System

Constipation	Lack of bulk to diet Laxative abuse Decreased fluid intake Poor dentition Prolonged immobilization Drugs, especially sedatives, tranquilizers, antihypertensives, narcotics	Dehydration Anorectal lesions, tumors Loss of defecation reflex Irritable colon
Atrophic gastritis		Potential predisposition to pernicious anemia and gastric carcinoma Decreased absorption of vitamin B_{12} and iron
Abdominal pain		Abdominal pathology Renal, gynecological, or genitourinary pathology
Heartburn or pyrosis	Hiatal hernia Spicy foods Medications including alcohol, calcium channel blockers, anticholinergics, nitrates	Ulcerative esophagitis Irritable colon Barrett's esophagus Food intolerance Poorly chewed food
Dysphagia	Decreased salivation Decreased esophageal peristalsis Medications, especially potassium chloride, quinidine, alendronate, tetracycline	Esophageal stricture Inflamed mouth or throat Achalasia Hiatal hernia Malignant tumor Hyperthyroidism Central nervous system dysfunction

Appendix continued on following page

COMMON SYMPTOMS OR SIGNS	CONTRIBUTING FACTORS	POTENTIAL SIGNIFICANCE
	Oropharyngeal dysfunction Enlarged aorta	Stroke Parkinson's disease Polymyositis hypothyroidism Zenker's diverticulum Osteophytic vertebrae Aortic dysphagia
Missing teeth	Malnutrition Poor oral hygiene Xerostomia	Insufficient nutritional intake, especially vitamins B and C Periodontal disease Bruxism (grinding)

Genitourinary System

COMMON SYMPTOMS OR SIGNS	CONTRIBUTING FACTORS	POTENTIAL SIGNIFICANCE
Benign prostatic hypertrophy		Mechanical obstruction
Dysuria		Inflammation Infection Stricture
Incontinence	Transient incontinence Precipitating factors: immobilization, acute confusional state, drugs (diuretics, sedatives, anticholinergics)	Stress incontinence Neurogenic bladder Mechanical obstruction Urinary tract infection Cognitive dysfunction

Neuromuscular System

COMMON SYMPTOMS OR SIGNS	CONTRIBUTING FACTORS	POTENTIAL SIGNIFICANCE
Limitation of range of motion	Osteoporosis (insufficient dietary calcium intake, inadequate hormones) Osteopenia Immobility	Osteoporosis Osteoarthritis Fracture Inflammation Contracture
Pain or stiffness with movement	Immobilization	Inflammation Osteoarthritis Disease atrophy
Weakness or paralysis		Neurological or systemic disorder
Gait disturbance	Deconditioning; disorders of eye, ear, and proprioception; hyperkeratotic toenails	Degenerative joint disease Neurological disorder
Insomnia	Decreased rapid eye movement sleep	Pain, depression, drug tolerance, or rebound Restless leg syndrome Sleep apnea
Decreased sensation in extremities Pathological reflexes		Peripheral vascular disease Neuropathies Central nervous system disease

COMMON SYMPTOMS OR SIGNS	CONTRIBUTING FACTORS	POTENTIAL SIGNIFICANCE
Altered mental status	Medications (e.g., anticholinergic) Stress—internal or external Sensory overload Deprivation	Delirium Dementia Depression
Tremors	Cold exposure Muscle weakness	Parkinson's disease Cerebellar disease Chronic alcoholism Vitamin B deficiency Familial Essential tremor

Sensory System

Loss of visual acuity		Glaucoma, cataract, macular degeneration, diabetes
Hearing loss	Environmental noise Previous middle ear disease Vascular disease Cerumen impaction	Occlusion of canal Sensorineural disturbance Otosclerosis Paget's disease Ototoxic medication Vascular or mass lesions
Diminished tactile sensation		Vascular diseases Diabetes Neurological disorder
Altered taste sensation	Poor oral hygiene Respiratory illness	Zinc deficiency Smoking Drugs may affect taste Brain tumor in the parietal lobe Diabetes neuropathy
Altered sensation of smell	Respiratory illness	Drugs Brain tumor

Hematological System

Anemia	Blood loss Chronic disease	Iron deficiency Malabsorption
Leukemia		

Laboratory Values in the Older Adult

LABORATORY TEST	NORMAL VALUES	CHANGES WITH AGE	COMMENTS
Urinalysis			
Protein	0–5 mg/100 mL	Rises slightly	May be due to kidney changes with age, urinary tract infection, renal pathology
Glucose	0–15 mg/100 mL	Declines slightly	Glycosuria appears after high plasma level; unreliable
Specific gravity	1.005–1.020	Lower maximum in elderly 1.016–1.022	Decline in nephrons impairs ability to concentrate urine
Hematology			
Erythrocyte sedimentation rate	Men: 0–20 Women: 0–30	Significant increase	Neither sensitive or specific in aged
Iron	50–160 µg/dL	Slight decrease	
Iron binding	230–410 µg/dL	Decrease	
Hemoglobin	Men: 13–18 g/100 mL Women: 12–16 g/100 mL	Men: 10–17 g/mL Women: none noted	Anemia quite common in the elderly
Hematocrit	Men: 45–52% Women: 37–48%	Slight decrease speculated	Decline in hematopoiesis
Leukocytes	4300–10,800/cu mm	Drop to 3,100–9,000/cu mm	Decrease may be due to drugs or sepsis and should not be immediately attributed to age
Lymphocytes	500–2400 T cells/cu mm 50–200 B cells/cu mm	T-cell and B-cell levels fall	Infection risk higher; immunization encouraged
Platelets	150,000–350,000/cu mm	No change in number	

LABORATORY TEST	NORMAL VALUES	CHANGES WITH AGE	COMMENTS
Blood Chemistry			
Albumin	3.5–5.0/100 mL	Decline	Related to decrease in liver size and enzymes; protein energy malnutrition common
Globulin	2.3–3.5 g/100 mL	Slight increase	
Total serum protein	6.0–8.4 g/100 mL	No change	Decreases may indicate malnutrition, infection, liver disease
Blood urea nitrogen	Men: 10–25 mg/100 mL Women: 8–20 mg/100 mL	Increases significantly up to 69 mg/100 mL	Decline in glomerular filtration rate; decreased cardiac output
Creatinine	0.6–1.5 mg/100 mL	Increases to 1.9 mg/100 mL seen	Related to lean body mass decrease
Creatinine clearance	104–124 mL/min	Decreases 10%/decade after 40 years of age	Used for prescribing medications for drugs excreted by kidney
Glucose tolerance	62–110 mg/dL after fasting; less than 120 mg/dL after 2 hours postprandial	Slight increase of 10 mg/dL/decade after 30 years of age	Diabetes increasingly prevalent; drugs may cause glucose intolerance
Triglycerides	40–150 mg/100 mL	20–200 mg/100 mL	
Cholesterol	120–220 mg/100 mL	Men: increase to 50 mg/100 mL then decrease Women: increase post-menopausally	Risk of cardiovascular disease
Thyroxine (T_4)	4.5–13.5 mcg/100 mL	No change	Changes suggest thyroid disease; may be seen in euthyroid patients with acute or chronic illness or caloric deficiencies
Triiodothryronine (T_3)	90–220 ng/100 mL	Decrease 25%	
Thyroid-stimulating hormone (TSH)	0.5–5.0 mcgu/mL	Slight increase	Sensitive indicator for diagnosing thyroid disease

Appendix continued on following page

LABORATORY TEST	NORMAL VALUES	CHANGES WITH AGE	COMMENTS
Alkaline phosphatase	13–39 iu/L	Increase by 8–10 iu/L	Elevations greater than 20% usually due to disease; elevations may be found with bone abnormalities, drugs (e.g., narcotics), and eating a fatty meal

Data from Cavalieri et al. (1992); Davis (1993); Garner (1989); Kelso (1990); and Melillo (1993a, 1993b, 1993c).

Cognitive Assessment

Marilyn P. Williams
Sally A. Salisbury

PROLOGUE

A hospital room. Early morning.

PSYCHIATRIST: How many children do you have?

FATHER: They're not children.

PSYCHIATRIST: Who is the President?

FATHER: Don't you know?

PSYCHIATRIST: Where is your home?

FATHER: In the country behind a cluster of beautiful Australian pine trees. You're invited.

PSYCHIATRIST: Who takes care of you?

FATHER: Who takes care of you?

Late afternoon of the same day.

DAUGHTER: Father, why did you fool that psychiatrist?

FATHER: What psychiatrist?

DAUGHTER: The man who was in here after breakfast.

FATHER: Him? He didn't say so. Such a silly kid. Who sent him, anyway?

DAUGHTER: I don't know. But, why didn't you cooperate?

FATHER: I wanted to have some fun with him. I confused him so. He couldn't figure it out.

DAUGHTER: Oh, father, you should see what he wrote down.

FATHER: Relax, dear. You're much like your mother. What could he write down? I gave him nothing.

The following case was presented during a multidisciplinary team conference on the geropsychiatric evaluation unit of an urban teaching hospital. The psychiatric resident, presenting the case of a 70-year-old patient admitted with diagnoses of depression and dementia, read the following excerpt from the neuropsychologist's evaluation:

The patient is adequately oriented to place and time. Attention span is within normal limits. Visual perceptual ability on a matching model task is within normal limits. Immediate visual memory is defective and copying shows multiple errors. Recall of brief stories shows mild confabulation with normatively adequate information recall overall. Current background information on screening items is average, but more complex testing shows retrograde amnesia with a temporal gradient. These findings are consistent with Korsakoff's syndrome. The patient's failure on visual memory items also is characteristic, as is the confabulatory reporting of recent history. The patient also exhibits lack of insight, which leads to difficulty with reasoning and judgment. While the patient is not frankly demented by psychometric standards, the criteria for a diagnosis of Alcohol Amnestic Disorder are met.

Following this erudite summation, the patient's primary nurse interjected, "Yes, that's all very interesting, but can he zip up his fly?" Although flippant in tone, the question is clinically relevant. If cognitive assessment is to be meaningful for the practicing clinician, it must relate to clinical concerns of function and disability, disease process, and treatment response. The identification of a memory deficit in isolation has limited relevance for the practitioner.

This chapter defines cognitive assessment and discusses the role of mental status testing within the context of a more global assessment. Specific areas of mentation are defined, and factors that influence elderly patients' test performances are discussed. Standardized instruments are presented that have been selected for their ease of administration and established psychometric properties in elderly populations. The application of cognitive assessment skills, including mental status testing, allows the gerontological nurse to answer the question "Can he zip up his fly?" by being able to relate the results of cognitive assessment to day-to-day functioning.

COMPREHENSIVE ASSESSMENT OF COGNITIVE STATUS

Just as a physical examination follows a prescribed outline, the assessment of cognitive function is also performed in a systematic way. *Cognitive function* refers to the performance of intellectual tasks, such as thinking, remembering, perceiving, communicating, orienting, calculating, and problem solving (Gurland & Cross, 1982; Trzepacz & Baker, 1993). The information gathered includes formal mental status testing as well as other factors such as the patient's past and current functional status, general appearance, level of consciousness, emotional state, flow of speech and thought, content of thought, insight, and judgment (Adams, 1985; Trzepacz & Baker, 1993). It is only within the context of this information that mental status test scores can be interpreted and a comprehensive assessment of cognitive status accomplished. The following section provides an overview of the data to be obtained as part of a comprehensive cognitive assessment.

Functional Status

Assessing a person's past and present functional status gives critical information regarding his or her self-care abilities (see Chapter 9), as deficits in cognition eventually affect these abilities (see Chapter 18). Many different scenarios can exist among the elderly: One patient may be able to independently perform the instrumental activities of daily living, whereas another patient may exhibit a pattern of deficits, beginning in the more cognitive-dependent tasks of shopping, cooking, or managing finances or medications. Clinical experience has shown that by the time a person presents for a dementia workup, according to relatives' recollections at the time of the examination, he or she has had difficulty with some of these activities for well over a year. If cognitive deficits are suspected, information regarding functional status may have to be gleaned from sources other than the patient.

General Appearance

General appearance is the impression of overall physical health and a person's ability to maintain grooming and hygiene and select appropriate clothing. Much information can be learned about a patient's self-care ability from the condition of his or her clothing, hair, nails, and other outward signs. Jones and Williams (1988) emphasized that this ability to "size up" the patient by carefully and systematically observing him or her is an obvious yet underreported dimension of assessment.

Clinicians observing a person over time may become aware of slightly soiled clothes, buttons missing, or hems unraveling on a patient who previously presented with a meticulous appearance. By looking at a patient's clothes or the general appearance of his or her feet at the time of admission, hospital nurses can gain considerable information about the patient prior to admission.

Level of Consciousness

A critical component of the mental status assessment is an accurate observation of the level of consciousness (LOC). Terms must be used to relate the individual's state of awareness as objectively as possible. This helps not only in differentiating between dementia and delirium but also in monitoring a person over time. Four

TABLE 7-1	
Terms Used to Describe Level of Consciousness	

Hypervigilant	Acutely aware of surroundings. May startle with noise. Decreased attention span or ability to concentrate. Difficult to get or maintain patient's attention.
Alert	Awake; aware of self and environment. When spoken to in a normal voice, patient looks at you and responds fully and appropriately to stimuli.
Lethargic	When spoken to in a loud voice, appears drowsy but opens eyes and looks at you, responds to questions, and then falls asleep.
Obtunded	Patient responds after much stimulation. Awareness and interest in environment is decreased.
Comatose	Despite repeated painful stimuli, remains unarousable, with eyes closed. No evident response to inner need or external stimuli.

Adapted from Bates, B. (1995). *A pocket guide to physical examination and history taking.* Philadelphia: J.B. Lippincott.

well-used terms are *alert*, *lethargic*, *obtunded*, and *comatose* (Table 7–1).

The term *hypervigilant* can be added to this list to describe the common presentation of a person in a state of delirium. Hypervigilance is being acutely aware of one's surroundings and startling at unpredictable noise; it is often accompanied by a decreased attention span or ability to concentrate, which can exacerbate nurses' efforts to get and keep the patient's attention (Bates, 1995). Patients with delirium often have an altered LOC that is either hypervigilant or hypersomnolent (lethargic or obtunded). This altered LOC can make mental status testing difficult and may lead the clinician to suspect delirium. Dementia, on the other hand, has been referred to as "intellectual impairment in clear consciousness" (p. 22); thus, clinicians noting any alteration in LOC should suspect something other than or in addition to a dementia (Gallo et al., 1994) (see also Chapter 18).

Emotional State

Emotional state is concerned with mood and affect. Table 7–2 provides a list of the terms

TABLE 7-2
Definition of Terms

Term	Definition
Mood	A pervasive and sustained emotion that may markedly color a person's perception of the world. Examples of moods are depression, anxiety, and elation.
Affect	A subjectively experienced feeling state or emotion that is expressed by observable behavior.
Speech	The use of language to express ideas and thoughts.
Thought content	The ideas, meaning, connection, and progression of a patient's mental process expressed by language.
Insight	The ability to observe oneself and one's situation and to interpret this observation in a way that is consistent with the perceptions of others.
Judgment	Social judgment (as used in this chapter), defined as the ability to recognize social situations and the socially appropriate response in such situations and to apply the correct response when faced with the real situation.
Memory	The intellectual function that registers stimuli, stores them as perceptions, and retrieves them at will.
Attention	The ability to focus in a sustained manner on one activity.
Concentration	The effortful, deliberate, and heightened state of attention in which irrelevant stimuli are deliberately excluded from conscious awareness.
Perception	The intellectual function that integrates sensory impressions into meaningful data and to memory. Perceptual functions include activities such as awareness, recognition, discrimination, patterning, and orientation.
Orientation	Awareness of where one is in relation to time, place, person, and situation.
Language	An expressive intellectual function through which information is communicated or acted on.
Constructional praxis	The capacity to draw or construct two- or three-dimensional figures or shapes. This complex function depends on accurate visual perception, integration of perception into kinesthetic images, and translating the kinesthetic images into fine-motor patterns that do the construction.

Data from American Psychiatric Association (1994). *Diagnostic and statistical manual of mental disorders* (4th ed., pp. 763–771). Washington, D.C.: American Psychiatric Association; Lezak, M. (1995). *Neuropsychological assessment* (pp. 17–45). New York: Oxford University Press; and Strub, R., & Black, F. W. (Eds.). (1985). *The mental status examination in neurology* (pp. 100–101, 126). Philadelphia: F. A. Davis.

and definitions used in cognitive assessment. *Mood* "may be thought of as an internal emotional climate" (Mueller & Fogel, 1996, p. 20). It is pervasive and lasting—not fleeting or transient, as is an emotional reaction. Well elderly individuals, like younger well people, have a mood that is neither depressed nor overly cheerful. When asked how they feel, they do not complain of depression, agitation, or anxiety. Although loneliness and isolation may be common in the elderly, healthy older adults acknowledge the existence of these feelings without dwelling on them. Well people describe an adaptation and a general satisfaction with daily life—a sense of peace with themselves. A prevailing mood that the patient describes as painful or troublesome, which is generally caused by depression, is termed *dysphoric*.

Affect is the term used in psychiatry to describe the range of emotions that a person demonstrates during an interview. It is the outward display of the inner emotion (Mueller & Fogel, 1996). Affect is more transient than mood and in the well person fluctuates with both subject content and situation. In assessing affect, the examiner should note whether there is a range of expression and whether the feelings expressed are expected and related to the content and circumstances. Patients expressing sadness, hopelessness, or "feeling blue" may indicate a depression and may need to be further evaluated. Depression can influence scores on mental status examinations and should be considered if cognitive impairment is of recent onset in patients with either family or personal histories of depression (Gallo et al., 1994).

Flow of Speech and Thought

Flow of speech and thought is the least precise area of assessment. Conflicting definitions exist for the terms commonly used in the assessment of speech and thought, such as *blocking, word salad,* and *circumstantiality.* It is best to describe what patients say by using a few brief quotations from their speech. In general terms, the nurse can listen and determine whether the speech is fluent or coherent. Do thoughts follow a logical progression or does the patient

cling to one idea of thought and repeat it over and over (perseveration)? One patient, for example, when asked why he had come to the hospital, succinctly replied that he had a coherence problem. In fact his self-assessment was most apt. Although verbally fluent and cognitively intact, he was floridly psychotic.

The patient's thoughts are most easily explored in the context of an informal interview. A good place to begin is to ask about events that led the patient to seek or require treatment. If the patient is reluctant to discuss major conflicts, the interviewer may begin by exploring more neutral topics and then moving gradually toward more difficult conflict areas. This is an opportune time to gain a brief history, ascertain who is living in the patient's household, and learn what the patient's lifestyle is like. If the patient describes what sounds like an ideal active life, it is important to ask specifically when, for example, the last visit to a friend, the last fishing trip, or the last visit from children occurred.

While assessing a patient's thought content, nurses can examine problem-solving ability by asking situation questions. Examples of these questions might include "What would you do if you woke up ill, home alone, in the middle of the night?" or "What would you do in an airport in a strange city on discovering that your money and airplane ticket were lost?" These questions can be woven into conversation or framed as routine questions that one asks all new patients. The concept of futurity indicates a person's level of optimism and ability to set goals and think abstractly. This can be ascertained by asking, "What would you like to be doing a year from now?" People who are very depressed are often unwilling to think in terms of the future, and people with cognitive impairment are often unable to do so.

Insight and Judgment

Insight and judgment are critical areas that are easily assessed during a free-flowing conversation. *Insight* signifies that patients realize they are ill (if they are) and that they understand the nature of their illness. It does not refer to the psychodynamics of the illness. Insight may be assessed by asking the following sorts of questions: "Are you sick in any way?," "What sort of illness do you have?," or "What do you think would be most helpful for your recovery?"

A common finding regarding insight in the frail elderly is a lack of awareness of functional deficits. It is unclear if this lack of awareness is caused by denial, a beginning dementia, or some other factor. It can make some elderly people resistant to accepting assistance; these individuals reason that if there is no problem, there is no reason to get help.

Judgment is often best determined through a patient history obtained from informants. It may also be approximated by asking patients how they have handled their life and what recent decisions they have made about their healthcare and living situation. Impaired insight and judgment may be found in patients with functional disorders or dementing illnesses, and the resultant behaviors may make patients seem more demented than they actually are. This is illustrated in the following case study.

Case Study

An elderly man was admitted to an acute care psychiatric service after repeatedly attempting to leave his nursing home and assaulting the staff members there. During one of his attempts to leave, the highway patrol picked him up traveling down the center of the interstate highway in his wheelchair. He had been diagnosed as having Alzheimer's disease and 6 months before had suffered a stroke, with right hemiparesis of upper and lower extremities. Shortly after admission to the nursing home, he fell while getting out of bed and broke his right foot. Staff members quickly became discouraged because he refused to actively participate in his own rehabilitation activities. His moods fluctuated between tearful despondency and irritability.

When tested, he scored 25 out of 30 on the Folstein Mini-Mental State Examination. When time was spent with him in informal conversation, it became apparent that although he knew where he was and recalled recent and remote events well, he had absolutely no perception of himself as disabled. The man was enraged at

his wife for not taking him home. He also could not understand why his wife, who was receiving radiation treatments for abdominal cancer, was unable to care for him, since in his perception he did not require care. He explained his wheelchair ride on the interstate as simply "going home" and could not understand why it had caused such a fuss. Rather than attempt to change these aberrant perceptions, the nurse focused on improving the patient's health status by using his intact cognition to bargain with him. The patient was allowed to miss group therapy, which he abhorred, if he would practice self-care activities and ambulation during that time. Once the patient was ambulatory with a walker and was able to dress, groom, and feed himself, he could be placed in a more independent, albeit locked, setting rather than in a skilled nursing home. The irony was that the more physically rehabilitated the patient became, the more of an escape risk he posed, as his insight and judgment remained severely impaired.

Perception and Interpretation

All the cognitive processes described thus far are dependent on accurate perception. Patients with posterior occipital lobe lesions have difficulty processing visual information, and patients with temporal lobe lesions may have impaired sound localization. Parietal lobe lesions may cause astereognosis, the inability to recognize objects through tactile stimulation, and tactile localization may also be affected.

Parietal lobe lesions or middle cerebral artery strokes may produce contralateral inattention, in which patients do not attend to stimuli from the affected side. Affected patients may be unaware of this deficit. They may fail to dress or groom the affected side, for example, but be unaware that anything is amiss in this task performance. Lesions of the posterior temporal lobe and the angular gyrus and supramarginal gyrus (the general interpretive area) may prevent patients from integrating sensory input from auditory, visual, or sensory receptive areas. Such patients may hear, read, and retain sensation but may not recognize thoughts conveyed or the meaning of sensory stimuli (Boss, 1984).

A patient with bilateral temporal and frontal lobe involvement is hyperreceptive to stimuli and easily distracted and has a short attention span, short-term and recent memory deficits, and mixed aphasia. In addition, if a patient lacks interpretive and mitigating ability, his or her behavior may be combative and impulsive. It is nonproductive to attempt reasoning or problem solving with such a patient; he or she will respond best to short sessions with input limited to concrete, discrete bits of information. The initial focus may be on limiting the assaultive behavior.

ASSESSMENT OF SPECIFIC COGNITIVE DOMAINS

Mental status tests typically evaluate a variety of intellectual functions, of which memory, language, attention, and visuospatial skills are the most common.

Memory

Memory can be divided into three specific types: immediate, recent (short term), and long term. Immediate memory is that which is first activated when a person recognizes and responds to a stimulus. This system has a very limited capacity; normal memory for an adult, for example, involves the immediate recall of nine forward digits. Immediate memory formation is partially dependent on rehearsal and is highly affected by distraction. A person with a deficit in immediate memory may be able to remember only one of five digits forward. In terms of functional status, this person will not remember just taking medication or eating a meal. If asked to sit on a chair and wait for assistance with ambulation, he or she may get up and fall in the time it takes a nurse to locate a wheelchair. A person in a delirium may have difficulty with immediate memory, owing to a decreased ability to concentrate.

Recent or short-term memory is not dependent on rehearsal. Information in short-term memory is stored for a few minutes to a few days. Short-term memory is dependent on both the storage and retrieval of information; thus, immediate memory must be intact or storage will not be accomplished. Short-term memory deficits are the hallmark of most types of dementia. Instructions to a newly admitted hospitalized patient to turn on the call light before getting up will be quickly forgotten if the patient has a dementia and is unable to remember.

Remote or long-term memory formation requires the establishment of a relatively permanent neuronal change in the brain, which transfers information into a stable protein anagram. Patients may be unable to form immediate or recent memories but may recall material that was learned before the onset of their illness. A patient with brain damage who previously enjoyed watching football, for example, may recognize the plays as they are being made and be able to follow the action, but he will not be able to recall which teams are playing or what the score is.

Memory can also be divided into concepts of abilities to learn, retain, and recall information. Any deficit in immediate or short-term memory affects learning. Learning and recall are tested on mental status examinations by presenting a list of three to five words and asking the patient to recite these words. Typically only patients in a profound delirium or with an aphasia are unable to immediately repeat the words. Later in the examination, the patient is asked to recall the words. Poor recall of the words can indicate difficulty with immediate or recent memory. If words are not recalled, clues or a multiple choice list can be given. If there is no recall even after assistance has been given, the information has not been retained. Accurate recognition with clues indicates retention but poor retrieval.

Orientation questions are part of memory assessment on most tests. Stating the date, year, and day of the week as well as one's age and current location (if outside of home) requires short-term memory and indicates that new information has been learned. People with a moderate dementia are unable to correctly state their age but will typically be accurate regarding their date of birth. In general, long-term memory remains intact until late in a dementia and is not comprehensively assessed in mental status testing.

Language

As used here, *language* refers to a system integrating sensory and motor cerebral centers that enables people to communicate verbally and in writing. Approximately 90% of people are right-handed and have a left hemisphere dominance for language. Left-handed individuals generally have a mixed pattern of cerebral dominance. An evaluation of the language system involves fluency (spontaneous speech), comprehension, repetition, naming, reading, and writing (Mueller & Fogel, 1996; Strub & Black, 1985).

Spontaneous speech can be evaluated by asking uncomplicated open-ended questions such as, "Tell me about why you are in the hospital" or "What do you do on an ordinary day?" The patient's ability to produce spontaneous speech should be evaluated, observing for mispronunciation and difficulty in word finding as well as the rate and rhythm of speech.

Repetition is assessed by having the patient repeat a phrase or a short list of words. Reading comprehension can be assessed by asking the patient to read and carry out a short written command. Writing is best tested by having the patient write sentences that are dictated or that follow a theme suggested by the examiner (Mueller & Fogel, 1996). Table 7–3 summarizes some of the more common language disorders.

In general, patients with aphasia cannot be tested with the screening tools described in this chapter. Once expressive aphasia has been determined, the patient should also be assessed for receptive aphasia, defined as an inability to comprehend. Comprehension, a person's ability to demonstrate understanding of spoken language, is best tested by asking patients to use a simple verbal or motor response to demonstrate that they understand the examiner. This can be accomplished by asking questions that can be answered "yes" or "no" or by having the patient point to common objects. If given more elaborate instructions, patients may fail because of apraxia or memory deficits rather than a lack of comprehension.

Attention

Attention, the ability to focus and sustain mental activity, involves both arousal and concentration. The prefrontal area of the cerebral cortex enables an individual to maintain a focus of attention, concentrate on a sequence of memories or thoughts, and encode and classify incoming sensory information. Without an ability to maintain one's focus of attention, a person becomes distracted and loses his or her train of thought. Such a person may be able to do a one-step arithmetic problem but unable to answer a complex or serial question. The prefrontal area and certain subcortical and right hemispheric areas enable one to maintain attention and effectively perform executive functions such as goal formulation, planning, and carrying out goal-directed plans (Lezak, 1995).

A change in LOC affecting attention and concentration is a hallmark of delirium; it also makes testing a person in a delirium difficult, leading to low test scores (Morency, 1990). LOC must therefore be taken into account when performing mental status tests. As previously noted, without a superimposed delirium most patients with a dementia do not exhibit an attention deficit.

Visuospatial Skills

This component of mental status testing follows a more traditional testing format, in that paper and pencil are needed. Typically, the patient is asked to copy a design or draw a clock (Folstein et al., 1975). Testing this component can give information regarding hemineglect, planning abilities, and the patient's understanding of spatial relationships within a certain space and among parts of the drawing (Sultzer, 1994). Visuospatial deficits are apparent in patients with Alzheimer's disease and certain types of strokes (see Figure 7–1 for examples of clock drawings).

FORMAL MENTAL STATUS TESTING

Providers often describe patients as confused, disoriented, or combative. The vagueness of such terms offers no help in determining the cause or extent of deficits or possible manage-

TABLE 7-3
Language Disorders

Type of Aphasia	Manifestation	Affected Brain Area
Global	Spontaneous speech absent or limited to a few stereotyped words Comprehension reduced to patient's name or few words	Posterior and anterior cortical areas
Nonfluent aphasia	Telegraphic speech, conjunctions and pronouns not used Repetition and reading aloud impaired Naming may show paraphasias Auditory and reading comprehension intact Frequent frustration, agitation, and depression	Anterior speech area Right-sided hemiplegia
Fluent aphasia	Severe disturbance in auditory comprehension Speech well articulated but lacks meaningful content, is unrelated to questions, has paraphasias Patient seems unaware he or she does not make sense; reading and writing are impaired	Posterior language area
Conduction aphasia	Fluent, halting speech, word-finding pauses, paraphasias Comprehension good, naming disturbed, reading unimpaired; writing shows errors in spelling, word choice, syntax	Supramarginal gyrus and arcuate fasciculus between anterior and posterior areas
Anomic aphasia	Word-finding difficulty, inability to name objects on confrontation; repetition good; may have alexia (inability to read) or agraphia (inability to write)	Can be caused by lesions in many parts of dominant hemisphere
Articulation disturbances (dysarthrias)	Buccofacial apraxia (inability to control muscles needed for speech) Dysfluency (stuttering or stammering)	Lesions between supramarginal gyrus and frontal lobe Etiology not known

Adapted from Strub, R., & Black, F. W. (Eds.). (1985). *The mental status examination in neurology.* Philadelphia: F. A. Davis.

ment strategies. Nurses can use brief, quantitative mental status examinations to assess the presence and severity of cognitive impairment in their patients. The tests are not intended for diagnostic purposes. However, when test results are interpreted according to the categories of information described in prior sections, mental status examinations can provide valuable objective data. These data allow practitioners to communicate findings in objective, measurable terms.

The frequency with which nurses working with the elderly use these mental status examinations is unknown. However, in a study of hospitalized patients older than 65 years of age, McCartney & Palmateer (1985) found that 79% of cognitive deficits were missed by examining physicians. Of the 394 examinations performed on 165 patients, only 4 mental status examinations were documented. Considering that clinicians revere objective data and would never guess a blood pressure or feel a forehead

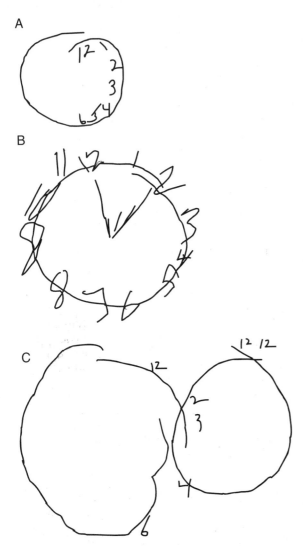

FIGURE 7-1. Examples of clock drawings. *A,* Left-sided neglect in a patient with a right hemispheric lesion. *B,* Poor visuospatial skills in a patient with multi-infarct dementia. *C,* Poor visuospatial skills in a patient with dementia of an unknown cause.

having blood drawn, and so forth. Even invasive testing often goes unchallenged. With the use of mental status testing, however, the clinician tests the ability of the person to think, often causing discomfort for the patient as well as the practitioner. The clinician's attitude is critical in setting the tone of the testing.

Some clinicians advise promoting a casual, nonthreatening atmosphere for a mental status examination by attempting to "sneak" the questions into conversation. In practice, however, it then becomes impossible to complete a formal test. Gurland (1992) suggested setting mental status questions within the context of doing a thorough health and social assessment. When the 5- to 10-minute tests (described later in this chapter) are administered with the same sense of routine as the taking of a blood pressure, the testing often becomes less threatening. Informal clinical experience has shown that fewer than 10% of patients have refused formal testing when approached in this manner.

The following are examples of ways of introducing mental status testing in different clinical situations:

- Establishing baseline mental status: "I'm going to ask you some questions to test your thinking. Some may seem dumb, some may be difficult, but I ask them of everyone so please bear with me."
- Establishing baseline mental status and monitoring a patient with a stroke over time: "You've had a stroke and sometimes it affects your thinking. I'm going to ask you some questions to see how you're doing right now."
- Ongoing assessment of patient in a possible delirium: "You're having some problems thinking right now, and we're trying to determine why. I'm going to ask you some questions to see how you're doing right now."

To alleviate further anxiety when administering the test, the advanced practice nurse must use experience, intuition, and common sense in deciding whether to pursue a question in which the wrong answer or no answer is given. Coaxing may improve performance in a patient with a probable depression but not in a patient

to document a fever, the reluctance to perform formal mental status testing is puzzling.

Introduction of Testing

People seeking healthcare take as a matter of course being weighed, having x-rays taken,

with a probable dementia. A patient who may be in a delirium may need constant refocusing to respond correctly to questions and will most likely fail any task requiring concentration. To develop this expertise, advanced practice nurses must perform tests routinely and become aware of the nuances of the various presentations.

Selection and Use of Instruments

Exponential growth in the fields of psychobiology (Restak, 1979) and neuropsychology (Lezak, 1995; Rao, 1996; Reitan & Davison, 1974) has greatly enhanced psychologists' ability to use formal testing to evaluate specific cerebral function. The tests used in this type of assessment are invaluable in assisting with diagnosis, identifying specific deficits, establishing normative values, and monitoring progression. Shorter tests have been developed for use by general healthcare professionals in clinical practice.

Mental status instruments are identified that have been age-adjusted and have shown validity and reliability in clinical settings. Care has been taken to select those tests that can be administered quickly in any setting. Methods that require elaborate instrumentation for their administration and scoring are intentionally omitted. The four instruments presented can be used by the advanced practice nurse to identify strengths and deficits and measure small increments of change either in a single patient or in a group of patients over time. The particular mental status test used is often dependent on the clinical setting and the clinician. There is, however, no doubt that formal testing beyond simple orientation questions must be used (Siu, 1991).

SHORT PORTABLE MENTAL STATUS QUESTIONNAIRE

Pfeiffer's Short Portable Mental Status Questionnaire (SPMSQ; 1975) consists of 10 questions that assess short-term memory, long-term memory, orientation to surroundings, and attention (Appendix 7–1). It was developed to test a range of intellectual performance from intact functioning to severe impairment. Ratings are made on the basis of errors: 0 to 2 (errors) = intact status, 3 to 4 = mild intellectual impairment, 5 to 7 = moderate intellectual impairment, and 8 to 10 = severe intellectual impairment.

Because the SPMSQ requires no special training and is quickly administered and scored, it is widely used. It does, however, have significant flaws. Nursing home residents or isolated elderly people may experience each day as just like another and be unaware of the day or date (Hays & Borger, 1985). Using a cutoff point of three errors, a Finnish study demonstrated its usefulness in screening for dementia in a medical inpatient, community-dwelling elderly sample. The same study found cutoff scores impossible to define for patients with delirium, owing to its variable presentation (Erkinjuntti et al., 1987). More recently, Moritz and colleagues (1995) used the SPMSQ to predict the onset of future limitations in the activities of daily living and found that four or more errors predicted limitations and could be used to forecast service needs.

Because of its brevity and simplicity, nurses may choose to use this tool to obtain baseline data on a population, to screen patients who are obviously severely demented or cognitively intact, or to assess and reassess a patient with a mental status change. A baseline SPMSQ performed during a person's optimal functioning provides invaluable information to a clinician who is seeing a patient for the first time. Finally, because this tool can be easily taught, it may be useful to advance practice nurses who are responsible for upgrading the assessment skills of others working with the elderly; its use and importance will become readily apparent to those providing hands-on care. People administering the test must use caution to avoid an overreliance on scores and to place the scores within the context of other assessment data previously obtained.

FOLSTEIN MINI-MENTAL STATE EXAMINATION

The Folstein Mini-Mental State Examination (MMSE) is a more comprehensive instrument that measures short-term memory, long-term memory, orientation, attention, calculation, registration, language, praxis, and copying of a design (Anthony et al., 1982; Folstein et al., 1975; Karuza et al., 1997) (Appendix 7–2). It can be administered in less than 10 minutes; additional time is needed if the person being tested has pronounced impairments (Zarit, 1997). The MMSE has demonstrated both reliability and validity, with test scores correlated with age-adjusted scores on the Wechsler Adult Intelligence Scale. Some specificity and sensitivity is lost when the test is used with minority or non–English speaking people (Zarit, 1997).

The advantage of this test is that it clearly tests short-term memory by asking the patient to recall three previously identified words. It also tests reading and writing ability and the ability to copy a design and follow a three-step command. A score of 23 points or less (out of 30) for a person with more than 8 years of formal education is indicative of cognitive impairment. Scores increase with educational level, and thus lower scores must take into account the extent of formal schooling (Crum et al., 1993).

As noted previously, the loss of short-term memory is the hallmark of a dementia. Consequently, in a person with Alzheimer's disease, items most likely to be missed are the recall of the three previously identified words, the date, and serial numbers. Although the orientation questions alone demonstrate low sensitivity in detecting dementia, they are most frequently used to test mental status (Ashford et al., 1989).

As nurses gain expertise in mental status testing, they should be aware of the typical pattern of deficits with dementia. Low scores without errors in recall, date, or serial numbers may indicate a diagnosis other than dementia. Dementia is a possible diagnosis when deficits follow a more typical pattern combined with a slow decline in functional status.

Nurses should be knowledgeable in administering both the SPMSQ and the Folstein MMSE for screening and monitoring purposes. If a patient has a limited attention span (e.g., a person who is in a delirium), the shorter test should be used. If deficits in the SPMSQ do not fit a pattern or do not explain serious functional deficits, the MMSE may be administered to further define cognitive deficits.

COGNITIVE CAPACITY SCREENING EXAMINATION

As with the MMSE, the Cognitive Capacity Screening Examination can be used to refine knowledge of suspected cognitive impairment (Jacobs et al., 1977). It contains 30 items and can be administered in 15 to 30 minutes by a healthcare professional; no special training is required. Each item is scored as one point, and a score of less than 20 (out of 30) indicates cognitive impairment (Karuza et al., 1997). This test measures orientation, concentration, attention, mental control, language functions of repetition and concept formation, and short-term memory. It has an advantage over other tests in that it contains guidelines for further exploration if cognitive impairment is present. Many of the items are repetitious, however, and, like the MMSE test, its strengths are reliability and validity, not sensitivity; false negatives are frequent (Nelson et al., 1986).

NEUROBEHAVIORAL COGNITIVE STATUS EXAMINATION

The Neurobehavioral Cognitive Status Examination (NCSE) independently assesses multiple domains of cognitive function: LOC, attention, concentration, constructions, memory, calculations, and reasoning (Appendix 7–3). Language is assessed in the areas of fluency, comprehension, repetition, and naming (Kiernan et al., 1987). The test has been validated and standardized using a geriatric population. Because it uses a screen and metric approach, it can be completed in 5 minutes by nonimpaired patients and in 20 minutes by most patients with impairments. The two-page test booklet is accompanied by a training manual and can be administered by professional healthcare providers after self-teaching. Although it is more difficult to use than other tests, the NCSE provides more patient information than the presence or absence of cognitive impairment (Kiernan et al., 1987). In addition, it has demonstrated more sensitivity than either the MMSE or the CCSE (Schwamm et al., 1987). The NCSE can be obtained from the Northern California Neurobehavioral Group, Inc., P.O. Box 460, Fairfax, California, 94978.

CLINICAL APPLICATION AND SUMMARY

Given the increasing incidence of cognitive impairment with age, its deleterious effects on functioning, and the possibility of identifying and treating reversible causes, the assessment of cognitive function should be an integral part of nurses' practice in working with the elderly. The process of cognitive assessment described here is intended to be a framework within which the practicing nurse interacts with patients and caregivers to gather data. The assessment is both systematic and deliberative, using interview and formal testing techniques.

Cognitive function is not static; it should be performed initially to establish a baseline and whenever a change in behavior, mental status, or level of functioning is a cause of concern. An accurate cognitive assessment constitutes an integral component of the practice of gerontological nursing.

REFERENCES

Adams, S. (1985). *Mental Status Examination: RN skills orientation to inpatient psychiatry*. Palo Alto, CA: Veterans Administration Medical Center.

Anthony, J. C., LeResche, L., Niaz, U., & von Korff, M. R. (1982). Limits of the Mini-Mental State as a screening test for dementia and delirium among hospital patients. *Psychological Medicine, 12*, 397–408.

Ashford, J. W., Kolm, P., Colliver, J., et al. (1989). Alzheimer patient evaluation and the Mini-Mental State: Item characteristic curve analysis. *Journal of Gerontology, 44*, 139–146.

Bates, B. (1995). *A pocket guide to physical examination and history taking*. Philadelphia: J. B. Lippincott.

Boss, P. S. (1984). Acute mood and behavior disturbances of neurological origin: Acute confusional states. *Journal of Neurosurgical Nursing, 14*, 61–68.

Crum, R., Anthony, J., Bassett, S., & Folstein, M. (1993). Population-based norms for the Mini-Mental State Examination by age and educational level. *Journal of the American Medical Association, 269*, 2386–2391.

Erkinjuntti, M. D., Sulkava, R., Wikstrom, J., & Autio, L. (1987). Short Portable Mental Status Questionnaire as a screening test for dementia and delirium among the elderly. *Journal of American Geriatrics Society, 35*, 412–416.

Folstein, M., Folstein, S. E., & McHugh, P. (1975). Mini-Mental State, a practical method for grading the cognitive state of patients for the clinician. *Journal of Psychiatric Research, 12*, 189–198.

Gallo, J., Reichel, W., & Andersen, L. (1994). *Handbook of geriatric assessment*. Gaithersburg, MD: Aspen Publications.

Gurland, B. J. (1992). The assessment of the mental health status of older adults. In J. E. Birren & R. B. Sloane (Eds.), *Handbook of mental health and aging* (pp. 220–248). Englewood Cliffs, NJ: Prentice-Hall.

Gurland, B. J., & Cross, P. (1982). The epidemiology of psychopathology in old age: Some clinical implications. *Psychiatric Clinics of North America, 5*(1), 11–26.

Hays, A., & Borger, F. (1985). A test in time. *American Journal of Nursing, 85*, 1107–1111.

Jacobs, J. W., Bernard, M. R., Delgado, A., & Strain, J. (1977). Screening for organic mental syndromes in the medically ill. *Annals of Internal Medicine, 86*, 40–46.

Jones, T., & Williams, M. (1988). Rethinking the approach to evaluating mental functioning of older persons: The value of careful observations. *Journal of the American Geriatrics Society, 36*, 1128–1134.

Karuza, J., Katz, P. K., & Henderson, R. (1997). Cognitive screening. In E. Andresen, B. Rothenberg & J. G. Zimmer (Eds.), *Assessing the health status of older adults* (pp. 143–179). New York: Springer.

Kiernan, R., Mueller, J., Langston, W. J., & Van Dyke, C. (1987). The Neurobehavioral Mental Status Examination: A brief but differential cognitive assessment. *Annals of Internal Medicine, 197*, 481–485.

Lezak, M. D. (1995). *Neuropsychological assessment* (3rd ed.). New York: Oxford University Press.

McCartney, J., & Palmateer, L. (1985). Assessment of cognitive deficit in geriatric patients: A study of physician behavior. *Journal of the American Geriatrics Society, 33*, 467–471.

Morency, C. (1990). Mental status change in the elderly: Recognizing and treating delirium. *Journal of Professional Nursing, 6*, 356–365.

Moritz, D. J., Berkman, L. F., & Kasl, S. V. (1995). Cognitive functioning and the incidence of limitation in activities of daily living in an elderly community sample. *American Journal of Epidemiology, 141*, 41–49.

Mueller, J., & Fogel, B. S. (1996). Neuropsychiatric examination. In B. S. Fogel & R. B. Schiffer (Eds.), *Neuropsychiatry* (pp. 11–28). Baltimore: Williams & Wilkins.

Nelson, A., Fogel, B. S., & Faust, D. (1986). Bedside cognitive screening instruments: A critical assessment. *Journal of Nervous & Mental Disease, 174*, 73–83.

Pfeiffer, E. (1975). A Short Portable Mental Status Questionnaire for the assessment of organic brain deficits in elderly patients. *Journal of the American Geriatrics Society, 23*, 433–441.

Rao, S. M. (1996). Neuropsychological assessment. In B. S. Fogel & R. B. Schiffer (Eds.), *Neuropsychiatry* (pp. 29–45). Baltimore: Williams & Wilkins.

Reitan, R. M., & Davison, L. A. (1974). *Clinical neuropsychology: Current status and applications*. New York: Winston/Wiley.

Restak, R. M. (1979). *The brain: The last frontier*. New York: Warner.

Schwamm, L. H., Van Dyke, C., Kiernan, R. J., et al. (1987). The Neurobehavioral Cognitive Status Examination: Comparison with the cognitive capacity screening examination and the mini-mental state examination in a neurological population. *Annals of Internal Medicine, 107*, 486–491.

Siu, A. (1991). Screening for dementia and investigating its causes. *Annals of Internal Medicine, 115,* 122–131.

Strub, R., & Black, P. W. (1985). *The mental status examination in neurology.* Philadelphia: F. A. Davis.

Sultzer, D. (1994). Mental status examination. In C. Coffey & J. Cummings (Eds.), *Textbook of geriatric neuropsychiatry* (pp. 111–127). Washington, D.C.: American Psychiatric Press.

Trzepacz, P. T., & Baker, R. W. (1993). *The psychiatric mental status examination.* New York: Oxford University Press.

Zarit, S. M. (1997). Brief measures of depression and cognitive function. *Generations, 21,* 41–43.

7-1

Short Portable Mental Status Questionnaire

1. What is the date today (month, day, year)?
2. What day of the week is it?
3. What is the name of this place?
4. What is your telephone number?
4A. What is your street address? (Ask only if the patient does not have a telephone.)
5. How old are you?
6. When were you born?
7. Who is the president of the United States now?
8. Who was president just before him?
9. What was your mother's maiden name?
10. Subtract 3 from 20 and keep subtracting 3 from each new number, all the way down.

INSTRUCTIONS FOR COMPLETION OF THE SHORT PORTABLE MENTAL STATUS QUESTIONNAIRE

Ask the subject questions 1 through 10 in this list and record all answers. All responses to be scored correct must be given by subject without reference to calendar, newspaper, birth certificate, or other aid to memory.

Question 1 is scored correct only when the exact month, exact date, and the exact year are given correctly.
Question 2 is self-explanatory.
Question 3 is scored correct if any correct description of the location is given. "My home," the correct name of the town or city of residence, or the name of hospital or institution if the subject is institutionalized are all acceptable.

Question 4 is scored correct when the telephone number can be verified or when the subject can repeat the same number at a different point in the conversation.
Question 5 is scored correct when the stated age corresponds to the date of birth.
Question 6 is to be scored correct only if the month, date, and year are all given.
Question 7 requires only the last name of the president.
Question 8 requires only the last name of the previous president.
Question 9 does not need to be verified. It is scored correct if a female first name plus a last name other than the subject's last name is given.
Question 10 is scored correct only when the entire series is performed correctly. Any error in the series or unwillingness to attempt the series is scored as incorrect.

SCORING OF THE SHORT PORTABLE MENTAL STATUS QUESTIONNAIRE

For the purposes of scoring, three educational levels have been established: (a) people who have only a grade school education; (b) persons who have had any high school education or who have completed high school; (c) persons who have had any education beyond the high school level, including college, graduate school, or business school.

For white subjects with at least some, but not more than, high school education, the following criteria have been established:

0–2 errors: Intact intellectual function
3–4 errors: Mild intellectual impairment

Adapted from Pfeiffer, E. (1975). A short portable mental status questionnaire for the assessment of organic brain deficit in the elderly patient. *Journal of the American Geriatrics Society, 23*(10), 433–441.

5–7 errors: Moderate intellectual impairment
8–10 errors: Severe intellectual impairment
Allow one more error if subject has had only a grade school education.

Allow one less error if subject has had education beyond high school.
Allow one more error for black subjects using identical education criteria.

APPENDIX 7 - 2

Mini-Mental State Examination

_____/30 correct

What is the year?	(1)
season?	(1)
month?	(1)
date (#1)?	(1)
day of the week?	(1)
part of the day?	
time of day (+1 hour)?	
What is the name of this place?	(1)
What street is it on?	
What floor are we on?	(1)
How long have we been here?	
What is the name of this city?	(1)
What is the name of this county?	(1)
What is the name of this state?	(1)

Please repeat the following three words. (shirt, brown, honesty)

I would like you to remember these three words.

What are they?   Immediate Recall _____ (111)

Repeat the three words until the patient learns all three.

What are they?   Number of trials _____

Spell the word "world" _____

Now spell the word "world" backwards _____ (11111)

From Folstein, M., Folstein, S. G., & McHugh, P. (1975). Mini-Mental State, a practical method for grading the cognitive state of patients for the clinician. _Journal of Psychiatric Research, 12,_ 189–198.

Do you remember the three words I gave you a few minutes ago?

_____   _____   _____ (111)

What is this called?   (Pencil) _____ (1)

(Watch) _____ (1)

Please repeat the following phrase.

I would like to go home _____

No ifs, ands, or buts _____ (1)

Listen carefully, I want you to: (111)

( ) Take the paper in your right hand

( ) Fold it in half, and

( ) Put it on the floor

Do what this says: "Close your eyes." (1)

Write a sentence. (1)

(If the patient cannot write a sentence spontaneously, dictate: "This is a very nice day.")

Copy a design: (1)

APPENDIX │ 7 - 3 │

Neurobehavioral Cognitive Status Examination

Name: _____   Occupational Status: _____

Age and Date of Birth: _____   Date: _____

Native Language: _____   Time: _____

Handedness (circle): L   R   Examiner: _____

Level of Education: _____   Examination Location: _____

COGNITIVE STATUS PROFILE*

	LOC	ORI	ATT	COMP	REP	NAM	CONST	MEM	CALC	SIM	JUD
				LANGUAGE						REASONING	
†AVERAGE RANGE							--6--			--8--	--6--
	--ALERT--	--12--	--(S)8--	--(S)6--	--(S)--	--(S)--	--(S)5--	--12--	--(S)4--	--(S)6--	--(S)5--
					--12--	--8--					
		--10--	--6--	--5--	--11--	--7--	--4--	--10--	--3--	--5--	--4--
MILD	--IMP--	--8--	--4--	--4--	--9--	--5--	--3--	--8--	--2--	--4--	--3--
MODERATE		--6--	--2--	--3--	--7--	--3--	--2--	--6--	--1--	--3--	--2--
SEVERE		--4--	--0--	--2--	--5--	--2--	--0--	--4--	--0--	--2--	--1--
Write in lower scores			X				X		X		

ABBREVIATIONS:

ATT — Attention
CALC — Calculations
COMP — Comprehension
CONST— Constructions
IMP — Impaired

JUD — Judgment
LOC — Level of Consciousness
MEM— Memory
NAM— Naming

ORI— Orientation
REP— Repetition
S — Screen
SIM— Similarities

*The validity of this examination depends on administration in strict accordance with the Neurobehavioral Cognitive Status Examination (NCSE) manual.

†For patients older than 65 years of age, the average range extends to the "mild impairment level" for Constructions, Memory, and Similarities.

Note: Not all brain lesions produce cognitive deficits that will be detected by the NCSE. Normal scores, therefore, cannot be taken as evidence that brain pathology does *not* exist. Similarly, scores falling in the mild, moderate, or severe range of impairment do not *necessarily* reflect brain dysfunction (see the section of the NCSE manual entitled "Cautions in Interpretation").

NEUROBEHAVIORAL COGNITIVE STATUS EXAMINATION

Record patient's responses verbatim.

I. LEVEL OF CONSCIOUSNESS

Alert _____ Lethargic _____ Fluctuating _____

Describe patient's condition: _____

II. ORIENTATION (Score 2, 1, or 0 points, as shown in parentheses.)

		Response	*Score*
A. Person	1. Name (0)	_____	____
	2. Age (2)	_____	____
B. Place	1. Current location (2)	_____	____
	2. City (2)	_____	____
C. Time	1. Date: mo (1) ____ day (1) ____ yr (2) ____		____
	2. Day of week (1)	_____	____
	3. Time of day within 1 hr (1)	_____	____

Total Score ____

III. ATTENTION

A. Digit Repetition
   1. Screen: 8-3-5-2-9-1   Pass ____   Fail ____
   2. Metric: Graded digit repetition (Score 1 or 0; discontinue after 2 misses at one level.)

	Score		*Score*		*Score*		*Score*
3-7-2	____	5-1-4-9	____	8-3-5-2-9	____	2-8-5-1-6-4	____
4-9-5	____	9-2-7-4	____	6-1-7-3-8	____	9-1-7-5-8-2	____

Total Score ____

B. Four-Word Memory Task
   Give the four unrelated words from Section VI: robin, carrot, piano, green. (Alternate list: table, lion, orange, glove.) Have patient repeat the four words twice correctly (see manual) and record the number of trials required to do this: ____.

IV. LANGUAGE

A. Speech Sample
   1. Fishing picture (Record patient's response verbatim.)

   _____

   _____

   _____

   _____

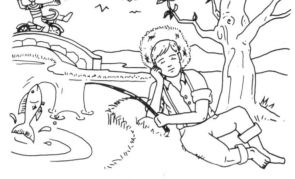

B. Comprehension (Be sure to have at least three other objects in front of the patient for this test.) If a, b, and c are successfully completed, praxis for these tasks is assumed normal.
   1. Screen: Three-step command: "Turn over the paper, hand me the pen, and point to your nose."

   Pass _____   Fail _____

   2. Metric: (Score 1 or 0.) If incorrect, describe behavior.

	Response	Score
a. Pick up the pen.	_____	____
b. Point to the floor.	_____	____
c. Hand me the keys.	_____	____
d. Point to the pen and pick up the keys.	_____	____
e. Hand me the paper and point to the coin.	_____	____
f. Point to the keys, hand me the pen, and pick up the coin.	_____	____
	Total Score	____

C. Repetition
1. Screen: The beginning movement revealed the composer's intention.

_____

Pass _____   Fail _____

2. Metric: (Score 2 if first try correct; 1 if second try correct; 0 if incorrect.)

Response   *Score*

a. Out the window.   _____ _____

b. He swam across the lake.   _____ _____

c. The winding road led to the village. _____ _____

d. He left the latch open.   _____ _____

e. The honeycomb drew a swarm of bees. _____ _____

f. No ifs, ands, or buts.   _____ _____

Total Score _____

D. Naming
1. Screen: a) Pen _____   b) Cap or top _____   c) Clip _____   d) Point, tip or nib _____

Pass _____   Fail _____

2. Metric: (Score 1 or 0.)

	Response	*Score*		*Response*	*Score*
a. Shoe	_____	___	e. Horseshoe	_____	___
b. Bus	_____	___	f. Anchor	_____	___
c. Ladder	_____	___	g. Octopus	_____	___
d. Kite	_____	___	h. Xylophone	_____	___

Total Score _____

A

B

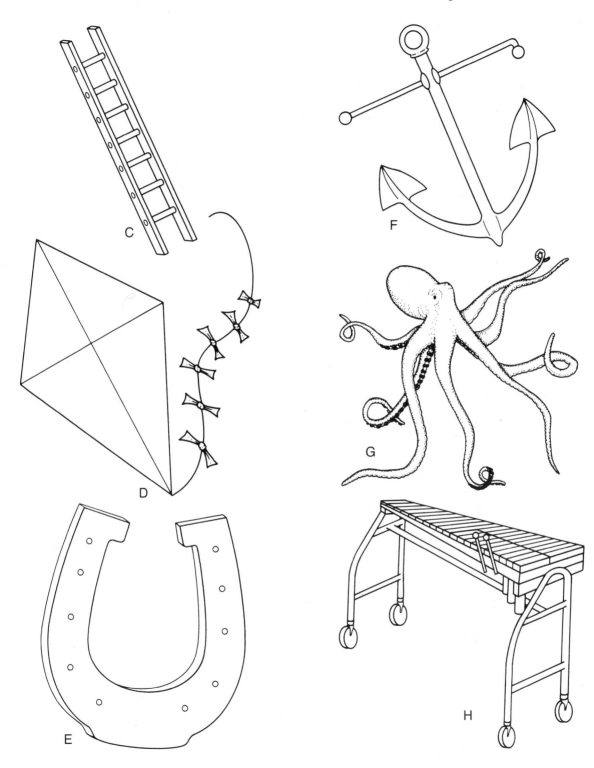

V. CONSTRUCTIONAL ABILITY

A. Screen: Visual Memory Task (Present stimulus sheet for 10 seconds, then have patient draw the two figures from memory. Must be perfect to pass. The examiner may wish to have patients who fail the screen copy the two figures.)

Pass _____   Fail _____

B. Metric: Design Constructions (Score 2 if correct in 0–30 seconds; 1 if correct in 31–60 seconds; 0 if correct in greater than 60 seconds or incorrect.)

		Record incorrect attempts below		*Time*	*Score*

Place squares in front of patient as shown here:

1. Design 1: _____ _____
2. Design 2: _____ _____
3. Design 3: _____ _____

Total Score _____

VI. MEMORY

(Score 3 if recalled without prompting; 2 if recalled with category prompt; 1 if recognized from list; 0 if not recognized.) Check if correct.

Words	*Check*	*Category Prompt*	*Check if Response*	*List (circle)*	*Score*
Robin	_____	Bird	_____	Sparrow, robin, bluejay	_____
Carrot	_____	Vegetable	_____	Carrot, potato, onion	_____
Piano	_____	Musical instrument	_____	Violin, guitar, piano	_____
Green	_____	Color	_____	Red, green, yellow	_____

Incorrect initial response: _____   Total Score _____

VII. CALCULATIONS

A. Screen: 5 × 13   Response: _____   Time: _____ (Must be correct within 20 seconds.)

Pass _____   Fail _____

B. Metric: (Score 1 point if correct within 20 seconds.) Problems may be repeated, but time runs continuously from first presentation.

	Response	Time	Score
1. How much is 5 + 3?	_____	_____	_____
2. How much is 15 + 7?	_____	_____	_____
3. How much is 39 ÷ 3?	_____	_____	_____
4. How much is 31 − 8?	_____	_____	_____

Total Score _____

VIII. REASONING

A. Similarities: (Explain "A hat and a coat are alike because they are both articles of clothing." If patient does not respond, encourage; if patient gives differences, score 0.)

1. Screen: Painting-music (Must be abstract—only "art," "artistic," or "forms of art" are acceptable.)

Pass _____   Fail _____

2. Metric: (Score 2 if abstract; 1 if imprecisely abstract or concrete; 0 if incorrect.) See manual for examples. Check if abstract.

	Check	Abstract Concept	Other Responses	Score
a. Rose-tulip	_____	Flowers	_____	_____
b. Bicycle-train	_____	Transportation	_____	_____
c. Watch-ruler	_____	Measurement	_____	_____
d. Corkscrew-hammer	_____	Tools	_____	_____

Total Score _____

B. Judgment

1. Screen: What would you do if you were stranded in the Denver airport with only $1.00 in your pocket?

_____

_____

Pass _____   Fail _____

2. Metric: (Score 2 if correct; 1 if partially correct; 0 if incorrect.)

a. What would you do if you woke up 1 minute before 8:00 A.M. and remembered an important appointment downtown at 8:00 A.M.?

_____

_____

Score _____

b. What would you do if you were walking beside a lake and you saw a 2-year-old child playing alone at the end of a pier?

_____

_____

Score _____

c. What would you do if you came home and found that a broken pipe was flooding the kitchen?

_____

_____

Score _____

Total Score _____

IX. MEDICATIONS

List *all* current medications and dosages:

1. _____   2. _____   3. _____   4. _____

5. _____   6. _____   7. _____   8. _____

X. GENERAL COMMENTS

Note any known or observed motor, sensory, or perceptual deficits that may affect test performance (e.g., impaired visual or auditory acuity, tremor, apraxia, dysarthria):

_____

_____

_____

Note "process features" such as distractability, frustration, exhaustion, and nature of cooperation. The patient's impression of his or her performance should also be noted here.

_____

_____

_____

_____

Space for Visual Memory Task

Assessment of Social Support

Linda R. Phillips

Humans, regardless of age, are social creatures, and for many reasons the structures and processes through which they give and receive social support are essential to human welfare. First, social support plays an essential role in promoting and maintaining mental health. It provides individuals with an affirmation of personhood, information and feedback, and opportunities for reciprocal intimacy and affection. Second, some evidence suggests that social support has an important role in alleviating stress and that mental and physical health are intimately linked through immune mechanisms. Thus, social support may be essential for promoting, maintaining, and restoring

physical health.* Last, at any age, dependency on others is part of the human condition; all humans depend on others for assistance on a daily basis and during times of trouble. Therefore, social support, the medium through which most dependency needs are met, is closely associated with continued survival.

Although social support is essential for a

---

*Excellent literature reviews and critiques on this topic include Berkman (1984), Cohen & Syme (1985), Cohen & Wills (1983), Dimond & Jones (1983), Gottlieb (1981), Gottlieb (1985), Greenblatt, Becerra, & Serafetinides (1982), Israel (1983), Leavy (1983), Mitchell & Trickett (1980), Norbeck (1982), Roberts (1984), Roberts (1988), and Thoits (1982).

person's survival regardless of age, its role for society's elderly is especially critical. The elderly have a greater number and intensity of dependency needs and, by virtue of physical and mental frailty, are more likely to require assistance with meeting even basic needs. In addition, resources have a natural tendency to shrink: Spouses and partners, friends and siblings die; opportunities for social involvement through natural mechanisms such as employment become reduced; family members move away. The elderly are therefore faced with intensified dependency needs *and* shrinking alternatives and resources for meeting these needs.

Understanding how social support is structured and what processes are involved in its formation, operation, and maintenance is directly related to survival in old age. This chapter describes social support for the aged, how it can be assessed, how nursing interventions might be affected by social support, and how nursing interventions might improve the operation of the social support system and sustain its function. It focuses on social support as both *structure* (including formal and informal social arrangements) and *process* (interactive, interpersonal mechanisms used for the elicitation, initiation, and maintenance of support).

COMPONENTS AND DEFINITIONS OF SOCIAL SUPPORT

Although definitions vary, *social support* is generally defined by three key activities: affirmation, affection, and aid (Kahn, 1979). *Affirmation* is evidenced by actions such as the provision of positive feedback (Barrera, 1981); validation behaviors (Caplan, 1974) such as encouragement, empathy, and the recognition of competence (Cobb, 1976; Porrit, 1979); and the endorsement of a person's behaviors, perceptions, or expressed views (Kahn & Antonucci, 1981). *Affection* is characterized by intimate interaction (Barrera, 1981); sharing and reciprocity (Cobb, 1976); and expressing positive feelings (House, 1981). *Aid* can be symbolic, informational, or instrumental. Symbolic aid involves activities that assist individuals in mobilizing personal resources and mastering emo-

tional burdens (Caplan, 1974). Informational aid includes actions such as providing advice, information, suggestions, directions, or information relevant to self-evaluation (House, 1981) as well as the provision of physical assistance, money, time, skills, and labor (Barrera, 1981; Caplan, 1974; House, 1981; Kahn & Antonucci, 1981). Thoits (1982) noted the literature support for a multidimensional definition of social support that considers all its facets, including the types of support, the amount of support perceived, and sources of support.

Although everyone needs each of these kinds of support, it is not necessary for a single person to provide them. For most people, the total need for social support is met by the individuals in their social network and the burden for total support is thus distributed among a number of individuals. The amount and type of available support is directly related to the overall size of the social network, the support required, and the accumulated resources of the individual. Thoits (1982) suggested that not all sources of support are equivalent in relieving distress. She identified the functional part of the social network as the *social support system* or the "subset of persons in the individual's social network upon whom he or she relies for socio-emotional aid, instrumental aid or both" (p. 148). This differentiation is particularly useful regarding the elderly because it does not define the system in terms of reciprocal exchange. Therefore, it can be used for describing social support systems that include family and friends for whom the exchange of support often follows norms of reciprocity, in contrast to professionals and other service providers for whom the exchange may not be symmetric.

Although most authors describe social support in positive terms, Tilden and Gaylen (1987) suggested that social support is fraught with costs and conflicts—in their words, "a dark side." It cannot be assumed that all individuals in a support system are providing support or that a person with a large support system is necessarily receiving the appropriate type and amount of support. In fact, if Tilden and Gaylen's assertions are correct, for some individuals, the support system itself is a source of distress, as in support systems in which there is considerable interpersonal conflict over the needs of the elderly person and how those needs should be met. Supporters also extract a cost in terms of acquiescence, compromise, and fulfilling their expectations, and maintaining support networks requires time, effort, and attention.

STRUCTURE OF SOCIAL SUPPORT SYSTEMS FOR THE ELDERLY

Social supports for the aged can be viewed as a matrix composed of subsystems, systems, and suprasystems crossed by formal and informal mechanisms (Fig. 8–1). The *subsystems* are composed of dyadic or triadic relationships characterized by intense mutual interdependence between the elderly person and significant others. These significant others do not necessarily have to be human; they can be companion animals, for example. These subsystems are embedded in *systems* composed of the interrelationships of the elderly person and more or less organized groups, such as the elderly person and his or her family unit or an elderly person and a group of care providers. Systems are embedded in *suprasystems,* which are composed of the interrelationships of the elderly and their social support systems within the context of the larger community. Examples of suprasystems include extended kinship systems, organized social service agencies, and government agencies such as social security.

The gerontological literature usually divides social supports into formal and informal support mechanisms. *Formal mechanisms* are organized and include institutions, government agencies, or private organizations. *Informal mechanisms* are those created by bonds of obligation or affection. These are not rigidly organized and do not usually involve the exchange of money. The support provided by family members, neighbors, and friends is an informal support mechanism.

Viewing social support from a matrix perspective is useful in gerontological nursing for a variety of reasons. First, it helps emphasize the inherent complexity of social support and permits the broadest possible range of supporters to be considered as part of the support system. Second, even when an elderly person appears to be totally devoid of interpersonal resources, it assists the nurse in identifying a range of possible supporters when the chosen intervention strategy is the mobilization of social supports to prevent premature institutionalization or functional decline. Last, this matrix view of social support allows the nurse to understand what the gerontological and long-term care literature calls the *care continuum* and its relationship to social support.

The care continuum is an abstract notion encompassing the provision of services and

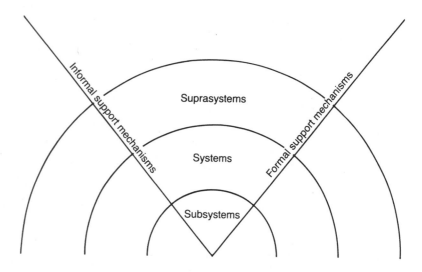

FIGURE 8–1. Social supports for the elderly form a matrix composed of subsystems, systems, and suprasystems crossed by formal and informal support mechanisms.

level of care needed to keep individuals healthy and functioning as independently as possible. It reflects the coupling of Leavell and Clark's (1958) levels of primary prevention with the delivery of healthcare services through formal and informal social support. Technically, health services for individuals of all age groups can be conceptualized as a care continuum in which primary prevention is required continuously and secondary and tertiary prevention are required episodically as illnesses occur. For the most part, younger people manage primary prevention independently provided that information and services are available and accessible. For these individuals, the illness trajectory is usually such that illness, function (self-care abilities), and symptoms vary together: When illness occurs, symptoms occur and function is impaired, and when the illness resolves, so do the symptoms; function returns to normal (Fig. 8–2). In fact, these three variables are so strongly associated in the young that they are often viewed as one and the same. The young generally need intense social support (particularly in the form of aid) only in times of acute illness or distress.

The situation for the elderly (see Fig. 8–2) is often quite different. Because many elderly people live with the presence of one or more chronic conditions, their illness trajectory is strikingly different from that of the young. Chronic conditions fluctuate markedly over time, and illness, function, and symptoms may not necessarily vary together. Chronic conditions may at times be present but asymptomatic, and function may be affected to a small degree or not at all. At other times, symptoms

may increase in intensity but still be manageable, with function scarcely affected. Yet at other times, the person may have an acute flair (or exacerbation) of the chronic condition or another acute illness superimposed, and symptoms may thus become difficult to manage and function greatly impaired. Function sometimes never returns to the preacute episode level. In addition, some chronic conditions have an unrelenting downhill effect on function even when symptoms are controlled and acute illnesses do not intervene.

Within this framework, the care continuum has a very different meaning for the elderly than for the young. The elderly may simultaneously need primary, secondary, and tertiary prevention. They may also need social support on a more or less continuous basis. The level and type of support needed may vary with the intensity of illness, symptoms, and functional impairment. The care continuum for the elderly, therefore, is equivalent to providing the least restrictive, most supportive care possible using various combinations of formal and informal support.

Formal Support Mechanisms

A wide variety of formal mechanisms exist in this country for providing social support to the elderly (Table 8–1). Although communities vary in their ability to deliver support services, most communities have some formal mechanisms designed to provide alternatives to meet elderly people's needs for assistance, improve their quality of life, prevent premature institu-

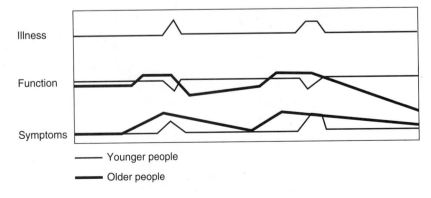

FIGURE 8–2. Comparison of the trajectory of illness in young and older people.

TABLE 8-1
Formal Support Mechanisms

In-Home Services

Social services
    Socialization centers (e.g., senior centers)
    Nutrition centers
    Transportation services
    Telephone reassurance
    Home-delivered meals
Home health services
    Chore services
    Home modification
    Durable medical equipment
    Instrumental services: shopping,
       transportation, laundry, meal preparation
    Personal care
    Supervisory services
    Respite care
    Hospice care
    Case management

Out-of-Home Services

    Adult daycare
    Respite care
    Foster care
    Boarding homes
    Supervisory care homes
    Skilled nursing and extended care facilities
    Acute care hospitals
    Transitional or subacute care facilities
    Rehabilitation services

tionalization, and augment family support. Although most such mechanisms are organized primarily to provide aid, they often also provide opportunities for affirmation and affection as relationships grow between the people being served and the people providing care.

The types of formal support mechanisms appropriate for an elderly person depend in part on the degree of functional impairment, the success of symptom management, and available social resources. For example, when elderly people are well, mobile, and independent and their needs for aid are minimal, they can use fairly unorganized, simple formal mechanisms such as churches and clubs to meet their needs for affirmation and affection as well as ambulatory care facilities or wellness centers to meet their healthcare needs. With increased disability, community-based short-term or long-term in-home services may be required,

as provided by social service or home health agencies. With prolonged disability and progressive deterioration, personal care and supervisory services are often required.

Out-of home services are similarly graded on the basis of needs and the amount of functional impairment. Protected care environments for the elderly may exist in which, for a fee, the elderly can be assured that they will receive the type of support needed at any given time. These environments usually consist of apartments (with some support services such as cleaning and meals) and an extended care facility. When individuals are capable of independent living, they live in the apartments, and when they need more intensive support, they move to the extended care facility.

The array of formal support for the elderly is extensive and complex. Obtaining the appropriate kind of formal support at the right time is becoming increasingly complicated, owing to current social and healthcare trends. Hospital stays are shorter than before, and extended care facilities are no longer viewed as permanent placements. As a consequence, most elderly people experience multiple transitions during illness episodes, and intensive care is more frequently provided in the home. In many communities, formal community-based or hospital-based systems exist to provide case management for older people and their families. Case managers arrange the necessary services, facilitate transitions and out-of-home placements, and coordinate the reentry of the elderly people back into the community through discharge planning from acute and extended care facilities. Whether or not formal case management services exist, however, the nurses in acute care facilities and ambulatory care settings are increasingly responsible for recognizing the need for support services, identifying the services available, and advocating on behalf of the elderly and families to ensure that formal support is provided when needed. Failure to assume this important role results in higher healthcare costs through acute care readmissions and greater suffering as the elderly and their families are faced with managing complicated health problems in the home without outside support.

Informal Support Mechanisms

Despite the presence of a more or less extensive formal support system in this country, most elderly people still receive the bulk of their support from their informal support networks. A large database derived from formal surveys documented that the informal network is the sole source of support for three fourths of all elderly living in the community, regardless of the type of support needed by the elderly person (affirmation, affection, or aid). These surveys included the 1982 Long-Term Care Survey (Select Committee on Aging, 1987; Stone et al., 1987), the National Health Interview Survey (Doty, 1986), the Channeling Demonstration Project (Stephens & Christianson, 1986), the Massachusetts Health Care Panel Study (Branch & Jette, 1983), and other smaller studies such as those by Cantor (1983), Horowitz and Dobrof (1982), Liu and colleagues (1985), and Tennestedt and McKinlay (1989).

Of the potential members of the informal network (friends, neighbors, or church members), family members clearly provide the vast majority of support. Aid, in the form of family caregiving, is the main type of support provided to the elderly by family members. Family members provide the elderly with a variety of instrumental support services, the most common being meals, shopping and errands, housekeeping, and transportation (Tennestedt & McKinlay, 1989). Family members may provide personal care services, including assistance with eating, dressing, toileting, or getting in and out of bed or moving around the house (Select Committee on Aging, 1987). Family members may also serve as case managers or care brokers (Archbold, 1983; McKinlay & Tennestedt, 1986; Select Committee on Aging, 1987).

Family members generally provide these support services for elderly family members regardless of the type or length of care needed. They provide aid to intensely ill and seriously disabled elderly people and generally seek the services of the formal support system or resort to institutional placement only when all other options are exhausted. The 1982 Long-Term Care Study, for example, showed that the duration of caregiving responsibilities varied greatly, but that most caregivers had provided care from 1 to 4 years and that about 20% had provided care over 5 years (Select Committee on Aging, 1987). Over 80% of the caregivers surveyed provided assistance 7 days a week. Another study reported that many caregivers devote from 50 to 60 hours a week to providing care (Tennestedt, 1984). Montgomery and colleagues (1985) developed a useful conceptualization of the intensity of family caregiving, reasoning that although caregiver responsibilities may extend over years, it is the constellation of tasks performed and not the duration of caregiving responsibilities that signifies the intensity of caregiving. They also suggested that the sequence in which caregiving tasks are assumed by family caregivers is fairly predictable and that stages can be differentiated based on the intimacy of tasks being performed and the frequency of contact. Using factor analysis, they confirmed seven categories or stages of caregiving that ranged from low intimacy, low frequency (e.g., walking, transportation, errands) to high intimacy, high frequency (e.g., feeding, toileting). Viewing caregiving in stages is useful for understanding that the intensity of caregiving responsibilities varies over time and is related to the elderly person's fluctuating needs (regarding illness, symptoms, and function) rather than to time in the role.

Studies have shown that family members generally provide care regardless of the elderly person's health status or intensity of need (Archbold, 1983); the family member's other responsibilities (Cantor, 1983), including employment status (Brody et al., 1987; Brody & Schoonover, 1986); whether the elderly person lives alone (Moss et al., 1985) or has female relatives (Horowitz, 1985); the family's ethnicity (Jenkins & Karno, 1992; Markides et al., 1986; Taylor, 1985); and geographical proximity to the elderly family member (Moss et al., 1985). Although there may be differences in the types of support offered by family members who live geographically close compared with those who live at a distance, extreme geographical distance does not substantially interfere with family members assuming caregiving support roles (Brody, 1985; Horowitz, 1985; Moss et al., 1985).

Some studies have focused on how family

caregivers come to be caregivers and how informal caregiving is organized. Shanas (1979) identified a hierarchical pattern of caregiver selection that is sequential and follows certain rules. If the elderly person in need of care is married and the spouse is physically able, most caregiving is provided by the spouse (regardless of age or gender) with or without the assistance of children, other relatives, or friends. If the spouse is no longer available or able, responsibility for support is assumed by the daughters (usually the eldest daughter first), daughters-in-law (if there is no daughter, the eldest son's wife is often expected to step in), and granddaughters (usually providing support to their mothers) (Shanas, 1979). If the individual has both daughters and sons, responsibilities for personal care and some kinds of instrumental support are often assumed by the females, while the males (sons, sons-in-law, or grandsons) assume responsibility of financial assistance and management (Horowitz, 1985).

The pattern described by Shanas is sometimes interpreted as being driven by strong social prescriptions and the *default principle.* The assumption under the default principle is that no one actually wants to be a caregiver, but since the social imperative to provide care to family members is strong, families organize in a structured way that eliminates the need for conscious decisions regarding who should act. It is almost as if families rigidly prescribe who will "get stuck" with the caregiving. In reality, however, even though caregiving can be burdensome and difficult, most family members see caregiving as a tangible way to show love, respect, and gratitude. Regardless of whether the elderly person is considered able to reciprocate in the present, family members often interpret their need to provide care in terms of his or her past actions and contributions. Caregivers are sometimes given special regard and status in the family and viewed by others as having a special bond with the elderly person. As opposed to being stuck with the role, family members sometimes compete for the role.

Other studies have found variations in or have elaborated on the pattern identified by Shanas (1979). Phillips (1984) defined several caregiving roles that could be assumed by family members. The *designated caregiver* role is given to the family member elected by the elderly person and other family members to assume the responsibility for the organization and implementation of support services. The election of the designated caregiver often follows the pattern identified by Shanas (1979) but can also be changed because of (1) special bonds between the elderly person and another child (other than the oldest daughter, with the elderly person trusting another child more); (2) the nature of the relationship between the elderly person and his or her spouse (because of past negative interactions, some elderly people trust their children or others more than their spouse and do not believe their spouse can or will provide good care); and (3) the relationship between the elderly person and the child's spouse (some spouses refuse to have the adult child involved in caregiving responsibilities, and some elderly people mistrust their child's spouse). The pattern may also be strongly influenced by ethnicity, with some ethnic groups (e.g., Hispanics) expecting the designated caregiver to be an adult child even if the spouse is alive and well (Phillips, 1985–1994).

The responsibility of the designated caregiver is to monitor the elderly person's behavior and physical and emotional well-being to determine the type and amount of support services needed. He or she is not responsible for meeting all the elderly person's needs but is responsible for mobilizing the social support system to ensure that these needs are met. The designated caregiver usually acts as the family spokesperson in times of decision making.

The *abdicator* role identified by Phillips (1984) identifies family members who are given the family's permission to not provide support for the elderly person. Abdicators are often "family ambassadors" who function to enhance the family's social status through their employment or other roles. The abdicator, rather than the designated caregiver, may be the elderly person's favorite, which can arouse great interpersonal conflict and resentment within the family.

The third role identified by Phillips is the *pretender,* who is a relative (often another adult child) with the potential and desire for being the designated caregiver. Often, pretenders feel they are best prepared to assume the caregiving role even though they are not the elderly person's elected choice.

According to Phillips (1984), two different caregiving structures exist that are differentiated by the degree to which the family accepts decisions about the designated caregiver role. In families with limited numbers of members or in which the election result is uncontested, the major role of the designated caregiver and others in the family is clear. These families experience little conflict and interact well with healthcare professionals, provided that professionals acknowledge the authority of the designated caregiver and do not attempt to negotiate care decisions with others in the family.

The second type of organizational structure exists in families in which more than one person has the potential for the designated caregiver position and other members disagree on who should assume this role. These families are characterized by considerable interpersonal conflict as individuals within the family compete for the favored position of designated caregiver, and this conflict is intensified during times of crisis. Even during times of relative calm, however, pretenders tend to criticize the activities of both the designated caregiver and the abdicators. Often the conflict among family members results in long delays between the onset of an elderly person's need for support and the mobilization of resources to meet the need.

Gross (1994) examined why certain individuals in families become caregivers and others do not. Using grounded theory, she identified the basic social process of *positioning* that "described the way in which parents and their children affect a mutually satisfying outcome relative to the dependence needs of aging parents" (p. 63). Positioning is a staged process that begins in the early life of the child and consists of four subcategories: education, preparation, reciprocation, and habitation. *Education* is the way through which elderly people transmit the family tradition of caregiving or the family's standard for assuming responsibility in a relationship of caring for dependent others in the family. *Preparation* involves the parent

assigning the caregiving responsibility to the child and endorsing the child's position to others in the family. Four types of responsibility are assigned; physical, emotional, social, and legal. *Reciprocation* represents the feelings of gratitude children learn in response to the contributions of their parents. *Habitation* involves children physically positioning themselves so they can easily assume caregiving responsibilities. It can involve moving closer to the elderly family member or vice versa, or moving in with the elderly person. The families described in this study by Gross (1994) were mostly free of conflict regarding who was the caregiver (Gross, 1994). Thus, they followed the first pattern previously identified by Phillips (1984).

Informal support is organized in complex and highly individual ways. When elderly people are in need, family members with actual or acquired kinship ties generally assume responsibility for maintaining and organizing the social support system. It is not uncommon, however, for other individuals within the elderly person's social network (lifelong friends, associates, neighbors) to serve as the designated caregiver. The development of new intimate relationships and remarriages late in life is not uncommon, which can lead to designated caregivers being chosen by individuals who are relatively new to the elderly person's social network. Often, these supportive relationships are assumed voluntarily. When the need for support becomes intense, roles are sometimes formalized through payment for services (sometimes this also occurs with adult children who have quit their jobs to provide care) or the assignment of a legal role (e.g., power of attorney, conservator). In addition, a formal supporter can on occasion become an informal supporter because of the intensity of the affective ties that has arisen from the intimacy of the caregiving relationship.

Relationships Between Formal and Informal Supports

Although the relationship between formal and informal supports has been little studied, it is clear that the current formal support networks alone—without the elderly's informal support networks—would fail to meet the needs of the elderly. Formal supporters supplement and augment the care provided by informal supporters and in many cases make it possible for families to continue to provide support despite other commitments and responsibilities. The relationship between formal and informal mechanisms is complementary. Formal support mechanisms existing alone would be immobilized by the demand for services in a system that could not financially absorb the burden. Owing to the variety of formal support mechanisms available, the elderly and their families have choices about the care mechanisms they use. The presence of formal supporters helps many elderly people remain at home despite progressive disability. When the elderly person is geographically separated from or devoid of informal supporters, formal social support mechanisms help prevent premature institutionalization by providing alternative methods for the provision of care.

There are two important factors regarding the relationship between formal and informal support networks of the elderly. First, conflict can arise between individuals in the two systems and serves only to make caring situations more difficult. Conflicts sometimes arise based on differing definitions about what kind of caregiving is needed. This point was well described by Bowers (1987) in her discussion of the five categories of caregiving that family members provide to elderly relatives in the community:

1. Anticipatory caregiving—support provided for the potential needs of the elderly
2. Preventive caregiving—support provided to prevent illness, injury, or physical and mental deterioration
3. Supervisory caregiving—care management support described by Archbold (1983), which includes activities such as arranging for, setting up, and checking out services
4. Instrumental caregiving—provision of all types of actual care, including meal preparation, physical care, transportation, property management, and socialization opportunities

5. Protective caregiving—activities performed to protect the elderly from damages to self-image and assaults to personal dignity

In discussing these five types of caregiving, Bowers (1987) noted that although members of the formal support systems usually value instrumental caregiving the most, informal support system members often value protective caregiving the most. Sharp differences of opinion may result about the kind and amount of support that is best for the elderly person at any given time. Most commonly, conflicts between the formal and informal system arise out of differences in expectations or values. Sometimes conflicts arise because the appropriate informal supporters are not consulted in care planning or because the knowledge of the informal supporters is not trusted or acknowledged by members of the formal system.

Second, the informal system does not cease to exist when the formal system is activated. In fact, although institutional placement often follows declines in the elderly person's functional status, it is not usually related to deteriorating family ties (Brody, 1966; Brody & Spark, 1966; Miller & Harris, 1965). Family relationships continue after placement and are often strengthened because family members are relieved of the heavy burden of care and have time and energy to provide and enjoy giving socioemotional support (Black & Bengston, 1977; Dobrof & Litwak, 1977).

Bowers (1988) examined the continuing relationships between family members and residents of long-term care facilities and discovered the strong need family members have to engage in *preservation caregiving*, which she defined as "care which is engaged in to maintain the older person's self, or more accurately, the adult offspring's perceptions of that self" (p. 362). Bowers identified four types of preservation caregiving: (1) maintaining family connectedness, (2) maintaining the elderly person's dignity, (3) maintaining the elderly person's hope, and (4) helping the elderly person control his or her environment. Similarly, Duncan and Morgan (1994) found that one of the responsibilities families described in relationship to institutional care was monitoring staff behavior to ensure that quality care was provided and that the resident was treated as a person rather than an object.

Both these studies demonstrated that (1) family relationships continue after institutionalization; (2) families evaluate the quality of care based on the relationships between the elderly person and staff members and the family and staff members; (3) family members believe they must be vigilant to prevent the damage institutional staff can do to older people's self-esteem and dignity; and (4) the relationship between staff and family members has the potential to be either beneficial and supportive or adversarial. Regardless of the setting in which the elderly family member is receiving care (e.g., homecare, daycare, acute care facility), it is important to be sensitive to the interpersonal issues involved in both formal and informal support systems and to plan the interface so that conflict is minimized.

SOCIAL SUPPORT AS PROCESS

Although social support is usually described in terms of structure (who does what and how much), this view suggests that support is static and predictable. In fact, social support is a dynamic, interactive process involving minute-to-minute, day-to-day interchanges among people. Understanding the dynamics of the social support process is important for understanding how social support systems can be mobilized and used to meet the needs of the elderly. The social support process is also *interactive*. All parties involved, including the elderly person, are active agents who think, feel, behave, plan, ascribe motives, make decisions, evaluate outcomes, and reflect. Therefore, a complete understanding of the social support process requires the consideration of at least two perspectives: those of the supporters and the elderly person. This section describes the dynamics from both perspectives.

Reciprocity is a key concept that accounts for the dynamics of social support systems from both perspectives. It refers to the exchange of goods, services, and sentiments within a relationship and the degree to which these are *perceived* to be distributed in a mutually satis-

fying manner (Homans, 1961). According to social exchange theory, as individuals interact over time, social norms dictate that each provides the other an equitable distribution of rewards and reinforcements. Among the chief rewards and reinforcements exchanged is mutual support in the form of aid, affirmation, and affection. Regardless of the nature of the relationship (e.g., spousal, filial, casual, formal), individuals interact only as long as their investments into the relationship are perceived as more or less equal to their profits or returns.

Dowd (1975) presented a succinct description of the effect aging can have on social exchange: As individuals age and disability becomes an issue, they become less able to reciprocate certain types of support and simultaneously require increasing support for themselves. The net result can be a reluctance on the part of elderly people to express their needs for all types of support and to consider the support they do receive as sufficient even when it is inadequate to maintain their sense of well-being and satisfaction with life. Conversely, they may continue to demand ever more support based on their perceptions of the significance of their past contributions. The supporters can thus experience resentment at the unequal exchange, a sense of failure that the elderly person appears to need more than they can provide, and a sense of frustration that their efforts are not met by "appropriate" expressions of gratitude. The ability of the elderly person to exchange money for support may intensify rather than diminish the inequity in the perspective of the supporter. When supporters perceive that the elderly person's only medium of exchange is money and that neither affirmation nor affection for the supporter is forthcoming, considerable resentment can be engendered.

Reciprocity is key in all forms of social exchange but operates differently depending on the nature of the relationship (formal vs. informal). The next section considers the dynamics of the two different types of social support.

Formal Supporters and the Social Support Process

The relationships between formal supporters and the elderly are ideal for describing how reciprocity works because formal relationships typically involve the exchange of money for services. Simply stated, the elderly person pays so much for a given level of support, and in return the supporter provides what is paid for. Unfortunately, the situations are never that simple, and many factors complicate the social support process in formal relationships. First, the exchange of money is rarely direct. Often third-party payers are involved, causing the elderly person to lose control over giving or withholding payment based on satisfaction. In some cases, the source of payment may be a gift over which the elderly person has almost no control. It can be difficult for either the elderly person or the supporter to comprehend the relationship between payment and service, and thus all sense of reciprocal exchange is lost. Admittedly, elderly people can gain some control over the exchange by providing other types of rewards (e.g., tips, gifts, warm sentiments) or terminating the relationship, but in many cases neither of these is a viable option based on the elderly person's resources or need for support.

Second, these situations are almost always complicated by power imbalances that significantly alter the nature of the relationships. When one person in the relationship is unable to reciprocate, the other gains a monopoly on rewards and can allocate rewards, services, or support regardless of what the elderly person does. Formal supporters have many sources of power with which they can exact compliance almost without consideration of what the elderly person thinks, feels, or wants.

The third complicating factor is that these relationships rarely involve only two people. The relationship between these two people typically operates in a context involving other individuals such as family members, other informal supporters, and a myriad of formal supporters. The influence of other people can be both positive and negative. In general, when groups of individuals interact with the same person over time, they develop a shared view of the individual and his or her needs and ability for self-care. When the shared view is positive, the treatment of the elderly person is likely to be supportive. However, when the shared view is negative, the elderly person's

situation can be very different. This point was well illustrated in Phillips and Van Ort's study (1995) on improvement of functional feeding in a dementia care unit. The contextual and behavior interventions used were largely successful in improving self-feeding behavior, but for a few subjects, the staff had a shared view a priori that the elderly patients were incapable of any self-feeding behaviors. As a result, despite evidence to the contrary, the staff overtly and covertly sabotaged the resident's feeding attempts, resulting in "no change" just as the staff had predicted.

Informal Supporters and the Social Support Process

Relationships between the elderly and their informal supporters are complex, and the effect of these relationships on the social support process is not reliably predictable. Unlike social support processes involving the elderly and the formal support system—which are likely to be greatly influenced by the norm of reciprocity—within the informal support system, the norm of reciprocity operates but is often secondary to other norms and influences. With informal supports, it is often difficult to know exactly which norms are most strongly influencing the social support process. Since these other norms are most readily apparent in family relationships, this section focuses on the complexities in the social support process that arise because the individuals are family members.

One factor that influences the social support process in families is the duration and history of the relationships. *Symbolic interactionism* (McCall & Simmons, 1976) suggests that as individuals interact over time, each person in the relationship develops a mental dossier that uniquely identifies the one person to the other. In aging families, the involved individuals have long histories. They may have interacted over years, often in excess of 50 or 60 years. As a result, their interaction dossiers are extensive and complex and include a vast store of experiences with and memories of the other person. Because these experiences and memories comprise the basis on which each individual's perceptions and expectations of the other person are formulated, they are also the basis for the individuals' behavior toward each other and interpretations of interpersonal feedback resulting from interaction (Phillips, 1990). To a large extent, it is the dossier that determines the type and amount of social support as well as interpretations of the responses to the support efforts.

A second factor influencing social support processes in aging families is the growing interdependence that exists among family members. This interdependence of course differs between spouse-spouse relationships and parent-child relationships. Many aging couples experience new levels of intimacy in the later years of marriage along with increased contentment, companionship, and satisfaction. The relationships between spouses become increasingly *symbiotic* (Clark & Anderson, 1967), with very elderly couples functioning almost as one person as each spouse accommodates for the frailties of the other. For many very elderly couples, survival in the community for either person literally depends on the survival of both. This is not to imply that relationships between aging spouses are idyllic, since conflicts do occur. As Pillemer (1987) documented, spouse abuse in old families is not only possible but is probably the most common form of abuse of the elderly. Nevertheless, very strong interdependence often characterizes the relationships between aging couples, which has implications for how social support is both given and received.

Interdependence is also evident in relationships between adult children and their parents. This interdependence is best described as *filial maturity* (Blenkner, 1969), a developmental stage in which the adult child is depended on for his or her adult capabilities. Troll (1971) believed filial maturity is achieved through a reciprocal process of social exchange between the parent and child during which the parent role models the nature of adult relationships and reinforces the adult child's appropriate role behaviors. This relationship is not to be mistaken as *role reversal*, however, in which adult children actually assume the supportive role of parent to the elderly person. In healthy families, the elderly person's perceptions of the adult child change, and vice versa. The child becomes a confidant valued by the elderly person as a mature significant other, and the elderly person becomes a friend valued by the adult child for his or her maturity and wisdom (Mutran & Reitzes, 1984). In many healthy aging families, filial maturity creates a new sense of reciprocity, with both parties recognizing and appreciating the unique contributions of the other.

Other factors that influence the social support process in families are best characterized as *family solidarity* or *familism* (when applied to adult children and parents, this is frequently called *intergenerational cohesion* or *solidarity*) (Atkinson et al., 1986; Bengtson et al., 1976; Markides & Krause, 1985; McChesney & Bengtson, 1988; Roberts & Bengston, 1990; Rossi & Rossi, 1990). Familism denotes the normative commitment of family members to family and family relationships (Heller, 1976). It denotes commitment that supersedes attention to individual contributions and rewards and also implies a strong value for the "exclusiveness" of the kinship structure. Burgess and Locke (1945) originally defined familism in terms of family members: dividing the social world into insiders (kin or family) and outsiders (all others); focusing activities on achieving familial, rather than individual goals; believing that family assets and resources belong to and should be used for the good of the whole; supporting other family members unconditionally; and believing in the need to perpetuate the family. Six dimensions of family solidarity are usually discussed: normative, structural, affectual, associational, consensual, and functional.

Normative solidarity refers to the behavioral standards within the family that govern expectations of individuals toward each other (Roberts et al., 1991). It reflects the "shoulds" of family interaction and exchange to which family members ascribe and is driven by a strong social norm (the norm of solidarity). According to George (1986), the norm of solidarity is a social imperative that involves an intense commitment to providing a loved one all the support and assistance he or she needs regardless of the costs to oneself.

The norm of solidarity is displayed as expressions of filial obligations by adult children and is usually quite strong. This solidarity not only influences the lengths to which adult children are willing to go to provide aid to their parents but also strongly influences the degree to which adult children and the elderly, particularly in certain ethnic groups, are willing to accept assistance from outside or formal sources (Guttman, 1979; Kahana & Kahana, 1984; Keefe et al., 1978, 1979; Markides et al., 1986; Mindel & Habenstein, 1981; Ramirez & Arce, 1981; Watson, 1982). Studies have investigated the relationship of filial obligation with other factors, including age (Rossi & Rossi, 1990), education (Finley et al., 1988), birth order (Hamon & Thiessen, 1989), religious affiliation (Guberman et al., 1992; Hamon & Theissen, 1989), and socioeconomic level (Finley et al., 1988; Lee, 1980; Leichter & Mitchell, 1967). Some research has shown that filial obligation toward the two parents can be different for the same adult child. Finley and colleagues (1988), for example, found that role conflict diminishes filial obligation of daughters to fathers but does not significantly affect obligations of daughters to mothers.

Structural solidarity is the pattern of role relationships enacted by family members over time (McChesney & Mangen, 1988). Gender strongly influences structural solidarity, and generally more helpful behaviors are exchanged between mothers and children than between fathers and children (Rossi & Rossi, 1990). Family size influences structural solidarity, with large families tending to limit the amount of help given by parents to children but to increase the amount of help given by children to parents (Rossi & Rossi, 1990). For example, larger family size increases the likelihood of elderly women living independently with informal support (Soldo et al., 1990). The marital status of the child also influences structural solidarity. Elderly people whose children are married typically receive less help from both their sons and daughters (Stoller, 1983).

Affectual solidarity relates to the extent of positive sentiments toward other family members (Mangen et al., 1988). One might assume that the greater the positive feelings toward a parent, the greater the likelihood of providing support; however, Jarrett (1985) found that the strength of filial obligation and an attitude of positive concern were better predictors of providing support or assistance than was affection.

Associational solidarity relates to the degree to which family members share activities and interact socially (Rossi & Rossi, 1990). Even though families in the United States are characterized by great mobility, distance does not substantially reduce adult children's propensity to offer support to their parents.

Consensual solidarity (sometimes also called *value consensus*) relates to the degree to which family members share beliefs, attitudes, and values (Roberts et al., 1991). In general, children put more store in similarity of values and beliefs than do parents (Rossi & Rossi, 1990). In Gross's study (1994), the degree to which children felt they shared beliefs and values with their parents was an important determinant for family members choosing the best caregiver in the family.

Functional solidarity refers to the extent to which family members exchange money, goods, or services (Roberts et al., 1991). The evidence for families exchanging aid with aging members is quite strong. In addition, the elderly appear to provide support to other family members, particularly in the areas of childcare and other domestic services. The entire concept of family caregiving rests on functional solidarity.

In summary, reciprocity is the basic mechanism that explains the process of social support between the elderly and their formal supporters (Fig. 8–3). It is also involved in the social support between the elderly and informal supporters, although other factors such as the history of the relationship, interdependence between the parties, and family solidarity are also influential (Fig. 8–4). The interaction of these three factors increases the complexity and unpredictability of the process, and as relationships between the elderly and their formal

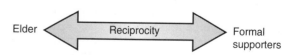

FIGURE 8–3. Social support process: elders and formal supporters.

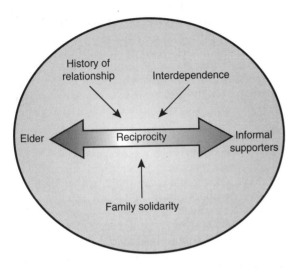

FIGURE 8–4. Social support process: elders and informal supporters.

supporters evolve over time—and as affectional bonds between the parties grow—they can also take on the complexity typical of relationships with informal supporters.

Social Support Process from the Perspective of the Elderly: Dependency Work

The recipients of support are sometimes viewed as passive recipients, dependent on the whims of others to get what they need. In fact, this is far from true. Gross's (1994) study showed that the elderly are active in positioning themselves and in role modeling certain behaviors to increase the likelihood that they will be given aid in old age. Phillips (1984) also made this observation and further noted the active role that the elderly played in the election and endorsement of a designated caregiver. Russell (1993) closely examined the ways in which the elderly elicit and sustain support. Using grounded theory, her data showed that even elderly people with cognitive impairments actively and volitionally seek aid through several strategies. She found that being dependent on others, rather than being a simple passive role, is like performing a difficult "dance" with a sometimes unwilling or insensitive partner. The dance takes planning, determination, cooperation, compromise, and a great deal of hard work (Russell, 1993).

Russell (1993) identified three facets of what she termed *dependency work*. The first was personal considerations that involve the elderly person working to resolve internal dependency issues. These considerations can be intrapsychic, with the elderly person struggling to reconcile a past self-image as an independent and autonomous adult with a new self-image of dependency and to deal with the implications of dependency for his or her self-esteem and feelings of self-worth. Personal considerations can be *pragmatic*, involving all the accommodations and compromises of incorporating new individuals and settings (e.g., change of residence, daycare, etc.) into daily life, and can also involve *covering*, in which the elderly person strategizes and acts to prevent becoming totally vulnerable, employing an information management strategy that requires active decisions about how much to tell to whom and when.

The second facet of dependency work identified by Russell (1993) is a consideration of others, involving asking, considering other's abilities, and expressing gratitude. Elderly people struggle with the balance of asking the right person for the right amount of assistance at the right time and often frame their requests so they include only what they need and not necessarily what they want. Other's abilities are also considered in these requests. Elderly people know that expressing gratitude for assistance is essential, and they therefore work hard to think of varied ways to do this.

The last aspect of dependency work is managing obligations that "reflected the work elders engaged in as they acted on and evaluated their beliefs and judgments of their, or their caregivers, sense of duty within care relationships" (Russell, 1993, p. 160). *Balancing the exchange*, which is grounded in reciprocity, is one aspect of managing obligations, as are *expectations of self*, which involve elderly people acting as they believe they should. The elderly believe that they should appear happy, contented, patient, appreciative, uncomplaining, and above all, should "get along" no matter what. Managing obligations also includes the *expectations of others:* consulting the elderly on decisions, providing them with up-to-date information, responding to their requests, and taking their preferences into consideration. The elderly evaluate supporter's behaviors according to these standards and strategize about how to get supporters to perform according to expectations.

Regardless of the individuals involved with the elderly, giving and receiving support is a delicate process that involves sensitivity and work. Many factors influence how and why support is given, how it is received, and how supportive relationships are sustained. The next section discusses how these many facets can be considered in an assessment of the elderly's social support systems.

ASSESSMENT OF SOCIAL SUPPORT FOR THE ELDERLY

Since social support has been the focus of considerable research, several excellent scales have been developed for its measurement. Two of these scales are discussed later to show strategies for gathering data and framing questions about social support. However, the reasons for collecting information in research and the types of information needed differ from those used in clinical practice. For practice only, these scales help define a way of thinking about social support and probably do not provide the type of information needed by clinicians for planning care.

The Norbeck Social Support Questionnaire (Norbeck et al., 1981, 1983), provides information about the size, density, and composition of the social network via three concepts: total functional support, total network, and total loss. The respondent first identifies up to 20 individuals who constitute his or her social network, such as a spouse or partner, relatives, friends, work or school associates, neighbors, healthcare providers, counselors or therapists, clergy, and others. The respondent answers nine questions about each individual that consider the amount of affirmation, affection, and potential to provide aid; the duration of relationship and frequency of contact; and relationships lost within the past year.

Barrera's Arizona Social Support Interview Schedule (ASSIS) elicits the names of network members and information about the size, density, and composition of the network (1981). For each person, it asks about the support available and actually used for material aid, physical assistance, intimate interaction, guidance, feedback, and social participation. It also elicits information about the *conflicted network*—namely, those individuals with whom the respondent has interpersonal conflict.

Neither scale is recommended for quantifying social support in clinical practice. Both scales are instead based on a certain logic that should be considered when assessing social support in clinical practice. First, they are specific in basing the assessment on the individuals and the support each individual provides rather than on some global notion of support. Second, they consider the size and composition of the network as well as the subjective perception of support provided by the network members. As a consequence, these scales help emphasize the idea that a large, dense network does not necessarily translate into strongly perceived support. Third, they include both informal and formal supporters in the network. Both scales also have their particular strengths. For example, the Norbeck Social Support Questionnaire addresses the issue of loss—an important concept when dealing with the elderly—and Barrera's ASSIS considers available versus used supporters and the conflicted network, both of which could be important for planning purposes (Barrera, 1981).

These scales provide a way of thinking about how social support can be assessed. They do not, however, consider all the factors that influence the ways in which social support is given and received. Table 8–2 suggests some of the other areas nurses should consider when assessing an elderly person's social support system. These include an assessment of what elderly people need in relationship to what they get; how they receive care or their dependency work; the norms, proscriptions, and history that influence the giving and receiving of support; and the potential network members who are not currently providing support.

Using this individual approach to assessing social support is time consuming and tedious

T A B L E 8 – 2
Assessment of Social Support Systems

Size, density, and diversity of the social support system,
    including formal and informal
    supporters—identification of the major role (e.g.,
    designated caregiver)
Types and amount of support provided and individuals
    involved in providing each type of support
Recent losses in the system and how these have
    influenced the type and amount of support available
Conflicts within the system, the people involved, and the
    nature of the conflicts
Types and amount of support needed by the elderly
    person, desired goals of the elderly person and
    caregiver, and the time constraints of need fulfillment
Issues involved in the elderly person receiving care,
    including effects on self-esteem and on the amount of
    support being offered
Degree to which the social support systems meet the
    elderly person's needs
Potential formal and informal social supports available to
    the elderly person
        Formal and informal supporters not being used
        Mechanisms currently in use that might be used in
            different ways
Existing structure of social relationships among the
    elderly and individuals in the social support system
        Distribution of rewards and reinforcements
        Past history of the relationship
        Norms and proscriptions that drive the system

but provides detailed information that can guide care planning and case management for the elderly and their families. The approach ultimely chosen depends on the nurse's goal, whether it be getting the elderly person into another setting or seriously attending to the elderly person's and his or her family's needs by developing a plan that accounts for continuity of care.

INTERVENTIONS BASED ON SOCIAL SUPPORT

Most nurses acknowledge the importance of social support, but few develop care plans that actually take into consideration how social support structures or processes affect quality of life. Nurses have a responsibility for the continued support of patients during care and after discharge. This responsibility involves understanding the complexity of the social support needed to maintain continued living and organizing the network so that care is provided. Because of changes in the healthcare delivery system toward shorter periods of formal support, particularly during the 1990s, this responsibility has become increasingly important.

There are five essential nursing interventions to be used in providing social support (Table 8–3).

1. Awareness—being sensitive to the social support needs of the elderly and the ways in which giving and receiving social support influence the short-term and long-term outcomes of care
2. Communication—gathering assessment data about the structure and organization of the elderly person's social support system and the needs of the elderly person and his or her family and sharing that information with others; advocating on behalf of the elderly and their families to other healthcare providers and third-party payers so the formal system accommodates, rather than ignores, the needs; sharing essential information with the elderly, family members, and other formal supporters to ensure continuity of care during transitions and times of need
3. Counseling—giving and receiving social support via interpersonal and intrapsychic processes; helping the elderly, family members, and other formal and informal supporters work through conflicts, articulate their expectations and frustrations, and provide feedback to each other (ignoring conflicts and unrealistic expectations only makes the situation worse)
4. Education—acquiring factual knowledge about what is available or still needed and

T A B L E 8 – 3
Interventions Based on Social Support
Awareness
Communication
Counseling
Education
Mobilization

what dependence and interdependence mean to the individuals involved; the elderly and their supporters are not born with knowledge about how to give and receive support graciously, and thus role modeling supportive behavior is probably one of the most powerful strategies nurses have to augment the learning process

5. Mobilization—identifying and mobilizing resources; the healthcare environment is evolving into a rushed, inhospitable environment that is basically insensitive to and unconcerned with the needs of the elderly other than reaching the goal of discharge. Social support and mobilization of support resources to meet needs should be the first—not the last—thing nurses consider when providing care to any elderly person in any setting

SUMMARY

Social support is essential to all human beings. In addition to making life pleasant and palatable for the elderly, social support is essential to survival. Given adequate social support, the elderly can often maintain life in the community long after their physical care needs would indicate the need for institutionalization. Without adequate social support, however, the elderly face premature institutionalization and premature decline. The organization of the social support for the elderly is often complex, involving a variety of informal and formal supporters. The interactions between an elderly person and his or her supporters can create turmoil and conflicts as well as intense burdens for the supporters who continue to remain within the often dwindling social support system. To achieve the best possible outcomes for elderly individuals, the assessment of social support should reflect the complexities of the support system and the needs of all individuals within the system as well as the complexity of the needs evidenced by the elderly person. Similarly, intervention strategies need to focus on upholding the existing system, augmenting it by formulating viable support alternatives, and maintaining the life of the elderly person beyond a marginal existence.

REFERENCES

Archbold, P. (1983). Impact of parent-caring on women. *Family Relations, 32,* 39–45.

Atkinson, M., Kivett, V., & Campbell, R. (1986). Intergenerational solidarity: An examination of a theoretical model. *Journal of Gerontology, 41,* 408–416.

Barrera, M. (1981). Social support in the adjustment of pregnant adolescents: Assessment issues. In B. H. Gottlieb (Ed.), *Social networks and social support* (pp. 69–96). Beverly Hills, CA: Sage Publications.

Bengtson, V., Olander, E., & Haddad, A. (1976). The "generation gap" and aging family members: Toward a conceptual model. In J. F. Gubrium (Ed.), *Times, roles, and the self in old age* (pp. 237–263). New York: Human Sciences Press.

Berkman, L. (1984). Assessing the physical health effects of social networks and social support. *Annual Review of Public Health, 5,* 413–432.

Black, K., & Bengston, V. (1977). Implications of telecommunications technology for old people, families and bureaucracies. In E. Shanas & M. Sussman (Eds.), *Family, bureaucracy, and the elderly* (pp. 174–195). Durham, NC: University Press.

Blenkner, M. (1969). The normal dependencies of aging. In R. Kalish (Ed.), *The dependencies of old people* (pp. 27–37). Ann Arbor, MI: Institute of Gerontology.

Bowers, B. (1987). Intergenerational caregiving: Adult caregivers and their aging parents. *Advances in Nursing Science, 9,* 20–31.

Bowers, B. (1988). Family perceptions of nursing home care. *Gerontologist, 28,* 361–368.

Branch, L., & Jette, A. (1983). Elder's use of informal long-term care assistance. *Gerontologist, 23,* 51–56.

Brody, E. (1966). The aging family. *Gerontologist, 6,* 201–206.

Brody, E. (1985). Parent care as a normative family stress. *Gerontologist, 25,* 19–29.

Brody, E., Kleban, M., Johnsen, P., et al. (1987). Work status and parent care: A comparison of four groups of women. *Gerontologist, 27,* 201–208.

Brody, E., & Schoonover, C. (1986). Patterns of parent care when adult daughters work and when they do not. *Gerontologist, 26,* 372–381.

Brody, E., & Spark, G. M. (1966). Institutionalization of the aged: A family crisis. *Family Process, 5,* 76–90.

Burgess, E., & Locke, H. (1945). *The family: From institution to companionship.* New York: American Book Company.

Cantor, M. (1983). Strain among caregivers: A study of experiences in the United States. *Gerontologist, 23,* 597–604.

Caplan, G. (1974). *Support systems and community mental health.* New York: Behavioral Publications.

Clark, M., & Anderson, B. (1967). *Culture and aging.* Springfield, IL: Charles C. Thomas.

Cobb, S. (1976). Social support as a moderator of life stress. *Psychosomatic Medicine, 38,* 300–314.

Cohen, S., & Syme, L. (1985). *Social support and health.* New York: Academic Press.

Cohen, S., & Wills, T. (1983). Stress, social support, and the buffering hypothesis. *Psychological Bulletin, 98,* 310–337.

Dimond, M., & Jones, S. (1983). Social support: A review and theoretical integration. In P. L. Chinn (Ed.), *Advances in nursing theory and development* (pp. 235–249). Rockville, MD: Aspen Publishers.

Dobrof, R., & Litwak, E. (1977). Guide to practice. In R. Dobrof & E. Litwak (Eds.), *Maintenance of family ties of long-term care patients: Theory and guide to practice* (pp. 1–79). (Department of Health and Human Services Publ. No. ADM81-400). Washington, D.C.: U.S. Government Printing Office.

Doty, P. (1986). Family care of the elderly: The role of public policy. *Millbank Memorial Fund Quarterly, 64,* 34–75.

Dowd, J. (1975). Aging as exchange: A preface to theory. *Journal of Gerontology, 35,* 596–602.

Duncan, M., & Morgan, D. (1994). Sharing the caring: Family caregivers' views of their relationships with nursing home staff. *Gerontologist, 34,* 235–244.

Finley, N., Roberts, M., & Banahan, B. (1988). Motivators and inhibitors of attitudes of filial obligation toward aging parents. *Gerontologist, 28,* 73–78.

George, L. (1986). Caregiver burdens: Conflict between norms of reciprocity and solidarity. In K. Pillemer & R. Wolf (Eds.), *Elder abuse: Conflict in the family* (pp. 67–92). Dover, MA: Auburn House.

Gottlieb, B. (1981). *Social network and social support.* Beverly Hills, CA: Sage Publications.

Gottlieb, B. (1985). Social networks and social support: An overview of research, practice, and policy implications. *Health Education Quarterly, 12,* 5–22.

Greenblatt, M., Becerra, R., & Serafetinides, E. (1982). Social networks and mental health: An overview. *American Journal of Psychiatry, 8,* 977–984.

Gross, P. (1994). *Motivators of adult child caregiving behaviors.* Unpublished doctoral dissertation. Tucson: University of Arizona.

Guberman, N., Maheu, P., & Maille, C. (1992). Women as family caregivers: Why do they care? *Gerontologist, 32,* 607–617.

Guttmann, D. (1979). Use of informal and formal supports by the white ethnic aged. In D. Gelfard & A. Kutzit (Eds.), *Ethnicity and aging: Theory, research and policy* (pp. 246–262). New York: Springer.

Hamon, R., & Thiessen, J. (1989). *What adult children do for their aging parents and why.* Unpublished paper presented at the 51st Annual Conference of the National Council on Family Relationships, New Orleans, LA.

Heller, P. (1976). Familism scale: Revalidation and revision. *Journal of Marriage and the Family, 38,* 423–429.

Homans, G. (1961). *Social behavior: Its elementary forms.* New York: Harcourt, Brace and World.

Horowitz, A. (1985). Sons and daughters as caregivers to older parents: Differences in role performances and consequences. *Gerontologist, 25,* 612–617.

Horowitz, A., & Dobrof, R. (1982). *The role of families in providing long-term care to the frail and chronically ill elderly living in the community.* Final report submitted to the Health Care Financing Administration. New York: Brookdale Center on Aging.

House, J. (1981). *Work, stress and social support.* Menlo Park, CA: Addison-Wesley.

Israel, B. (1983). Social networks and health status: Linking theory, research and practice. *Patient Counseling Education, 4,* 65–79.

Jarrett, W. (1985). Caregiving within kinship systems: Is affection really necessary? *Gerontologist, 25,* 5–10.

Jenkins, J., & Karno, M. (1992). The meaning of expressed emotion: Theoretical issues raised by cross-cultural research. *American Journal of Psychiatry, 149,* 9–21.

Kahana, E., & Kahana, B. (1984). Jews. In E. Palmore (Ed.), *Handbook of the aged in the United States* (pp. 155–180). Westport, CT: Greenwood.

Kahn, R. (1979). Aging and social support. In M. W. Riley (Ed.), *Aging from birth to death* (pp. 77–91). New York: Westview Press.

Kahn, R., & Antonucci, T. (1981). Convoys over the life course: Attachment, roles and social support. In P. B. Baltes & O. Bream (Eds.), *Life span development and behavior* (pp. 253–286). New York: Academic Press.

Keefe, S., Padilla, A., & Carlos, M. (1978). The Mexican-American extended family as an emotional support system. In J. Casas & S. Keefe (Eds.), *Family and mental health in the Mexican-American community* (pp. 49–67). Monograph No. 7, Spanish Speaking Mental Health Research Center, University of California at Los Angeles.

Keefe, S., Padilla, A., & Carlos, M. (1979). The Mexican-American extended family as an emotional support system. *Human Organization, 38,* 144–152.

Lee, G. (1980). Kinship in the seventies: A decade review of research and theory. *Journal of Marriage and the Family, 42,* 193–204.

Leavell, H., & Clark, E. (1958). *Preventive medicine for the doctor in his community.* New York: McGraw-Hill.

Leavy, R. (1983). Social support and psychological disorder: A review. *Journal of Community Psychology, 11,* 3–21.

Leichter, H., & Mitchell, W. (1967). *Kinship and casework.* New York: Russell Sage.

Liu, K., Manton, K., & Liu, B. (1985). Home care expenses for noninstitutionalized elderly with ADL and IADL limitations. *Health Care Financing Review, 7,* 51–58.

Mangen, D., Bengtson, V., & Landry, P. (Eds.). (1988). *Measurement of intergenerational relations.* Newbury Park, CA: Sage Publications.

Markides, K., Boldt, J., & Ray, L. (1986). Sources of helping and intergenerational solidarity: A three-generations study of Mexican Americans. *Journal of Gerontology, 41,* 506–511.

Markides, K., & Krause, E. (1985). Intergenerational solidarity and psychological well-being among older Mexican Americans: A three-generations study. *Journal of Gerontology, 40,* 390–392.

McCall, G., & Simmons, J. (1976). *Identities and interactions.* New York: Free Press.

McChesney, K., & Bengtson, V. (1988). Solidarity, integration, and cohesion in families: Concepts and theories. In D. Mangen, V. Bengtson & P. Landry (Eds.), *Measurement of intergenerational relations* (pp. 15–30). Newbury Park, CA: Sage Publications.

McChesney, K., & Mangen, D. (1988). Measuring family structure. In D. Mangen, V. Bengtson & P. Landry (Eds.), *Measurement of intergenerational relations* (pp. 65–73). Newbury Park, CA: Sage Publications.

McKinlay, J., & Tennestedt, S. (1986). *Social networks and the care of frail elders.* Final Report to the National Institute of Aging (Grant No. AGO3869). Boston: Boston University.

Miller, M., & Harris, A. (1965). Social factors and family

conflicts in a nursing home population. *Journal of the American Geriatrics Society, 13,* 845–851.

Mindel, C., & Habenstein, R. (1981). *Ethnic families in America.* New York: Elsevier.

Mitchell, R., & Trickett, E. (1980). Task force report: Social network as mediators of social support. *Community Mental Health Journal, 16,* 27–44.

Montgomery, R., Gonyea, J., & Hooyman, N. (1985). Caregiving and the experience of subjective and objective burden. *Family Relations, 34,* 19–26.

Moss, M., Moos, S., & Moles, E. (1985). The quality of relationships between elderly parents and their out-of-town children. *Gerontologist, 25,* 134–140.

Mutran, E., & Reitzes, D. (1984). Intergenerational support activities and well-being among the elderly: A convergence of exchange and symbolic interaction perspectives. *American Sociological Review, 49,* 117–130.

Norbeck, J. (1982). The use of social support in clinical practice. *Journal of Psychosocial Nursing and Mental Health Services, 20,* 22–29.

Norbeck, J., Lindsey, A., & Carrieri, V. (1981). The development of an instrument to measure social support. *Nursing Research, 30,* 264–269.

Norbeck, J., Lindsey, A., & Carrieri, V. (1983). Further development on the Norbeck social support questionnaire normative data and validity testing. *Nursing Research, 32,* 4–9.

Phillips, L. (1984). On becoming a caregiver. Paper presented at the 13th annual Nursing Research Conference, University of Arizona, Tucson.

Phillips, L. (1990). Elder-family caregiver relationships: Determining appropriate nursing interventions. *Nursing Clinics of North America, 24,* 795–807.

Phillips, L. (1985–1994). Causal factors affecting the quality of family caregiving. Project supported by National Center of Nursing Research, National Institutes of Health Report No. RO1 NU01323. In progress.

Phillips, L., & Van Ort, S. (1995). Issues in conducting intervention research in long-term care settings. *Nursing Outlook, 43,* 249–253.

Pillemer, K. (1987). Maltreatment of the elderly at home and in institutions: Extent, risk factors, and policy recommendations. *Legislative Agenda for An Aging Society: 1988 and Beyond.* Proceedings of a Congressional Forum by the Select Committee on Aging, House of Representatives, and the Special Committee on Aging, United States Senate. Washington, D.C.: U.S. Government Printing Office Publ. No. 100-664, pp. 145–169.

Porrit, D. (1979). Social support in crisis: Quantity or quality? *Social Science Medicine, 13A,* 715–721.

Ramirez, O., & Arce, C. (1981). The contemporary Chicano family: An empirically based review. In A. Baron (Ed.), *Explorations in Chicano psychology* (pp. 3–28). New York: Prager.

Roberts, S. (1984). Social support—meaning, measurement, and relevance to community health nursing practice. *Public Health Nursing, 1,* 158–167.

Roberts, S. (1988). Social support and help seeking: Review of the literature. *Advances in Nursing Science, 10,* 1–11.

Roberts, R., & Bengston, V. (1990). Is intergenerational solidarity a unidimensional construct? A second test of a formal model. *Journal of Gerontology, 45,* 12–20.

Roberts, R., Richards, L., & Bengston, V. (1991). Intergenerational solidarity in families: Untangling the ties that bind. *Marriage and Family Review, 16,* 1–20.

Rossi, A., & Rossi, P. (1990). Of human bonding: Parent-child relationships across life course. New York: Aldine de Gruyter.

Russell, C. (1993). *Care seeking and elders' dependency work: "My time is occupied trying to live."* Unpublished doctoral dissertation. Tucson: University of Arizona.

Select Committee on Aging (1987). *Exploding the myths: Caregiving in America.* A study by the Subcommittee on Human Services of the Select Committee on Aging, House of Representatives (Comm. Publ. No. 99-611).

Shanas, E. (1979). The family as a social support system in older age. *Gerontologist, 19,* 169–174.

Soldo, B., Wolf, D., & Agree, E. (1990). Family households, and care arrangements of older women: A structural analysis. *Journal of Gerontology, 45,* 238–249.

Stephens, S., & Christianson, J. (1986). *Informal care of the elderly.* Lexington, MA: Lexington Books.

Stoller, E. (1983). Parental caregiving by adult children. *Journal of Marriage and the Family, 45,* 851–858.

Stone, R., Carrerate, G., & Sangi, J. (1987). Caregivers of the frail elderly: A national profile. *Gerontologist, 27,* 616–626.

Taylor, R. (1985). The extended family as a source of support to elderly blacks. *Gerontologist, 25,* 488–495.

Tennestedt, S. (1984). *Informal care of frail elders in the community.* Unpublished doctoral dissertation. Boston: Boston University.

Tennestedt, S., & McKinlay, J. (1989). Informal care for frail older persons. In M. Ory & K. Bond (Eds.), *Aging and health care* (pp. 145–166). London: Routledge.

Thoits, P. (1982). Conceptual, methodological, and theoretical problems in studying social support as a buffer against life stress. *Journal of Health and Social Behavior, 23,* 145–159.

Troll, L. (1971). The family of late life: A decade review. *Journal of Marriage and the Family, 33,* 263–270.

Tilden, V., & Gaylen, R. (1987). Cost and conflict: The darker side of social support. *Western Journal of Nursing Research, 9,* 9–18.

Watson, W. (1982). *Aging and social behavior: An introduction to social gerontology.* Belmont, CA: Wadsworth.

Functional Assessment

Yvonne Browne Sehy
Marilyn P. Williams

Functional well-being significantly influences an elderly person's quality of life. A multidimensional functional approach that is patient oriented and focuses on those acts that a patient can or cannot do has been advocated as an essential component of geriatric assessment. Generally, this is divided into three major categories: physical, psychological, and social function.

Physical function includes the following domains: (1) general physical health; (2) activities of daily living (ADL), defined as those activities needed for self-care, such as bathing, dressing, or walking; and (3) instrumental activities of daily living (IADL), defined as those activities needed to support independent living, such as cooking, shopping, and laundry. Domains of *psychological function* include cognitive and affective status. *Social function* includes social interactions and resources, subjective well-being and coping, and the fit between person and environment (Kane & Kane, 1981).

This chapter provides information on the assessment of physical and social function, instruments to assess function in each of these categories, and instruments for a multidimensional functional assessment. (Chapter 7 focuses on cognitive function, Chapter 8 on the assessment of social support, and Chapter 17 on affective status.)

REASONS FOR FUNCTIONAL ASSESSMENT

There are several reasons for incorporating systematic assessment of functional status into advanced nursing practice. First, the assessment of functional status identifies patient concerns. For most people, illness is characterized not by pathology or medical diagnosis but by the restriction of activity or the presence of discomfort. Illness, then, is defined by the patient as restricted activity or pain. Conversely, the medical definition of illness is viewed in terms of biological or psychological dysfunction. Thus, the patient's definition of illness—patient-perceived morbidity—may or may not correlate with the medical definition of illness—clinical morbidity (Wilson-Barnett & Foraham, 1982). This helps explain why the vast majority of elderly people, despite multiple chronic conditions, continue to consider themselves healthy if they can still do what they have always done.

Figure 9–1 illustrates the relationship between clinical morbidity and patient-perceived morbidity. The goal in most traditional settings is to move patients from group I to group IV; that is, from a state in which both the patient and the healthcare professional acknowledge an illness to a state of complete wellness. When working with the chronic problems of the elderly population, however, the goal is often to move patients from group I to II; that is, people still may have multiple health problems but regard themselves as healthy because they can still function as before.

Second, functional deficits may represent a manifestation of disease. Unlike ill younger people, older adults rarely present with a single specific complaint that points to the system or organ in which disease occurs. Often, vague complaints such as feeling weak or tired lead to an impaired functional status and are the first indicators of a disease process, whether it is an acute illness or an exacerbation of a chronic disease (Besdine, 1995). Although the reasons are not well understood for disease presenting first as loss of function in older patients, it appears that disease causes a disruption in the homeostasis within the most vulnerable systems. Difficulties in ambulation, cognition, nutrition, and continence can therefore signal disease in almost any system in the elderly (Besdine, 1995).

Third, the assessment of functional status may support the decision of whether to treat a patient. Given little or no functional limitation, the treatment of abnormal laboratory test results may be withheld if the treatment carries with it substantial risk and greater discomfort (Besdine, 1995). Similarly, conservative treatment may be continued if it can be documented that the condition has not caused a decline in functioning.

Fourth, the monitoring of functional status tracks changes in untreated conditions. If a decision has been made to not treat, functional status must be monitored to determine changes that may indicate a need for reassessment. The patient with previously untreated mitral stenosis, for example, may become a candidate for surgery when fatigue or activity intolerance interferes with functioning. Similarly, the removal of cataracts may or may not be indicated, depending on how much the condition interferes with the person's normal functioning: The nurse using functional assessment to

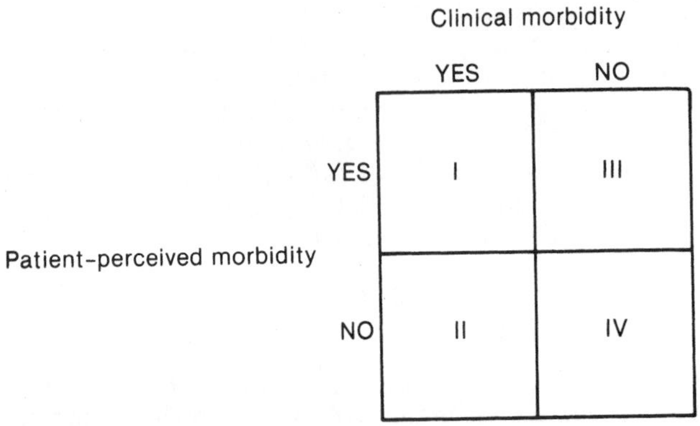

FIGURE 9–1. The relationship between clinical morbidity and patient-perceived morbidity. (From Wilson-Barnett, J., & Foraham, M. [1982]. *Recovery from illness.* New York: John Wiley & Sons.)

monitor change may advocate for cataract removal based on different sets of data in the 80-year-old man who can no longer find his golf ball on the fairway and in the 75-year-old resident of a skilled nursing facility who can no longer find his room owing to poor vision.

Fifth, describing remediable functional deficits assists in setting realistic goals. Cure as a goal is often not appropriate when caring for the elderly person with chronic, irreversible conditions and can lead to a sense of therapeutic impotence. An assessment of functional status can indicate strengths and define problem areas for further assessment. A return to or maintenance of functional status can then be reflected in the care plan, with appropriate interventions aimed at the source of the deficit. Knowledge of patients' functional ability prior to the acute illness will help the nurse determine what the patients can and should be doing for themselves as well as the appropriate discharge goals. Nowhere is this more pertinent than in an acute care setting in which the treatment of illness and maintenance of functional states must take place concurrently.

Sixth, the focus on functional status decreases fragmentation within healthcare teams or in institutional settings by organizing the care plan according to functional status. Since the cause of functional deficits in the elderly is frequently multifactorial, expertise from a variety of disciplines is often required to plan and implement interventions aimed at the source of the deficits. Discipline-specific jargon not only hampers communication but also interferes with the coordination of care, leading to fragmented, discipline-specific goals. Terms such as *degrees of independence in feeding, transfer*, and *ambulation* are patient oriented, measurable, and easily communicated within multidisciplinary settings.

Seventh, the assessment of functional deficits assists in determining the need for services. Maddox (1981) emphasized that services often do not benefit older adults. He cited the key issue as matching the care provided by the service to the specific impairment of the individual; this need for services is not determined by diagnosis alone but rather by specific functional deficits. Equally important to defining the specific functional deficit is determining the causes of the defined deficits. A process of first defining the functional deficit and then determining its cause gives direction when attempting to locate appropriate community service.

Eighth, the assessment of functional status assists in determining the need for placement. The decision to institutionalize an elderly person, particularly one who is cognitively impaired, is often made within the acute care hospital when family members are most vulnerable to the suggestions of healthcare professionals (Johnson & Grant, 1986). If discharge summaries are reflective of the information used to determine placement, the decision to institutionalize appears to be based solely on a list of diagnoses. Yet many older people with numerous problems still function independently within the community. Medical diagnosis alone is therefore an inadequate indicator of the need for placement (Falcone, 1983); rather, a patient's deteriorating physical and functional status and a lack of available social support are most often associated with placement decisions.

Finally, the assessment of deficits in function can assist in ethical decision making. Knowing the person's functional capacity and deficits prior to the illness provides valuable information on quality of life issues when deciding whether to initiate or terminate treatment.

CONDUCTING A FUNCTIONAL ASSESSMENT

In almost any setting, the nurse is the healthcare professional who spends the most time with the elderly patient and is therefore in an ideal position to obtain data regarding functional ability. The nurse in the skilled nursing facility, acute care, or homecare setting can obtain valuable information by simply taking the time to watch a person eat, dress, walk, or bathe. Even slight decrements in functioning may be significant in the frail elderly client. Functional assessment of the elderly has improved with the use of measurement instruments involving observation, self-administered questionnaires, and interviews.

Both observation and self-report methods of

assessing function in the elderly may be problematic. Rubenstein and colleagues (1984) reported that patients tend to overrate, and family members underrate, the patient's functional abilities when compared with findings obtained from direct observation by a nurse. Physicians were found to have poor abilities to detect moderate to mild functional impairments (Pinholt et al., 1987) and were less accurate in assessing physical function than the elderly patients themselves or family members (Elam et al., 1989). Similarly, Ward-Griffin and Bramwell (1990) reported discrepancies between nurses' and elderly individuals' perceptions of self-care abilities and health status.

Whether relying on report or observation to assess an individual's functional abilities, the nurse must be aware of the conditions surrounding the assessment process and how they might influence an elderly person's responses. Although direct observation, as used in performance tests, avoids many subjective biases in judgment, it is still influenced by the observer's ability to elicit the individual's best or usual performance (Applegate et al., 1990; George, 1997). Reuben and colleagues (1995) found that the relationships between commonly used self-administered, interview-administered, and performance-based measures of physical function were inconsistent and weak, suggesting that the instruments were not measuring the same construct.

Guralnik and colleagues (1989) suggested that the assessment of physical functioning status would be improved if objective physical performance measures were used to supplement traditional self- and proxy-reported measures. Despite the limitations inherent in measurements of function, established assessment instruments to evaluate functional status allow the nurse and other care providers to more accurately validate, monitor, and clearly communicate clinical impressions to other members of the healthcare team.

Functional Assessment Instruments

Instruments that measure function in the elderly have been developed for use in a variety of settings for several purposes. These instruments may be divided into *norm-referenced* and *criterion-referenced* measures. Norm-referenced tests compare the performance of individuals with each other and therefore discriminate among individuals regarding a specific behavior or attribute. These instruments are further divided into standardized and nonstandardized tests. Standardized tests are designed for widespread and consistent use in a variety of settings and have been constructed, tested, revised, and administered under specific conditions. In contrast, nonstandardized tests are usually designed for a specific setting and are flexible so that content may be updated frequently and adapted to accommodate minor changes (Waltz et al., 1991).

Criterion-referenced tests have a different focus. They determine whether an individual is able to perform or attain a specific behavior or level of functioning without comparison with the performance of others. Criterion-referenced tests such as the Katz ADL Index (Katz et al., 1970) are more prevalent than norm-referenced tests in functional assessment of the elderly, because it is often important to determine whether an individual can function at a level that supports independence and self-care.

Selecting an Instrument

The use of easily administered, reliable, and well-validated instruments that encompass the major functional domains improves the efficiency and comprehensiveness of health assessment in the elderly. Cautious selection of assessment instruments should be based on the purpose of the measurement and its inherent value assumptions (Applegate, 1987; George, 1997). For example, an assessment of ADL for a terminally ill individual may not serve a useful purpose or be relevant if the goal of care is to provide comfort and emotional support rather than to encourage improved functional abilities.

An assessment instrument may be selected based on its use for screening, assessment, or monitoring. Screening for clinical purposes or case finding, for example, focuses on the likely population at risk and a threshold value, such as eligibility for certain services. The *specificity*—the extent to which individuals lacking a characteristic are accurately classified—is more important in screening than is *sensitivity*—the extent to which individuals who truly manifest a characteristic are accurately classified. This avoids falsely labeling those elderly people who do not require interventions (Applegate, 1987). A screening tool should be brief, inexpensive, and appropriate for administration by nonprofessionals as well as professionals.

An assessment instrument used to diagnose or describe a condition should be capable of detecting increments of change in function. Those self-report measures that do not clearly define the activity being assessed or have response categories that are open to misperception and inaccurate responses impair clinicians' abilities to detect changes in the subsequent administration of the test. Categories of response that are too large or inclusive may not capture small but clinically important changes in functioning (Guralnik et al., 1989).

Monitoring involves rescreening or retesting specific problem areas at specified intervals, especially following interventions. The frequency of monitoring is based on the expected frequency of change or the signs of actual change. For example, patients in a stroke rehabilitation setting may have ADL assessed every 2 weeks to measure improvement related to the rehabilitation services.

RELIABILITY AND VALIDITY

High reliability and validity are desirable characteristics of these instruments. *Reliability* is the degree to which results of repeated measures of an instrument are consistent or reproducible. *Validity* is the degree to which an instrument measures what it claims to measure. Because reliability is a necessary prerequisite for validity, weaknesses in the reliability of a measuring instrument also weaken its validity. Conversely, an instrument may have high reliability but low validity; its measurements are consistent but it fails to measure the attribute of interest (Waltz et al., 1991).

Ware (1984) recommended attaining instrument reliability scores of at least 0.90 to make clinical decisions, although few assessment tools attain scores this high. Reliability of self-report assessment measures used with the elderly may be adversely affected by factors such as misunderstanding the meaning of questions or items, difficulty with accurate recall and reporting, physical frailty, or proxy reporting by family members or others (Applegate, 1987). Although the actual observation of functional abilities in the elderly is probably a more accurate measurement than self-reporting, it is often impractical because of time and resource limitations. Observation is most useful for areas of function that can be quickly assessed in the clinical setting or in the home.

CRITERIA FOR SELECTION

Functional assessment instruments must be considered acceptable by clients, family members, and healthcare providers. A summary of criteria to be considered in selecting a functional assessment instrument is presented in Table 9–1.

TABLE 9-1
Criteria for Selecting an Assessment Instrument

Issue	Rationale
Relevance and usefulness	Assessment data are useful for their intended purpose
Reliability and validity	Instrument is a reliable and valid measure of the domain or attribute of interest as reported by previous users and is capable of tracking change over time
Patient acceptability	Respondents' willingness and ability to participate in assessment improves the usefulness, reliability and validity of the instrument
Resources required	Amount of time, number of personnel, and amount of training needed to administer the instrument all affect its usefulness
Accessibility	Instrument and collected data are readily accessible to all providers for planning, monitoring, and evaluating care

The functional assessment instruments presented in this chapter address the needs of nurses specializing in care of the elderly in a variety of settings. They include physical, social, and multidimensional assessment instruments that are relatively brief and useful in clinical practice and have acceptable levels of reliability and validity. The measurement categories or scales used should be able to place individuals accurately on a continuum from poor to excellent health or functioning (Rubenstein et al., 1988). Most of the instruments included have proved clinically useful over time. A few new instruments are also included that appear promising for clinical use.

There is an obvious overlap of abilities needed to function in different domains, such as the cognitive abilities necessary for performing ADL. The delineation of functional assessment domains or categories is meant to provide organizational and conceptual clarity; however, it may change as our understanding and development of geriatric assessment progresses (Reuben & Solomon, 1989).

There are no specific training recommendations for administering most of the functional assessment instruments included in this chapter. Some instruments include minimum criteria to be met by individuals performing the assessment, such as knowledge of medical terminology or participation in a brief training session. Specific information and questions about the administration of assessment instruments should be directed to the developers of the instruments. Practice, supervised by those who are experienced and competent in use of these instruments, is highly recommended to strengthen the reliability of the tests and, indirectly, their validity.

Although functional assessment is often targeted to specific groups, general recommendations for clinical practice are being developed. Rubenstein and colleagues (1988) recommended evaluating each home-dwelling client older than age 65 years with a clinical interview, a depression scale, and a review of IADL at least once every 3 years. Patients older than age 75 years, those older than age 65 years in hospitals or nursing homes, or any elderly person with problems performing the IADL should have an additional evaluation of mental status and basic ADL. Evaluation of IADL, ADL, and mental status should be performed on anyone suspected of having a disability or dementia. It is hoped that by integrating functional assessment into clinical practice, the use of appropriate measuring instruments will grow, enhance nursing practice, and improve care of the elderly.

ASSESSMENT OF PHYSICAL FUNCTION

Measurements of physical health or functioning are generally hierarchical. The assessment of physical function falls into four categories: general physical health, basic self-care activities or ADL, more complex activities associated with independent living or IADL, and a new category, advanced activities of daily living (AADL). AADL include activities beyond those needed to maintain independent living but which contribute significantly to quality of life, such as recreational, occupational, and community activities (Reuben & Solomon, 1989). New difficulty in performing a higher-level function, such as playing golf, may be the first indication of a more serious functional decline.

Instruments of General Physical Health

General physical health has been determined via medical diagnoses, physical measurements of health (such as various laboratory indices), the evaluation of impairments, professional ratings of an individual's health, the use of health services, and self-ratings of health. Although none of these methods gives a complete picture of an individual's health status, two instruments that measure physical health have been reported to have acceptable levels of reliability and validity.

The Index of Illness (Shanas, 1962) is a 5-minute, scored, self-report interview in which respondents use a body systems checklist to report about illnesses experienced during the preceding 4-week period as well as current health problems. It includes an open-ended assessment of past health problems and the degree to which activities have been restricted during the past 12 months. According to the test, "sicker" respondents from a national sample of noninstitutionalized elderly had more complaints about health and were more likely to be recipients of public welfare as a main source of income; this result supports the validity of the Index of Illness (Stahl, 1984).

The Older Americans Resources and Services (OARS) Center instrument developed at Duke University (1978) is a 1-hour multidimensional test comprising five domains, including physical health. A global rating of physical health is obtained using descriptive anchors. It is the most widely used assessment tool to measure physical health for a community sample without data from a physical examination or physiological tests (Kane & Kane, 1981). The OARS has high test-retest and interrater reliability. In one study, criterion-related validity was based on high correlations between professional judgments and results from the test. Construct validity was supported by the OARS' ability to discriminate among elderly populations in the community, outpatient clinics, and institutional settings (Ernst & Ernst, 1984).

Instruments of Activities of Daily Living

ADL include those activities needed for self-care: dressing, bathing, toileting, mobility, eating, and continence. Scores on ADL instruments are based on definitions of the degree of independent functioning for each activity or the degree and type of assistance needed for a given activity. ADL scales are useful in describing baseline functioning, setting goals, and monitoring abilities. These instruments differ somewhat in the specific physical functioning assessed as well as their ability to detect change.

The Katz Index of ADL (Katz et al., 1963) is a Guttman scale that allows the observation and rating of six ADL functions (Fig. 9–2). This index, which may be self-administered or administered by an interviewer in about 5 minutes, has been adapted as a Likert-type scale to better define the degree of dependence for each function measured. It was found to be

highly reliable in the elderly in homecare and sheltered-housing groups (Sherwood et al., 1977). The index's construct validity is supported by its paralleling of human physical development. Overall ADL scores correlate with range of motion and cognitive function (Katz et al., 1970). The Katz Index is appropriate for patients in acute or long-term care or in community settings.

The OARS ADL section, which includes information on bathing, dressing, toileting, transfers, continence, feeding, walking, and grooming, relies on information from the patient or a relative. A global score is obtained for both ADL and IADL function, which prohibits comparison with other ADL instrument scores. The OARS has been widely used in community-based gerontological research (Duke University, 1978). A shorter, 30-minute version of the OARS instrument, the Functional Assessment Inventory, distinguishes among elderly respondents in nursing homes, adult living facilities, adult daycare centers, and senior centers. This shorter test has reliability and validity similar to the OARS instrument if it is administered by trained interviewers (Pfeiffer et al., 1980).

The Timed "Up & Go" test (Podsiadlo & Richardson, 1991) provides significant objective data in a short time. The elderly person is asked to rise from a chair, walk 3 meters (approximately 10 feet), turn around, and return to and sit in the chair. This activity is timed and recorded. The time required appears to correlate inversely with functional status; that is, increased time implies increased dependence (Guralnik et al., 1995). This test may prove useful in settings such as the office where it is impractical to actually observe ADL. The Timed "Up & Go" test may eventually prove useful in predicting levels of disability in people older than the age of 70 years (Guralnik et al., 1995).

The Physical Performance Test (PPT) (Reuben & Siu, 1990) assesses multiple domains of physical function that extend across a wide range of difficulties (Fig. 9–3). It includes timed, observed performances of nine tasks that simulate ADL (a seven-item version does not include stairs). The test requires a few simple props and can be administered in less than 10 minutes by a layperson with minimal training. Items are

Index of Independence in
Activities of Daily Living

The Index of Independence in Activities of Daily Living is based on an evaluation of the functional independence or dependence of patients in bathing, dressing, going to the toilet, transferring, continence, and feeding. Specific definitions of functional independence and dependence appear below the index.

A   Independent in feeding, continence, transferring, going to toilet, dressing, and bathing.
B   Independent in all but one of these functions.
C   Independent in all but bathing and one additional function.
D   Independent in all but bathing, dressing, and one additional function.
E   Independent in all but bathing, dressing, going to toilet, and one additional function.
F   Independent in all but bathing, dressing, going to toilet, transferring, and one additional function.
G   Dependent in all six functions.
Other   Dependent in at least two functions, but not classifiable as C, D, E, or F.

Independence means without supervision, direction, or active personal assistance, except as specifically noted below. This is based on actual status and not on ability. A patient who refuses to perform a function is considered as not performing the function, even though he is deemed able.

BATHING (sponge, shower, or tub)
Independent: assistance only in bathing a
   single part (as back or disabled extremity)
   or bathes self completely
Dependent: assistance in bathing more than
   one part of body; assistance in getting in
   or out of tub or does not bathe self

TRANSFER
Independent: moves in and out of bed independently and moves in and out of chair
   independently (may or may not be using
   mechanical supports)
Dependent: assistance in moving in or out
   of bed and/or chair; does not perform
   one or more transfers

DRESSING
Independent: gets clothes from closets and
   drawers; puts on clothes, outer garments,
   braces; manages fasteners; act of tying
   shoes is excluded
Dependent: does not dress self or remains
   partly undressed

CONTINENCE
Independent: urination and defecation entirely self-controlled
Dependent: partial or total incontinence in
   urination or defecation, partial or total
   control by enemas, catheters, or regulated
   use of urinals and/or bedpans

GOING TO TOILET
Independent: gets to toilet; gets on and off
   toilet; arranges clothes, cleans organs of
   excretion; (may manage own bedpan used
   at night only and may or may not be using mechanical supports)
Dependent: uses bedpan or commode or receives assistance in getting to and using
   toilet

FEEDING
Independent: gets food from plate or its
   equivalent into mouth; (precutting of
   meat and preparation of food, as buttering bread, are excluded from evaluation).
Dependent: assistance in act of feeding (see
   above); does not eat at all or parenteral
   feeding.

FIGURE 9–2 *See legend on opposite page*

scored on a five-point scale (0–4), and a protocol for administering the PPT is provided. Reuben and colleagues (1992) found that both the nine- and seven-item versions of the PPT demonstrate high internal consistency and interrater reliability. Concurrent validity was demonstrated with self-reported measures of physical function. Scores on the PPT were highly correlated with other tests of ADL and were moderately or weakly correlated with health status, cognitive and mental health status, and age, thus demonstrating construct validity. The PPT was

Evaluation Form

Name _____ Date of Evaluation _____

For each area of functioning listed below, check description that applies. (The word *assistance* means supervision, direction of personal assistance.)

BATHING—either sponge bath, tub bath, or shower

☐ Receives no assistance (gets in and out of tub by self if tub is usual means of bathing)

☐ Receives assistance in bathing only one part of body (such as back or a leg)

☐ Receives assistance in bathing more than one part of body (or not bathed)

DRESSING—gets clothes from closets and drawers—including underclothes, outer garments, and using fasteners (including braces, if worn)

☐ Gets clothes and gets completely dressed without assistance

☐ Gets clothes and gets dressed without assistance except for assistance in tying shoes

☐ Receives assistance in getting clothes or in getting dressed, or stays partly or completely undressed

TOILETING—going to the "toilet room" for bowel and urine elimination; cleaning self after elimination and arranging clothes

☐ Goes to "toilet room," cleans self, and arranges clothes without assistance (may use object for support such as cane, walker, or wheelchair and may manage night bedpan or commode, emptying same in morning)

☐ Receives assistance in going to "toilet room" or in cleansing self or in arranging clothes after elimination or in use of night bedpan or commode

☐ Doesn't go to room termed "toilet" for the elimination process

TRANSFER—

☐ Moves in and out of bed as well as in and out of chair without assistance (may be using object for support such as cane or walker)

☐ Moves in or out of bed or chair with assistance

☐ Doesn't get out of bed

CONTINENCE—

☐ Controls urination and bowel movement completely by self

☐ Has occasional "accidents"

☐ Supervision helps keep urine or bowel control; catheter is used or is incontinent

FEEDING—

☐ Feeds self without assistance

☐ Feeds self except for getting assistance in cutting meat or buttering bread

☐ Receives assistance in feeding or is fed partly or completely by using tubes or intravenous fluids

FIGURE 9–2. Katz Index of Activities of Daily Living. (From Katz, S., Ford, A. B., Moskowitz, R. W., et al. [1963]. Studies of illness in the aged. The Index of ADL: A standardized measure of biological and psychosocial function. *Journal of the American Medical Association, 185,* 914–919. Copyright 1963 by the American Medical Association.)

PHYSICAL PERFORMANCE TEST SCORING SHEET

	Physical Performance Test		Score
	Time	Scoring	
1. Write a sentence (whales live in the blue ocean)	_____ sec*	≤10 sec = 4 10.5–15 sec = 3 15.5–20 sec = 2 >20 sec = 1 unable = 0	_____
2. Simulated eating	_____ sec	≤10 sec = 4 10.5–15 sec = 3 15.5–20 sec = 2 >20 sec = 1 unable = 0	_____
3. Lift a book and put it on a shelf	_____ sec	≤2 sec = 4 2.5–4 sec = 3 4.5–6 sec = 2 >6 sec = 1 unable = 0	_____
4. Put on and remove a jacket	_____ sec	≤10 sec = 4 10.5–15 sec = 3 15.5–20 sec = 2 >20 sec = 1 unable = 0	_____
5. Pick up penny from floor	_____ sec	≤2 sec = 4 2.5–4 sec = 3 4.5–6 sec = 2 >6 sec = 1 unable = 0	_____
6. Turn 360 degrees	discontinuous steps 0 continuous steps 2 unsteady (grabs, staggers) 0 steady 2		_____
7. 50-foot walk test	_____ sec	≤15 sec = 4 15.5–20 sec = 3 20.5–25 sec = 2 >25 sec = 1 unable = 0	_____
8. Climb one flight of stairs†	_____ sec	≤5 sec = 4 5.5–10 sec = 3 10.5–15 sec = 2 >15 sec = 1 unable = 0	_____
9. Climb stairs†	Number of flights of stairs up and down (maximum 4)		_____
TOTAL SCORE (maximum 36 for 9-item, 28 for 7-item)			_____ 9-item _____ 7-item

*For timed measurements, round to nearest 0.5 seconds.
†Omit for 7-item scoring.

FIGURE 9–3 *See legend on opposite page*

PHYSICAL PERFORMANCE TEST PROTOCOL

Administer the Physical Performance Test as outlined below. Subjects are given up to two chances to complete each item. Assistive devices are permitted for tasks 6 through 8.

1. Ask the subject, when given the command "go," to write the sentence "whales live in the blue ocean." Time from the word "go" until the pen is lifted from the page at the end of the sentence. All words must be included and legible. Period need not be included for task to be considered completed.

2. Five kidney beans are placed in a bowl, 5 inches from the edge of the desk in front of the patient. An empty coffee can is placed on the table at the patient's nondominant side. A teaspoon is placed in the patient's dominant hand. Ask the subject, on the command "go," to pick up the beans, one at a time, and place each in the coffee can. Time from the command "go" until the last bean is heard hitting the bottom of the can.

3. Place a Physician's Desk Reference or other heavy book on a table in front of the patient. Ask the patient, when given the command "go," to place the book on a shelf above shoulder level. Time from the command "go" to the time the book is resting on the shelf.

4. If the subject has a jacket or cardigan sweater, ask him or her to remove it. If not, give the subject a lab coat. Ask the subject, on the command "go" to put the coat on completely such that it is straight on his or her shoulders and then remove the garment completely. Time from the command "go" until the garment has been completely removed.

5. Place a penny approximately 1 foot from the patient's foot on the dominant side. Ask the patient, on the command "go," to pick up the penny from the floor and stand up. Time from the command "go" until the subject is standing erect with penny in hand.

6. With subject in a corridor or in an open room, ask the subject to turn 360 degrees. Evaluate using scale on PPT scoring sheet.

7. Bring subject to start on 50-foot walk test course (25 feet out and 25 feet back) and ask the subject, on the command "go," to walk to 25-foot mark and back. Time from the command "go" until the starting line is crossed on the way back.

8. Bring subject to foot of stairs (nine to 12 steps) and ask subject, on the command "go," to begin climbing stairs until he or she feels tired and wishes to stop. Before beginning this task, alert the subject to possibility of developing chest pain or shortness of breath and inform the subject to tell you if any of these symptoms occur. Escort the subject up the stairs. Time from the command "go" until the subject's first foot reaches the top of the first flight of stairs. Record the number of flights (maximum is four) climbed (up and down is one flight).

FIGURE 9–3. Physical performance test scoring sheet and protocol. (From Reuben, D. B., & Sui, A. L. [1990]. An objective measure of physical function of elderly persons: The physical performance test. *Journal of the American Geriatrics Society, 38,* 1111–1112. Copyright by the American Geriatrics Society.)

reported to be predictive of mortality and nursing home placement (Reuben et al., 1992), although further testing in various populations and settings is needed to establish its usefulness in detecting, monitoring, and predicting functional changes in the elderly.

Instruments of Instrumental Activities of Daily Living

IADL—those activities needed to support independent living—generally include housekeeping, food preparation, use of the telephone, doing laundry, using public transportation, taking medicine, handling finances, shopping, mobility, and home maintenance. The same limitations of measuring physical functioning apply to IADL as to ADL.

Long-term care settings usually do not encourage IADL performance by the elderly. The choice of an IADL assessment tool should be based on expected performance in the least restrictive setting for the individual. Supportive organizations such as homemaker services or Meals on Wheels may allow an individual with other instrumental skills to live in the home.

An eight-item IADL scale developed at the Philadelphia Geriatric Center (Lawton & Brody, 1969) is based on the interview of an informant and focuses on instrumental activities of the elderly necessary for successful community living (Fig. 9–4). A five- or six-item scale omitting food preparation, housekeeping, and sometimes doing laundry has been used for men to avoid sex bias. Lawton and Brody (1969) reported a reproducibility of 0.94 (Guttman scales) as well as high interrater reliability. Discriminant validity was supported by moderately high correlations of the scale with four other measures of functioning in a sample of applicants to the Philadelphia Geriatric Center (Eustis & Patten, 1984).

A brief version of the IADL scale from the

ACTION	SCORE
A. Ability to Use Telephone	1
1. Operates telephone on own initiative—looks up and dials numbers, etc.	1
2. Dials a few well-known numbers	1
3. Answers telephone but does not dial	0
4. Does not use telephone at all	
B. Shopping	
1. Takes care of all shopping needs independently	1
2. Shops independently for small purchases	0
3. Needs to be accompanied on any shopping trip	0
4. Completely unable to shop	0
C. Food Preparation	
1. Plans, prepares, and serves adequate meals independently	1
2. Prepares adequate meals if supplied with ingredients	0
3. Heats and serves prepared meals, or prepares meals but does not maintain adequate diet	0
4. Needs to have meals prepared and served	0
D. Housekeeping	
1. Maintains house alone or with occasional assistance (e.g., "heavy work-domestic help")	1
2. Performs light daily tasks such as dishwashing, bedmaking	1
3. Performs light daily tasks but cannot maintain acceptable level of cleanliness	1
4. Needs help with all home maintenance tasks	1
5. Does not participate in any housekeeping tasks	0
E. Laundry	
1. Does personal laundry completely	1
2. Launders small items—rinses socks, stockings, etc.	1
3. All laundry must be done by others	0
F. Mode of Transportation	
1. Travels independently on public transportation or drives own car	1
2. Arranges own travel via taxi, but does not otherwise use public transportation	1
3. Travels on public transportation when assisted or accompanied by another	1
4. Travel limited to taxi or automobile with assistance of another	0
5. Does not travel at all	0
G. Responsibility for Own Medications	
1. Is responsible for taking medication in correct dosages at correct times	1
2. Takes responsibility if medication is prepared in advance in separate dosages	0
3. Is not capable of dispensing own medication	0
H. Ability to Handle Finances	
1. Manages financial matters independently (budgets, writes checks, pays rent and bills, goes to bank), collects and keeps track of income	1
2. Manages day-to-day purchases, but needs help with banking, major purchases, etc.	1
3. Incapable of handling money	0

FIGURE 9–4. Instrumental activities of daily living scale. (From Lawton, M. P., & Brody, E. [1969]. Assessment of older people: Self-maintaining and instrumental activities of daily living. *Gerontologist, 9*, 181. Reprinted with permission).

OARS multidimensional tool may be used to screen the elderly for functional impairment and their need for more comprehensive assessment (Fillenbaum, 1985) (Fig. 9–5). The five items from the OARS IADL section include handling personal finances, meal preparation, shopping, travel, and housework. These items constitute a Guttman scale (hierarchical in levels of functioning) and are rated as (1) performed unaided, (2) performed with some help, or (3) unable to be performed at all (Fillenbaum, 1985). The instrument may be self-administered or administered by a trained interviewer in less than 5 minutes. Concurrent, discriminant, and predictive validity as well as reliability have been reported.

1. Can you get to places out of walking distance . . .
   1 Without help (can travel alone on buses, taxis, or drive your own car)?
   0 With some help (need someone to help you when traveling), or are you unable to travel unless emergency arrangements are made for a specialized vehicle like an ambulance?
   —Not answered
2. Can you go shopping for groceries or clothes (assuming she or he has transportation) . . .
   1 Without help (taking care of all shopping needs yourself, assuming you had transportation)?
   0 With some help (need someone to go with you on all shopping trips), or are you completely unable to do any shopping?
   —Not answered
3. Can you prepare your own meal . . .
   1 Without help (plan and cook full meals yourself)?
   0 With some help (can prepare some things but unable to cook full meals yourself), or are you completely unable to prepare any meals?
   —Not answered
4. Can you do your housework . . .
   1 Without help (can scrub floors, etc.)?
   0 With some help (can do light housework but need help with heavy work), or are you completely unable to do any housework?
   —Not answered
5. Can you handle your own money . . .
   1 Without help (write checks, pay bills, etc.)?
   0 With some help (manage day-to-day buying but need help with managing your checkbook and paying your bills), or are you completely unable to handle money?
   —Not answered

FIGURE 9–5. The five instrumental activities of daily living items, adapted from the Older Americans Resources and Services (OARS) multidimensional functional assessment questionnaire. (From Fillenbaum, G. G. [1995]. Screening the elderly: A brief instrumental activities of daily living measure. *Journal of the American Geriatrics Society, 33,* 706. Copyright by the American Geriatrics Society.)

Advanced Activities of Daily Living

AADL was defined by Reuben and Solomon (1989) as voluntary, typically culturally defined, and individual activities. Deficits in these activities significantly precede deficits in ADL or IADL. Examples of AADL are golfing, participation in church groups, and volunteer work. As much as ADL alone fail to track the activities of community-dwelling elderly people, so do IADL. Thus, in the very active elderly, the AADL play an important role.

The goal of healthcare professionals is often that of returning a person to premorbid functional status as measured by ADL and IADL—not by the patient's ability to play 18 holes of golf or to drive to other activities. The inability to perform personally valuable AADL could explain why Becker and Kaufman found in their study of 102 patients who had a stroke that after 12 months, none considered themselves "recovered" despite the documentation of such by various disciplines (Becker & Kaufman, 1995).

ASSESSMENT OF SOCIAL FUNCTION

Social function has been defined as the degree to which people function as members of the community (Donald et al., 1978). More specifically, Kane and colleagues (1985) defined it as adaptation or "the way a person meets social expectations and responsibilities" through various activities and relationships (role performance, social behavior, and social skills) (p. 5). In contrast, Kane and colleagues defined *social support,* a related but distinct concept, as "the way a person is anchored in a social milieu or network so as to receive information, protection, assistance, and a sense of belonging and worth" (p. 5). These two concepts are closely related, since the ability to develop and maintain a support system is a part of healthy social functioning.

Since there are numerous concepts and issues that may be considered in the social domain, there is little consensus on the description and measurement of social functioning.

Norms have not been measured for many of the tests, and there are few longitudinal studies that correlate social scale scores with later outcomes (Kane & Kane, 1981). Culture and socioeconomic background and the patient's environment define and limit social activities and relationships, making generalizability of social functioning measures questionable.

Characterizing social functioning as either good and adaptive or bad and maladaptive presupposes a societal consensus about acceptable social behavior or an association between certain social behaviors and perceived well-being, neither of which is firmly supported by research at this time (Kane et al., 1985). Consequently, Kane and colleagues (1985) recommended selecting social function instruments that measure the minimum social involvement, opportunity to exchange confidences, and social stimulation that is necessary for any individual's well-being as well as identifying negative behaviors that signal social maladaptation. More specifically, Kane and Kane (1981) identified the assessment of social interactions and resources, subjective well-being and coping, and the fit between a person and his or her environment as important indicators of social functioning. Selected instruments from the first two categories are reviewed subsequently.

Instruments of Social Interactions and Resources

Measures of social interactions and resources include intergenerational support, professional ratings of social functioning, self-reported activity questionnaires, and diaries of daily activities. The instruments included in this section use self-report and interviews.

The OARS Social Resources Scale (Duke University, 1978) is the best-known general social functioning measure for the elderly. This brief scored and structured interview may be used for community-dwelling or institutionalized elderly people to rate social resources, including family structure; patterns of friendship and visiting; the availability of a confidant; and the availability of a helper if needed.

The Rand Social Health Measure (Donald &

Ware, 1982) was developed as part of a large study of the effects of health insurance on healthcare use and health status. The instrument consists of 11 self-report items about contacts with friends and family as well as the quality of relationships and involvement in groups. Reliability estimates range from 0.16 to 0.75, and face, content, discriminant, and construct validities have been reported.

Instruments of Subjective Well-Being and Coping

Well-being is difficult to define. Carp (1977) described it as the inner aspect of coping, adaptation, or adjustment, and other measures of well-being have included subjective well-being, happiness, morale, life satisfaction, contentment, and personal adjustment. Because subjective well-being is associated with positive mental health, similar items may measure these two domains (Sauer & Warland, 1982).

Subjective well-being has frequently been assessed using measures of life satisfaction. Life satisfaction has been criticized as a superficial measure of well-being that is overly concerned with situational factors such as activity, health, and socioeconomic level (Euler, 1992). Euler instead recommended using the Measure of Psychosocial Development (MPD) (Hawley, 1988) based on Erik Erikson's adult stages of the life cycle to assess psychological adjustment and well-being. Although the MPD, a 56-item test, may not be appropriate for screening in many clinical situations, there is a need for assessment instruments that measure psychodynamic development in the elderly.

Coping, or active problem solving, has been measured with projective tests and responses to hypothetical situations; however, difficulty with interpretation and a lack of longitudinal data make validity difficult to establish. The ability to cope depends on environmental demands for coping, personality traits, and social role modeling. An accurate predictor of an elderly person's ability to cope would enable a more appropriate allocation of supportive resources (Kahana et al., 1982).

The Philadelphia Geriatric Center Morale Scale (Lawton, 1975), a 17-item scale interview or self-administered questionnaire, measures agitation, attitudes toward aging, and lonely dissatisfaction. The instrument has been shown to have predictive validity. High morale is correlated with variables such as physical health, participation in activities, satisfaction with social interaction, and mobility. Construct validity needs further testing, however. Reliability was high for large samples of institutional, public housing, and community residents (Kozma et al., 1991; Okun & Stock, 1987; Sauer & Warland, 1982).

The Life Satisfaction Index (Neugarten et al., 1961), both 15- and 20-item versions, measures mood tone, zest, and congruence to assess both psychological and physical dimensions of subjective well-being. Estimates of reliability have ranged from 0.72 to 0.87 for various forms of the index and 0.75 for internal consistency (Kozma et al., 1991; Okun & Stock, 1987). The Philadelphia Geriatric Center Morale Scale and the Life Satisfaction Index have a correlation of 0.74.

MULTIDIMENSIONAL ASSESSMENT INSTRUMENTS

Multidimensional assessment measures provide information about functioning across a variety of domains to characterize the overall status of the individual. These screening instruments generally require 30 to 90 minutes to complete as well as adequate staff training to ensure correct administering and interpretation (Applegate, 1987).

Shorter comprehensive functional assessment instruments have more recently been developed to improve the acceptability and efficiency of functional assessment for the respondents and assessors, as well as to maintain the reliability and validity of the measures. Although these shorter tools do not provide as much information about functional abilities as the longer comprehensive assessment tools, they may prove to be practical and efficient clinical screening tools that indicate the need to assess an area of function in more depth and detail (Rubenstein et al., 1988).

Kane and Kane (1981) recommended the use of assessment instruments that use self-report

and systematic observation over caregiver judgment ratings such as those found in the Stockton Geriatric Rating Scale (Meer & Baker, 1966), the Parachek Geriatric Rating Scale (Parachek & Miller, 1974), and the Physical and Mental Impairment-of-Function Evaluation Scale (PAMIE) (Gurel et al., 1972). Some of the more recent brief comprehensive functional assessment instruments included in this review use self-report rather than caregiver judgment to rate an individual's functional status. Clinical assessments that combine self-report with an observation of functional abilities show promise for improving the efficiency and usefulness of functional assessments performed in the ambulatory setting (Fleming et al., 1995; Lachs et al., 1990).

The OARS (Duke University, 1978) was developed for use in clinical research and program evaluation using a multidimensional functional assessment questionnaire with 105 questions to be administered in about 1 hour. The OARS assesses function in five domains: social resources, economic resources, mental health, physical health, and ADL. Judgment is then made on an impairment score for each domain, and a cumulative impairment score is then calculated. Reliability has been variable, depending on the domain tested, although there was good agreement among raters in the assignment of comparative levels of functioning and specific numerical ratings (Fillenbaum, 1978). Consensual validity was claimed by the authors and the OARS has been shown to discriminate among different populations (Duke University, 1978). A 30-minute version of the OARS, the Functional Assessment Inventory (Pfeiffer et al., 1980), yields ratings on the same five domains with reported acceptable reliability and validity if administered by trained interviewers.

The Sickness Impact Profile (SIP) (Gilson et al., 1975) has been used widely to measure healthcare outcomes and functional health status. It is recognized as one of the best validated multidimensional health measures (Parkerson et al., 1990). The SIP, which contains 136 items measuring sleep and rest, emotional behavior, body care and movement, home management, mobility, social interaction, ambulation, alertness behavior, communication, work, recre-

FUNCTIONAL STATUS QUESTIONNAIRE

Category	Item

PHYSICAL FUNCTION
Basic activities of daily living

During the past month, have you had difficulty
    taking care of yourself; that is, eating, dressing, or bathing?
    moving in and out of a bed or chair?
    walking indoors, such as around your home?

Intermediate activities of daily living

    walking several blocks?
    walking one block or climbing one flight of stairs?
    doing work around the house, such as cleaning, light yard work?
    home maintenance?
    doing errands, such as grocery shopping?
    driving a car or using public transportation?
    doing vigorous activities, such as running, lifting heavy objects, or
    participating in strenuous sports?

Responses: usually did with no difficulty (4), usually did with some difficulty (3), usually did with much difficulty (2), usually did not do because of health (1), usually did not do for other reasons (0)

PSYCHOLOGICAL FUNCTION
Mental health

During the past month
    have you been a very nervous person?
    have you felt calm and peaceful?*
    have you felt downhearted and blue?
    were you a happy person?*
    did you feel so "down in the dumps" that nothing could cheer you up?

Responses: all of the time (1), most of the time (2), a good bit of the time (3), some of the time (4), a little of the time (5), none of the time (6)

SOCIAL ROLE FUNCTION
Work performance (for those employed during the previous month)

During the past month, have you
    done as much work as others in similar jobs?*
    worked for short periods of time or taken frequent rests because of your health?
    worked your regular number of hours?*
    done your job as carefully and accurately as others with similar jobs?*
    worked at your usual job, but with some changes because of your health?
    feared losing your job because of your health?

Responses: all of the time (1), most of the time (2), some of the time (3), none of the time (4)

Social activity

During the past month, have you had difficulty
    visiting relatives or friends?
    participating in community activities, such as religious services, social activities, or volunteer work?
    taking care of other people, such as family members?

Responses: usually did with no difficulty (4), usually did with some difficulty (3), usually did with much difficulty (2), usually did not do because of health (1), usually did not do for other reasons (0)

Quality of interaction

During the past month, did you
    isolate yourself from people around you?
    act affectionate towards others?*
    act irritable toward those around you?
    make unreasonable demands on your family and friends?
    get along well with other people?*

Responses: all of the time (1), most of the time (2), a good bit of the time (3), some of the time (4), a little bit of the time (5), none of the time (6)

Single-item questions

Which of the following statements best describes your work situation during the past month? *Responses:* working full-time, working part-time, unemployed, looking for work, unemployed because of my health, retired because of my health, retired for some other reason.

During the past month, how many days did illness or injury keep you in bed all or most of the day? *Response:* 0–31 days.

During the past month, how many days did you cut down on the things you usually do for one-half day or more because of your illness or injury? *Response:* 0–31 days.

During the past month, how satisfied were you with your sexual relationships? *Responses:* very satisfied, satisfied, not sure, dissatisfied, very dissatisfied, did not have any sexual relationships.

How do you feel about your own health? *Responses:* very satisfied, satisfied, not sure, dissatisfied, very dissatisfied.

During the past month, about how often did you socialize with friends or relatives, that is, go out together, visit in each other's homes, or talk on the telephone? *Responses:* every day, several times a week, about once a week, two or three times a month, about once a month, not at all.

FIGURE 9–6 *See legend on opposite page*

Sample functional status report

PHYSICAL FUNCTION   WARNING ZONE = *******************
1. Basic activities of daily living   0 . . . . 56 -------------------------- 100

                                 ****
2. Intermediate activities of daily
   living   0 . . . . . 7 ---100

                                 ****
PSYCHOLOGICAL FUNCTION
Mental health   0 . . . . 36 ----------------------------------- 100

                                 ****
ROLE FUNCTION
1. Employment status   Retired because of health
2. Work performance   Not applicable
SOCIAL FUNCTION
1. Social activity   0 --- 100

                                 ****
2. Quality of interaction   0 . . . . 56 ----------------------- 100

                                 ****
3. Frequency of contact   Everyday
BED REST DAYS   0
RESTRICTED DAYS   31
SEXUAL RELATIONSHIPS   Did not have any sexual relationships
FEELING ABOUT HEALTH   Very satisfied

SUMMARY
The patient scored in the acceptable range of the following scales: none
Responses to the functional status questionnaire reveal the following general areas of concern: basic ADL, intermediate
   ADL, mental health, social activity, quality of interaction.
The patient reported significant problems with the following activities: eating, dressing, bathing, walking one block,
   working around house, doing errands, driving a car, visiting relatives or friends, participating in community activities,
   taking care of other people, doing vigorous activities.

FIGURE 9–6. Functional status questionnaire. Asterisk (*) indicates scores are reversed. (Reprinted from Jette, A. M., & Cleary, P. D. [1987]. Functional disability assessment. *Physical Therapy, 67,* 1857–1858, with the permission of the APTA.)

ation and pastimes, and eating, may be self-administered or administered by interview in about 30 minutes. It was developed and tested on sample groups with a majority age 55 years and older, including those with and those without health problems. The SIP can be reported as an overall score or as separate scores for each of the 12 dimensions. Its reliability is reportedly high, and there is positive correlation with instruments measuring similar dimensions (Stahl, 1984).

The Functional Independence Measure (FIM) was developed to assess functional independence in individuals with disability and is a commonly used measure in rehabilitation settings. It consists of 18 items that are scored on a Likert-type scale from 1 (complete dependence) to 7 (complete independence). The areas assessed include self-care, sphincter control, ability to transfer, locomotion, communication, and social cognition. There is evidence of high interrater reliability and concurrent validity (Ottenbacher et al., 1994).

The Minimum Data Set (MDS) for Resident Assessment and Care Screening was developed in response to the Omnibus Reconciliation Act of 1987, which mandated a national resident assessment system for nursing facilities. The MDS systematizes the assessment of each resident's functional, medical, mental, and psychosocial status on admission and at regular intervals thereafter. The intent is to determine

SF-36 Questions

1. In general, would you say your health is:

2. *Compared to 1 year ago,* how would you rate your health in general now?

3. The following items are about activities you might do during a typical day. Does *your health now limit you* in these activities? If so, how much?
   a. *Vigorous activities,* such as running, lifting heavy objects, participating in strenuous sports
   b. *Moderate activities,* such a moving a table, pushing a vacuum cleaner, bowling, or playing golf
   c. Lifting or carrying groceries
   d. Climbing *several* flights of stairs
   e. Climbing *one* flight of stairs
   f. Bending, kneeling, or stooping
   g. Walking *more than a mile*
   h. Walking *several blocks*
   i. Walking *one block*
   j. Bathing or dressing yourself

4. During the *past 4 weeks,* have you had any of the following problems with your work or other regular daily activities *as a result of your physical health?*
   a. Cut down the *amount of time* you spent on work or other activities
   b. *Accomplished less* than you would like
   c. Were limited in the *kind* of work or other activities
   d. Had *difficulty* performing the work or other activities (for example, it took extra effort)

5. During the *past 4 weeks,* have you had any of the following problems with your work or other regular daily activities *as a result of any emotional problems* (such as feeling depressed or anxious)?
   a. Cut down the *amount of time* you spent on work or other activities
   b. *Accomplished* less than you would like
   c. Didn't do work or other activities as *carefully* as usual

6. During the *past 4 weeks,* to what extent has your physical health or emotional problems interfered with your normal social activities with family, friends, neighbors, or groups?

7. How much *bodily* pain have you had during the *past 4 weeks?*

8. During the *past 4 weeks,* how much did *pain* interfere with your normal work (including both work outside the home and housework)?

9. These questions are about how you feel and how things have been with you *during the past 4 weeks.* For each question, please give the one answer that comes closest to the way you have been feeling. How much of the time during the *past 4 weeks*
   a. Did you feel full of pep?
   b. Have you been a very nervous person?
   c. Have you felt so down in the dumps that nothing could cheer you up?
   d. Have you felt calm and peaceful?
   e. Did you have a lot of energy?
   f. Have you felt downhearted and blue?
   g. Did you feel worn out?
   h. Have you been a happy person?
   i. Did you feel tired?

FIGURE 9–7 *See legend on opposite page*

whether a person is appropriate for placement in a skilled nursing facility and to provide a comprehensive assessment for newly admitted residents. It is assumed that this comprehensive assessment leads to improved care planning and care provision.

Like the OARS, certain items on the MDS have higher reliability than others. Generally, however, items have a minimum reliability of 0.40 with a range of up to 0.75 for some of the ADL items. Depending on the number of times a resident has been assessed and the assessor's knowledge of the resident, the time required to administer the tool is 80 to 120 minutes (Morris et al., 1990). A revised MDS for use in homecare populations is currently being tested.

The Functional Status Questionnaire (FSQ) (Jette & Cleary, 1987; Jette et al., 1986), which

10. During the *past 4 weeks,* how much of the time has your *physical health or emotional problems* interfered with your social activities (like visiting with friends, relatives, etc.)?

11. How TRUE or FALSE is *each* of the following statements for you?
    a. I seem to get sick a little easier than other people
    b. I am as healthy as anybody I know
    c. I expect my health to get worse
    d. My health is excellent

SF-36 Response Choices
 1. Excellent, very good, good, fair, poor
 2. Much better now than one year ago; somewhat better now than one year ago; about the same as one year ago; somewhat worse now than one year ago; much worse than one year ago
 3. Yes, limited a lot; yes, limited a little; no, not limited at all
 4. a–d Yes, No
 5. a–c Yes, No
 6. Not at all, slightly, moderately, quite a bit, extremely
 7. None, very mild, mild, moderate, severe, very severe
 8. Not at all, a little bit, moderately, quite a bit, extremely
 9. All of the time, most of the time, a good bit of the time, some of the time, a little of the time, none of the time
10. All of the time, most of the time, some of the time, a little of the time, none of the time
11. Definitely true, mostly true, don't know, mostly false, definitely false

FIGURE 9–7. The 36-item Short-Form Health Survey (SF-36). (From Ware, J. E., & Sherbourne, C. D. [1992]. The MOS 36-item Short-Form Health Survey [SF-36]. *Medical Care, 30,* 482–483. Copyright by the Medical Outcomes Trust, Inc.)

was designed to screen for disability and to monitor clinical changes in functional performance, differentiates impaired functional performance on the basis of uniform scoring of progressively more difficult activities (Fig. 9–6). It measures physical, psychological, and social functioning and may be administered in about 15 minutes. Thirty-four items are scored by computer, producing six summary scale scores and six single-item scores. Warning zones for each functional scale score indicate problem areas of functioning for each individual. Reliability estimates based on internal consistencies for the six FSQ scale scores range from 0.64 to 0.82, and predicted correlations between scales with similar and dissimilar content support convergent validity.

The Medical Outcomes Study Health Status Short Form (SF-36) is a 36-item multidimensional instrument designed for use in clinical practice, research, health policy evaluations, and population surveys (Ware & Sherbourne, 1992). (One form of the SF-36 is in Figure 9–7.) The health concepts surveyed include physical functioning, role limitations due to physical problems, social functioning, bodily pain, mental health role limitations due to emotional problems, vitality, and general health percep-

tions. Most of the 36 questionnaire items were adapted from older instruments. The questionnaire requires 10 to 15 minutes to administer and is available in a variety of formats suitable for self-administration, telephone administration, or personal interview with elderly clients. Internal consistency and construct validity have been reported (Lyons et al., 1994). The SF-36 scoring manual and questionnaire forms can be obtained by completing a user agreement with the senior author (International Resource Center for Health Care Assessment, 1992).

The Duke Health Profile (DUKE) is a 17-item measure of health as an outcome of medical intervention and health promotion derived from the 63-item Duke University of North Carolina Health Profile (Parkerson et al., 1981, 1990, 1995, 1996) (Fig. 9–8). The self-report instrument includes six health measures (physical, mental, social, general, perceived health, and self-esteem) and four dysfunction measures (anxiety, depression, pain, and disability). The original instrument data were gathered from ambulatory primary care patients, including those more than 65 years of age. Internal consistency and test-retest reliability were found to be acceptable. The authors claimed face, construct, and clinical validity of the

Date today: _____ Date of birth: _____ Female: ___ Male: ___ ID number: _____

DUKE HEALTH PROFILE (The DUKE)

Copyright© 1989 and 1994 by the Department of Community and Family Medicine,
Duke University Medical Center, Durham, N.C., U.S.A.

INSTRUCTIONS:

Here are a number of questions about your health and feelings. Please read each question carefully and check (√) your best answer. You should answer the questions in your own way. There are no right or wrong answers. (Please ignore the small scoring numbers next to each blank.)

	Yes, describes me exactly	Somewhat describes me	No, doesn't describe me at all
1. I like who I am..	12	11	10
2. I am not an easy person to get along with..................	20	21	22
3. I am basically a healthy person	32	31	30
4. I give up too easily..	40	41	42
5. I have difficulty concentrating	50	51	52
6. I am happy with my family relationships....................	62	61	60
7. I am comfortable being around people......................	72	71	70

TODAY would you have any physical trouble or difficulty:

	None	Some	A lot
8. Walking up a flight of stairs.......................................	82	81	80
9. Running the length of a football field..........................	92	91	90

DURING THE PAST WEEK: How much trouble have you had with:

	None	Some	A lot
10. Sleeping...	102	101	100
11. Hurting or aching in any part of your body...............	112	111	110
12. Getting tired easily..	122	121	120
13. Feeling depressed or sad.......................................	132	131	130
14. Nervousness...	142	141	140

DURING THE PAST WEEK: How often did you:

	None	Some	A lot
15. Socialize with other people (talk or visit with friends or relatives)...	150	151	152
16. Take part in social, religious, or recreation activities (meetings, church, movies, sports, parties).............	160	161	162

DURING THE PAST WEEK: How often did you:

	None	1–4 days	5–7 days
17. Stay in your home, a nursing home, or a hospital because of sickness, injury, or other health problem..	172	171	170

FIGURE 9–8 *See legend on opposite page*

SCORING THE DUKE HEALTH PROFILE*

Copyright © 1994 by the Department of Community and Family Medicine,
Duke University Medical Center, Durham, N.C., U.S.A.
(Revised October 1994)

Item	Raw Score	
8	= _____	
9	= _____	
10	= _____	PHYSICAL HEALTH SCORE
11	= _____	
12	= _____	
Sum	= _____	× 10 = ☐

Item	Raw Score	
1	= _____	
4	= _____	
5	= _____	MENTAL HEALTH SCORE
13	= _____	
14	= _____	
Sum	= _____	× 10 = ☐

Item	Raw Score	
2	= _____	
6	= _____	
7	= _____	SOCIAL HEALTH SCORE
15	= _____	
16	= _____	
Sum	= _____	× 10 = ☐

GENERAL HEALTH SCORE

Physical health score = _____
Mental health score = _____
Social health score = _____
Sum = _____ ÷ 3 = ☐

PERCEIVED HEALTH SCORE

Item	Raw Score	
3	= _____	× 50 = ☐

Item	Raw Score	
1	= _____	
2	= _____	
4	= _____	SELF-ESTEEM SCORE
6	= _____	
7	= _____	
Sum	= _____	× 10 = ☐

To calculate the scores in this column the raw scores must be revised as follows:
If 0, change to 2; if 2, change to 0; if 1, no change.

Item	Raw Score	Revised	
2	= _____	→ _____	
5	= _____	→ _____	
7	= _____	→ _____	
10	= _____	→ _____	ANXIETY SCORE
12	= _____	→ _____	
14	= _____	→ _____	
Sum	= _____	× 8.333 = ☐	

Item	Raw Score	Revised	
4	= _____	→ _____	
5	= _____	→ _____	
10	= _____	→ _____	DEPRESSION SCORE
12	= _____	→ _____	
13	= _____	→ _____	
Sum	= _____	× 10 = ☐	

Item	Raw Score	Revised	
4	= _____	→ _____	
5	= _____	→ _____	
7	= _____	→ _____	ANXIETY-DEPRESSION
10	= _____	→ _____	(DUKE-AD) SCORE
12	= _____	→ _____	
13	= _____	→ _____	
14	= _____	→ _____	
Sum	= _____	× 7.143 = ☐	

PAIN SCORE

Item	Raw Score	Revised	
11	= _____	→ _____	× 50 = ☐

DISABILITY SCORE

Item	Raw Score	Revised	
17	= _____	→ _____	× 50 = ☐

*Raw score = last digit of the numeral adjacent to the blank checked by the respondent for each item. For example, if the second blank is checked for item 10 (blank numeral = 101), then the raw score is "1," because 1 is the last digit of 101.

Final score is calculated from the raw scores as shown and entered into the box for each scale. For physical health, mental health, social health, general health, self-esteem, and perceived health, 100 indicates the best health status, and 0 indicates the worst health status. For anxiety, depression, anxiety-depression, pain, and disability, 100 indicates the worst health status, and 0 indicates the best health status.

Missing values: If one or more responses is missing within one of the eleven scales, a score cannot be calculated for that particular scale.

FIGURE 9–8. The DUKE Health Profile (DUKE) and scoring the DUKE. (From Parkerson, G. R., Broadhead, W. E., & Tse, C. J. [1994]. The Duke Health Profile. *Medical Care, 33,* 53–56.)

DUKE based on correlations with other well-established instruments as well as differences between the health scores of patients with clinically different health problems.

Table 9–2 lists additional assessment instruments that are more problem specific or disease specific than those described in this chapter or may otherwise prove to be clinically useful. The disease-specific instruments typically focus on those activities directly related to the disease in question, such as hand function in arthritis. Additional brief multidimensional functional assessment instruments are included (presented as procedures or guidelines) that have been developed for use in ambulatory settings. A more complete listing of assessment instruments may be found in the *Clear-*

inghouse on health indexes (National Center for Health Statistics, 1994). Several comprehensive reviews on assessment instruments are also available (Geron, 1997; Lawton & Teresi, 1994; McDowell & Newell, 1996).

SUMMARY

If healthcare is to truly meet the needs of the elderly, the assessment of functional abilities must become a required component of holistic health assessment. Observational measures of physical functioning when used alone or in combination with self-report and proxy report are well suited to clinical use with elderly individuals; however, self-report functional assess-

TABLE 9–2		

Additional Functional Assessment Instruments

Instrument	Authors	Target Population
Physical		
Physical Performance and Mobility Examination	Winograd et al. (1994)	Hospitalized, frail elderly
Performance Test of Activities of Daily Living (PADL)	Kuriansky & Gurland (1976)	Frail elderly in variety of settings
Functional Vital Signs	Williams et al. (1982)	Elderly women outpatients
Tinetti Balance and Gait Evaluation	Tinetti (1986); Tinetti et al. (1986)	Elderly at risk for falls
Karnofsky Performance Scale	Karnofsky et al. (1948); Crooks et al. (1991)	Elderly outpatients
Functional Status Questionnaire	Jette et al. (1986)	Elderly outpatients
Disease or Problem Specific		
Arthritis Impact Measurement Scales (AIMS)	Meenan (1988); Meenan et al. (1984)	Individuals with arthritis
Health Assessment Questionnaire Disability Score (HAQ)	Fries et al. (1982)	Individuals with arthritis
Visual Analogue Pain Scale	McDowell & Newell (1996)	Individuals with pain
Social		
Life Satisfaction in the Elderly Scale	Salamon & Conte (1984)	Healthy elderly
Multidimensional		
Yale Functional Assessment Screening Instrument	Lachs et al. (1990)	Elderly outpatients
Sickness Impact Profile Short Form	Bergner et al. (1976)	Patients in variety of settings
Dartmouth Primary Care Cooperative Information Project (COOP Chart)	Nelson et al. (1987)	Ambulatory office, clinic patients
Summary of Practical Functional Assessment in Elderly Patients	Fleming et al. (1995)	Elderly office patients
Comprehensive Older Persons' Evaluation	Campbell & Thompson (1990); Pearlman (1987)	Frail elderly in variety of settings

ment measures are more appropriate for large-scale population studies or screening tools. The observation of performing a function is considered a more accurate measurement than self-report or report offered by others. Even so, Kane and Kane (1981) cautioned that functional limitations can be overestimated because of restricted environments with limited opportunity to perform as well as a person's unwillingness to perform a function, for whatever reason.

No single assessment instrument is ideal for every situation. The user is advised to select an instrument that has been used in a similar setting and that is both reliable and valid for measuring the attributes under evaluation.

The recent developments of brief multidimensional functional assessment instruments, clinical assessment guidelines that include observation of function, and the use of computers to score and report assessments hold promise for the future (Kane, 1997). Nevertheless, the need for skilled interviewers and professional judgment in geriatric assessment will likely continue.

REFERENCES

Applegate, W. (1987). Use of assessment instruments in clinical settings. *Journal of the American Geriatrics Society, 35*, 45–50.

Applegate, W. B., Blass, J. P., & Williams, T. F. (1990). Instruments for the functional assessments of older patients. *New England Journal of Medicine, 322*, 1207–1214.

Becker, G., & Kaufman, S. (1995). Managing an uncertain trajectory in old age: Patients' and physicians' views of stroke. *Medical Anthropology Quarterly, 9*, 169–187.

Bergner, M., Bobbitt, R., Pollard, W., et al. (1976). The sickness impact profile: Validation of a health status measure. *Medical Care, 14*, 57–67.

Besdine, R. (1995). A problem-oriented approach. Introduction. In W. B. Abrams, M. H. Beers & R. Berkow (Eds.), *The Merck manual of geriatrics* (2nd ed., pp. 5–7). Whitehouse Station, NJ: Merck & Co., Inc.

Campbell, L. A., & Thompson, B. L. (1990). Evaluating elderly patients: A critique of comprehensive functional assessment tools. *Nurse Practitioner, 15*(8), 11–18.

Carp, F. M. (1977). Morale: What questions are we asking of whom? In C. S. N. Nydegger (Ed.), *Measuring morale: A guide to effective assessment*. Washington, D.C.: Gerontological Society.

Crooks, V., Waller, S., Smith, T., et al. (1991). The use of the Karnofsky performance scale in determining outcomes and risk in geriatric outpatients. *Journal of Gerontology, 46*(4), M139–M144.

Donald, C. A., & Ware, J. E. (1982). *The quantification of*

social contacts and resources, R-2937-HHS. Santa Monica, CA: Rand Corporation.

Donald, C. A., Ware, J. E., Brook, R. H., & Avery, A. D. (1978). *Conceptualization and measurement of health for adults in the Health Insurance Study, vol. 4.* Social Health (R-1978-4-HEW). Santa Monica, CA: Rand Corporation.

Duke University Center for the Study of Aging and Human Development (1978). *Multidimensional functional assessment: The OARS methodology.* Durham, NC: Duke University.

Elam, J. T., Beaver, T., El Derwi, D., et al. (1989). Comparison of sources of functional report with observed functional ability of frail older persons [abstract]. *Gerontologist, 29* (Suppl.), 308A.

Ernst, M., & Ernst, N. S. (1984). Functional capacity. In D. J. Mangen & W. A. Peterson (Eds.), *Research instruments in social gerontology, vol. 3* (pp. 9–84). Minneapolis: University of Minnesota Press.

Euler, B. L. (1992). A flaw in gerontological assessment: The weak relationship of elderly superficial life satisfaction to deep psychological well-being. *International Journal of Aging and Human Development, 34*(4), 229–310.

Eustis, N. N., & Patten, S. K. (1984). The effectiveness of long-term care. In D. J. Mangen & W. A. Peterson (Eds.), *Research Instruments in Social Gerontology, vol. 3* (pp. 217–316). Minneapolis: University of Minnesota Press.

Falcone, A. (1983). Comprehensive functional assessment as an administrative tool. *Journal of the American Geriatrics Society, 31*, 642–650.

Fillenbaum, G. G. (1978). Validity and reliability of the multidimensional functional assessment questionnaire. In Duke University Center for the Study of Aging and Human Development, *Multidimensional Functional Assessment: The OARS Methodology* (pp. 39–50). Durham, NC: Duke University.

Fillenbaum, G. G. (1985). Screening the elderly: A brief instrumental activities of daily living measure. *Journal of the American Geriatrics Society, 33*(10), 698–706.

Fleming, K. C., Evans, J. M., Weber, D. C., & Chuatka, D. S. (1995). Practical functional assessment of elderly persons: A primary-care approach. Symposium on Geriatrics, part III. *Mayo Clinic Proceedings, 70*, 890–910.

Fries, J. F., Spitz, P. W., & Young, D. Y. (1982). The dimensions of health outcomes: The Health Assessment Questionnaire, disability and pain scales. *Journal of Rheumatology, 9*, 789–793.

George, L. (1997). Choosing among established assessment tools: Scientific demands and practical constraints. *Generations, 21*(1), 32–36.

Geron, S. M. (Ed.). (1997). Using assessment to improve practice: New developments and measures. *Generations, 21*(1).

Gilson, B. S., Gilson, J. S., Bergner, M., et al. (1975). The Sickness Impact Profile: Development of an outcome measure of health care. *American Journal of Public Health, 65*, 1304–1310.

Guralnik, J. M., Branch, L. G., Cummings, S. R., et al. (1989). Physical performance measures in aging research. *Journal of Gerontology, 44*(5), M141–M146.

Guralnik, J. M., Ferruci, L., Simonsick, E., et al. (1995). Lower extremity function in persons over the age of 70 years as a predictor of subsequent disability. *New England Journal of Medicine, 332*, 556–561.

Gurel, L., Linn, M. W., & Linn, B. S. (1972). Physical and mental impairment-of-function evaluation in the aged: The PAMIE scale. *Journal of Gerontology, 27*, 83–90.

Hawley, G. A. (1988). Measures of Psychosocial Development [test]. Odessa, FL: Psychological Assessment Resources, Inc.

International Resource Center for Health Care Assessment (1992). *How to score the SF-36 Short-Form Health Survey.* Boston: The Health Institute.

Jette, A. M., & Cleary, P. D. (1987). Functional disability assessment. *Physical Therapy, 67*(12), 1854–1859.

Jette, A. M., Davis, A. R., Cleary, P. D., et al. (1986). The functional status questionnaire: Reliability and validity when used in primary care. *Journal of General Internal Medicine, 23*, 143–151.

Johnson, C., & Grant, S. (1986). *The nursing home in American Society.* Baltimore: Johns Hopkins University Press.

Kahana, E., Fairchild, T., & Kahana, B. (1982). Adaptation. In D. J. Mangen & W. A. Peterson (Eds.), *Research instruments in social gerontology, vol. 1* (pp. 145–160). Minneapolis: University of Minnesota Press.

Kane, R. A., & Kane, R. L. (1981). *Assessing the elderly: A practical guide to measurement.* Lexington, MA: Lexington Books.

Kane, R. A., Kane, R. L., & Arnold, S. (1985). *Measuring social functioning in mental health studies: Concepts and instruments.* National Institute of Mental Health, DHHS Publ. No. ADM85-1384, Series DN, No. 5. Washington, D.C.: U.S. Government Printing Office.

Kane, R. L. (1997). Using technology to enhance assessment. *Generations, 21*(1), 55–58.

Karnofsky, D. A., Abelman, W. H., Craver, L. F., et al. (1948). The use of nitrogen mustards in the palliative treatment of carcinoma. *Cancer, 1*, 634–656.

Katz, S., Downs, T. D., Cash, H. R., & Grotz, R. C. (1970). Progress in development of the index of ADL. *Gerontologist, 10*, 20–30.

Katz, S., Ford, A. B., Moskowitz, R. W., et al. (1963). Studies of illness in the aged: The Index of ADL, a standardized measure of biological and psychosocial function. *Journal of the American Medical Association, 185*, 914–919.

Kozma, A., Stones, M. J., & McNeil, J. K. (1991). *Psychological well-being in later life.* Toronto, Canada: Butterworths.

Kuriansky, J., & Gurland, B. (1976). The performance test of activities of daily living. *International Journal of Aging and Human Development, 7*, 343–352.

Lachs, M. S., Feinstein, A. R., Cooney, L. M., Jr., et al. (1990). A simple procedure for general screening for functional disability in elderly patients. *Annals of Internal Medicine, 112*(9), 699–706.

Lawton, M. P. (1975). The Philadelphia Geriatric Center Morale Scale: A revision. *Journal of Gerontology, 30*, 85–89.

Lawton, M. P., & Brody, E. (1969). Assessment of older people: Self-maintaining and instrumental activities of daily living. *Gerontologist, 9*, 179–186.

Lawton, M. P., & Teresi, J. A. (Eds.). (1994). *Annual Review of Gerontology and Geriatrics, 14.*

Lyons, R. A., Perry, H. M., & Littlepage, B. N. (1994). Evidence for the validity of the Short-Form 36 Questionnaire (SF-36) in an elderly population. *Age and Ageing, 23*, 182–184.

Maddox, G. (1981). Measuring the well-being of older adults. In A. R. Somers & D. R. Fabian (Eds.), *The geriatric imperative* (pp. 117–136). New York: Appleton-Century-Crofts.

McDowell, I., & Newell, C. (Eds.). (1996). *Measuring health: A guide to scales and questionnaires* (2nd ed.). New York: Oxford University Press.

Meenan, R. F. (1985). New approaches to outcome assessment: The AIMS Questionnaire for arthritis. *Advances in Internal Medicine, 31*, 167–185.

Meenan, R. F., Anderson, J. J., Kazis, L. E., et al. (1984). Outcome assessment in clinical trials: Evidence for the sensitivity of a health status measure. *Arthritis and Rheumatology, 27*(12), 1344–1352.

Meer, B., & Baker, J. A. (1966). The Stockton Geriatric Rating Scale. *Journal of Gerontology, 21*, 392–403.

Morris, J., Hawes, C., Fries, B., et al. (1990). Designing the national resident assessment instrument for nursing homes. *Gerontologist, 30*(3), 293–307.

National Center for Health Statistics (1994). *Clearinghouse on Health Indexes.* Hyattsville, MD: U.S. Dept. of Health and Human Services, Public Health Service, National Center for Health Statistics.

Nelson, E., Wasson, J., Kirk, J., et al. (1987). Assessment of function in routine clinical practice: Description of COOP Chart method and preliminary findings. *Journal of Chronic Diseases, 40*(suppl. 1), 55S–63S.

Neugarten, B. L., Havighurst, R. J., & Tobin, S. S. (1961). The measurement of life satisfaction. *Journal of Gerontology, 16*, 134–143.

Okun, M. A., & Stock, W. A. (1987). The construct validity of subjective well-being measures: An assessment via quantitative research syntheses. *Journal of Community Psychology, 15*, 481–492.

Ottenbacher, K. J., Mann, W. C., Granger, C. V., et al. (1994). Inter-rater agreement and stability of functional assessment in the community-based elderly. *Archives of Physical Medicine and Rehabilitation, 75*, 1297–1301.

Parachek, J. F., & Miller, E. R. (1974). Validation and standardization of a goal-oriented quick-screening geriatric scale. *Journal of the American Geriatrics Society, 22*, 278–283.

Parkerson, G. R., Jr., Broadhead, W. E., & Tse, C. J. (1990). The Duke Health Profile. *Medical Care, 28*(11), 1056–1072.

Parkerson, G. R., Jr., Gehlbach, S. H., Wagner, E. H., et al. (1981). The Duke-UNC Health Profile: An adult health status instrument for primary care. *Medical Care, 19*, 806–828.

Parkerson, G. R., Jr., Tse, C. K., & Broadhead, W. E. (1995). Health status and severity of illness as predictors of outcomes in primary care. *Medical Care, 33*, 53–66.

Parkerson, G. R., Jr., Tse, C. K., & Broadhead, W. E. (1996). Anxiety and depressive symptom identification using the Duke Health Profile. *Journal of Clinical Epidemiology, 49*, 85–93.

Pearlman, R. (1987). Development of a functional assessment questionnaire for geriatric patients: The Comprehensive Older Persons' Evaluation (COPE). *Journal of Chronic Diseases, 40*(56), 85S–94S.

Pfeiffer, E., Johnson, T. M., & Chiofolo, R. C. (1980, November). *Functional assessment of elderly subjects in four service settings.* Paper presented at the Annual Scientific Meeting of the Gerontological Society of America, San Diego, CA.

Pinholt, E. M., Kroenke, K., Hanley, J. F., et al. (1987). Functional assessment of the elderly: A comparison of standard instruments with clinical judgment. *Archives of Internal Medicine, 147,* 484–488.

Podsiadlo, D., & Richardson, S. (1991). The Timed "Up & Go": A test of basic functional mobility for frail elderly persons. *Journal of the American Geriatrics Society, 39,* 142–148.

Reuben, D. B., & Siu, A. L. (1990). An objective measure of physical function of elderly persons: The physical performance test. *Journal of the American Geriatrics Society, 38,* 1105–1112.

Reuben, D. B., Siu, A. L., & Kimpau, S. (1992). The predictive validity of self-report and performance-based measures of function and health. *Journal of Gerontology, 47*(4), M106–M110.

Reuben, D. B., & Solomon, D. (1989). Assessment in geriatrics: Of caveats and names [editorial]. *Journal of the American Geriatrics Society, 37,* 570.

Reuben, D. B., Valle, L. A., Hays, R. D., et al. (1995). Measuring physical function in community-dwelling older persons: A comparison of self-administered, interviewer-administered, and performance-based measures. *Journal of the American Geriatrics Society, 43*(1), 17–23.

Rubenstein, L. V., Calkins, D. R., Greenfield, S., et al. (1988). Health status assessment for elderly patients: Report of the Society of General Internal Medicine task force on health assessment. *Journal of the American Geriatrics Society, 37,* 562–569.

Rubenstein, L., Schairer, C., Wieland, G., & Kane, R. (1984). Systematic biases in functional status assessment of elderly adults: Effects of different data sources. *Journal of Gerontology, 39,* 686–691.

Salamon, M. J., & Conte, V. A. (1984). *Manual for the Salamon and Conte Life Satisfaction in the Elderly Scale.* Psychological Assessment Resources, Inc.

Sauer, W. J., & Warland, R. (1982). Morale and life satisfaction. In D. W. Mangen & W. A. Peterson (Eds.), *Research instruments in social gerontology, vol. 1* (pp. 195–201). Minneapolis: University of Minnesota Press.

Shanas, E. (1962). *The health of older people.* Cambridge, MA: Harvard University Press.

Sherwood, S. J., Morris, J., Mor, V., & Gutkin, C. (1977). *Compendium of measures for describing and assessing long-term care populations.* Boston: Hebrew Rehabilitation Center for the Aged.

Stahl, S. M. (1984). Health. In D. J. Mangen & W. A. Peterson (Eds.), *Research instruments in social gerontology, vol. 1* (pp. 85–116). Minneapolis: University of Minnesota Press.

Tinetti, M. E. (1986). Performance-oriented assessment of mobility problems in elderly patients. *Journal of the American Geriatrics Society, 34,* 119–126.

Tinetti, M. E., Williams, T. F., & Mayewski, R. (1986). Fall risk index for elderly patients based on number of chronic disabilities. *American Journal of Medicine, 80,* 429–434.

Waltz, C. F., Strickland, O. L., & Lenz, E. R. (1991). *Measurement in nursing research* (2nd ed.). Philadelphia: F. A. Davis.

Ward-Griffin, C., & Bramwell, L. (1990). The congruence of elderly client and nurse perceptions of the client's self-care agency. *Journal of Advanced Nursing, 15,* 1070–1077.

Ware, J. E. (1984). Methodologic considerations in the selection of health status assessment procedures. In N. K. Winger, M. E. Matteson, C. D. Furberg, & J. Elinson (Eds.), *Assessment of quality of life in clinical trials of cardiovascular therapies* (pp. 87–111). New York: Le Jacq Publishing.

Ware, J. E., & Sherbourne, C. D. (1992). The MOS 36-item Short-Form Health Survey (SF-36). *Medical Care, 30*(6), 473–481.

Williams, M. E., Hadler, N. M., & Earp, J. A. (1982). Manual ability as a marker of dependency in geriatric women. *Journal of Chronic Diseases, 35,* 115–122.

Wilson-Barnett, J., & Foraham, M. (1982). *Recovery from illness.* New York: John Wiley & Sons.

Winograd, C. H., Lemsky, C. M., Nevitt, M. C., et al. (1994). Development of a physical performance and mobility examination. *Journal of the American Geriatrics Society, 42,* 743–749.

Nursing Management of Common Clinical Problems

Urinary Incontinence

Jean F. Wyman

Urinary incontinence is a common problem for older adults that has significant physical, psychological, social, and economic consequences. Incontinence is associated with skin irritation, pressure ulcers, urinary tract infections, and falls. The embarrassment and fear of having an accident can cause a person to restrict daily activities and social contacts, thereby contributing to social isolation, depression, a loss of self-esteem, and a reduced quality of life. Reactions to being incontinent, however, are unique to each individual and are not predictable based on the severity of the urine loss (Wyman et al., 1990). Caregiver burden and stress in family members and nursing staff members in long-term care settings can lead to a *burn-out syndrome* (Noelker, 1987; Ory et al., 1986; Yu et al., 1991). The costs associated with incontinence are enormous, having risen 60% during a recent 5-year period (Fantl et al., 1996). Hu (as cited by Fantl et al., 1996) estimated the annual direct costs of caring for incontinence for all age groups to be $16.4 billion (based on 1994 dollars); of this, $11.2 billion is spent in the community and $5.2 billion in nursing homes.

This chapter provides an overview of urinary incontinence, including the epidemiology of incontinence, the mechanism of continence, age-related changes that affect continence status, and the types and causes of incontinence.

The evaluation and management of incontinence are discussed along with the implications for the advanced practice nurse (APN) across a variety of care settings.

EPIDEMIOLOGY

Urinary incontinence is defined as the involuntary loss of urine that is sufficient to be a problem (Fantl et al., 1996). Prevalence estimates range from 15 to 35% among community-dwelling older adults; 21 to 53% among homebound older adults; 19 to 23% among elderly people admitted to acute care hospitals; and 38 to 55% among elderly people institutionalized in long-term care settings (Dey, 1996; Diokno et al., 1986; Herzog & Fultz, 1990; Mohide, 1986; Noelker, 1987; Palmer et al., 1991, 1992; Sullivan & Lindsey, 1984). Urinary incontinence among nursing home residents is more severe than in community-dwelling populations and is more commonly associated with fecal incontinence (Ouslander & Schnelle, 1995).

In community-dwelling older populations, women are twice as likely as men to be incontinent (Herzog & Fultz, 1990); however, the female-to-male ratio is lower in frail elderly home-bound and institutionalized populations (Dey, 1996; Palmer, 1988). Because most of the epidemiological research has been conducted in white populations, relatively little is known about racial differences in the prevalence and etiology of incontinence.

Although there is a trend of increased prevalence of incontinence with age, age alone is not a risk factor. Risk factors associated with incontinence include immobility, cognitive impairment (e.g., delirium), medications, smoking, morbid obesity, fecal impaction, low or excessive fluid intake, environmental barriers, high-impact physical activities, diabetes mellitus, stroke, hypoestrogenism, pelvic muscle weakness, pregnancy, vaginal delivery, episiotomy, childhood enuresis, and possibly race (Fantl et al., 1996).

MECHANISM OF CONTINENCE

Normal Micturition

The lower urinary tract, consisting of the bladder and the urethra, is considered a single functional unit. Micturition is divided into two distinct phases: a *storage phase*, consisting of bladder filling and urine storage, and an *expulsion phase*, consisting of bladder emptying and urine evacuation. The storage phase of micturition is dependent on a stable detrusor muscle (the contractile portion of the bladder), which inhibits contractions as the bladder distends and accommodates increasing volumes of urine. In addition to a stable detrusor that does not contract involuntarily, the storage phase requires a competent sphincter mechanism. This mechanism is considered physiological rather than anatomical in nature and consists of three parts: (1) an intrinsic urethral smooth muscle sphincter that extends from the bladder neck or outlet through the pelvic floor; (2) a distal (external to the bladder neck) intrinsic urethral striated muscle sphincter that surrounds the urethra and is separate from the pelvic floor; and (3) an extrinsic (external to the urethra) periurethral striated musculature located at the urogenital diaphragm (also known as the pelvic floor muscles) (Fig. 10–1) (Gosling, 1979).

Micturition, a complex event that is not fully understood, is coordinated through the central, autonomic, and somatic nervous systems. Both the bladder and urethra are enervated by the sympathetic and parasympathetic fibers of the autonomic nervous system. The sympathetic division controls urine storage, and the parasympathetic division initiates bladder emptying. Stimulation of beta receptor sites in the bladder body and outlet causes smooth muscle relaxation. Stimulation of the alpha-adrenergic receptor site causes contraction of the smooth muscle in the bladder neck, which in turns causes increased tone and resistance at the bladder outlet. The pudendal nerve, part of the somatic nervous system, enervates the periurethral striated musculature, also known as the extrinsic sphincter mechanism (Wall et al., 1993).

Micturition is primarily a reflex activity controlled by the central nervous system and mediated through the sacral micturition center, which allows urine storage and emptying even when cortical micturition centers are not intact. Evidence for this mechanism is seen in infants who have not sufficiently developed neurologi-

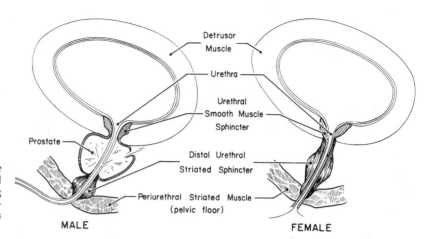

FIGURE 10–1. Anatomy of the lower urinary tract. (Adapted from Wyman, J. [1988]. Nursing assessment of the geriatric outpatient population. *Nursing Clinics of North America, 22,* 170.)

MALE FEMALE

cally and in patients with spinal cord injuries. As the bladder fills with urine, it stimulates stretch receptors in the bladder wall that send a signal to the sacral micturition center and brain via autonomic pathways. Centers in the brain can either facilitate or inhibit voiding. A pontine micturition center coordinates detrusor contraction with sphincter relaxation so that these occur synchronously and voiding results. Centers in the basal ganglia and frontal lobes inhibit reflex detrusor contraction so voiding can be delayed (Fig. 10–2). Diseases involving the central nervous system (e.g., Parkinson's disease, which affects the basal ganglia) can cause detrusor hyperactivity (Wein & Barrett, 1988).

Continence is maintained as long as the intraurethral pressure is higher than the intravesical pressure. Under normal conditions, 150 to 250 mL of urine can be stored before bladder pressure begins to increase and the first sensation of the urge to void is perceived. During this time, the sphincter mechanism increases its resistance, and central nervous system inhibition allows the bladder to continue to fill to a maximum capacity of 400 to 600 mL. Voiding results when intravesical pressure exceeds intraurethral pressure. Central nervous system inhibition is released, thereby causing sphincter relaxation. Parasympathetic stimulation causes the bladder to contract and empty.

Age-Related Changes

Although age-related changes can alter bladder and urethral function (Table 10–1), their impact

on the maintenance of continence is unclear. None of these changes alone causes incontinence, but any can place a person at risk for its development. In women, the most influential change is a reduction in estrogen level. Estrogen receptors are located in the epithelium and tissues lining and surrounding the bladder,

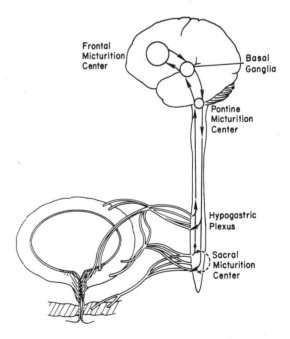

FIGURE 10–2. Neuroanatomy of lower urinary tract function. (From Wyman, J. [1988]. Nursing assessment of the geriatric outpatient population. *Nursing Clinics of North America, 22,* 171.)

TABLE 10-1

Age-Related Changes Affecting Bladder Function

Change	Potential Effect on Bladder Function
Decreased bladder capacity	Frequency
Increased residual urine volume	Risk of urinary tract infection
Uninhibited bladder contractions	Urgency, frequency, incontinence
Increased nocturnal urine production	Nocturia, enuresis
Decreased estrogen	Atrophic vaginitis, urgency, frequency, urinary tract infection, risk of pelvic organ prolapse
Lower urethral pressure (women)	Stress incontinence
Benign prostatic hyperplasia (men)	Urgency, frequency, straining, urinary retention, overflow incontinence
Decreased immune function	Risk of urinary tract infection

urethra, and vagina. Hypoestrogenism causes atrophy of these tissues, resulting in friability, inflammation, diminished periurethral blood flow, susceptibility to infection, weakened pelvic floor muscles, and pelvic prolapse, all of which can cause urinary symptoms. In men, the most influential change is prostatic hyperplasia, which can affect bladder storage and emptying. Although evidence for age-related changes in bladder capacity and residual urine is limited, uninhibited bladder contractions in continent, neurologically normal men and women have been well documented (Diokno et al., 1986).

Other age-associated changes that affect mobility, dexterity, and vision may make it more difficult to locate and reach a toilet or toileting aid and to disrobe in time for voiding. Changes in the pattern of fluid excretion whereby more than half of the daily fluid is excreted at night cause nocturia in 70% of community-dwelling older adults. (Diokno et al., 1986; Kirkland et al., 1983). Age-related changes in immune function can also increase the susceptibility to urinary tract infections (Ouslander, 1992).

TYPES AND CAUSES OF URINARY INCONTINENCE

Urinary incontinence involves dysfunctions occurring in either the filling and storage phase or the emptying phase of micturition (Fig. 10–3). Failure to store urine may be caused by increased bladder contractility, also known as detrusor instability, by decreased outlet resistance, or by a combination of both. Failure to empty urine can be caused by increased outlet resistance, which obstructs the passage of urine, by decreased detrusor contractility, or by a combination of both. In frail elderly patients, detrusor hyperactivity with impaired bladder contractility (DHIC) may also cause incontinence (Resnick & Yalla, 1987). Patients with DHIC have involuntary detrusor contractions yet must strain to empty their bladders. Table 10–2 indentifies common causes associated with these types of dysfunctions.

Urinary incontinence has been broadly categorized into two types: (1) acute or transient incontinence and (2) persistent or established incontinence. Acute incontinence can occur from several potentially reversible causes, which can be remembered by the acronym

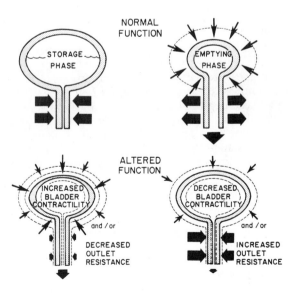

FIGURE 10–3. Normal and abnormal lower urinary tract function.

TABLE 10-2
Types and Causes of Urinary Incontinence

Type	Description	Pathophysiology	Characteristics	Common Causes
Stress	Urethral sphincter failure usually associated with increased intraabdominal pressure	Urethral hypermobility due to anatomic changes or defects such as fascial detachments Intrinsic urethral sphincter deficiency (ISD) failure of the sphincter at rest	Small amounts of urine loss during coughing, sneezing, laughing, or other physical activities; usually daytime only Continuous urine loss at rest or with minimal exertion (postural changes)	Pelvic prolapse in women, childbirth damage Prostatectomy, anti-incontinence surgery in women, radiation therapy, childbirth damage, trauma, congenital weakness, epispadias
Urge	Involuntary loss of urine associated with a strong sensation of the need to void	Involuntary bladder (detrusor) contractions (detrusor instability) Detrusor hyperactivity with impaired bladder contractility (DHIC) Involuntary sphincter relaxation	Loss of urine with an abrupt and strong desire to void; usually loss of urine on way to bathroom; urine loss varying from moderate to large amount; associated with frequency, nocturia, and possible suprapubic discomfort; DHIC-elevated post-void residual volume	Central nervous system damage due to stroke, Alzheimer's disease, Parkinson's disease; interference with spinal inhibitory pathways owing to spondylosis or metastasis; local bladder disorder such as cancer, stone, radiation effects, cystitis, interstitial cystitis; outlet obstruction
Mixed	Combination of stress and urge incontinence	Combination of stress and urge features as above	Combination of stress and urge symptoms as above; one symptom (urge or stress) often more bothersome to the patient than the other	Combination of causes of stress and urge incontinence, as above
Overflow	Urine loss resulting from obstruction and/or overdistention of bladder	Acontractile, hypotonic, or underactive detrusor	Variety of symptoms, including frequent or constant dribbling, urge or stress incontinence symptoms, urgency, frequency	Drugs, fecal impaction, diabetes, lower spinal cord injury, or disruption of the motor innervation of the detrusor muscle; may be idiopathic In men, prostatic hyperplasia, prostatic carcinoma, or urethral stricture In women, obstruction due to severe genital prolapse or surgical overcorrection of urethral detachment
Functional	Urine leakage associated with inability or unwillingness to toilet appropriately	Normal lower urinary tract function; caused by nongenitourinary factors	Chronic cognitive and physical impairments; may be complicated by iatrogenic causes	Dementia, pain, and other conditions impairing mobility status; inaccessible caregivers; toilets, or toileting substitutes; psychiatric illness; hostility; environmental barriers
Unconscious or reflex	Urine loss without any warning or sensory awareness	Neurological dysfunction most common; although can occur in patients without overt neurological dysfunction	Postmicturitional or continual (dribbling) incontinence; occurs without warning or sensory awareness May have severe urgency with bladder hypersensitivity (sensory urgency)	Neuropathic conditions such as paraplegia; secondary to radiation cystitis, inflammatory bladder conditions, radical pelvic surgery, or myelomenigocele

DIAPPERS coined by Resnick (Urinary Incontinence Guideline Panel, 1992):

Delirium, an acute confusional state, interferes with a person's awareness of the need to void and his or her ability to reach a toilet in time. Often the first sign of acute illness in the elderly patient is urinary incontinence secondary to confusion.

Infection of the urinary tract may precipitate incontinence; however, the incontinence may continue even if the infection is treated. It is less clear whether asymptomatic bacteriuria is associated with incontinence (Ouslander, 1992). Asymptomatic bacteriuria occurs in 15 to 30% of older women and 5 to 12% of older men in community-dwelling populations; 25 to 50% of women and 15 to 25% of men in nursing home populations; and 30% of elderly patients in acute care hospitals. Although the results from several studies differ regarding the role of bacteriuria in the cause of incontinence, Ouslander (1992) recommended that incontinent elderly patients with significant bacteriuria be considered symptomatic rather than asymptomatic and that eradication of the bacteriuria be completed before pursuing further evaluation.

Atrophic vaginitis or urethritis resulting from low estrogen levels in postmenopausal women may cause reversible incontinence.

Pharmaceuticals such as caffeine, diuretics, sedatives/hypnotics (including alcohol), narcotics, anticholinergics, alpha- and beta-adrenergic agonists, alpha-antagonists, and calcium channel blockers can contribute to the development and exacerbation of incontinence (Table 10–3).

Psychological causes, such as depression, anger, hostility toward caregivers, and regression in psychiatric patients, have been linked to incontinence.

Excess fluid from a high fluid intake (especially caffeinated beverages) or from volume overload with venous insufficiency or congestive heart failure may precipitate incontinence. Endocrine problems such as hyperglycemia and hypercalcemia, both of which cause polyuria, may also trigger incontinence.

Restricted mobility, especially when urinary frequency and urgency are present, is a common cause of incontinence in the elderly. It may be associated with neurological disease, or it may result from a recent fracture or other injury; arthritic pain; or the use of physical restraints, intravenous therapy, or other treatments restricting movement.

Stool impaction, which causes outlet obstruction, has been cited as a primary cause of incontinence occurring in 5 to 10% of frail nursing home patients (Resnick, 1984).

Established incontinence is classified into six types: stress, urge, mixed, overflow, functional, and unconscious or reflex (see Table 10–2) (Fantl et al., 1996). These are not necessarily exclusive, and many older patients with incontinence experience two or more types together. Patients with acute incontinence also present with these symptom types.

Stress Incontinence. Stress incontinence is characterized by the loss of a small amount of urine in the absence of a detrusor contraction usually during sudden increases in intraabdominal pressure, such as with coughing, sneezing, laughing, lifting, or bending. The underlying cause is an inability of the urethra to sustain pressure that exceeds that of the bladder, particularly under exertional events. Patients with intrinsic sphincteric deficiency usually lose urine continuously with minimal exertion. Stress incontinence is the most common type of incontinence in women, and it occurs less frequently in men (Diokno et al., 1986; Fantl et al., 1991; Makinen et al., 1992).

Urge Incontinence. This type of incontinence is characterized by a strong urge to void immediately prior to the loss of urine. Affected individuals relate that they cannot make it to the toilet before leakage occurs or that they have "key in the lock" syndrome; that is, they lose urine on arriving home and unlocking their door. Urine is usually lost in moderate to large amounts. Many of these patients also report urinary frequency and nocturia. The underlying cause is uninhibited bladder contractions usually described as unstable bladder or detrusor function. When a causative neurologic lesion is identified, the detrusor instability is

TABLE 10-3

Medications Associated with Urinary Incontinence

Drug Type	Effect
Caffeine	Polyuria, urgency, frequency
Alcohol	Polyuria, frequency, urgency, sedation, delirium, immobility
Diuretics	Polyuria, urgency, frequency
Sedatives/hypnotics	Sedation, decreased awareness of need to void, delirium, immobility, muscle relaxation

Anticholinergics
  Antidepressants
  Antipsychotics
  Antiparkinsonian
  Antispasmodics
  Antihistamines
  Antiglaucoma
	Decreased bladder contractility, urinary retention, fecal impaction, overflow incontinence
	
	Antipsychotics can also cause sedation, rigidity, and immobility

Alpha-adrenergic agonists (present in many over-the-counter cold and diet preparations)	Decreased bladder contractility, urinary retention, overflow incontinence
Beta-adrenergic agonists	Decreased bladder contractility, urinary retention, overflow incontinence
Alpha-adrenergic antagonists	Decreased outlet resistance, stress incontinence
Calcium channel blockers	Decreased bladder contractility, urinary retention, overflow incontinence
Narcotic analgesics	Urinary retention, fecal impaction, sedation, delirium

Data from Fantl et al. (1996) and Wyman (1991).

called *detrusor hyperreflexia* (Abrams et al., 1988). Urge incontinence is most common in older people (Diokno et al., 1986).

Mixed Incontinence. Both stress and urge symptomatology are characteristic of mixed incontinence. The underlying cause can be urethral and/or bladder dysfunction. Mixed incontinence occurs most frequently in older women. One of the two symptoms is usually more prevalent or bothersome to the patient, and treatment is tailored to this symptom.

Overflow Incontinence. Overflow incontinence is associated with overdistension of the bladder resulting from outlet obstruction or an underactive detrusor. Outlet obstruction is more common in men than in women, owing to prostatic hyperplasia and, less frequently, to prostatic cancer and urethral stricture. Although outlet obstruction occurs rarely in women, it can result as a complication from antiincontinence surgery and severe pelvic organ prolapse. Symptoms are quite variable, ranging from frequent leakage to continuous

dribbling with stress or urge symptoms. Patients typically void in small volumes, have a diminished urine stream, complain of incomplete bladder emptying, or have an impaired sensation of bladder fullness.

Functional Incontinence. This pattern of urine loss is precipitated by factors outside the lower urinary tract, rather than abnormal bladder or urethral function. It is associated with cognitive and physical impairments, psychological causes, and environmental factors that influence appropriate toileting. Functional incontinence can be caused by inaccessible toilets or toileting substitutes, a lack of caregivers to assist in toileting, confusional states, and psychiatric illness. The diagnosis of functional incontinence is one of exclusion, because patients with cognitive or mobility impairments may have other types and causes of incontinence (Skelly & Flint, 1995). In older patients, functional incontinence tends to coexist with the other types of incontinence (Wyman et al., 1993).

Unconscious or Reflex Incontinence. This type of incontinence occurs without any warning or sensory awareness (Fantl et al., 1996); urine loss occurs either postmicturition or as continual dribbling. The underlying cause is usually neurogenic, resulting in decreased bladder compliance, although nonneurogenic factors may also cause decreased bladder compliance. Other factors include inflammatory bladder conditions, neurological bladder disorders following radical pelvic surgery, and myelomeningocele.

MANAGEMENT OF URINARY INCONTINENCE

Urinary incontinence in the elderly results from multiple interacting causes, including physiological, psychological, social, and environmental factors. The following steps should be taken for successful management of incontinence:

- Conduct a thorough evaluation that characterizes the type of incontinence and precipitating causes and, if possible, identifies the underlying cause
- Identify and correct potentially reversible causes that may be contributing to the incontinence
- Involve the patient and family (if appropriate) in the treatment decision-making process
- Start with the least invasive, lowest-risk therapy
- In institutional settings, target intensive treatment to those patients most likely to benefit
- Treat intractable incontinence with supportive interventions that will preserve skin integrity and maintain comfort and dignity
- Refer for specialist evaluation in complex situations, including those requiring surgical intervention, or when a behavioral or pharmacological trial has failed

Assessment

Even when directly questioned during health examinations, many older adults fail to report incontinence. When asked if they have this problem, they may not understand the term *incontinence,* or they may not perceive that they are having bladder difficulties because they use a collection device that controls their urine loss. An initial approach at screening for incontinence might be to ask questions such as "Are you having any problems with your bladder?," "Do you ever have trouble holding your urine (water)?," "Do you ever accidentally lose urine when you don't want to?," or "Do you ever leak urine when you cough, sneeze, or do any activity?" If the initial question is answered negatively, a good follow-up question is "Do you wear any type of pad or protective device to collect your urine?"

An assessment should be conducted when incontinence is reported by the patient, his or her family, or a staff member or if the clinician detects an odor or actual leakage. The basic evaluation includes a history and physical examination, a voiding record, a cough stress test, postvoid residual (PVR) volume determination, and urinalysis (Fantl et al., 1996). Additional laboratory tests such as blood chemistry determination, urodynamic evaluation, and endoscopic and imaging studies may be indicated in selected patients based on findings in the initial evaluation. Key aspects of a comprehensive evaluation of urinary incontinence are presented in Table 10–4.

HISTORY

The patient history includes (1) an assessment of continence status; (2) relevant genitourinary, neurological, medical, and psychological data; (3) medications; (4) functional abilities; (5) social factors; and (6) environmental characteristics (see Table 10–4 for greater detail). The first part of the history focuses on identifying the type of incontinence—stress, urge, mixed, overflow, functional, unconscious, or reflex—and determining the symptom(s) most bothersome to the patient. It is important to ascertain the effect of incontinence on daily activities and its impact on quality of life. Normal voiding patterns should be determined. Although these are variable among individuals, the frequency of diurnal micturition usually ranges from six to eight voidings per day, and noctur-

TABLE 10-4

Comprehensive Evaluation of Urinary Incontinence

History

Continence history
  Onset, duration, and frequency of incontinence
  Precipitating circumstances (cough, sneeze, laugh, lifting, bending, exercise; on way to bathroom or "key in the lock" syndrome; position change; washing hands; sexual intercourse or orgasm in women; surgery, trauma, injury; recent illness; new medication)
  Associated symptoms (urgency, frequency, nocturia, enuresis, postmicturition dribbling, lack of sensation of bladder fullness; sensation of incomplete bladder emptying; obstructive symptoms such as hesitancy, slow or interrupted stream, straining; dysuria; hematuria; suprapubic or pelvic pain)
  Most bothersome symptom(s) to patient
  Timing and pattern (diurnal or nocturnal or both) of incontinent episodes and continent voids
  Ability to delay voiding
  Amount and type of loss (spurt and/or stream; continuous dribbling)
  Use of pads, briefs, and protective devices (type and number of pads or clothing changes/day)
  Bowel habits (constipation, impaction, fecal incontinence)
  Daily fluid intake (amount, caffeine and alcohol use)
  Current and past management strategies and outcomes (behavioral, drug, surgical intervention; preventive toileting; other)
  Effect of incontinence on quality of life
  Motivation for continence
  Treatment preferences and expectations
Genitourinary history
  Childhood enuresis
  Women—past childbirth(s) (number of vaginal deliveries, any traumatic delivery)
  Recurrent urinary tract infections (≥3 in past year)
  Past surgery (pelvic, prostatectomy, or other lower urinary tract surgery)
  Bladder cancer
  Past pelvic radiation therapy
  Renal disease
Other medical history
  Acute illness
  Cardiovascular disease (hypertension, congestive heart disease)
  Neurological disease (stroke, Parkinson's disease, dementia, multiple sclerosis, spinal cord lesions)
  Musculoskeletal disease (arthritis)
  Cancer
  Psychiatric disorders (depression, schizophrenia, other)
  Smoking history
Medication review
  Prescription and over-the-counter (OTC) medications
Functional assessment
  Mobility (gait speed, ability to toilet)
  Dexterity (ability to disrobe)
Environmental characteristics
  Accessible toilets or toileting aids
  Distance to toilet
  Need and use of toileting substitutes
  Chairs and bed allow ease when rising
Social characteristics
  Living arrangements
  Identified caregiver and degree of caregiver involvement
  Caregiver's perceptions of cause, severity, and treatment preferences; willingness to assist with treatment; and expectations of treatment

Table continued on following page

nal micturition is usually not more than twice a night in older people (Abrams et al., 1983). It is important to identify how long a patient can delay voiding once the first urge to void has been perceived. This is critical in older adults with impaired mobility.

Functional assessment of mobility and dexterity is important, as is an evaluation of the environment—the accessibility of and distance to the bathroom, the availability of caregivers, and the need for and use of toileting substitutes. Social factors that are essential in developing the treatment plan include living arrangements, the availability of a caregiver, and the caregiver's perception of the problem and willingness to assist with toileting and other

TABLE 10-4

Comprehensive Evaluation of Urinary Incontinence *(Continued)*

Physical Examination

Neurological examination
  Mental status
  Mood
  Neurological abnormalites (focal signs, signs of Parkinson's disease, balance impairment, other)
  Gait and walking speed
Abdominal examination
  Diastasis recti
  Organomegaly
  Masses
  Peritoneal irritation
  Distended bladder
Genital examination
  Skin condition
  Women—atrophic vaginitis, pelvic organ prolapse, pelvic masses, perivaginal muscle tone, other abnormalities
  Men—abnormalities of the foreskin, penis, and perineum
Rectal examination
  Sphincter tone (resting and active)
  Perineal sensation
  Fecal impaction
  Masses
  Men—prostate size, consistency, and contour
Other
  Signs of congestive heart failure
Cough stress test (direct observation of urine loss with full bladder)
Postvoid residual volume determination
Voiding record (kept for 3–7 days)
Laboratory tests
  Urinalysis
  Urine culture and sensitivity (if indicated)
  Urine cytology (if indicated)
  Blood test (glucose, blood urea nitrogen, creatinine, calcium for polyuria in the absence of diuretics or for suspected compromised renal
    function)
Specialized evaluation (selected cases only)
  Urodynamic tests
    Cystometry
    Uroflowmetry
    Women—urethral pressure profilometry or leak point pressures
  Cystourethroscopy
  Imaging tests

Data from Fantl et al. (1996) and Wyman (1991).

interventions. An assessment of the patient's treatment preferences and expectations as well as his or her motivation for achieving continence can help the clinician determine the appropriate treatment approach.

PHYSICAL EXAMINATION

The physical examination includes abdominal, genital, rectal, and neurological evaluations. A mental status evaluation using a standardized instrument (see Chapter 7) should also be used to screen for cognitive impairments that may be contributing to the incontinence. For patients with cognitive or mobility impairments,

an important part of the examination is observing their ability to use a toilet or a toileting substitute.

The physical examination should focus on detecting neurological abnormalities such as focal and parkinsonian signs, abnormal sensation, diabetic neuropathy, lumbar and cervical spondylosis, normal pressure hydrocephalus, and congestive heart failure. An abdominal examination should be completed to identify bladder distention, suprapubic discomfort or tenderness, organomegaly, diastasis recti (separation of the rectus muscles of the abdominal wall), and the presence of masses.

The pelvic examination should include an inspection of the genitalia, noting perineal skin condition and signs of atrophic vaginitis or infection, and palpation for pelvic organ prolapse, which can include cystocele, uterine prolapse, rectocele, enterocele, and vaginal vault prolapse. Women with prolapse beyond the introitus or who are symptomatic should be referred to a gynecologist. However, the presence of pelvic organ prolapse is a nonspecific finding that may not be related to the cause of the incontinence but may still require immediate surgical repair (Ouslander, 1992). The examiner should assess the female patient's ability to correctly contract the pelvic floor muscles and determine the strength and endurance of pelvic muscle contraction. The pelvic floor muscles are located approximately 5 cm inside the vaginal introitus at the 5 o'clock and 7 o'clock positions. Generally, the patient is asked to perform a pelvic muscle contraction against the examiner's finger(s) that is placed within the vagina. The examiner can also place a hand across the patient's abdomen to assess for simultaneous abdominal contraction and observe use of accessory muscles (e.g., buttocks, thighs) or straining during pelvic muscle contraction.

In the male, the genitalia should be inspected to note skin condition and any abnormalities of the foreskin, penis, and perineum. The prostate should be palpated to determine size, contour, and consistency. Men with severe obstructive symptoms and an enlarged or hard, nodular prostate should be referred to a urologist. Pelvic muscle strength should be examined in patients with postprostatectomy incontinence with a digital examination of the rectum. Table 10–5 outlines an example of a simple clinical scale that can be used to assess pelvic muscle strength in women and men (Wyman, 1994). The rectal examination should also include an assessment for fecal impaction.

VOIDING RECORD

One of the most helpful assessment techniques is the voiding record (Figs. 10–4 and 10–5). This should be used for a 3- to 7-day period to document the severity of incontinence, to determine the presence of any associated irrita-

---

TABLE 10-5

Clinical Rating Scale for Pelvic Muscle Contraction

0   No palpable muscle contraction

1   Flicker (e.g., barely able to detect)

2   Weak but clearly perceived

3   Moderate pressure but short duration

4   Good pressure, finger(s) firmly gripped with increased duration

5   Strong pressure, finger(s) forcefully gripped and pulled inward with long duration

---

tive symptoms (e.g., frequency and nocturia), and to identify precipitating events. Several variations of a voiding record have been described for use in institutions (Autry et al., 1984; Ouslander et al., 1986), outpatient settings (Wyman, 1988; Wyman & Burgio, 1988), and with homecare patients (McDowell, 1994). Voiding record data are helpful in characterizing the pattern of incontinence, determining the clinical diagnosis of incontinence type, examining the relationship between fluid intake and voiding patterns, and establishing the appropriate management approach. Voiding records are also critical in establishing a baseline measure for assessing treatment outcome.

LABORATORY TESTS

A clean-catch urine specimen should be collected for urinalysis. Evidence of urinary tract infection (≥ 2 bacteria/high-power field on microscopic urinalysis or positive leukocyte esterase and nitrites on urine dipstick testing) or symptoms that strongly suggest infection warrant urine culture and sensitivity testing (Wall et al., 1993). Hematuria without bacteriuria may be indicative of prostate or bladder cancer, a bladder or kidney stone, or prostatitis; patients with any of these symptoms should be referred. Patients with urine glucose and protein results may have undetected or poorly controlled diabetes or renal disease and should also be referred. Blood testing (e.g., blood urea nitrogen, creatinine, glucose, and calcium) is recommended if compromised renal function

Time	Did you urinate in the toilet?	Did you have a leaking episode? L = large; S = small	Activity at time of leakage	Urge present	Amount/type fluid intake
12–1 AM					
1–2 AM					
2–3 AM					
3–4 AM					
4–5 AM					
5–6 AM					
6–7 AM					
7–8 AM					
8–9 AM					
9–10 AM					
10–11 AM					
11–12 N					
12–1 PM					
1–2 PM					
2–3 PM					
3–4 PM					
4–5 PM					
5–6 PM					
6–7 PM					
7–8 PM					
8–9 PM					
9–10 PM					
10–11 PM					
11–12 PM					

FIGURE 10–4. Voiding record for use in ambulatory care. (From Wyman, J. [1988]. Nursing assessment of the geriatric outpatient population. *Nursing Clinics of North America, 22,* 182.)

INSTRUCTIONS: EACH TIME THE PATIENT IS CHECKED:

1) Mark one of the circles in the BLADDER section at the hour closest to the time the patient is checked.
2) Make an X in the BOWEL section if the patient has had an incontinent or normal bowel movement.

✔ = Incontinent, small amount	◡ = Dry	x = Incontinence BOWEL
● = Incontinent, large amount	Δ = Voided correctly	x = Normal BOWEL

PATIENT NAME _____ ROOM # _____ DATE _____

TIME	BLADDER			BOWEL			
	Incontinence of urine	Dry	Voided correctly	Incontinence	Normal	Initials	Comments
12 am	• ●	○	Δ cc ____				
1	• ●	○	Δ cc ____				
2	• ●	○	Δ cc ____				
3	• ●	○	Δ cc ____				
4	• ●	○	Δ cc ____				
5	• ●	○	Δ cc ____				
6	• ●	○	Δ cc ____				
7	• ●	○	Δ cc ____				
8	• ●	○	Δ cc ____				
9	• ●	○	Δ cc ____				
10	• ●	○	Δ cc ____				
11	• ●	○	Δ cc ____				
12 pm	• ●	○	Δ cc ____				
1	• ●	○	Δ cc ____				
2	• ●	○	Δ cc ____				
3	• ●	○	Δ cc ____				
4	• ●	○	Δ cc ____				
5	• ●	○	Δ cc ____				
6	• ●	○	Δ cc ____				
7	• ●	○	Δ cc ____				
8	• ●	○	Δ cc ____				
9	• ●	○	Δ cc ____				
10	• ●	○	Δ cc ____				
11	• ●	○	Δ cc ____				
TOTALS:							

FIGURE 10–5. Voiding record for institutional care. (From Ouslander, J. G., Urman, H. N., & Uman, G. C., [1986]. Development and testing of an incontinence monitoring record. *Journal of the American Geriatrics Society, 34*, 83–90.)

is suspected or if polyuria in the absence of diuretic use is present (Fantl et al., 1996).

Treatment of asymptomatic bacteruria with or without pyuria in older patients has been controversial. In chronic nursing home patients, eradication of bacteriuria has not had a significant effect on incontinence (Boscia et al., 1986).

BLADDER FUNCTION TESTS

PVR should be determined either through straight catheterization or the use of bladder ultrasonography. The patient should void immediately prior to PVR determination. Voiding can be observed at this time to detect signs of hesitancy, straining, or slow or interrupted stream, which may indicate outlet obstruction or bladder contractility. PVRs less than 50 mL are considered normal bladder emptying. Repetitive PVRs of 100 to 200 mL or higher are signs of inadequate bladder emptying; these patients may need referral to help determine the significance of these symptoms. Because PVR volumes can vary for numerous reasons, obtaining at least two PVRs is important when interpreting clinical significance, especially in the 50 to 199 mL range (Fantl et al., 1996).

The cough stress test is useful in diagnosing stress incontinence. It is performed by asking the patient to cough with a full bladder and then documenting the presence of urine loss in supine and standing positions. If leakage occurs at the height of the cough exertion, then stress incontinence is present; if leakage is delayed or persists after the cough, then detrusor instability should be suspected.

Referrals for specialized tests are necessary in the following situations (Fantl et al., 1996):

- Uncertain clinical diagnosis
- Failure of a simple trial of behavioral or pharmacological therapy
- Consideration of surgical intervention
- Hematuria without infection
- Presence of comorbid conditions, including recurrent urinary tract infection, previous antiincontinence or radical pelvic surgery, symptomatic or severe genital prolapse, prostate abnormalities suggestive of prostate cancer, abnormal PVR urine, and neurological conditions (e.g.,

multiple sclerosis, spinal cord lesions, and injuries)

Although gerontological APNs are not expected to conduct specialized tests without additional training, they should be familiar with the various diagnostic tests that can be used to further evaluate incontinence.

Urodynamic evaluation is used to determine the anatomical and functional status of the bladder and urethra. Procedures used include a voiding cystometrogram or pressure flow study, uroflowmetry, cystometry, urethral pressure profilometry, abdominal leak point pressures, and electromyography (descriptions given in Wall et al., 1993). Cystoscopy or visualization of the bladder and urethra is recommended when (1) there is sterile hematuria or pyuria; (2) urodynamics fail to duplicate symptoms; or (3) there is a new onset of irritative voiding symptoms, bladder pain, recurrent cystitis, or a suspected foreign body. Imaging studies using radiographic and ultrasonographic techniques are recommended only when the evaluation of anatomical conditions associated with incontinence is clinically necessary (Fantl et al., 1996). *Videourodynamics* combines the various urodynamic tests with simultaneous fluoroscopy and is used in the assessment of complex incontinence.

STANDARDIZED ASSESSMENT IN NURSING HOMES

Nursing homes are required by federal statute (Omnibus Budget Reconciliation Act, 1987) to perform a standardized comprehensive assessment of residents on admission to the facility, quarterly, and when there is a significant change in condition. These assessments should be performed using the Resident Assessment Instrument, which includes the Minimum Data Set (MDS). Using the MDS, the detection of incontinence or the use of an indwelling catheter should trigger the use of the Resident Assessment Protocol (RAP) for incontinence. The RAP provides a similar assessment to the clinical practice guideline on urinary incontinence recommended by the Agency for Health Care Policy and Research (Fantl et al., 1996); however, it should be supplemented with a voiding record to aid the treatment decision-making process. A similar assessment procedure is being developed for use in home health agencies.

Intervention

All potentially reversible causes of incontinence should be treated (Table 10–6). A variety of approaches are used in the management of incontinence; these include lifestyle, behavioral, pharmacological, surgical, and supportive interventions (Table 10–7). In the treatment decision-making process, the APN should consider the following factors:

- Type(s) of incontinence
- Severity and life impact of incontinence
- Patient's cognitive and physical functioning status
- Patient's and/or family caregiver's preferences, expectations, and level of motivation
- Cost-benefit factors

Realistic, mutually agreed on goals should be set for care, with the overall objective that each individual attain his or her optimal potential for continence, whether it is full or partial control. For those who cannot achieve complete control, most conditions can be improved and comfort increased.

LIFESTYLE MANAGEMENT

Strategies targeted toward reducing risk factors may be helpful in preventing and managing urinary incontinence. Especially in cases of stress incontinence, weight reduction in obese individuals may help decrease the abdominal pressure placed on the bladder during exertional events. Smoking cessation may be effective in reducing a chronic cough that precipitates stress incontinence. In individuals prone to constipation, a bowel program that incorporates adequate fiber, fluid, and activity can prevent a fecal impaction that may lead to overflow incontinence (see Chapter 11). Elimination

TABLE 10-6
Management of Transient Causes of Incontinenece

Cause	Intervention
Delirium	Treat underlying cause of confusion
Infection (e.g., urinary tract)	Appropriate antibiotic therapy
Atrophic vaginitis or urethritis	Estrogen replacement therapy
Pharmaceuticals	
Caffeine	Eliminate caffeine intake; switch to decaffeinated products
Alcohol	Eliminate alcohol use
Diuretics	Discontinue or change therapy if possible; modify dosing schedule
Anticholinergics	Discontinue use if possible or reduce dosage
Sedatives or hypnotics	Discontinue use if possible; switch to short-acting agents
Alpha-adrenergics	Discontinue use if possible
Calcium channel blockers	Discontinue use or switch drug class if possible
Narcotic analgesics	Switch to nonnarcotic analgesic if possible; use alternative methods to control pain (e.g., TENS unit); treat constipation by concurrent use of laxative regimen if chronic narcotic use required
Psychological	Treat depression or other psychiatric illness
Endocrine problems (e.g., uncontrolled diabetes mellitus)	Institute appropriate treatment
Excess fluid	Treat underlying condition, alter diuretic dosing schedule if possible
Restricted mobility	Treat underlying cause; increase toilet accessibility with toileting aids or availability of caregivers
Stool impaction	Disimpact; implement bowel regimen

TABLE 10-7

Management of Established Incontinence

Type of Incontinence	Intervention
Stress	Scheduling regimen Pelvic muscle exercises Biofeedback Vaginal cones Electrical stimulation Pelvic organ support device Estrogen replacement therapy Alpha-adrenergic agonist drugs Tricyclic antidepressant agents Periurethral bulking injections Surgery Urethral inserts (women only) External patches (women only) Absorbent products
Urge	Scheduling regimen Pelvic muscle exercises Biofeedback Electrical stimulation Anticholinergic agents Tricyclic antidepressant agents Estrogen replacement therapy Surgery in selected cases (e.g., removal of irritating lesion or with severe refractory incontinence) Absorbent product
Overflow	Credé method to assist voiding Intermittent catheterization Indwelling or suprapubic catheterization Pelvic organ support device (women with prolapse only) Absorbent products
Functional	Scheduling regimen Toileting substitutes Environmental alterations Physical therapy Absorbent products External collection devices Indwelling catheterization (selected patients only)
Unconscious or reflex	Depends on cause; similar to urge incontinence

Data from Fantl et al. (1996) and Wyman (1994).

of caffeine (a diuretic) and alcohol (a central nervous system depressant and bladder irritant) may improve continence status. Nutrasweet, citrus foods, and carbonated beverages have also been associated with urgency, frequency, and incontinence. Ensuring adequate fluid intake (1500 mL/day) is important in maintaining renal function (National Research Council, Food and Nutrition Board, 1990). Both extremes of fluid intake (i.e., too much or too little) have been associated with the development of incontinence (Colling et al., 1994; Smith & Smith, 1987). If nocturia (two or more times per night) or enuresis is present, limiting fluid intake after 8:00 or 9:00 P.M. may help reduce these problems. If patients have peripheral edema, elevating their legs during the late afternoon and early evening hours may help control nocturia and nocturnal enuresis. Patients may also benefit from taking diuretic medications so they will achieve a peak effect at the time most convenient for toileting.

Correcting faulty habits in voiding behavior may be helpful. Because many continent and incontinent individuals have infrequent voiding patterns, the use of regular voidings on a 2- to 3-hour schedule may be useful. Another important strategy is to teach patients to empty their bladder completely. Poor habit patterns often involve fast and incomplete bladder emptying. Thus, it may be useful for a patient to take his or her time when voiding, to wait a minute after voiding is completed, and then to attempt to empty the bladder further. For those patients with the sensation of incomplete bladder emptying, use of the Credé method may be beneficial.

BEHAVIORAL MANAGEMENT

Behavioral therapy is recommended as the first line of treatment in managing urinary incontinence (Fantl et al., 1996). It has few side effects and is effective in controlling urine loss associated with bladder and urethral dysfunction. Behavioral therapy includes scheduling regimens and pelvic muscle rehabilitation techniques (Table 10–8), which can be used in combination with each other or with other types of intervention (multimodality treatment). Some techniques require caregiver implementation when there are cognitive or physical impairments, whereas others can be implemented by patients who are cognitively intact but may have physical deficits. Behavioral therapy requires a motivated patient or caregiver, and continual involvement is usually necessary to maintain an optimal treatment outcome. Even the most frail elderly patients can benefit from these interventions.

Scheduling Regimens

Scheduling regimens include timed voiding, habit training, prompted voiding, and bladder training. Each of these is associated with good improvement rates but relatively low cure rates. Success of scheduling regimens used with institutionalized patients relies on staff members' training, compliance, and incentives for active participation. Thus, it is important to develop management procedures to monitor staff implementation of toileting interventions and to provide feedback about performance (Schnelle, 1990).

Timed Voiding. This fixed voiding schedule—usually every 2 hours—is used for stress, urge, overflow, functional, and reflex incontinence. Although it is typically employed with institutionalized or impaired populations, timed voiding can also be effective in treating outpatient populations without impairments when infrequent voiding patterns are present (i.e., less than 5 voidings per waking hours). In uncontrolled studies, institutionalized male patients improved by 85% (Sogbein & Awad, 1982) and outpatient women by 79% (Godec, 1994).

Habit Training. This individually prescribed toileting schedule involves voiding intervals adjusted to the patient's voiding pattern. It is used for stress, urge, functional, and reflex incontinence. Although it is usually used in institutionalized or homebound populations, it is also effective in cognitively intact outpatient populations when a consistent pattern of incontinence is observed, such as with diuretic usage. *Patterned urge response toileting* (PURT), a specialized type of habit training that has been tested in nursing home and homebound elderly populations, involves the use of an electronic monitoring device to identify the timing of incontinent episodes. In a randomized controlled study of nursing home patients, 86% showed a significant reduction in their incontinence, one third of which showed a 25% or greater improvement over baseline incontinence (Colling et al., 1992).

Prompted Voiding. Prompted voiding consists of three elements used by caregivers: (1) monitoring the patient on a regular basis, (2) prompting the patient to try to use the toilet, and (3) praising the patient for maintaining continence and trying to toilet (Table 10–9; see Schnelle, 1991, for details). This technique is used to treat cognitively or physically impaired homebound or institutionalized patients with incontinence. Monitoring the patient involves the caregiver approaching the patient and asking if he or she is dry or wet and checking to

TABLE 10-8
Behavioral Therapy for Urinary Incontinence

Intervention	Description	Patient Characteristics
Scheduling Regimens		
Timed voiding	Fixed scheduled toileting that does not change, usually 2-hr intervals; usually caregiver dependent	Used for stress, urge, and functional incontinence in patients with cognitive or physical impairments; patients without impairments who have infrequent voiding patterns; and as an adjunct in patients with mild to moderate incomplete bladder emptying
Habit retraining	Scheduled toiletings with adjustments of voiding intervals (longer or shorter) based on patient's voiding pattern; usually caregiver dependent	Used for stress, urge, and functional incontinence in patients with cognitive or physical impairments; as an adjunct in patients with mild to moderate incomplete bladder emptying; and in patients without impairments who have diuretic-induced incontinence
Prompted voiding	Scheduled toiletings that require prompts to void from caregiver, usually on a 2-hr interval; patient assisted in toileting only if response is positive	Used for stress, urge, and fuctional incontinence in patients who are functionally able to use toilet or toileting substitute; able to feel urge sensation; able to request toileting assistance; and who have availability of a caregiver
Bladder training	Scheduled voidings with progressive voiding intervals; systematic ability to delay voiding through use of urge inhibition; patient education and use of reinforcement techniques	Used for stress and urge incontinence in patients who are cognitively intact; able to toilet (alone or with assistance); motivated to comply with training program
Pelvic Muscle Rehabilitation		
Pelvic muscle exercises	Regular practice of pelvic muscle contractions; use of pelvic muscle contraction for urge inhibition; patient education	Used for stress and urge incontinence in patients who are able to identify and contract pelvic muscles; cognitively intact; and motivated to comply with exercise program
Vaginal weight training	Active retention of increasing vaginal weights; used in combination with pelvic muscle exercises and patient education	Used primarily for stress incontinence in patients who are cognitively intact; able to stand; able to contract pelvic muscles; who have sufficient vaginal vault and introitus to retain cone or sufficient pelvic muscle strength to retain lightest cone; and who are motivated to comply; contraindicated in patients with pelvic organ prolapse
Biofeedback	Use of electronic or mechanical instruments to display visual or auditory information about neuromuscular or bladder activity; used to teach pelvic muscle contraction and urge inhibition; patient education	Used for stress and urge incontinence in patients who are able to understand analog or digital signals and are motivated and able to learn voluntary control through observation
Electrical stimulation	Application of electrical current to sacral and pudendal afferent fibers through vaginal, anal, or surface electrodes; used to inhibit detrusor instability and improve awareness, contractility, and efficiency of pelvic muscle contraction; patient education	Used for stress and urge incontinence in patients who are motivated to comply; contraindicated in patients with diminished sensory perception, moderate or severe pelvic organ prolapse, urinary retention, history of cardiac arrhythmia or demand cardiac pacemaker

Data from Fantl et al. (1996) and Wyman & Burgio (1988).

verify the patient's answer. Positive feedback is provided if the individual provides a correct response. The patient is regularly (typically every 2 hours) prompted or asked if he or she needs to use the toilet; 3-hour prompts have also been used effectively (Burgio et al., 1994). Positive feedback is again given for appropriate toileting. Prompted voiding is recommended for patients who can ask for assistance, respond when prompted to toilet, or

TABLE 10-9
Prompted Voiding Protocol

Assessment Period (3–5 days)

1. Contact residents every 2 hours from 7 A.M. to 7 P.M. for 2–3 days, then every 2 hours for 2–3 days.
2. Focus their attention on voiding by asking them whether they are wet or dry.
3. Check them for wetness, record on bladder record, and give feedback on whether their response was correct or incorrect.
4. Whether wet or dry, ask residents if they would like to use the toilet or urinal. If they say yes:
   • Offer assistance.
   • Record results on bladder record.
   • Give positive reinforcement by spending an extra minute or two talking with them.
   If they say no:
   • Inform them that you will be back in 2 hours and request that they try to delay voiding until then.
   • If there has been no attempt to void in the last 4 hours, repeat the request to use the toilet once or twice more before leaving.
5. Measure voiding volumes as often as possible:
   • Place a measuring "hat" in the commode.
   • Preweigh and then reweigh incontinence pads or garments.

Targeting

1. Prompted voiding is more effective in some residents than in others. The best candidates for continuing an effective prompted voiding program are those who show the following characteristics during the assessment period:
   • Correct assessment of their wet or dry status
   • Voiding in the toilet, commode, or urinal (as opposed to being incontinent) more than half the time
   • Maximum voiding volume of 200 mL or more
   • Lower voiding frequencies
2. Residents who do not show any of the characteristics should be considered for either further evaluation to determine the specific type of incontinence or supportive management (e.g., using urine collection devices for selected patients or a checking and changing protocol).

Prompted Voiding (ongoing protocol)

1. Check the resident every 2 hours from 7 A.M. to 7 P.M.
2. Use the same procedures as those for the assessment period.
3. For nighttime management, use either a modified prompted voiding schedule or a urine collection device.
4. If a resident who has been responding well begins to show an increase in incontinence frequency despite adequate staff implementation of the protocol, they should be evaluated for reversible factors.

Adapted from Ouslander, J. G., & Schnelle, J. F. (1995). Incontinence in the nursing home. *Annals of Internal Medicine.* 122, 438–448.

learn to recognize some degree of bladder fullness or the need to void (Fantl et al., 1996). Randomized controlled trials of prompted voiding in nursing home residents found an average daily reduction of 0.8 to 1.8 incontinent episodes per patient (Burgio et al., 1994; Creason et al., 1989; Hu et al., 1989; Schnelle, 1990).

Bladder Training. This technique consists of a program of patient education in combination with a progressive voiding schedule and positive reinforcement techniques. It is used primarily to treat those outpatients who are cogni-tively intact and have symptoms of urge, stress, or mixed incontinence or who are experiencing urgency-frequency symptoms without incontinence. The goals of treatment include correcting habit patterns of frequent urination, improving the ability to control urgency, prolonging voiding intervals, increasing bladder capacity, reducing incontinent episodes, and building patients' confidence in their ability to control lower urinary tract function. Randomized controlled clinical trials in female outpatient populations indicated cure rates of 12 to 18%, with significant improvement rates of associated symptoms such as urgency, frequency, and nocturia (Fantl et al., 1991; Wyman et al; in press).

Table 10–10 summarizes the scheduling regimen used in a bladder training program (see Wyman & Fantl, 1991, for details). The protocol involves a 6-week outpatient program with weekly office visits to monitor progress, adjust the voiding interval, and provide positive reinforcement and support. Patient education, a critical component to the success of the program, includes a discussion of normal bladder control, the pathophysiology underlying incontinence, and a description of the bladder training protocol. Emphasis is placed on the development of urgency inhibition techniques that use distraction, relaxation, and affirmations (self-statements). A behavioral contract is used

---

TABLE 10–10
Scheduling Regimen Used in Bladder Training

1. An initial voiding interval is assigned based on the voiding pattern observed in a 1-week voiding record. If urinary frequency is ≥60 minutes, a 1-hour interval is assigned; if frequency is <60 minutes, a 30-minute interval is assigned.
2. Voidings are assigned during waking hours only.
3. Patients must void as scheduled whether they feel the need to void or not. Emphasis is placed on the effort to void and *not* the amount of urine voided.
4. Patients must make every effort *not* to void between assigned voidings by using urge inhibition techniques (e.g., distraction, relaxation, and affirmations or self-statements).
5. If voiding does occur at an unscheduled time, patients must get back on schedule at the next assigned time.
6. If the schedule is well tolerated (i.e., fewer than 25% of the voiding intervals are interrupted) and a decrease of the incontinence frequency occurs, the voiding interval is increased by 30 minutes.
7. If the schedule is not well tolerated (i.e., an increase in incontinence frequency occurs or more than 25% of the voiding intervals are interrupted), the voiding interval either is decreased by 30 minutes or remains the same.
8. A daily treatment log is kept to record adherence to the voiding schedule, unscheduled voidings, and incontinent episodes.
9. If no improvement is shown after 3 weeks, the patient should be reevaluated and the treatment plan revised.

Adapted from Wyman, J. F. (1993). Managing urinary incontinence with bladder training: A case study. *Journal of ET Nursing, 20,* 121–126.

to encourage optimal commitment to the program. Daily logs are used to monitor progress and adherence.

Pelvic Muscle Rehabilitation

Pelvic muscle rehabilitation includes four methods: (1) pelvic muscle exercises (PME) alone, (2) PME augmented with biofeedback, (3) PME augmented with vaginal weight training, and (4) pelvic floor electrical stimulation. APNs who subspecialize in continence management are more likely to use the latter three methods. Pelvic muscle rehabilitation is used to treat motivated patients with stress and urge incontinence. Each method is effective in significantly improving or curing incontinence but requires continual use to maintain treatment outcomes.

Pelvic Muscle Exercises. PME, also known as *Kegel's exercises,* involve voluntary contraction and relaxation of the levator ani muscle complex. The goals of PME are to strengthen and build endurance in the periurethral and perivaginal muscles, increase urethral closure pressure, improve the support of the pelvic organs, provide reflex bladder inhibition, and reduce incontinent episodes. Improvement rates in clinical trials of PME in women with stress incontinence range from 62 to 77% (Dougherty et al., 1993; Wells et al., 1991).

Pelvic muscle training involves completing a pelvic muscle assessment as previously described, teaching muscle awareness, and conducting muscle training (Table 10–11). Teaching correct pelvic muscle contraction is critical to the success of the intervention. Fewer than 50% of women can correctly contract their pelvic floor muscles on verbal coaching alone (Bump et al., 1991). Errors made in contracting the pelvic muscles include the use of Valsalva effort as well as contracting abdominal, gluteal, and thigh muscles. Incorrect PME can potentially worsen incontinence. Generally, patients with weak muscles and difficulty isolating pelvic floor muscles should be referred to a continence nurse specialist or a physical therapist for special training with the use of biofeedback and/or electrical stimulation.

During PME training, patients are instructed to contract or squeeze their pelvic floor mus-

TABLE 10-11
Pelvic Muscle Exercises

Muscle Awareness

1. Have the patient identify his or her pelvic floor muscles using any of the following techniques:
   - Try to stop your urine stream while paying attention to the muscles that are moving to cut off the urine flow. Place a hand on the lower abdomen to feel if any tightening occurs. (This technique is not recommended as a training procedure.) The patient should feel a pulling in and lifting up of the pelvic floor muscles without any tightening of the abdominal muscles.
   - Imagine that you are in a crowded room and have to pass abdominal gas. Try to stop the passage of flatus or push off the need to have a bowel movement.

2. If the patient continues to have difficulty, insert a finger(s) into the vagina or rectum, keeping a hand on the abdomen. Have the individual try to squeeze and pull in your finger. The patient can also practice by placing her/his own finger in the vagina or rectum to feel the muscle contraction.

Muscle Training (only after correct pelvic muscle contraction achieved)

1. Instruct the patient to squeeze or tighten the pelvic muscles holding the contraction strong and steady for 10 seconds, followed by a 10 second relaxation period.

2. Repeat 25 times. Perform this exercise set twice a day for a total of 50 contractions per day.

3. If muscles get tired during practice sessions, instruct the patient to perform a fewer number of contractions per exercise set. Encourage him or her to try to work up to the required number of contractions per day, even if it takes more exercise sets to achieve this goal.

4. Instruct a patient with weak pelvic floor muscles who has difficulty holding a contraction to perform a pelvic muscle contraction for fewer seconds and to gradually work up to the 10 second contraction. Maintain the 10 second relaxation period following each contraction.

5. The exercises can be performed in any position. Initially, the patient should practice them in a lying position with knees flexed and feet flat. As the patient's skill in performing the contraction improves, he or she can do them in a sitting or standing positions. However, it is recommended to complete one exercise set in the lying position each day.

6. Instruct the patient in using pelvic muscle contraction as a prevention strategy (e.g., prior to and during exertional events such as sneezing, coughing, lifting or bending to prevent urine leakage).

7. Instruct a patient with urgency problems to do several quick, strong contractions to quiet the bladder down. Often, the feeling of urgency will pass. He or she can then walk calmly at a normal pace to the bathroom to void.

8. It takes 4 to 6 weeks to achieve a training effect in the pelvic muscles and another 4 to 6 weeks to judge the effectiveness of the exercise program. Thus, the patient should be instructed to expect little progress in the first several weeks of exercising while the muscles are becoming stronger.

9. If the exercises work effectively, the patient will need to continue to practice them indefinitely. The number of exercises needed to maintain a treatment effect is unknown; however, after 3 to 6 months of exercise, the patient may be able to maintain the same benefit while performing 25 contractions once daily or 50 contractions three days a week.

cles by "drawing in" or "lifting up," as if to cut off their urine stream or to stop themselves from passing flatus, while keeping their abdominal, gluteal, and thigh muscles relaxed. The muscle training program consists of home practice of 50 to 80 sustained (10-second) contractions with an equal relaxation period every day, performed in 2 to 4 exercise sets (20–25 contractions per set) over a 12- to 24-week period. Patients with weak muscles, however, may need an individualized exercise prescription based on their ability to perform a pelvic muscle contraction (i.e., their duration and strength). As endurance builds in the pelvic muscles, the contraction time is gradually increased to 10 seconds. Ongoing supervision and patient support are essential to achieving optimal treatment outcomes.

Biofeedback Training. *Biofeedback* is a teaching technique that uses electronic or mechanical equipment to provide visual and/or auditory feedback regarding a patient's physiological response. It has been used to help patients learn correct pelvic muscle contraction and to inhibit bladder contractions. Biofeedback can involve single or multiple measurement using electromyography or manometric methods with surface, vaginal, or anal probes. Multiple feedback methods involve the simultaneous measurement of pelvic and abdominal muscle contraction and may also include monitoring detrusor activity. Biofeedback therapy is usually provided on an intensive basis, with treatment sessions held weekly or even more frequently. Home biofeedback training devices are also available, although third-party reimbursement for these devices has been problematic. Improvement rates associated with biofeedback training range from 54 to 87% (Fantl et al., 1996). In a controlled clinical trial, biofeedback-augmented PME was superior to PME alone in treating women with severe stress urinary incontinence, whereas no differences were noted in patients with mild to moderate incontinence (Burns et al., 1993).

Vaginal Weight Training. This program is used to treat women with stress incontinence. The patient wears a specially designed vaginal cone (20–100 g) while ambulatory and/or while performing PME for 15 minutes twice a day. As muscle strength increases, the cone weight is increased. The sustained contraction required to retain the cone weight is thought to increase the strength of the pelvic muscles, and the weight is thought to provide heightened proprioceptive feedback of pelvic muscle contraction. In premenopausal women, improvement rates are 68 to 80% (Fantl et al., 1996). Vaginal weight training has not been evaluated in postmenopausal women, with or without estrogen replacement therapy, or in those with pelvic organ prolapse.

Electrical Stimulation. Electrical stimulation involves the use of a vaginal or anal electrode that passes a low dose of electrical current and thereby produces a passive contraction of the pelvic muscles and reflex inhibition of the bladder. It is used to treat male and female patients with stress, urge, and mixed incontinence. Stimulation therapy is helpful in teaching patients how to correctly contract their pelvic muscles, particularly those patients who have weak muscles or who lack muscle awareness. Contraindications to electrical stimulation depend on whether rectal or vaginal stimulation is provided. In general, stimulation therapy should not be used in patients with diminished sensory perception, moderate to severe pelvic organ prolapse, urinary retention, a history of cardiac arrhythmia, or a demand cardiac pacemaker. Adverse effects include pain and discomfort that are usually minimal and subside with treatment. Office and home stimulators are available. Office stimulation may occur intensively over a short period or may be conducted over several weeks. Home stimulation therapy is usually prescribed at two 15- to 30-minute sessions a day. Improvement rates are 48 to 76% in women with stress incontinence (Fantl et al., 1996). Further research is needed to establish the ideal parameters for stimulation and to determine the efficacy of electrical stimulation used alone or in combination with other treatments in older adults.

PHARMACOLOGICAL MANAGEMENT

Drug therapy is used in the management of stress and urge incontinence in older adults. Medications are used to decrease bladder contractility and increase urethral resistance. Because of the risk of adverse effects, medications are generally used as a second line of therapy in incontinence management, frequently in combination with behavioral methods. Studies have shown no difference in treatment outcomes between a particular medication and a behavioral therapy. Comparisons tested include phenylpropanolamine versus pelvic muscle exercises (Wells et al., 1991); propantheline, oxybutynin, or flavoxate and imipramine versus bladder training (Columbo et al., 1995; Fantl et al., 1981; Jarvis, 1981); and oxybutynin versus habit training (Ouslander et al., 1988). Table 10–12 presents the recommended drugs for incontinence. When prescribing medication

TABLE 10-12
Drug Management of Urinary Incontinence

Type of Incontinence	Drug	Dosage	Mechanism of Action	Adverse Effects
Urge	Anticholinergic agents *Oxybutynin Propantheline Dicyclomine	 2.5–5 mg t.i.d. or q.i.d. 7.5–30 mg b.i.d., t.i.d., or q.i.d. 10–20 mg t.i.d.	Decrease bladder contractility; increase bladder capacity	Dry mouth, blurred vision, elevated intraocular pressure, constipation, urinary retention, tachycardia, drowsiness, delirium; should not be used with outlet obstruction
Stress	Alpha-adrenergic agonist agents *Phenylpropanol-amine *Pseudoephedrine	 25–100 mg sustained release b.i.d. 15–30 mg t.i.d.	Increase urethral resistance	Hypertension, irritability, nervousness, dizziness, headaches, insomnia, tachycardia, arrhythmias, sweating, respiratory difficulties, anorexia, urinary retention; should not be used with outlet obstruction or hypertension
Stress or urge	Tricyclic antidepressant agents Imipramine Doxepin Desipramine Nortriptyline	10–25 mg initially, q.d. to t.i.d.; sustained release form available	Decrease bladder contractility; increase urethral resistance	Nausea, insomnia, weakness, fatigue, postural hypotension, cardiac condition disturbances, anticholinergic effects (see above); should not be used with outlet obstruction
Stress or urge	Conjugated estrogen	Topical: 0.5 gm/application 1–3 times/week Oral: 0.3–.625 mg q.d. for 21 days each month Progesterone 5 mg q.d. for 10 days each month should be given if the patient has not had a hysterectomy	Improve periurethral vascularity, tone, and coaptation; decrease bladder contractility, increase urethral resistance	Breast tenderness, increased vaginal discharge, nausea, headache, hypertension, depression, thrombophlebitis or thrombolism, pulmonary embolism, myocardial infarction, oily skin, gallstones, weight gain, fluid retention

*Recommended as first line of drug therapy.
b.i.d., twice daily; q.d., every day; q.i.d., four times a day; t.i.d., three times a day.
Adapted from Wyman, J. F. (1994). Level 3: Comprehensive assessment and management of urinary incontinence by continence nurse specialists. *Nurse Practitioner Forum, 5,* 177–185.

for the elderly, the lowest dose should be used initially and the dosage slowly titrated upward until the desired effect is reached.

SURGICAL MANAGEMENT

Surgical intervention is appropriate in carefully selected older patients whose incontinence has become so bothersome that it is significantly affecting their quality of life. Recent advances in the development of less invasive techniques hold promise for use in the elderly. Surgery is indicated in the treatment of stress incontinence, overflow incontinence secondary to anatomical obstruction, and urge incontinence secondary to lower urinary tract pathology (e.g., bladder stone, tumor, diverticulum). Although less common, surgery is also used for urge incontinence associated with severe refractory detrusor instability. The type of surgery used depends on the underlying pathophysiology (see Fantl et al., 1996, for recommendations on the surgical management of urinary incontinence).

All patients anticipating surgery should receive a thorough preoperative assessment that includes a urodynamic evaluation. Preoperative teaching is essential to prepare patients for the procedure itself, the recovery period (with details about activity limitations), and expected outcomes, including potential complications and their treatment (e.g., pelvic floor defects in women, urinary retention, wound infection, and new onset of detrusor instability).

SUPPORTIVE INTERVENTION

Supportive interventions include the use of environmental alterations, such as toileting substitutes, absorbent products, catheters or other urine collection devices, occlusive and pelvic support devices, physical therapy, and skin care. These interventions are essential in managing incontinence in patients with cognitive and physical impairments, moderate to severe outlet obstruction, and chronic intractable incontinence.

Environmental Alterations

Environmental modifications that facilitate efficient access to a toilet or a toileting substitute may prevent or reduce functional incontinence and also enhance treatment outcomes for urge incontinence. Patients may benefit from consulting an occupational or physical therapist for the best way to modify the environment. A clear path that is free from obstacles and well lit is critical for reaching a toilet safely and quickly. Wearing loosely fitting clothes with elastic waistbands or snap or Velcro fasteners facilitates disrobing for those patients with manual dexterity problems. For women, a dress or skirt may be easier to manage than slacks that have a zipper. Toilets should be a sufficient height, at least 17 inches from the floor (Fantl et al., 1996). For patients with musculoskeletal pain or weakness, the use of grab-bars near the toilet seat and a raised toilet seat can make toileting easier. For patients who use wheelchairs, access can be improved by removing the bathroom door and using a curtain or saloon doors.

Toileting substitutes are devices used as a toilet when the toilet is inaccessible. They include urinals, bedpans, and commodes. A variety of male and female urinals are available, including some that are spill proof. If a bedpan is required, it should be carefully selected. The use of a bed trapeze should be considered for patients with adequate upper-extremity strength. A fracture bedpan may be more appropriate for women. Use of an inflatable bedpan is helpful for the bedbound patient who is obese or who has pain or difficulty moving. A commode chair is beneficial for patients with mobility impairments, nocturia, and nocturnal enuresis. There are several different types of commodes available; some can be placed over the toilet, whereas others have drop arms and adjustable heights. Call lights or bells should be placed within easy reach and made more visible by using a dark-colored call cord (Long, 1991).

An important environmental alteration is to set positive expectations for continence. Continence behavior may be improved by requiring residents in long-term care facilities to be dressed in proper daytime clothing rather than in nightclothes. Similarly, it is important to establish administrative guidelines that continence is an important goal of care and to provide incentives to help motivate staff members.

Absorbent Products

A wide variety of disposable and reusable absorbent products are available, ranging in cost. These include the following (Fantl et al., 1996):

- Thin pads
- Shields (wider and longer than pads)
- Guards (heavier pads, often with foam outer shell)
- Undergarments (full-length pads usually held in place by waist straps)
- Combination pad-briefs (can be worn instead of underwear)
- Bed pads

The National Association for Continence (1997) publishes an annual resource guide of continence products and services, which is helpful in selecting an appropriate product (Appendix 10–1). Absorbent products are essential for treating refractory incontinence and are also useful as an adjunct to other interventions. However, early dependency on these products may be a deterrent to patients seeking proper evaluation and treatment. Adverse effects associated with the improper use of absorbent products include contact dermatitis, skin infections, pressure ulcers, and urinary tract infections. Thus, good skin care and frequent changes of the absorbent product are necessary.

The spiraling cost of incontinence has resulted, in part, from the increased availability and use of disposable products. These products tend to be more costly to use than reusable products but offer greater absorptive capability and convenience. Although reusable products are less expense to purchase, they can be costly to wash and maintain and have been associated with more skin breakdown (Hu et al., 1990).

Catheters and Other Urine Collection Devices

Several types of catheters and urine collection devices are used in incontinence management; these include external collection devices, intermittent catheters, indwelling urethral catheters, and suprapubic catheters. The use of intermittent catheterization is necessary in patients with outlet obstruction, but the long-term use of the other types of catheters is controversial. Generally, they are recommended for use in patients who have intractable incontinence or overflow incontinence caused by obstruction and for whom other interventions are not feasible.

External condom catheters should be used only when there are mobility impairments, intact genital skin, sufficient penis length, and no bladder obstruction. Condom catheters vary in the type of material used (e.g., latex rubber, polyvinyl, or silicone) and their design. Although condom catheters are preferable to indwelling catheters, with improper or prolonged use they can cause complications such as abrasion, dermatitis, ischemia, necrosis, edema, maceration of the penis, and urinary tract infection (Ouslander et al., 1987).

Prior to catheter placement, the penile skin should be inspected, cleaned, and shaved if necessary. A skin product such as a skin sealant can be used to protect skin integrity and enhance the adhesion of the sheath to the skin. An appropriately sized condom should be carefully applied to prevent constriction, and the tubing of the collection system should be free of kinks. A smaller leg bag is preferable to a large leg bag because the collected urine can put too much weight on the catheter and pull it off. Condom catheters should be removed at least daily. If a complication occurs, the external catheter should not be used again until the problem has been resolved. A urinary pouch may be useful for a retracted penis that cannot be fitted with a condom catheter. Patient and caregiver education is essential for ensuring the proper application of external devices and subsequent inspection for complications. Female external urine collection devices exist but have not proved successful.

Intermittent catheterization (IC) is the treatment of choice for patients with spinal cord injury and overflow incontinence secondary to an underactive or partially obstructed bladder. Sterile technique is recommended with elderly patients (Fantl et al., 1996). The procedure can be performed by caregivers or the patients themselves if they have adequate manual dexterity. Bladder emptying should be performed on a schedule, typically every 3 to 6 hours.

Adverse effects associated with IC include urethral inflammation, stricture, false passage, infection, hydronephrosis, and epididymitis. Although no comparison studies have been conducted, the long-term use of IC is preferred over indwelling catheterization.

Because of the high risk of complications, indwelling urethral catheterization is recommended only in selected patients (Table 10–13). Virtually all patients develop bacteriuria after 2 to 4 weeks of catheterization (Warren, 1990). Other complications include obstruction secondary to encrustation, unprescribed removal by the patient, pain, bladder spasms, urethral erosion, stones, epididymitis, urethritis, periurethral abscess, chronic renal inflammatory changes, fistula formation, hematuria, urinary leakage, urinary tract infection, urosepsis, and death.

There has been limited research to guide catheter selection and management. Several types of catheters are available (e.g., latex, silicone, Teflon, and silicone- or Teflon-coated latex). Latex catheters are prone to encrustation and may cause urethral irritation and possibly allergic reactions in patients with latex sensitivity (Kinney et al., 1980). Silicone catheters are associated with less cytotoxicity and urethral stricture than those with latex and are preferable for long-term use. Silicone or Teflon coating of latex catheters may disintegrate within a few hours after catheter placement, thus exposing the urethral epithelium to direct contact with the latex (Woods & Bender, 1989). Newer catheters that are silver coated, antimicrobial, or lubricous coated may decrease the risk of complications (Johnson et al., 1990; Liedberg et al.,

1990). The catheter size should be as small as possible; typically, 14- and 16-French catheters are used with a 5 cc balloon filled with 10 cc of sterile water.

No information exists on the optimal frequency of changing an indwelling catheter; however, the usual practice is every 30 days unless there is encrustation, blockage, or symptomatic urinary tract infection (Fantl et al., 1996). Routine catheter irrigation is not recommended; it is ineffective in eradicating bacteriuria and may also increase the risk of infection. Neither disinfecting collection bags to prevent infection nor clamping the catheter prior to removal have proved effective (Fantl et al., 1996). Leakage around the catheter may be an indication of catheter blockage from encrustations or bladder spasms caused by catheter irritation. The patient should be checked for fecal impaction or chronic constipation, which might trigger a spasm, and for urinary tract infection. Use of anticholinergic drugs to decrease bladder contractility may be necessary (Gray et al., 1991); however, the routine use of antibiotic suppression therapy to prevent bacteriuria is not recommended (Ouslander, 1992).

The use of indwelling catheterization to monitor fluid output during acute illnesses or as short-term therapy carries the risk of leading to long-term use; nurses must therefore be vigilant about identifying the purpose of catheter placement and removing the catheter once the purpose has been achieved. Patients in acute care settings are often discharged to a long-term care facility or their home with an unnecessary catheter because staff members assumed it was required. Table 10–14 provides a protocol for removing catheters from patients who have had them for several weeks or more.

Suprapubic catheters can be used following gynecological, urological, and other surgery or as an alternative to long-term urethral catheterization for patients with urethral closure. Suprapubic catheters are contraindicated in patients with detrusor instability (Fantl et al., 1996). Complications associated with their use include bladder stones, symptomatic urinary tract infection, hematoma, skin erosion, leakage around the catheter, and recurrent catheter blockage.

TABLE 10-13

Indications for Indwelling Catheterization

Overflow incontinence with obstruction in patients for whom intermittent catheterization is not feasible

Acutely ill patients in whom incontinence interferes with necessary monitoring of fluid balance

Short-term management of stage III or IV pressure ulcers

Seriously impaired or terminally ill patients in whom bed and clothing changes are painful and disruptive

Data from Fantl et al. (1996) and Warren (1990).

TABLE 10-14
Protocol for Removal of an Indwelling Catheter

Note: This protocol should not be used in patients with established overflow incontinence.

Prior to Removal of Catheter (1–2 days)

1. Review drug use. If possible, discontinue or reduce those drugs that are likely to cause urinary retention.
2. Monitor intake and output every 8 hours.
3. The therapeutic benefit of antibiotic therapy in the bladder retraining process following catheterization has not been determined. Some clinicians have found it beneficial to initiate a 5 to 14 day course of a broad spectrum antibiotic (e.g., trimethroprim and sulfamethoxazole [Bactrim], ciprofloxacin [Cipro]) beginning 2 days prior to catheter removal.

Catheter Removal

4. Remove the indwelling catheter (clamping the catheter before removal is not necessary).

Following Catheter Removal

5. Initiate a 2-hour toileting schedule during waking hours.

   Instruct the patient on techniques to trigger voiding (such as running water, stroking inner thigh, putting hands in warm water) and to help completely empty bladder (such as bending forward, applying suprapubic pressure, and double voiding).

   Note: The patient may void every 15 to 20 minutes for the first 6 to 12 hours after catheter removal, while the bladder is adjusting to storing urine.

6. If the patient has not voided in 6 to 8 hours, request that he or she attempt to void. Perform a postvoid residual (PVR) volume determination by straight catheterization or bladder ultrasonagraphy. Continue to monitor output and PVRs until PVRs are consistently less than 200 mL.

   If the PVR is greater than 400 mL, continue to monitor for 2 more days. If the PVR does not decrease, reinsert the indwelling catheter and refer for specialist evaluation.

7. If the patient is voiding frequently (i.e., greater than every 2 hours), encourage him or her to delay voiding as long as possible. Instruct the patient in urge inhibition techniques (distraction, relaxation, and pelvic muscle contraction, if able) and techniques to help empty bladder completely.

8. If the patient continues to have incontinence, he or she should be reevaluated to rule out reversible causes and to determine whether referral to a specialist is necessary for further evaluation.

Occlusive and Pelvic Organ Support Devices

Occlusive devices designed for women and men may be useful in treating stress incontinence. Recent innovations in the treatment of female stress incontinence include intraurethral devices (e.g., Reliance Urinary Control Insert [UroMed, Needham, MA]) and external soft devices worn at the urinary meatus (e.g., Impress Softpatch [UroMed] and Fem Assist [Insight Medical, Bolton, MA]). These devices must be sized appropriately and changed with each voiding. Complications with intraurethral devices include infection, migration into the bladder, and discomfort. External devices may cause infection, skin irritation, and discomfort.

Penile compression devices have been used to treat stress incontinence by mechanically closing the urethra. Both penile clamps and cuff compression devices are available, with the Cunningham Clamp (Bard, Murray Hill, NJ) the most commonly used. These devices must be released at 2- to 3-hour intervals to allow for bladder emptying and the maintenance of tissue integrity, and they should not be worn at night (Fantl et al., 1996; Gray et al., 1991). They should be used only by cognitively intact, motivated, and manually dextrous patients and are most successful when used for short periods during exertional activities such as tennis or golf (Gray et al., 1991). Complications include pain, penile and urethral erosion, penile edema, and obstruction.

Women with stress or overflow incontinence associated with pelvic organ prolapse may be helped by the use of a pessary. *Pessaries* are rubber or silicone devices inserted into the vagina that are designed to reduce pelvic prolapse and restore normal functioning. They should not be used in patients with vaginal prolapse or vaginitis or in women who cannot remove or insert the device without routine access to a healthcare provider (Fantl et al., 1996). Pessaries are made in a variety of shapes and sizes and should be properly fitted by a trained healthcare provider. Patients should be monitored every 3 months to check vaginal mucosal integrity. Complications related to misuse or neglect include discomfort, ulceration of the vagina, rectovaginal and vesicovaginal fistula, and voiding difficulties. Patients should be shown how to insert, remove, and clean the pessary and should be educated about the need for frequent monitoring.

Physical Therapy

Patients with functional incontinence caused by mobility impairments may benefit from physical therapy aimed at strengthening muscles and improving gait and balance. Several studies have indicated that mobility improvement is associated with a reduction in incontinence (Jirovec, 1991; Palmer et al., 1991). The use of a mobility aid such as a cane, walker, or wheelchair might also be beneficial.

Skin Care

Good skin care is essential for all incontinent patients but especially for those with continuous or large-volume leakages or who have mobility impairments. Ideally, the skin should be cleaned without rubbing, preferably using a perineal cleanser, and patted or air dried after each incontinent episode (Fiers, 1996). Perineal cleansers in rinse and no-rinse formulations are less irritating to the skin than soap and water. A moisturizing lotion or cream can be applied if necessary. If skin irritation is present or at risk, a moisture barrier product should be used. Skin sealants that provide a clear, copolymer film to the skin need to be reapplied every 12 to 24 hours. Moisture barrier creams and ointments should be reapplied after each incontinent episode. Skin problems such as a monilial infection (*Candida albicans*), which appears as a patch of erythema containing macules and papules, can be treated with an over-the-counter antifungal cream or ointment. A variety of skin care products are available from different manufacturers. Fiers (1996) provided an excellent review of the different products and the criteria to be used in their selection.

ROLE OF THE ADVANCED PRACTICE NURSE

The APN can make a significant difference in the quality of life of incontinent older adults across all care settings. APNs play a key role in the prevention, early detection, diagnosis, and management of urinary incontinence. Health promotion efforts should be targeted to all adults and should include strategies to maintain good bladder health. Nurses should become involved in multidisciplinary efforts targeted toward educating the public about incontinence. These efforts can include health lectures, participation at health fairs, television or radio interviews or talk shows, help lines, public service announcements, and multimedia educational materials (Fantl et al., 1996). APNs can also initiate support groups for people with incontinence and their family members. Because most health professional and paraprofessional programs provide limited education on incontinence care, APNs should be involved in planning continuing education for these healthcare providers. The need for staff development is especially great in home health, acute care, and long-term care settings. APNs should also be involved in developing incontinence protocols tailored to specific practice settings, which could incorporate quality improvement techniques for the successful implementation of continence programs. By presenting an optimistic attitude about the management of incontinence, APNs can help set positive expectations for staff members and patients.

An increasing number of APNs are subspecializing in the management of patients with incontinence. Continence nurse specialists are involved in collaborative, consultative, and independent practice across multiple settings. These nurse specialists are likely to use more sophisticated assessment procedures and a greater variety of treatment approaches than are available to APNs in generalist practice.

A relatively recent development in incontinence care is the introduction of continence clinics located in community settings, which offer comprehensive assessment and management programs. Shipes (1991) provided recommendations for developing and marketing a continence clinic. In some institutional settings, a continence team or continence nurse specialist is available to evaluate and provide treatment recommendations for incontinent patients. Nurses interested in starting an independent practice in continence management should review Newman and Palumbo's (1994) article for guidelines on establishing this type of practice.

SUMMARY

Urinary incontinence is a prevalent and costly health problem in the elderly. Research-based clinical practice guidelines are now available to guide the diagnosis and management of patients with urinary incontinence. These guidelines should be incorporated into advanced nursing practice across all care settings. APNs should take an active role in health promotion and the early detection, assessment, and management of older adults with incontinence. An increasing number of APNs are assuming leadership roles as continence nurse specialists in the provision of continence care. Through quality nursing care, patients with incontinence can achieve a significant reduction of symptoms, leading to an improved quality of life.

REFERENCES

Abrams, P., Blaivas, J. G., Stanton, S. L., et al. (1988). Standardization of terminology of lower urinary tract function. *Scandinavian Journal of Urology and Nephrology, 114*(suppl.), 5–19.

Abrams, P., Feneley, R., & Torrens, M. (1983). *Urodynamics.* New York: Springer-Verlag.

Autry, P., Lauzon, F., & Holliday, P. J. (1984). The voiding record: An aid to decrease incontinence. *Geriatric Nursing, 5,* 22–25.

Boscia, J. A., Kobasa, W. D., Abrutyn, E., et al. (1986). Lack of association between bacteriuria and symptoms in the elderly. *American Journal of Medicine, 81,* 979–982.

Bump, R. C., Hurt, W. G., Fantl, A., et al. (1991). Assessment of Kegel pelvic exercise performance after brief verbal instruction. *American Journal of Obstetrics and Gynecology, 165,* 322–329.

Burgio, L. D., McCormick, K. A., Scheve, A. S., et al. (1994). The effects of changing prompted voiding schedules in the treatment of incontinence in nursing home residents. *Journal of the American Geriatrics Society, 42,* 315–320.

Burns, P. A., Pranikoff, K., Nochajski, T. H., et al. (1993). A comparison of effectiveness of biofeedback and pelvic muscle exercise treatment of stress incontinence in older community-dwelling women. *Journal of Gerontology, 48,* 167–174.

Colling, J. C., Ouslander, J. G., Hadley, B. J., et al. (1992). The effects of patterned urge response toileting (PURT) on urinary incontinence among nursing home residents. *Journal of the American Geriatrics Society, 40,* 135–141.

Colling, J. C., Owen, T. R., & McCreedy, M. R. (1994). Urine volumes and voiding patterns among incontinent nursing home residents. Residents at highest risk for dehydration are often the most difficult to track. *Geriatric Nursing, 15(4),* 188–192.

Columbo, M., Zanetta, G., Scalamgrino, S., et al. (1995). Oxybutynin and bladder training in the management of female urinary urge incontinence: A randomized study. *International Urogynecology Journal, 6,* 63–67.

Creason, N. S., Grybowski, J. A., Burgener, S., et al. (1989). Prompted voiding therapy for urinary incontinence in aged female nursing home residents. *Journal of Advanced Nursing, 14,* 120–126.

Dey, A. N. (1996). *Characteristics of elderly home health care users: Data from the 1993 National Home and Hospice Care Survey. Advance data from Vital and Health Statistics No. 272.* Hyattsville, MD: National Center for Health Statistics.

Diokno, A. C., Brock, B. M., Brown, M. B., et al. (1986). Prevalence of urinary incontinence and other urological symptoms in the noninstitutionalized elderly. *Journal of Urology, 136,* 1022–1025.

Dougherty, M., Bishop, K., Mooney, R., et al. (1993). Graded pelvic muscle exercise. Effect on stress urinary incontinence. *Journal of Reproductive Medicine, 39,* 684–691.

Fantl, J. A., Hurt, W. G., & Dunn, L. J. (1981). Detrusor instability syndrome: The use of bladder retraining drills with and without anticholinergics. *American Journal of Obstetrics and Gynecology, 140,* 885–890.

Fantl, J. A., Newman, D. K., Colling, J., et al. (1996). *Urinary incontinence in adults: Acute and chronic management*. Clinical Practice Guideline No. 2: Update. Agency for Health Care Policy and Research Publication No. 96-0682. Rockville, MD: U.S. Department of Health and Human Services, Public Health Service, Agency for Health Care Policy and Research.

Fantl, J. A., Wyman, J. F., McClish, D. K., et al. (1991). Efficacy of bladder training in older women with urinary incontinence. *Journal of the American Medical Association, 265*, 609–613.

Fiers, S. A. (1996). Breaking the cycle: The etiology of incontinence dermatitis and evaluating and using skin care products. *Ostomy/Wound Management, 42(3)*, 32–43.

Godec, C. J. (1994). Timed voiding: A useful tool in the treatment of urinary incontinence. *Urology, 23*, 97–100.

Gosling, J. (1979). The structure of the bladder and urethra in relation to function. *Urologic Clinics of North America, 6*, 31–38.

Gray, M., Siegel, S., Troy, R., et al. (1991). Management of urinary incontinence. In D. B. Doughty (Ed.), *Urinary and fecal incontinence: Nursing management* (pp. 95–150). St. Louis, MO: Mosby–Year Book.

Herzog, A. G., & Fultz, N. H. (1990). Prevalence and incidence of urinary incontinence in the community-dwelling population. *Journal of the American Geriatrics Society, 38*, 273–281.

Hu, T. W., Igou, J. F., Kaltreider, D. L., et al. (1989). A clinical trial of a behavioral therapy to reduce urinary incontinence in nursing homes. *Journal of the American Medical Association, 261*, 2656–2662.

Hu, T. W., Kaltreider, D. L., & Igou, J. F. (1990). The cost-effectiveness of disposable versus reusable diapers. *Journal of Gerontological Nursing, 16(2)*, 19–24.

Jarvis, G. J. (1981). A controlled trial of bladder drill and drug therapy in the management of detrusor instability. *British Journal of Urology, 53*, 565–566.

Jirovec, M. M. (1991). The impact of daily exercise on the mobility, balance, and urine control of cognitively impaired nursing home residents. *International Journal of Nursing Studies, 28*, 145–151.

Johnson, J. R., Roberts, P. L., Olsen, R. J., et al. (1990). Prevention of catheter-associated urinary tract infections with silver oxide–coated urinary catheter. *Journal of Infectious Diseases, 162*, 1145–1150.

Kinney, A. B., Blout, M., & Dowell, M. (1980). Urethral catheterization. *Geriatric Nursing, 1*, 258–263.

Kirkland, J. L., Lye, M., Levy, D. W., et al. (1983). Patterns of urine flow and electrolyte excretion in healthy elderly people. *British Medical Journal, 287*, 1665–1667.

Liedberg, H., Lundeberg, T., & Eckman, P. (1990). Refinements in the coating of urethral catheters reduces the incidence of catheter-associated bacteriuria. *European Urology, 17*, 236–240.

Long, M. L. (1991). Managing urinary incontinence. In C. Chenitz, J. Takano-Stone & S. A. Salisbury (Eds.), *Clinical gerontological nursing: A guide for advanced practice* (pp. 203–214). Philadelphia: W. B. Saunders.

Makinen, J. I., Gronroos, M., Kiiholma, P. J. A., et al. (1992). The prevalence of urinary incontinence in a randomized population of 5237 adult Finnish women. *International Urogynecology Journal, 3*, 110–113.

McDowell, B. J. (1994). Care of urinary incontinence in the home. *Nurse Practitioner Forum, 5*, 138–146.

Mohide, A. (1986). The prevalence and scope of urinary incontinence. *Clinics in Geriatric Medicine, 2*, 639–656.

National Association for Continence (1997). *Resource guide: Products and services for incontinence* (8th ed.). Union, SC: National Association for Continence.

National Research Council, Food and Nutrition Board (1990). *Recommended dietary allowances* (10th ed.). Washington, D.C.: National Academy Press.

Newman, D. K., & Palumbo, M. V. (1994). Planning an independent nursing practice for continence services. *Nurse Practitioner Forum, 5*, 190–193.

Noelker, L. (1987). Incontinence in elderly cared for by family. *Gerontologist, 27*, 194–200.

Omnibus Budget Reconciliation Act (1987). Subtitle C, Nursing Home reform. Public Law No. 100–203. Washington, D.C.: U.S. Government Printing Office.

Ory, M. G., Wyman, J. F., & Yu, L. (1986). Psychosocial factors in urinary incontinence. *Clinics in Geriatric Medicine, 2*, 657–672.

Ouslander, J. G. (1992). Geriatric urinary incontinence. *Disease-a-Month, 38(2)*, 67–149.

Ouslander, J. G., Blaustein, J., Connor, A., et al. (1988). Habit training and oxybutynin for incontinence in nursing home patients: A placebo-controlled trial. *Journal of the American Geriatrics Society, 36*, 40–46.

Ouslander, J. G., Greengold, B., & Chen, S. (1987). External catheter use and urinary tract infections among incontinent male nursing home residents. *Journal of the American Geriatrics Society, 35*, 1063–1070.

Ouslander, J. G., & Schnelle, J. F. (1995). Incontinence in the nursing home. *Annals of Internal Medicine, 122*, 438–449.

Ouslander, J. G., Urman, H. N., & Uman, G. C. (1986). Development and testing of an incontinence monitoring record. *Journal of the American Geriatrics Society, 34*, 83–90.

Palmer, M. H. (1988). Incontinence: The magnitude of the problem. *Nursing Clinics of North America, 23*, 139–157.

Palmer, M. H., Bone, L. R., Fahey, M., et al. (1992). Detecting urinary incontinence in older adults during hospitalization. *Applied Nursing Research, 5*, 174–180.

Palmer, M. H., German, P. S., & Ouslander, J. G. (1991). Risk factors for urinary incontinence one year after nursing home admission. *Research in Nursing and Health, 14*, 405–412.

Resnick, N. M. (1984). Urinary incontinence in the elderly. *Medical Grand Rounds, 3*, 284–289.

Resnick, N. M., & Yalla, S. V. (1987). Detrusor hyperactivity with impaired contractile function: An unrecognized but common cause of incontinence in elderly patients. *Journal of the American Medical Association, 257*, 3076–3081.

Schnelle, J. F. (1990). Treatment of urinary incontinence in nursing home patients by prompted voiding. *Journal of the American Geriatrics Society, 38*, 356–360.

Schnelle, J. F. (1991). *Managing urinary incontinence in the elderly*. New York: Springer.

Shipes, E. (1991). Continence clinics. In D. B. Doughty (Ed.), *Urinary and fecal incontinence: Nursing management*. (pp. 151–168). St. Louis, MO: Mosby–Year Book.

Skelly, J., & Flint, A. J. (1995). Urinary incontinence associated with dementia. *Journal of the American Geriatrics Society, 43*, 286–294.

Smith, P. S., & Smith, L. J. (1987). Fluid intake. In P. S. Smith & L. J. Smith (Eds.), *Continence and incontinence:*

Psychological approaches to development and treatment (pp. 95–99). London: Croom Helm.

Sogbein, S. K., & Awad, S. A. (1982). Behavioral treatment of urinary incontinence in geriatric patients. *Canadian Medical Association Journal, 127*, 863–864.

Sullivan, D. H., & Lindsey, R. W. (1984). Urinary incontinence in the geriatric population of an acute care hospital. *Journal of the American Geriatrics Society, 32*, 646–650.

Urinary Incontinence Guideline Panel (1992). *Urinary incontinence in adults: Clinical practice guideline.* AHCPR Publication No. 92-0038. Rockville, MD: Agency for Health Care Policy and Research, Public Health Service, U.S. Department of Health and Human Services.

Wall, L. L., Norton, P. A., & DeLancey, J. O. L. (1993). *Practical Urogynecology.* Baltimore: Williams & Wilkins.

Warren, J. W. (1990). Urine-collection devices for use in adults with urinary incontinence. *Journal of the American Geriatrics Society, 38*, 364–367.

Wein, A. J., & Barrett, D. M. (1988). *Voiding: Function and dysfunction.* Chicago: Year Book Medical Publishers, Inc.

Wells, T., Brink, C., Diokno, A., et al. (1991). Pelvic muscle exercise for stress urinary incontinence in elderly women. *Journal of the American Geriatrics Society, 39*, 785–791.

Woods, D. R., & Bender, B. S. (1989). Long-term urinary tract catheterization. *Medical Clinics of North America, 73*, 1441–1453.

Wyman, J. F. (1991). Incontinence and related problems. In C. Chenitz, J. Takano-Stone & S. A. Salisbury. (Eds), *Clinical gerontological nursing: A guide to advanced practice* (pp. 181–202). Philadelphia: W. B. Saunders.

Wyman, J. F. (1988). Nursing assessment of the geriatric outpatient population. *Nursing Clinics of North America, 22*, 169–187.

Wyman, J. F. (1993). Managing urinary incontinence with bladder training: A case study. *Journal of ET Nursing, 20*, 121–126.

Wyman, J. F. (1994). Level 3: Comprehensive assessment and management of urinary incontinence by continence nurse specialists. *Nurse Practitioner Forum, 5*, 177–185.

Wyman, J. F., & Burgio, K. L. (1988). Advances in urinary incontinence management in the elderly. *Advances in Clinical Rehabilitation, 2*, 82–107.

Wyman, J. F., Elswick, R. K., Ory, M. G., et al. (1993). Influence of functional, urological, and environmental characteristics on urinary incontinence in community-dwelling older women. *Nursing Research, 42*, 270–275.

Wyman, J. F., & Fantl, J. A. (1991). Bladder training in ambulatory care management of urinary incontinence. *Urologic Nursing, 11(3)*, 11–17.

Wyman, J. F., Fantl, J. A., McClish, D. K., et al. (in press). Comparative efficacy of behavioral interventions in the management of female urinary incontinence. *American Journal of Obstetrics and Gynecology.*

Wyman, J. F., Harkins, S. W., & Fantl, J. A. (1990). Psychosocial impact of urinary incontinence in the community-dwelling population. *Journal of the American Geriatrics Society, 38*, 282–288.

Yu, L. C., Johnson, K., Kaltreider, D. L., et al. (1991). Urinary incontinence: Nursing home staff reaction toward residents. *Journal of Gerontological Nursing, 17(11)*, 34–41.

APPENDIX $\boxed{\textbf{10-1}}$

Resources

PRINT MATERIALS

Burgio, K. L., Pearce, K. L., & Lucco, A. J. (1989). *Staying dry: A practical guide to bladder control*. Baltimore: John Hopkins University Press.

Fantl, J. A., Newman, D. K., Colling, J., et al. (1996). *Urinary incontinence in adults: Acute and chronic management*. Clinical Practice Guideline, No. 2; Update. Agency for Health Care Policy and Research Publication No. 96-0682. Rockville, MD: U.S. Department of Health and Human Services, Public Health Service, Agency for Health Care Policy and Research. Note: Several versions are available: the Clinical Practice Guideline, the Quick Reference Guide for Clinicians, and the Consumer Version (available in English and Spanish). To order, call 800-358-9295 or write to AHCPR Publications Clearinghouse, P.O. Box 8547, Silver Springs, MD 20907.

National Association for Continence (1997). *Resource guide: Products and services for incontinence*. 8th ed. Union, SC: National Association for Continence.

Newman, D. K., & Dzurinko, M. (1997) *The urinary incontinence sourcebook*. Los Angeles: Lowell House.

Wound, Ostomy, and Continence Nurses Society (1992). *Standards of care: Patients with urinary incontinence*. Costa Mesa, CA: Wound Ostomy Continence Nurses Society.

CONSUMER ADVOCACY ORGANIZATIONS

National Association for Continence
P.O. Box 544
Union, SC 29379
(803) 585-8789
National clearinghouse and patient advocacy organization; provides a variety of patient education and resource materials, including a quarterly newsletter.

The Simon Foundation
P.O. Box 835K
Wilmette, IL 60091
(800) 23-SIMON
Nonprofit organization promoting research and public education; provides a variety of patient education and resource materials, including lecture series called "I Can Manage" and a quarterly newsletter.

SPECIALTY ORGANIZATIONS

American Urogynecological Society
401 N. Michigan Avenue
Chicago, IL 60611
(312) 644-6610

American Urological Association
1120 North Charles Street
Baltimore, MD 21201
(410) 727-1100

Association of Rehabilitation Nurses
4700 W. Lake Avenue
Glenview, IL 60025
(800) 229-7530
(847) 375-4710

International Continence Society
Werner Schafer
Membership Secretary
Urologische Klinik der RWTH Aachen
52062 Aachen, Germany
Telephone: 49 (241) 808-9828
Fax: 49 (241) 888-8452

Society for Urologic Nurses and
Associates
East Holly Avenue
P.O. Box 56
Pittman, NJ 08071
(609) 256-2335

Wound, Ostomy, and Continence Nurses
Society
2755 Bristol Street
Suite 110
Costa Mesa, CA 92626
(714) 476-0268
122, 438–448.

Constipation, Diarrhea, and Fecal Incontinence

Joyce Takano Stone
Jean F. Wyman

Constipation, diarrhea, and fecal incontinence are bowel-related problems of major concern in geriatric care because of the frequency of their occurrence, the discomfort and distress they cause, the potential complications that can arise, and the additional cost in time and materials necessary for their treatment. This chapter discusses the possible causes of these conditions as well as their prevention, assessment, and management.

NORMAL BOWEL FUNCTION

Normal bowel function is dependent on (1) physical activity, (2) regular meals and the intake of adequate fluids and fiber in the diet, and (3) either consistent toileting time or a prompt response to the urge to defecate (Hogstel & Nelson, 1992; Kubalanza-Sipp & French, 1990; Mahan & Escott-Stump, 1996).

Physical Activity. Exercise and activity are

essential to maintain the musculoskeletal system and the physiological bowel response. Activity enhances peristalsis, and decreased activity slows colonic transit (Wald, 1990). In a large study, inactivity in all age groups was associated with self-reported constipation, independent of dietary intake (Sandler et al., 1990).

Fluids and Fiber. Drinking sufficient amounts of fluid and eating a well-balanced diet rich in high-fiber foods help maintain normal bowel function. One and a half to 2 L of fluids a day are recommended for older people (Harari et al., 1993; Hogstel & Nelson, 1992). The decreased thirst response in the elderly, a fear of incontinence, an inability of cognitively impaired people to recognize or express their need for fluids, or hot weather may result in the inadequate intake of fluids and thus dehydration (Castle, 1989; Cheskin & Schuster, 1994).

The frequency and consistency of stool is determined by the foods consumed (Davies et al., 1986). The typical diet in western countries tends to be low in fiber; the average daily fiber intake of 11 g for women and 17.5 g for men is less than the optimal 20 to 30 g (Bliss & Murray, 1991; Burkitt, 1982; Schneeman & Tietyen, 1994; Williams, 1992). The amount of fiber needed to keep the stool soft and to prevent constipation varies considerably among individuals. The stimulation of the urge to defecate was previously attributed to the water-holding capacity of fiber, leading to an increase in stool bulk and its stretching effect on the colon. However, the urge stimulation is now attributed to the volatile short-chain fatty acids produced by the action of colonic bacteria on fiber (Mahan & Escott-Stump, 1996).

Toileting

Routine or Schedule. Bowel evacuation occurs every day or every other day in most people and every 3 days in others. A timely response to the urge to defecate and establishing a consistent routine or schedule for elimination are important. Periods of high gut motility occur on arising and after meals (Castle, 1989). Thirty to 40 minutes after a meal is often the best time for toileting, as this takes advantage of the gastrocolic and duodenocolic reflexes (Harari et al., 1993; Leslie, 1990).

Position. Proper positioning is important for defecation. The squatting position is the natural, optimal physiological position for defecation (Leslie, 1990).

Time and Privacy. Sufficient time should be allowed for the older person to not feel rushed or hurried. However, the length of time the patient is left on the toilet, commode, or bedpan should not exceed 20 to 30 minutes (Stryker, 1977). Visual and auditory privacy helps the patient relax and avoid embarrassment from the sounds and odors associated with defecation.

Equipment and Special Products. For frail older patients, a toilet with a padded seat and backrest and side handrails allows for ease in transfer and provides support and comfort. An elevated toilet seat may facilitate getting on and off the toilet. A footstool can also be used with an elevated toilet seat to support the feet and raise the knees slightly higher than the hips, allowing for a natural squatting position (Cannon, 1981).

Disposable undergarments and pads are available to provide ease of care and to protect the patient from soiling clothes and bedding during the bowel training period. Skin irritation can be prevented with prompt cleansing and the application of a moisture barrier skin cream or spray. A fecal incontinence bag provides the necessary skin protection when there is diarrhea or a frequent discharge of feces. However, the use of rectal tubes or indwelling catheters with inflated balloons as an internal drainage system for fecal incontinence or diarrhea is contraindicated. Their use may result in a decreased responsiveness of the rectal sphincters as well as damage to the rectal mucosa (Halpin, 1986; Mowlam et al., 1986).

Patient and Family Education. Patients and their families often have misconceptions resulting from incorrect or limited information about bowel function. Questions that clinicians should address include (1) what is a normal bowel pattern?, (2) what causes elimination problems?, and (3) how should these problems be treated? Patient education should include a discussion of the consequences of inappropriate or prolonged laxative use and the undesirable addition or deletion of certain foods in the diet. Other factors affecting bowel function (e.g., activity and exercise, diet, and medications) should be discussed, with emphasis given to their role in preventing elimination problems (Cannon, 1981).

CONSTIPATION

Definition

The definition of constipation is highly subjective, and as a result, elderly people may define constipation differently than their healthcare providers (Cheskin & Schuster, 1994; Sandler et al., 1990). *Constipation* has been defined as insufficient frequency of defecation, insufficient quantity of stool, abnormally hard and dry stools, difficulty with defecation (dyschezia), or a sense of incomplete evacuation (Kumar et al., 1992; Talley et al., 1992; Wald, 1993). It is difficult to determine what constitutes insufficient frequency. A normal bowel pattern may range from three stools a day to a comfortable bowel movement once every 3 to 5 days (Devroede, 1993; Koch, 1995; Shafik, 1993). Among elderly people complaining of constipation, dyschezia and long periods between bowel movements are the most commonly reported symptoms (Talley et al., 1992; Whitehead et al., 1989).

Scope of the Problem

Constipation is a common complaint of older adults. Although it is perceived to be an age-related problem, the frequency of bowel movements does not differ between healthy old people and young people (Johanson et al., 1989; Sandler et al., 1990; Wald, 1990), and transit time through the intestinal tract in mobile older people is similar to that in younger people (Brocklehurst, 1992). However, elderly people complain of constipation more frequently than do younger people, and as many as 30% of healthy older people use laxatives regularly (Harari et al., 1993; Sandler et al., 1990; Wald, 1993).

Types and Causes of Constipation

Constipation is a symptom caused by numerous diseases and other factors such as diet and the environment (Table 11–1). If the cause is unknown, the condition is referred to as *primary* or *idiopathic constipation* (Koch, 1995; Kumar et al., 1992; Shafik, 1993).

Primary or idiopathic constipation has been associated with immobility or decreased levels of physical activity, inadequate intake of fluids and dietary fiber, failure to respond to the urge to defecate, chronic use of stimulant laxatives, and increased serum progesterone levels in women (Koch, 1995). Studies are questioning the effects—if any—of dietary fiber, exercise, serum progesterone levels in women, and chronic use of laxatives on stool weight, colonic transit time, or colonic nerves. Studies comparing constipated subjects with healthy, age- and sex-matched controls, for example, have not demonstrated causal relationships (Cheskin & Schuster, 1994; Koch, 1995). Several studies on constipation and the elderly suggest that constipation is related to psychological distress and caloric intake, rather than to fiber and other dietary factors such as liquid intake. Some of these studies did show that nonconstipated subjects consume more fiber and/or fluids; however, these differences were not statistically significant (Sandler et al., 1990; Stewart et al., 1992; Towers et al., 1994; Whitehead et al., 1989).

Idiopathic constipation can be divided into two types, based on the underlying mechanism. The first type, colonic inertia or slow-transit constipation, develops from a diffuse motility disorder of the colon, in which either colon hyperactivity with back-and-forth movements of colonic contents or colon hypoactivity causes a slowed colonic transit. The second type of idiopathic constipation is caused by a rectal outlet disorder (anismus or spastic pelvic floor syndrome), in which the individual is not able to expel stool from the rectum because of paradoxical contractions of the pelvic floor (Koch, 1995; Kumar et al., 1992; Wald, 1993). The rectal outlet disorder may also be due to a hyperactive rectosigmoid junction or abnormal anorectal motility (Devroede, 1993).

Age-associated changes predispose older

TABLE 11-1
Causes of Constipation

Decreased physical activity
  Weakness
  Immobility
Inadequate intake of fluids and fiber
  Use of convenience foods, which are highly
    refined and low in fiber
  Poor dentition
  Blunted taste and smell
  Impaired thirst sensation
Poor toileting habits
  Voluntary suppression of the urge to
    defecate
  Not allowing adequate time
Psychological factors
  Anxiety
  Depression
  Stress
  Confusion
Environmental factors
  Unavailable or inaccessible toilet
  Lack of privacy
  Lack of uninterrupted time; being rushed
  Having to use bedpan or commode
  Dependence on others to meet toileting
    needs
Disorders
  Colorectal disorders
    Hemorrhoids
    Anal fissures
    Colitis
    Obstructions due to
      ischemia, tumors, diverticulitis, polyps,
      or strictures

Disorders *Continued*
  Neuromuscular disorders—generalized muscle
    weakness or incoordination
  Parkinson's disease
  Dementia
  Stroke
  Multiple sclerosis
  Spinal cord abnormalities
  Stretch injury to pudendal nerve
  Endocrine or metabolic disorders
  Diabetes
  Hypokalemia
  Hypercalcemia
  Hypothyroidism
  Hyperparathyroidism
Medications
  Chronic use of laxatives and enemas
  Anticholinergics
    Antidepressants (e.g., tricyclics, monoamine
      oxidase inhibitors)
    Antiparkinsonian drugs
    Antiarrhythmics, antihypertensives (e.g.,
      calcium channel blockers, diuretics)
    Antipsychotics (e.g., phenothiazines)
    Antispasmodics
    Antihistamines
  Antacids (e.g., aluminum, calcium)
  Analgesics, narcotics
  Iron, bismuth
  Nonsteroidal antiinflammatory drugs

Data from Brocklehurst (1992); Castle (1989); Cheskin & Schuster (1994); Devroede (1993); Kane et al. (1994); and Wald (1995).

people to problems with elimination. An age-related decline in inhibitory nerve-mediated response can decrease the relaxation of the colonic circular muscle, leading to segmental motor incoordination and functional partial obstruction of the colon (Koch, 1995). Weakened abdominal muscles make it difficult to apply adequate pressure during defecation. Reduced internal sphincter tone with impaired rectal sensation can also place the elderly at risk for constipation (Brocklehurst, 1992; Harari et al., 1993). Less active elderly people have decreased intestinal motility, which causes a delayed transit time. Other factors contributing to the development of constipation include (1) diet alterations caused by poor dentition and changes in smell and taste, (2) inadequate fluid intake related to decreased feelings of thirst, (3) the use of easily prepared foods that are highly refined and low in fiber, and (4) anorexia. Psychological factors such as anxiety, stress, and depression, which can accompany the many personal losses encountered by older people, may also affect nutritional intake (Resnick, 1985).

Assessment of Constipation

The assessment of constipation includes a patient history, a physical examination, and a bowel record (Table 11–2). The history includes

TABLE 11-2

Assessment of Constipation

Bowel History and Associated Symptoms

Characteristics of bowel function
   Frequency of defecation
   Stool consistency and color
   Straining, pain with defecation, sensation of incomplete
     evacuation
   Incontinence
     Fecal soiling
     Incontinence of feces and urine
   Onset and duration of constipation
   Other symptoms: Headache, foul breath, furred tongue,
     fatigue, irritability, insomnia
Medications, including laxative use
Dietary pattern
   Adequacy of fiber and fluid intake
   Recent changes in dietary patterns
   Meal pattern and food preferences
Activity pattern
Emotional state

Physical Examination

Palpation of thyroid gland
Abdominal examination
   Bowel sounds
   Distended abdomen
   Abdominal tenderness or pain
   Mass
Rectal examination
   Cutaneous sensation
   Perineal descent
   Internal and external sphincter tone
   Anal fissures or hemorrhoids
   Mass

Laboratory and Other Tests

Serum potassium, calcium, glucose
Creatinine and thyrotropin levels
Urine culture
Stool for occult blood
Abdominal x-ray
Flexible proctosigmoidoscopy
Barium enema
Specialized studies
   Colonic transit study
   Anorectal manometry
   Anorectal electromyography
   Defecography

Data from Cheskin & Schuster (1994); Devroede (1993); Koch (1995); and Wald (1995).

pation should be noted. The onset, nature, duration, and severity of constipation should be determined. Most elderly people report having been constipated for years. A fairly sudden alteration in bowel function is usually caused by an underlying disease (Cheskin & Schuster, 1994). The clinician should ascertain what strategies are used by the patient to manage the constipation. Relevant information is collected on past and present medical problems that could have influenced the development of constipation. A review of medications focuses on drugs known to cause constipation. A careful diet history is obtained and analyzed for adequacy of fiber and fluid intake. Information on food preferences, meal patterns, and any recent changes in dietary pattern should be obtained. Activity patterns and recent changes in life should also be noted. The emotional state of the patient is evaluated to determine if stress or depression is a contributing factor (Wald, 1995).

The physical examination includes both abdominal and rectal examinations. When performing the abdominal examination, the clinician should check for the presence of any increased or absent bowel sounds, abdominal distention or tenderness, or palpable masses. Absent or increased bowel sounds are associated with bowel obstruction; tenderness may indicate diverticulosis; and a palpated mass in the descending colon may be feces. The presence of an enlarged liver could be suggestive of a neoplastic process. During the rectal examination, which is a critical part of the evaluation, the clinician should note the presence of any anal fissures, hemorrhoids, or impaction and should assess anal sphincter tone. The type of constipation may be determined by the amount and consistency of stool in the rectum. If stool is found in the rectal vault, this may indicate a failure of the defecation mechanism. The absence or presence of a small amount of stool is usually indicative of colonic atony (Cheskin & Schuster, 1994). A stool test for occult blood should be performed (Harari et al., 1993).

If simple causes for constipation cannot be determined or if the clinical evidence (e.g., recent severe weight loss) is suggestive of a pathological process, the patient should be re-

the patient's definition of constipation along with his or her characterization of normal bowel function and associated symptoms. Other symptoms that often accompany consti-

ferred for further medical evaluation (Wald, 1990). This evaluation may incorporate additional tests, such as a complete blood count and electrolyte determination, abdominal x-ray studies, a barium enema, and a proctoscopy or colonoscopy examination. For patients with infrequent defecation, colonic transit and motility tests may be indicated, and for patients with possible functional anorectal abnormalities, an anorectal manometry may be performed (see Table 11–2) (Cheskin & Schuster, 1994; Devroede, 1993).

Management of Constipation

The major points in the prevention and treatment of constipation are summarized using the letters F-E-C-E-S (adapted from Rousseau, 1988a).

F—Fluid and fiber intake
E—Education on normal bowel function and good bowel habits
   Exercise and activity program
   Environmental factors reviewed
C—Cathartics discontinued; used only if necessary and on a temporary basis
   Creation of individualized bowel program
   Consistent, routine toileting schedule
E—Elimination of causative factors
   Elimination of constipating medications
   Evaluation of efficacy and effectiveness of measures taken
S—Stimulation of gastrocolic reflex
   Stabilization with a good bowel program

A phase-in management approach to constipation begins with treating any underlying disease. If no specific cause is identified, attention should be given to preventing its recurrence by modifying or eliminating the factors that place the older person at risk for constipation (Castle, 1989; Cheskin & Schuster, 1994) (Table 11–3). Treatment goals include the following (Wald, 1993):

1. The older person will pass a soft, formed stool without difficulty

2. The range of frequency will be three

TABLE 11-3
Management of Constipation

Acute Constipation

Determine underlying cause and initiate appropriate treatment
Nonpharmacological approach
   Education about normal bowel habits
   Toileting timed with gastrocolic reflex
   Dietary adjustment to include adequate fluids and fiber in diet
   Regular exercise
Pharmaceutical preparations to rapidly reduce symptoms—use one of the following:
   Enema—tap water, saline, or small bulk sodium phosphate and biphosphate enema
   Polyethylene glycol electrolyte solution (GoLYTELY)
   Short course of stimulant laxative

Chronic Constipation

Determine underlying cause and initiate appropriate treatment
Nonpharmacological approach (same as shown previously for acute constipation)
If nonpharmacological approach is ineffective, introduce pharmaceutical preparations
Mildest oral preparation at the lowest effective dose
   Bulk-forming agents
   Hyperosmotic laxatives if bulk-forming agents are ineffective or poorly tolerated
   Irritant or stimulant laxatives as required
Suppositories and enemas if previous measures are not successful
   Glycerin suppository
   Tap water, saline, or small bulk enemas

Data from Castle (1989); Cheskin & Schuster (1994); Kot & Pettit-Young (1992); McEvoy (1998); Rousseau (1988a); and Wald (1993).

movements per day to one movement every 3 to 5 days

3. Complications such as abdominal distention, fecal impaction, idiopathic megacolon, and stercoral ulceration will be prevented

NONPHARMACOLOGICAL MEASURES

Nonpharmacological interventions, the first step and mainstay of treatment, include (1) education about normal bowel habits; (2) toileting with emphasis on comfort, privacy, and timing to take advantage of the gastrocolic reflex; and (3) ensuring regular exercise as well as adequate fluids and fiber in the diet (Harari et al., 1993). The gastrocolic response can be initiated by drinking warm fluids or eating a warm meal in the morning (Koch, 1995; Williams & DiPalma, 1990). Fruit juices, especially orange, lemon, and prune juice, can be included in the diet to keep the stool soft (Cannon, 1981; Stryker, 1977).

A high-fiber diet enlarges and softens the stools, distends the rectum, and elicits the urge to defecate (Koch, 1995). Foods high in dietary fiber include whole-grain cereals and breads and, to a lesser degree, fresh fruit, green vegetables, and nuts (Williams, 1992). Fiber should be introduced into the diet slowly to prevent flatulence and abdominal cramping. Initially, small amounts of whole-grain bread and cereal, such as 1 teaspoon of flaked bran or one high-fiber cracker (e.g., Wasa), can be added to the diet. The amount of cooked fruits and vegetables can be increased before raw fruits and vegetables are added to the diet (Robinson et al., 1986; Williams, 1992; Winograd & Jarvik, 1986).

Bran has been promoted as an effective alternative or complement to laxatives in treating constipation. Several bowel program studies have reported success in decreasing constipation and maintaining bowel function with the use of bran in the diet (Battle & Hanna, 1980; Behm, 1985; Miller, 1985; Pattee & West, 1988; Resnick, 1985). The usefulness of bran as a treatment for constipation is limited, however, because it is difficult to administer in a palatable manner (Sandman et al., 1983). Ways to make bran more acceptable include adding it to bread, meatloaf, casserole, applesauce, juices, and other foods (Hogstel & Nelson, 1992; Miller, 1985). Caution should be used in giving bran to constipated, bedfast patients, as adding bulk to the distended colon may worsen the constipation (Rousseau, 1988a).

The full effect of adding fiber to the diet may not be evident for 4 to 5 days, and a trial period of 4 to 6 weeks should be allowed (Bliss & Murray, 1991). Fiber is contraindicated in patients with obstructive lesions, megacolon or megarectum disorders, or neurogenic constipation. These patients should be treated by reducing colonic contents and with periodic timed evacuations (Cheskin & Schuster, 1994; Wald, 1993).

In some older patients, fluid and dietary adjustments may be sufficient changes to achieve good elimination. A nutritionist or dietitian may be consulted to evaluate the diet and provide suggestions for improvement. Recommendations will have a greater chance of acceptance if the older person's food preferences, cultural beliefs, lifestyle, and economic resources are taken into consideration.

PHARMACOLOGICAL MEASURES

If the previous measures are insufficient treatment for constipation, pharmacological therapy can be instituted along with the continuation of nonpharmacological interventions.

Laxatives. Laxatives are often self-prescribed and overused by older adults living in the community. They are also one of the most frequently prescribed medications in hospitals and long-term care facilities. At least one type of laxative is prescribed for 76% of hospitalized elderly patients and 74% of nursing home residents (Harari et al., 1993). Laxatives should be used infrequently, and their use should be viewed as temporary. When laxatives are indicated to achieve stool consistency or to establish a schedule, the mildest oral laxative is the best choice for treatment. The lowest effective dose is given for a duration not to exceed 1 week (Alterescu, 1986; McEvoy, 1998; Moriarity & Irving, 1992).

The laxative used is determined by the type of elimination problem that is present. Bulk-forming laxatives, for example, are indicated for the initial treatment of simple constipation in active, ambulatory older people. Irritant laxatives are indicated in people with severe abdominal and perineal muscle weakness, loss of rectal reflex, or severe constipation. They may also be used when the use of a constipating medication is required (Castle, 1989). Stool softeners are often prescribed to prophylactically treat constipation in institutionalized elderly people. However, their effectiveness in preventing and treating constipation is unclear, and there is little evidence to support their routine use (Castle et al., 1991; Harari et al., 1993).

The time for administering laxatives is determined by the time planned for the evacuation. If a bowel movement is planned in the morning, the laxative should be given in the evening, and if the bowel movement is planned for the evening, the laxative should be taken in the morning (McEvoy, 1998). If laxatives are used for 1 week or less at the appropriate dosages, the incidence of adverse side effects, such as diarrhea and fluid and electrolyte depletion, is rare. See Table 11–4 for a summary of oral laxative preparations and their actions, doses, precautions, and side effects.

Initial pharmacological interventions begin with bulk agents. Caution should be used with fiber supplements, however. If there is any impaction, the impaction must be removed before introducing additional fiber to the diet. As mentioned earlier, the efficacy of stool softeners in treating constipation is controversial. They may be helpful when used for a short period in patients with excessive straining during defecation; however, they are of questionable value for the long-term treatment of chronic constipation.

Saline laxatives containing salts of magnesium and sodium are the most favored and commonly prescribed laxatives for hospitalized elderly people. Osmotic agents such as magnesium salts increase the water content of fecal material. The laxatives have a rapid onset of action: 1 to 3 hours after administration. However, a more gradual means for catharsis is recommended to restore regular bowel habits (Harari et al., 1993). Saline laxatives containing magnesium should be avoided in older people with renal impairment because of the danger of magnesium toxicity (Tedesco & DiPiro, 1985).

Hyperosmolar agents, such as lactulose and sorbitol, are effective for the long-term treatment of constipation if fiber supplements are ineffective or poorly tolerated or if patients have decreased renal function (Harari et al., 1993; Koch, 1995; Lederle et al., 1990; Wald, 1993). They are indicated for treating chronic constipation and are used to prevent fecal impaction in bedridden or institutionalized people taking bulk-forming agents (Castle, 1989; Donatelle, 1990). Compared with lactulose, sorbitol 70% is less expensive and equally effective and is associated with fewer uncomfort-

able side effects (Harari et al., 1993; Koch, 1995). Polyethylene glycol solutions (Golytely) at doses of 225 to 450 g (8–16 oz.) daily have been found effective in treating chronic constipation (Andorsky & Goldner, 1990). For refractory, constipated elderly people, hyperosmotic agents should be used with a local agent such as glycerin suppositories. Blood glucose levels should be monitored in diabetic patients taking hyperosmolar agents.

Irritant or stimulant laxatives are added to the treatment program if other measures have been ineffective. Stimulant laxatives such as phenolphthalein and bisacodyl are not recommended for use over an extended period, as increased doses are required to produce the desired results (Koch, 1995). In addition, the long-term use of these stimulant preparations leads to abdominal cramps, fluid and electrolyte disturbances, malabsorption, and cathartic colon (Harari et al., 1993). Phenolphthalein has been found to be potentially carcinogenic and unsafe for self-medication and chronic use (Artymowicz et al., 1997; Dunnick & Hailey, 1996; McEvoy, 1998).

Suppositories and Enemas. These treatments are indicated when oral preparations are ineffective and there is difficulty expelling soft stool (Donatelle, 1990). Suppositories initiate the reflexes that stimulate peristalsis of the lower colon and rectum, resulting in relaxation of the external anal sphincter. They are helpful during the initial phase of a bowel management program and should be stopped once a regular pattern has been established. Most suppositories work in 30 minutes and should be inserted 30 minutes before results are desired. Proper insertion is important if the suppository is to be effective: Suppositories should be inserted beyond the internal and external sphincters and placed against the rectal wall. They are ineffective if inserted into the fecal mass (Basch & Jensen, 1991).

Enemas are indicated when several days have passed since the last bowel movement or when there is an impaction. A small amount of tap water (2 to 3 ounces given with a rubber syringe) is often enough to promote a bowel response. If the stool is firm, sodium phosphate and biphosphate or an oil-retention enema should be administered. In patients who lack

TABLE 11-4

Laxatives

Type	Action	Preparation	Dose	Precautions/Side Effects
Bulk	Absorbs water to form gelatin-like mass in the intestine, which distends the colon Distention serves as a stimulus for intestinal activity Onset of action: usually within 12–24 hr; full effect may take 2–3 d	Dietary bran Psyllium (Metamucil) Methylcellulose (Citrucel)	10–20 g/d 3.4 g or 1 tsp, 1–3 times/d 2 g or 1 tbsp, 1–3 times/d	Flatulence and bloating may be experienced in first few days of treatment Can harden stools and lead to intestinal obstruction Should not be used in patients with swallowing difficulty Should be mixed with 240 mL of fluid, followed by drinking an additional 240 mL of fluid
Stool softener	Lowers surface tension; permits water and lipids to penetrate fecal material Softens stool to make passage easier Laxative action is thought to result from stimulation of electrolyte and water secretion in the colon Onset of action: 24–72 hr	Docusate salts Docusate calcium (Surfak) Docusate potassium (Diocto-K) Docusate sodium (Colace)	15–360 mg at bedtime	Dosage varies widely; doses should only be large enough to produce softening of the stools May enhance absorption of coadministered drugs Action enhanced if used with mineral oil; combination should be used only for severe cases; should not be used for prolonged periods Ensure adequate fluid intake
Lubricant	Retards absorption of water in intestines Lubricates fecal matter and intestinal mucosa Minimizes discomfort or effort to defecate Onset of action: 6–8 hr	Mineral oil	15–45 mL	Risk of aspiration in debilitated patients, especially those with impaired gag reflex Chronic usage may cause malabsorption of fat-soluble vitamins Avoid routine, regular use

Table continued on following page

245

TABLE 11-4 *Continued*

Laxatives

Type	Action	Preparation	Dose	Precautions/Side Effects
Saline	Exact mechanism not clear; current thought, although unproved, is that nonabsorbable salts hold sufficient water in the small intestine to maintain isotonic concentration Increased volume of intestinal contents indirectly stimulates stretch receptors and increases peristalsis Onset of action: 1–3 hr	Magnesium citrate Magnesium hydroxide (Milk of magnesia) Magnesium sulfate Sodium phosphate Dibasic Monobasic	11–25 g 2.4–4.8 g 30–60 mL 10–30 g 3.42–7.56 g 9.1–20.2 g	Produces a semifluid or watery stool; may cause electrolyte imbalance, abdominal cramps, dehydration Minimum effective dose of magnesium preparations is 80 mEq of magnesium Hypermagnesemia may occur in people with decreased renal function
Hyperosmotic	Draw water from tissues into feces by exerting a hygroscopic and/or local irritating action	Sorbitol	15–30 mL of 70% solution	High oral doses required for laxative action
	Breakdown of synthetic sugar in colon; produces lactic and pyruvic acids, which stimulate colonic secretions and motility; osmotic effect of organic acid metabolites results in increased water content and softening of stool Onset of action: 24–48 hr	Lactulose (Chronulac)	15–30 mL, 1–2 times/d	Sweet taste of lactulose solution can be made more palatable by diluting with water or fruit juice Frequent problem with abdominal discomfort, gaseous distention, belching, and flatulence during first few days of treatment Diarrhea indicates a need for dose reduction Serum electrolytes should be checked if the older person uses drug for more than 6 months
	Onset of action: 1 hr	Polyethylene glycol (GoLYTELY)	240–480 mL	More potent; effective for bowel preparation and treatment of fecal impaction

	Mechanism of action	Examples	Dose	Comments
Irritant or stimulant	Alters fluid and electrolyte transport; results in fluid accumulation Some stimulate peristalsis Onset of action: 6–10 hr			Dose-dependent diarrhea and cramping Ensure adequate fluid intake Excessive purgation may result in dehydration and electrolyte disturbances Chronic use may lead to laxative dependence and loss of normal bowel function; years of abuse may cause cathartic colon with atony and dilation
1. Anthraquinone	Mild laxative (except aloe); 6–8 hr required for absorption and excretion Acts on colon to stimulate peristalsis	Cascara sagrada aromatic fluid extract Cascara tablet Senna Aloe	2–6 mL/d 0.3–1 g 0.5–2 g 120–250 mg	Discoloration of urine (pink to red or brown to black) may occur
2. Dehydrocholic acid	Mild laxative	Dehydrocholic acid (Decholin)	250–300 mg, 3 times/d	
3. Diphenylmethane	Powerful stimulant of large bowel Acts directly or reflexively; increases activity of small intestine Onset of action: 6–8 hr	Bisacodyl (Dulcolax) Phenolphthalein	5–15 mg at bedtime 30–270 mg	To prevent gastric irritation, enteric-coated tablets should be taken whole—not crushed or chewed—or taken within 1 h of taking antacids or milk Discoloration of urine (pink to red) may occur Considered a potential carcinogen Single dose may produce laxation for several days
4. Castor oil	Strong purgative; extent of gastrointestinal absorption unknown Onset of action: 2–6 hr	Castor oil	15 mL	High risk of malabsorption and dehydration Use should be reserved for total colonic evacuation Emulsion preparation should be shaken before administering Mix with 120–240 mL of fluid

Data from Castle (1989); Cheskin & Schuster (1994); Donatelle (1990); Harari et al. (1993); McEvoy (1998); Rousseau (1988a); and Wald (1995).

anal sphincter tone, backflow from an enema can be prevented by using a cone tip for colostomy irrigations or a baby bottle nipple fitted around the tip of the catheter (Basch & Jensen, 1991; Halpin, 1986).

Large-volume enemas should be avoided in bowel management programs, as total cleansing results in too little stool for defecation. Several days are then required for the accumulation of stool to stimulate elimination. For older patients, small-bulk enemas have been found to be as effective as large-volume enemas (Brocklehurst, 1992). Tap water and saline enemas can also be administered. It is recommended that no more than 1 pint of fluid be infused at a time (Rousseau, 1988a). Soapsud or large-volume enemas should not be used because they cause discomfort, electrolyte imbalances, and fluid shifts and may lead to shock and death (Resnick, 1985). Acute colitis is a serious adverse effect of soapsud enemas (Rousseau, 1988b).

Table 11–5 lists the suppository and enema preparations used to treat constipation, along with the action, dose, precautions, and side effects of each preparation.

DIARRHEA

Definition

Diarrhea is defined as an increase in daily stool weight of more than 200 g, an increase in frequency to more than three stools per day, and an increase in fluidity (Friedman & Isselbacher, 1994). Abnormal sensations such as urgency and pain often accompany the change in bowel pattern and consistency (Wald, 1995).

Scope of the Problem

Diarrhea poses a serious health problem for elderly people, as diarrheal diseases are associated with increased morbidity and mortality in this age group. Diarrhea is one of the most common sources of infections in nursing homes. Half of the deaths caused by diarrhea in the United States occur in people older than 74 years of age (Bennett & Greenough, 1994).

Although diarrhea is usually self-limiting, lasting 24 to 48 hours, the consequences in the elderly can be severe because significant fluid losses can occur in a relatively short period. Age-related changes affect the normal response mechanisms that compensate and correct fluid and electrolyte deficits. These changes include a decreased ability of the aging kidney to respond to disturbances in volume and a decreased function in the mechanism whereby hyperosmolarity caused by volume depletion leads to thirst. In addition, dementia and impaired mobility or communication may affect older people's ability to respond to thirst and to obtain fluids (Bennett & Greenough, 1994).

Delayed or inadequate treatment of diarrhea may result in intravascular depletion as well as electrolyte imbalance caused by a loss of water and salts. This result may lead to silent atherosclerosis, causing partial occlusion of blood vessels and hypoperfusion of vital organs. Congestive heart failure, mental status changes, or a worsening of renal failure may also occur (Bennett & Greenough, 1994).

Types and Causes of Diarrhea

Diarrhea is generally categorized as *acute*, with a duration of less than 2 to 3 weeks, or *chronic*, with a duration either greater than 3 weeks, whether constant or intermittent (Fine et al., 1993; Friedman & Isselbacher, 1994) (Table 11–6).

ACUTE DIARRHEA

Acute diarrheas are usually caused by infectious agents. The person presents with watery stool that may contain blood. If nausea and vomiting occur several hours after eating, food poisoning may be the cause. If there is high fever, bloody diarrhea, and abdominal pain, an invasive bacteria such as *Clostridium difficile,* *Salmonella,* or *Shigella* may be the underlying cause (Friedman & Isselbacher, 1994).

In older patients, acute diarrhea may also be caused by complications of medications, fecal impaction, and high-osmolarity supplemental feedings (Bennett & Greenough, 1994). Fecal impaction often presents as diarrhea with the

TABLE 11-5
Suppositories and Enemas

Type	Action	Preparation	Dose	Precautions/Side Effects
Lubricant	Lubricates fecal matter and intestinal mucosa	Mineral oil	120 mL/enema	Pruritus ani may result from leaking oil
Saline	Produces evacuation within 2–5 min	Sodium phosphate (Fleet enema) Dibasic Monobasic	6.84–7.56 g 18.24–20.16 g	Given as a single dose
Hyperosmotic	Reflexively stimulates emptying of rectum Local irritant Onset of action Suppository: 15–30 min Enema: 15–30 min	Sorbitol solution (25–30%) Glycerin	120 mL/enema 2–3 g suppository 5–15 mL/enema	Adverse effects are rare Glycerin may cause rectal discomfort, irritation, cramping, pain
Irritant or stimulant	Strong stimulant that acts on mucous membrane to stimulate reflexes resulting in peristalsis Onset of action: 15–60 min	Bisacodyl Dulcolax Fleet Bisacodyl Enema	10 mg/suppository 10 mg/30 mL solution	Proper administration is important; suppository should be inserted beyond the internal and external sphincters and placed sideways against the colon wall; contact with colon wall is critical Daily use may cause rectal burning

Data from Harari et al. (1993); McEvoy (1998); Rousseau (1988a); Shafik (1993); and Wald (1995).

TABLE 11-6

Types and Causes of Diarrhea

Type	Clinical Features	Examples of Conditions
Acute		
Fecal-oral transmission (water or food contamination)	Dehydration	Infectious agents
Person-to-person transmission (aerosolization, hands or surface contamination, sexual activity)	Protein-calorie malnutrition	*Clostridium difficile*
	Nausea, vomiting, abdominal pain, or fever, depending on cause	*Escherichia coli*
	Diarrhea—watery or bloody	*Salmonella*
		Adenovirus
		Astrovirus
		Norwalk agent
		Giardia
		Ingestion of drugs
		Chemotherapy
		Resumption of enteral feeding following a prolonged fast
		Fecal impaction
Chronic: Inflammatory or Exudative		
Inflammation and ulceration of the intestinal mucosa	Discharge of mucus, serum proteins, and blood into bowel lumen	Ulcerative colitis
Damaged epithelium	Increased fecal water and electrolyte excretion	Crohn's disease
Mucosal injury	Fever, abdominal pain, blood and/or leukocytes in stool	Radiation enterocolitis
		Shigella
		Salmonella
		Campylobacter
		Viral gastroenteritis
		Clostridium difficile
		Escherichia coli
		Infections associated with acquired immune deficiency syndrome
		Ischemia

Chronic: Osmotic or Malabsorptive

Mechanism	Clinical Manifestations	Causes
Poorly absorbed or nonabsorbable solute causing retention of fluid in intestinal lumen Reduced absorptive surface	Diarrhea stops when person fasts or does not ingest poorly absorbable solute Bulky, greasy, foul-smelling stools; weight loss Nutrient deficiencies Stool analysis reveals osmotic gap	Magnesium antacids and laxatives containing citrate Carbohydrate malabsorption (fructose, sorbitol) Pancreatic insufficiency Lactase deficiency Diffuse mucosal disease Extensive resection of intestine

Chronic: Secretory

Mechanism	Clinical Manifestations	Causes
Inhibition of sodium chloride absorption or stimulation of chloride secretion Bacterial enterotoxins Enteroviruses Dihydroxyl bile acids Fatty acids Laxatives Hormonally mediated Defective neural control	Dehydration Metabolic acidosis Diarrhea usually persists when person fasts; exception is when cause is fatty acid, malabsorption, or laxative Absent or small osmotic gap	Disease or resection of distal ileum Infection with bacterial enterotoxins Use or abuse of stimulant laxatives Bile acid or fatty acid malabsorption Idiopathic inflammatory bowel disease Hyperthyroidism Small intestinal lymphoma

Chronic: Motility Disturbance

Mechanism	Clinical Manifestations	Causes
Increased motility Decreased contact time of chyme with absorptive surfaces of the intestinal lumen Decreased rectal compliance	Exclude secretory and osmotic diarrhea Fecal electrolyte pattern resembles that of secretory diarrhea Alternating diarrhea and constipation	Chronic diarrheal diseases such as irritable bowel syndrome, malignant carcinoid syndrome, postvagotomy, postcholecystectomy, postgastrectomy diarrhea Diarrhea due to diabetic neuropathy, hyperthyroidism

Data from Ammon (1995); Bennett & Greenough (1994); Fine et al. (1993); Friedman & Isselbacher (1994); and Kowlessar (1995).

overflow of watery stool around the impacted mass (Cheskin & Schuster, 1994). Enteral feedings can cause diarrhea if they are administered to patients who are malnourished or who have received nothing by mouth. In these patients, edema of the gut wall and atrophy of the intestinal villi result in decreased absorptive surface and capacity (Basch & Jensen, 1991; Fine et al., 1993).

CHRONIC DIARRHEA

Chronic diarrhea is categorized as inflammatory or exudative diarrhea, osmotic or malabsorption diarrhea, secretory diarrhea, or diarrhea caused by a disturbance in intestinal motility (Friedman & Isselbacher, 1994).

Inflammatory diarrhea presents with fever, abdominal tenderness, and blood or leukocytes in the stool. Inflammatory lesions are evident on intestinal mucosal biopsy.

Osmotic diarrhea occurs with the ingestion of a poorly absorbed or nonabsorbable solute, which causes water influx into the intestinal lumen. It is characterized by an increase in stool volume. The diarrhea begins abruptly and stops when the person fasts or does not ingest the offending solute (Kowlessar, 1995).

Secretory diarrhea is caused by abnormal fluid and electrolyte transport, which results directly from the effect of an offending agent on the enterocyte or from the release of extracellular regulators of secretion (neurohumoral mechanisms, endocrine-paracine mediators, and mediators of immune or inflammatory responses). In patients with secretory diarrhea, there is a large output of watery stool. The diarrhea persists with fasting because the ingestion of food is not necessarily the cause of the abnormal fluid and electrolyte transport (Friedman & Isselbacher, 1994).

Disturbance in intestinal motility results from a decreased contact time of chyme with the absorptive surfaces of the intestinal lumen. With such an absorption problem in the small intestine, large amounts of fluids are delivered to the colon, which is unable to absorb the extra fluid, resulting in diarrhea. The diarrhea may alternate with constipation. Other signs and symptoms include abdominal pain, mucus

in the stool, and a sense of incomplete evacuation.

Assessment of Diarrhea

A summary of the clinical evaluation for diarrhea is provided in Table 11–7. Identifying volume depletion in the elderly person is critical. Signs that normally guide the clinician in evaluating younger patients are not helpful when evaluating volume depletion in older adults. Poor skin turgor and dry tongue, for example, are not good indicators because they are frequently seen in older adults. An orthostatic change in blood pressure is an important but late clinical indicator of volume depletion; it can indicate a loss of up to 6 to 10% of the extravascular volume, with the possibility of hypoperfusion of vital organs. A sudden loss of 5 to 10% of body weight signifies moderate to severe dehydration. Total plasma protein or plasma-specific gravity provides more helpful information on intravascular and extravascular fluid volume than do serum electrolyte levels (Ammon, 1995; Bennett & Greenough, 1994).

A thorough history, which is the most important diagnostic tool, helps determine the appropriate workup for a patient. When evaluating an older person with diarrhea, the clinician should consider intestinal obstruction, appendicitis, diverticulitis, and vascular insufficiency, as they are common in this age group (Bennett & Greenough, 1994).

Diarrhea may present with various signs and symptoms. Specific information should be obtained on the mode of onset, the duration, and the severity of symptoms. Acute diarrhea should be differentiated from chronic diarrhea. (Chronic diarrhea may have an acute onset.) The character of the stools and the location and quality of any accompanying pain may provide information about the site and cause of the diarrhea.

The physical examination includes an abdominal examination for masses, bruits, ascites, hepatosplenomegaly, and gaseous distention. A rectal examination is performed for the presence of a perianal fistula or abscess, reduced sphincter tone, or a rectal mass or impaction. In addition, the clinician should check

TABLE 11-7
Evaluation of Diarrhea

History

Characteristics of the diarrhea
  Onset, duration, frequency
  Character of stool—amount, color, odor, presence of
    blood, pus, mucus
  Location and quality of pain
Relevant medical history
  Past gastrointestinal surgery
  Radiation
  Gastrointestinal disorders
  Neurologic disorders
  Metabolic disorders
Medication review of drugs inducing diarrhea (including
    nonprescriptive drugs)
  Antacids, laxatives
  Antibiotics
  Colchicine
  Diuretics, antihypertensives
  Neuroleptics—lithium, fluoxetine (Prozac)
  Sorbitol-containing syrups
  Digitalis, quinidine
Diet history
  Food additives or supplements
  Food intolerances
Activity
  Social gatherings
  Recent travel abroad

Physical Examination

Abdominal
  Presence of mass, bruit, ascites
  Gaseous distention
Rectal
  Perianal fistula or abscess
  Reduced sphincter tone
Neurological
  Evidence of peripheral neuropathy

Laboratory and Other Tests (if indicated)

Spot stool test: White blood cells, occult blood, Sudan
  stain for fat, culture for enteric pathogens, ova, and
  parasites
Blood: Complete blood count, serum electrolytes
Radiographic studies: Small bowel studies, abdominal
  and pelvic sonograms
Special procedures: Sigmoidoscopy with biopsies,
  colonoscopy with biopsies

Data from Ammon (1995); Fine et al. (1993); Friedman &
Isselbacher (1994); and Kowlessar (1995).

for fever, edema, postural hypotension, signs of anemia, and lymphadenopathy. The diagnostic tests to be used should be determined from the history, the physical examination, and

an inspection of the stool specimen (Fine et al., 1993). If a patient presents with severe and bloody diarrhea, fever, systemic toxicity, and dehydration, a stool culture to identify an infectious agent is indicated (Friedman & Isselbacher, 1994).

Management of Diarrhea

The treatment of diarrhea is threefold: (1) correction of fluid and electrolyte deficits, (2) symptomatic therapy of diarrhea and associated symptoms, and (3) specific treatment aimed at the cause (Ammon, 1995).

CORRECTION OF FLUID AND ELECTROLYTE DEFICITS

Acute watery diarrhea is the most common type of diarrhea seen in the elderly. In most situations, it has a self-limiting course lasting 2 to 5 days. In the elderly, immediate attention must be given to correct fluid and electrolyte deficits before complications occur. Isotonic formulas and formulas containing bulk agents are recommended (Basch & Jensen, 1991; Bennett & Greenough, 1994).

Oral rehydration therapy (ORT) should be employed as soon as diarrhea is noted. Inexpensive and simple to administer, it is the treatment of choice for dehydration associated with diarrhea. An electrolyte solution can be made at home (Basch & Jensen, 1991), or one of several commercially prepared solutions can be used (Bennett & Greenough, 1994) (Table 11–8). The rate of replacement intake should equal the output through stool, urine, and insensible water losses (Ammon, 1995). If the loss is severe, the person should be offered sips of the ORT solution every 3 to 5 minutes to replace the fluid loss. Intravenous therapy is indicated when oral intake is not possible, owing to nausea and vomiting, or when there is profound dehydration, metabolic acidosis, or shock (Ammon, 1995).

During hydration, the older patient should be observed for signs indicating overhydration and cardiac failure, such as rales at the lung bases, jugular vein distention, and sacral or peripheral edema. Adequate treatment is indicated by urination occurring every 3 to 4 hours

TABLE 11-8
Oral Hydration Therapy

Homemade Electrolyte Solution*

1 tbsp salt
1 tbsp baking soda
1 tbsp corn syrup
1 can (6 oz) frozen orange juice concentrate

Add water to make one quart of liquid.

Replace fluid volume lost through diarrhea with equivalent volume of solution. If unable to estimate volume of fluid loss, replace with 8 oz of solution for every bowel movement.

Analysis of 6 Commercially Available Oral Rehydration Therapy Solutions and a Prepared Rice-Based Solution†

Oral Rehydration Therapy Solution	Na (mEq)	K (mEq)	Cl (mEq)	Base‡ (mEq)	Carbohydrate§ (g)	Calories (kcal)
ORS¶ (Jianas Bros.)	90	20	80	30	20	80
Pedialyte (Ross)	45	20	35	30	25	100
Pediatric Electrolyte (NutraMax Products)	45	20	35	30	25	100
ElderLyte (NutraMax Products)	45	20	35	30	25	100
Rehydralyte (Ross)	75	20	65	30	25	100
Infalyte (Mead Johnson)	50	25	45	34	30	126
Rice-based	90	20	80	30	80	320

*From Basch, A., & Jensen, L. (1991). Management of fecal incontinence. In D. B. Doughty (Ed.), *Urinary and fecal incontinence: Nursing management* (p. 246). St. Louis, MO: Mosby-Year Book. Copyright 1991 by Mosby-Year Book.

†From Bennett, R. G., & Greenough, W. B. (1994). Diarrhea. In W. R. Hazzard, E. L. Bierman, J. P. Blass et al. (Eds.), *Principles of geriatric medicine and gerontology* (p. 117). New York: McGraw-Hill. Reproduced with permission of The McGraw-Hill Companies.

‡ HCO_3 or citrate.

§ ORS, Pedialyte, Pediatric Electrolyte, ElderLyte, and Rehydralyte contain glucose. Infalyte contains rice syrup solids. Rice-based oral rehydration therapy can be made from precooked instant rice cereal (e.g., Gerber's Rice Cereal for Baby).

¶ This is the World Health Organization-UNICEF formula.

and a urine specific gravity of less than 1.015. More precise evaluation can be obtained through plasma specific gravity or plasma protein levels. In patients with a protracted illness, the daily measurement of body weight provides some information about hydration. In addition to ORT, continued and early feeding typically facilitates a less severe, shorter disease course, a more rapid recovery period, and fewer complications (Bennett & Greenough, 1994).

SYMPTOMATIC THERAPY

Dietary measures can be taken to improve stool consistency and reduce stool volume. Foods that absorb fluid from the stool include apple, banana, yogurt, cheese, rice, and some wheat products. Fatty foods are poorly digested in diarrheal conditions, whereas carbohydrate digestion and absorption are the least impaired (Basch & Jensen, 1991).

Antibiotic therapy is contraindicated in the elderly unless the pathogen has been identified and its antibiotic resistance pattern determined (Ammon, 1995; Bennett & Greenough, 1994). Antisecretory drugs are recommended to counteract the inflammation and concomitant loss of fluids through the secretion of prostaglandin and other substances. Although adsorbents and antimotility drugs may shorten the course of illness, they are not effective in preventing fluid loss. Anticholinergic drugs may be prescribed to relieve cramping. Opiates may help slow gastric transit; suppress gastric, pancreatic, and biliary secretions; and improve water and electrolyte absorption (Ammon, 1995). Anticholinergic drugs and opiates are contraindicated if an enteroinvasive organism is suspected, owing to the possibility of prolonging colonization or causing an ileus (Friedman & Isselbacher, 1994). In all cases of diarrhea in the elderly, Bennett and Greenough (1994) recommended an early use of ORT, administration of the antisecretory drug bismuth subsalicylate (Pepto-Bismol), and avoidance of all other antidiarrheal drugs. Drugs used primarily to treat diarrhea are listed in Table 11–9.

SPECIFIC TREATMENT

The treatment for diarrhea is determined by the underlying cause. For example, if diarrhea is caused by bacterial toxins, medications, or specific foods, the causative agent should be removed. Surgery may be indicated when there is intestinal obstruction, diverticulosis, or vascular insufficiency (Bennett & Greenough, 1994).

FECAL INCONTINENCE

Definition and Impact of the Problem

Fecal incontinence is the involuntary passage of stool, ranging from fecal soiling to complete emptying of the rectum (Schiller, 1993). It is a distressing problem for older people, who suffer indignity, rejection, shame, and embarrassment from soiling as well as discomfort from skin irritation. The increased burden for caregivers may lead to the elderly individual being placed in a nursing home (Noelker, 1987; Schiller, 1993). The costs to hospitals, nursing homes, and other healthcare centers are high in terms of expenses for supplies, laundry, and nursing time. Fecal incontinence can, for the most part, be prevented. If it does occur, it can be alleviated or controlled (Kane et al., 1994; Tobin & Brocklehurst, 1986).

Prevalence

Prevalence studies of fecal incontinence reveal that it occurs in 3 to 4% of community-dwelling elderly people (Barrett, 1992; Campbell et al., 1985; Schiller, 1993; Thomas et al., 1984), 10 to 25% of hospitalized older patients, and 32 to 62% of the elderly residents residing in nursing homes (Brocklehurst, 1992; Madoff et al., 1992; Wald, 1990). Fecal incontinence is usually associated with urinary incontinence (Barrett, 1992). The prevalence of double incontinence (fecal and urinary incontinence) is estimated to be 10 to 13% of noninstitutionalized elderly people (Thomas et al., 1984) and 20% of elderly people residing in institutions (Isaacs & Walkey, 1964). Fecal incontinence in older adults is often associated with cognitive impairments, impaired mobility, and fecal impaction (Brocklehurst, 1992; Schiller, 1993).

Mechanism of Continence

Fecal continence occurs through the functioning of the internal and external sphincter and the puborectalis and levator ani muscles in combination with nervous system control. Although the act of defecation is a reflex activity independent of the central nervous system, the desire to defecate and the ability to inhibit defecation are under voluntary control through a center in the medulla.

Fecal continence is dependent on four factors: (1) rectal sensation—the ability to perceive rectal distention and to distinguish the nature of rectal contents (gas, liquid, or solid), (2) an ability to contract the external anal sphincter and puborectalis muscle to control the timing of defecation, (3) motivation to make the appropriate response, and (4) an ability of the rectum and distal colon to serve as a reservoir for feces through adaptive compliance and accommodation (Wald, 1990). Age-related changes that may increase the susceptibility of older people to incontinence include decreased resting and sphincter pressures; decreased rectal volumes required to inhibit anal sphincter tone; and a less compliant rectum (Bannister et al., 1987; Schiller, 1993). The majority of fecal incontinence cases in the elderly are caused by

TABLE 11-9
Drugs to Treat Diarrhea

Action	Preparation/Dose	Precautions/Side Effects
Bismuth Subsalicylate		
Antisecretory Coating and astringent effect	30 mL every 1 hr up to 8 doses, then 30–60 mL, 4 times/d	Few side effects Increased risk of salicylate toxicity with decreased renal function
Opium Preparations		
Delays gastrointestinal transit Suppresses gastric, pancreatic, and biliary secretion Stimulates water and electrolyte absorption Reduces stool volume and frequency	Paregoric: 5–10 mL, 1 to 4 times/d Opium tincture: 0.6 mL, 4 times/d Codeine phosphate: 15–60 mg every 6 hr	For all types of chronic diarrhea Contraindicated in acute infectious diarrhea; increases contact time between bacteria and mucosal wall Opium tincture contains 25 times more morphine than does paregoric Depressive effect Dose-related abdominal cramps, ileus Addictive potential with prolonged use Prescribe at specified intervals rather than per loose bowel movement to avoid overdosing Opiate withdrawal symptoms
Diphenoxylate Hydrochloride		
Acts on smooth muscle of intestinal tract Inhibits gastrointestinal motility and propulsion Onset of action: 45–60 min Duration of action: 3–4 hr	Diphenoxylate hydrochloride and atropine sulfate (Lomotil): 5 mg 4 times/d	Action similar to opioids Not for use in diarrhea caused by poisoning and infections Cautions applicable to atropine should be observed in commercially available preparations Contraindicated in liver disease and glaucoma Withdrawal and addictive potential with high dosage and prolonged use
Loperamide Hydrochloride		
Acts on nerve endings and/or intramural ganglia of the intestinal wall Slows intestinal motility Prolongs intestinal transit time, resulting in reduced fecal volume, increased fecal viscosity and bulk density, and decreased loss of fluid and electrolytes	Loperamide hydrochloride (Imodium): 2–4 mg every day or twice/d	Should not be used for infectious, acute diarrhea Monitor for central nervous system toxicity in patients with hepatic dysfunction

Data from Altman (1995); Ammon (1995); Basch & Jensen (1991); Friedman & Isselbacher (1994); Kowlessar (1995); and McEvoy (1998).

marked changes in fecal contents or by alterations in the sphincter mechanism or in cognitive function (Wald, 1993).

Causes of Fecal Incontinence

Causes of fecal incontinence include (1) fecal impaction, (2) gastrointestinal disorders, (3) neurological disorders, and (4) iatrogenic causes (Brocklehurst, 1992; Kane et al., 1994) (Table 11–10). The most common cause in the elderly is fecal stasis and impaction, which often results from chronic constipation (Brocklehurst, 1992). These individuals usually present with continuous incontinence and loose stools. The loose stool that leaks around the impaction is caused by mucus and fluid being produced from the irritation of hard stool on the rectum (Read & Abouzekry, 1986). In addition to the

---

TABLE 11–10
Causes of Fecal Incontinence

Fecal impaction
  Chronic constipation
    Decreased dietary fiber and fluids
    Decreased exercise
    Immobility

Gastrointestinal disorders
  Diarrhea
  Diverticulitis
  Infections
  Ulcerative colitis
  Crohn's disease
  Short-gut syndrome
  Proctitis
  Rectal prolapse
  Postoperative complications
  Tumors of colon or rectum
  Radiation enteritis

Neurological disorders
  Dementia
  Multiple sclerosis
  Autonomic neuropathy (e.g., diabetes mellitus)
  Inefficient local inhibitory reflexes
  Spinal cord injury
  Cerebrovascular accident

Environmental and iatrogenic causes
  Chronic laxative or enema use
  Drug-induced
  Changes and barriers in the environment

---

paradoxical watery diarrhea, other symptoms of fecal impaction include anorexia, nausea, vomiting, and abdominal distention and pain. The consistency of stool may range from soft to hard and from a single mass to multiple pellets (Koch, 1995; Wrenn 1989). Although impaction can occur anywhere in the colon, the majority of fecal impactions occur in the rectal vault and can be easily diagnosed by digital examination. However, in a study by Smith and Lewis (1990), 30% of the subjects with an empty rectum had a large amount of feces in the rectosigmoid area. If fecal impaction is suspected, an x-ray film of the abdomen should be obtained (Koch, 1995; Wrenn, 1989).

Gastrointestinal disorders that cause diarrhea can contribute to the development of incontinence, particularly in patients with reduced mobility, rectal sensory impairment, or internal and external sphincter weakness (Barrett, 1992). Diarrhea can result from acute bowel infections, irritable bowel syndrome, and nonspecific inflammatory bowel conditions.

Neurological causes for fecal incontinence can be local or central in origin. Central causes are more common in the elderly and are related to a loss of inhibition of the defecation reflex, which occurs in patients with severe cognitive impairments (Brocklehurst, 1992). These patients typically pass a formed stool into their bed or clothing once or twice daily, usually when the gastrocolic reflex is stimulated following the intake of food. This type of incontinence can be more successfully managed than other types. Fecal incontinence can also occur in patients with inefficient local inhibitory reflexes that make it difficult to constrict the sphincter adequately. Long-term laxative abuse, which can damage the colonic mesenteric plexus, is a major contributing factor.

Iatrogenic causes for fecal incontinence are related to an excessive use of enemas or drugs known to produce diarrhea or constipation. Sedatives, hypnotics, narcotics, and muscle relaxants decrease an older person's awareness of the urge to defecate and ability to get to the toilet on time. An illness or an admission to a hospital or nursing home can disrupt an older person's usual level of exercise and activity, owing to bedrest or immobility, and can also cause a decrease in dietary and fluid intake and a change in the usual manner and time of toileting.

Assessment of Fecal Incontinence

Fecal incontinence tends to be underreported and accepted as a way of life for elderly patients (Leigh & Turnberg, 1982). Unless a direct question is asked regarding incontinence, patients may not volunteer information that they have this problem. For this reason, clinicians should include specific questions related to bowel function when assessing older adults, such as "Do you ever notice any staining or soiling on your underpants (undershorts)?" or "Do you ever have a bowel movement before you are able to get to a toilet?"

Assessment of the patient with fecal incontinence involves a careful history to identify possible contributing causes, a physical examination, a bowel record, and a functional assessment. The prognosis for patients with double incontinence of long duration is worse than for patients with a recent onset of fecal incontinence associated with drug use or gastrointestinal symptoms such as diarrhea, abdominal colic, and tenesmus. Table 11–11 summarizes key aspects used in the evaluation of fecal incontinence.

HISTORY

The patient history includes a characterization of the incontinence, such as its onset, duration, frequency, timing, amount, and consistency, and associated symptoms, such as urgency, lack of warning, presence of blood, diarrhea, constipation, and straining to defecate. The clinician should gather information on the patient's normal bowel patterns and laxative use prior to the incontinence as well as relevant information on anorectal surgery or trauma, neurological disease, multiple childbirths, inflammatory bowel disease, and past pelvic radiation or trauma. The clinician should conduct a medication review, focusing on the identification of drugs known to induce constipation or diarrhea; a diet history, with particular attention given to adequacy of fiber and

fluids; and an activity history. The patient's environment should be assessed for access to toileting facilities and the availability of caregivers to assist in toileting. Any difficulty the patient experiences with clothing fastenings should be noted. The patient's motivation to be continent and the attitudes of the caregiver, if present, are also important considerations in determining the management of incontinence.

PHYSICAL EXAMINATION

This includes abdominal palpation to determine the presence of feces and a rectal examination to detect hemorrhoids or painful fissures, rectal prolapse, prostatic enlargement, fecal impaction or a rectal mass, anal deformity or disease, or anal gaping. Anal gaping, or the failure of the anal canal to contract after digital examination, indicates sphincter damage. In general, an estimation of anal sphincter tone and strength on digital examination correlates poorly with objective tests (Schiller, 1993). Any excoriation of the perineum should be noted. Abnormal sphincter tone, rectal prolapse, or significant pelvic prolapse warrant further evaluation.

The clinician should conduct a mental status examination along with an exploration of the patient's awareness of the problem and motivation to become continent. Patients with severe dementia most likely have concomitant urinary incontinence and no awareness of either problem. A neurological examination to screen for underlying contributory neuropathies or an absent bulbocavernous reflex should also be completed. Mobility status and the ability to toilet oneself should be determined.

BOWEL RECORD

Figure 11–1 is an example of a bowel record, which helps clinicians assess stool characteristics in relationship to variables known to influence bowel patterns. Data obtained from the bowel record are helpful in characterizing the pattern and frequency of incontinence and the relationships among fluid and food intake, activity patterns, laxative use, and the timing of

TABLE 11-11
Evaluation of Fecal Incontinence

History	**Environmental characteristics**
	Accessible bathrooms
Characteristics of the incontinence	Use of bedside commode
Onset, duration, frequency	Restrictive clothing
Stool consistency (loose, formed, hard) and	Availability of caregivers
amount	
Timing (diurnal or nocturnal, or both; associated	**Physical Examination**
with meals)	
Associated symptoms (urgency, lack of warning,	Abdominal examination
alternating bouts of diarrhea and constipation,	Presence of masses
straining to defecate, blood in stool)	Neurological examination
Normal bowel patterns (daily pattern, habits	Mental status
associated with defecation)	Evidence of peripheral neuropathies
Laxative (cathartics, suppositories) and enema	Rectal examination
use	Condition of perineum (excoriation)
Relevant medical history	Anorectal conditions (fissures, hemorrhoids,
Past surgery (anorectal, intestinal, laminectomy)	prolapse, anal deformity)
Past childbirths (number, traumatic delivery)	Presence of anal gaping
Past pelvic trauma or radiation	External anal sphincter tone and voluntary
Gastrointestinal disorders (bowel infection,	contraction
irritable bowel syndrome, diverticulitis,	Fecal mass or impaction
ulcerative colitis, Crohn's disease, carcinoma,	Prostatic enlargement
anorectal conditions)	Bulbocavernous reflex
Neurologic disorders (dementia, stroke, brain	Stool occult blood
tumor, multiple sclerosis)	
Metabolic disorders (diabetes mellitus)	**Functional Assessment**
Concomitant urinary incontinence	
Medication review (including nonprescription	Mobility status; ability to toilet self
drugs)	
Drugs inducing constipation	**Bowel Record**
Drugs inducing diarrhea	
Diet history	Keep 1 week
Adequacy of fiber intake	**Laboratory and Other Tests (if indicated)**
Adequacy of fluid intake	
Activity patterns	Stool culture
Active versus inactive	Abdominal x-ray
Patient's or caregiver's perceptions	Barium enema
Perception of cause and severity	Proctoscopy/sigmoidoscopy
Interference with daily activities	Anoscopy
Motivation for continence	Anorectal ultrasound
Burden on caregiver	Anorectal manometry/electromyography
	Defecography

Data from Basch & Jensen (1991); and Schiller (1993).

bowel movements. This record helps determine the appropriate management approach.

LABORATORY AND OTHER TESTS

If the incontinence is of sudden onset and short duration and is associated with diarrhea, laboratory investigations may include tests for occult blood in the feces and a stool culture. Other tests might be indicated to rule out causes of contributory diarrhea or constipation.

If indicated, patients may be referred for further medical evaluation, including radiographic studies of the abdomen and lower gastrointestinal tract, defecography, anorectal manometry, anal electromyography, and sigmoidoscopy.

Management of Fecal Incontinence

As common and familiar as the fecal incontinence problem is, ignorance, negative atti-

DATE: _____

| TIME | BOWEL | | STOOL CONSISTENCY (Hard, Soft, Fluid) & Amount (Large, Small) | USE OF SUPPOSITORY (Number) or ENEMA | URINE | | FLUID INTAKE | FOOD INTAKE (Poor, Fair, Good) | PHYSICAL ACTIVITY (None, Poor, Fair, Good) |
	Incontinent	Normal			Incontinent	Normal			
12–1 AM									
1–2 AM									
2–3 AM									
3–4 AM									
4–5 AM								Breakfast	
5–6 AM									
6–7 AM									
7–8 AM									
8–9 AM									
9–10 AM									
10–11 AM								Lunch	
11–12 AM									
12–1 PM									
1–2 PM									
2–3 PM									
3–4 PM								Dinner	
4–5 PM									
5–6 PM									
6–7 PM									
7–8 PM									
8–9 PM									
9–10 PM									
10–11 PM									
11–12 PM									

FIGURE 11–1. Bowel record.

tudes, confusion, and treatment inconsistencies are associated with this condition in the clinical setting (Davis et al., 1986). Advanced practice nurses are often called on as consultants to assist in the management of fecal incontinence.

The treatment of fecal incontinence begins with a careful assessment of the condition. Once the cause has been determined and other contributing factors identified, a management plan can be developed and implemented. The goal of the treatment program is to assist older people in achieving fecal continence. If this is not possible, the goal should be to manage the problem so the person will have predictable, planned eliminations. The likelihood of success for any treatment program is increased when the patient's personal needs, lifestyle, finances, resources, and environment are considered (Alterescu, 1986).

Careful documentation in the patient's chart or bowel record is essential. Key information to record for a bowel program includes (1) medications, equipment, and techniques used and their results; (2) the consistency and amount of stool; (3) the time of elimination; and (4) incontinent episodes. Evaluation is based on the results, and changes in the plan are made accordingly. A plan should be tried for a week before any changes are made, and only one aspect of the program should be changed at a time (Alterescu, 1986; Kubalanza-Sipp & French, 1990). Any problems that arise, such as diarrhea or constipation, should be addressed immediately.

SUPPORTIVE MANAGEMENT

Absorbent products and fecal containment devices are available for stool containment in patients with transient incontinence caused by severe diarrhea, intractable fecal incontinence, prolonged immobility, or altered levels of consciousness. Fecal containment devices include both external collection devices and internal drainage systems. External devices consist of a drainable pouch attached to a synthetic adhesive skin barrier constructed to conform to the perianal area and buttocks. Guidelines for applying an external device include shaving perianal hair, applying a skin barrier paste to the gluteal fold, using a contact skin adhesive, and using two people to apply the device (one person supports the patient's buttocks and the other person applies the pouch) (Basch & Jensen, 1991). An internal drainage system is used whenever there is extensive skin breakdown or lack of adherence of an external device. The system involves the use of a large-bore catheter (e.g., size 30 French) that is connected to a bedside drainage bag. Because of safety concerns, internal drainage systems are recommended for short-term use only and are contraindicated in patients with rectal disease or who are immunocompromised (Basch & Jensen, 1991). Deodorants are available to help with odor control. The National Association for Continence (P.O. Box 544, Union, SC, 29379; telephone 803-585-8789) publishes an annual resource guide of continence products, which is helpful in selecting an appropriate product.

The remainder of this section describes the treatment for each type of incontinence. A summary of treatment approaches is presented in Table 11–12.

FECAL IMPACTION

Older people with fecal incontinence caused by impaction with overflow typically experience frequent staining from liquid or semiformed stools (Barrett, 1992; Winograd & Jarvik, 1986). The basic approach to treating this problem is to remove the impaction and initiate a bowel regimen to reestablish normal bowel function (Tobin & Brocklehurst, 1986; Wald, 1990). Clearance of the lower bowel is accomplished with a course of small bulk enemas. The enemas should be discontinued when there is no return, which usually occurs within 7 to 10 days (Brocklehurst, 1992; Goldstein et al.,

1989). Another approach consists of multiple oil and saline enemas, giving one of each both in the morning and evening. This treatment should be continued for 5 days and then changed to once a day for 1 to 2 weeks (Devroede, 1993). Some treatment programs use purgatives such as a nightly or morning insertion of a glycerin or irritant suppository to set a planned time for elimination.

Concurrent measures should be taken to prevent the recurrence of constipation. These measures include the intake of adequate dietary fiber and a minimum of 1.5 to 2 L of fluids per day, exercise, and timely response to the urge to defecate. In ambulatory elderly patients, bulk laxative preparations may be used to obtain the appropriate stool consistency, which is a soft, moist, formed stool. Sorbitol (15–30 mL) or lactulose (15–30 mL) has been found effective in relieving constipation in frail, immobile elderly patients and in patients for whom bulking agents are ineffective or not tolerated. When long-term therapy is required, the bowel program should consist of the basic elements of fiber, fluids, activity, and suppositories taken two to three times a week or daily (Harari et al., 1993; Winograd & Jarvik, 1986).

Bowel habit training is also an effective approach to manage overflow fecal incontinence secondary to fecal retention (McCormick & Burgio, 1984). Regular toileting is achieved by using the gastrocolic reflex that occurs after meals, usually following breakfast. The patient is instructed to attempt a bowel movement immediately after breakfast every day, and an enema is administered to stimulate a bowel movement if one does not occur for 2 consecutive days (McCormick & Burgio, 1984).

In resistant cases of fecal impaction, manual disimpaction or total gut irrigation may be required (Brocklehurst, 1992; Devroede, 1993). Manual removal of the impaction may be necessary to prevent mucosal necrosis or an ulcer caused by the hardened fecal mass (Devroede, 1993). This procedure should be used as a last resort, as irritation to the anus and rectum or damage to the anal sphincter can occur. Removal starts with softening the intestinal contents with oil-retention enemas (Kubalanza-Sipp & French, 1990). Soap and hydrogen per-

TABLE 11–12

Treatment of Fecal Incontinence

Gastrointestinal Disorders

1. Recognize change in bowel function as the presenting sign of a number of disorders
2. Diagnose disorder
3. Treat underlying cause (e.g., antibiotics, surgery, biofeedback, diet modification)

Fecal Impaction

1. Clear lower bowel
   a. Course of small bulk enemas daily (7–10 d)
   b. Nightly or morning insertion of suppository
   c. In resistant cases, perform manual disimpaction or total gut irrigation
2. Prevent recurrence of constipation
   a. Bowel maintenance program
      1. Adequate dietary fiber
      2. 2 L of fluids daily
      3. Activity and exercise
      4. Encourage timely response to the urge to defecate
3. For long-term therapy
   a. Bowel maintenance program
   b. Add if indicated
      1. Bulk-forming agent
      2. Hyperosmotic laxative
      3. Suppositories and enemas
4. For the cognitively impaired
   a. Bowel maintenance program
   b. Habit training (see under neurogenic disorders)

Neurogenic Disorders

1. Initiate bowel program
   a. Adequate dietary fiber
   b. 2 L of fluids daily
   c. Activity and exercise
   d. Consistent toileting time
2. Introduce habit training
   a. Increase awareness of the urge to defecate
   b. Note elimination pattern; plan scheduled toileting based on identified pattern of regular toileting after breakfast, taking advantage of the gastrocolic reflex

Neurogenic Disorders *Continued*

   c. Position in normal posture for defecation; instruct to contract abdominal muscles and lean forward to increase intraabdominal pressure
   d. If necessary, use suppositories or digital stimulation to heighten rectal sensations and to increase awareness of the defecation reflex
   e. Enemas to stimulate bowel movement if one does not occur for 2 consecutive days
3. For severely demented patients, induce constipation with planned periodic evacuation
4. Consider biofeedback for selected patients

Environmental or Iatrogenic Causes

1. Identify cause and take necessary measures to correct the situation
   a. Prevent prolonged bedrest, immobility
   b. Ensure intake of adequate fluids and fiber
   c. Encourage timely response to urge to defecate
2. Check medications
   a. Note time of administration
   b. Monitor medications
      1. Sedatives, hypnotics
      2. Laxatives
      3. Narcotics
      4. Antacids
      5. Muscle relaxants
3. Monitor environmental and other factors
   a. Timely response to call light
   b. Accessible toilet (commode, bedpan)
   c. Comfortable room temperature
   d. Privacy
   e. Unhurried, relaxed atmosphere
   f. Clothing that is easy to manipulate
   g. Use of restraints avoided

Data from Basch & Jensen (1991); Brocklehurst (1992); Winograd & Jarvik (1986).

oxide enemas may irritate the rectal mucosa and should be avoided (Wrenn, 1989).

A topical anesthetic such as lidocaine ointment (5%) may be applied 5 to 10 minutes prior to removing the impaction. The anesthetic lubricates the anorectal tissue and decreases the discomfort caused by the manual removal of hard stool (Mager-O'Conner, 1984). Disimpaction should be completed in stages, as sudden evacuation of the large bulk of stool lowers intraabdominal pressure and may cause transient hypotension and dizziness. In the final step, a small retention enema or a suppository should be administered to complete the evacuation (Mager-O'Conner, 1984; Wrenn, 1989).

Whole-gut irrigation for marked fecal retention has been successful using 1 to 2 L of polyethylene glycol (GoLYTELY) for 2 days, given orally or by nasogastric tube (Brocklehurst, 1992; Harari et al., 1993; Wald, 1993).

GASTROINTESTINAL DISORDERS

In patients with gastrointestinal disorders, the underlying disease needs to be diagnosed and the appropriate treatment initiated. Diverticular diseases, for example, are treated with a high-fiber diet and bulk-forming agents (Schneeman & Tietyen, 1994; Williams, 1992). Surgical approaches may be indicated when medical therapy fails or when there are alterations in anorectal anatomy and continence mechanisms. However, the success rate and the quality of continence after surgery vary among the procedures (Madoff et al., 1992; Schiller, 1993; Wald, 1990).

NEUROLOGICAL DISORDERS

A bowel program for people with neurological fecal incontinence consists of steps to promote bowel regularity, including physical exercise, high fluid intake, a diet including high-fiber foods, and consistent toileting. Habit training should be initiated and measures taken to increase the patient's level of awareness of the urge to defecate. The time of elimination should be noted and subsequent toileting scheduled according to the observed pattern.

In settings with numerous patients requiring care, it may be difficult to provide optimal scheduling routines. More staff time is required with the habit training approach, and patients tend to rely on staff members unless self-toileting is rewarded (McCormick & Burgio, 1984).

Another approach in habit training is to toilet the patient 30 minutes after each meal, when a response is likely. Rectal suppositories, which increase the rectal sensation and aware-

ness of the urge to eliminate, can be used to establish a consistent toileting time (Basch & Jensen, 1991; Goldstein et al., 1989). The use of suppositories should be only temporary and gradually discontinued while the patient establishes regularity through exercise, diet, and regular toileting (Turner, 1987). Digital stimulation can also be used to heighten rectal sensation. In this technique, a gloved, lubricated finger is inserted into the anal canal and moved in a circular motion for 30 seconds to 2 minutes, until the sphincter relaxes (Basch & Jensen, 1991; Kubalanza-Sipp & French, 1990).

Neurogenic incontinence in severely demented older people is treated by inducing constipation and planned periodic evacuations (Kane et al., 1994; Tobin & Brocklehurst, 1986; Winograd & Jarvik, 1986). Winograd and Jarvik (1986) recommended the use of a planned evacuation program in which a phosphate enema given in the morning two or three days a week is alternated with a constipating agent such as diphenoxylate (Lomotil) on the other days. Brocklehurst's (1992) approach includes the use of a constipating drug, such as codeine phosphate given daily, and enemas or suppositories for a planned evacuation twice a week.

Biofeedback therapy may be beneficial for patients with idiopathic fecal incontinence or fecal incontinence caused by peripheral and autonomic neuropathies or for patients who have had anal sphincter surgery or trauma (Basch & Jensen, 1991; Wald, 1995). Studies examining biofeedback that included older people in the sample reported a success rate of 63% and higher (MacLeod, 1987; Whitehead et al., 1985). Biofeedback is appropriate for people who are motivated, cognitively intact, and have at least minimal rectal sensation and the ability to contract their external sphincter (Schiller, 1993; Wald, 1995). The most common techniques of biofeedback use a manometric catheter or an electromyographic (EMG) sensor placed in the anal canal along with surface EMG electrodes placed on the abdomen or gluteus maximus to identify activity in those muscle groups. Patients are taught to isolate and contract the external sphincter with visual feedback of their responses provided through a computer monitor (Jensen, 1997). Another method is to create rectal distention by administering a small volume of air in a rectal balloon until the patient senses distention. Smaller volumes of air are subsequently administered until the patient shows no further improvement in response (Wald, 1993). This biofeedback method uses operant conditioning to improve the older person's conscious threshold for sensation of rectal distention and to increase control of internal anal sphincter contraction (Schiller, 1993). Biofeedback can be conducted in outpatient, inpatient, and home health settings (Jensen, 1997).

Biofeedback therapy is usually performed in conjunction with a home pelvic muscle exercise program similar to that used in the management of urinary incontinence (see Chapter 10). Once it has been determined that the patient can correctly contract his or her pelvic floor muscles without the use of accessory muscles, instructions are given to perform a total of 50 10-second pelvic muscle contractions broken down into several exercise sets per day (e.g., 10 to 25 contractions per exercise set) (Whitehead et al., 1985). Each contraction should be followed by a 10-second rest period. Because of weakened muscles, patients may initially only be able to hold a contraction for a few seconds. As the muscles strengthen and build endurance, however, most patients will gradually become able to achieve longer contractions.

Electrical stimulation through the use of anal, vaginal, or surface electrodes may be used as an adjunct to biofeedback and home pelvic muscle exercises or as the sole therapy in the treatment of fecal incontinence. Office and home stimulators are available. Typically, home electrical stimulation therapy is prescribed at one to two 15- to 30-minute sessions a day.

ENVIRONMENTAL OR IATROGENIC CAUSES

If fecal incontinence is caused by environmental or iatrogenic factors, removing the cause or changing the situation will resolve this temporary incontinence problem (see Chapter 16).

SUMMARY

Constipation, diarrhea, and fecal incontinence are problems frequently managed by the ad-

vanced practice nurse. For the most part, these conditions can be prevented. When they do occur, effective measures are available to increase patient comfort, prevent complications, make life easier for the caregivers, and lower the expenses involved in care. The successful management of bowel problems is dependent on thoroughly evaluating the problem, identifying the underlying cause, and initiating prompt, appropriate treatment.

REFERENCES

Alterescu, V. (1986). Theoretical foundations for an approach to fecal incontinence. *Journal of Enterostomal Therapy, 13,* 44–48.

Altman, D. F. (1995). Drugs used in gastrointestinal diseases. In B. Katzung (Ed.), *Basic and clinical pharmacology* (6th ed., pp. 949–961). Norwalk, CT: Appleton & Lange.

Ammon, H. V. (1995). Part 1: Diarrhea. In W. S. Haubrich & F. Schaffner (Eds.) & J. E. Berk (Consult. Ed.), *Bockus' Gastroenterology, vol. 1* (5th ed., pp. 87–102). Philadelphia: W. B. Saunders.

Andorsky, R. I., & Goldner, F. (1990). Colonic lavage solution (polyethylene glycol electrolyte lavage solution) as a treatment for chronic constipation: A double-blind, placebo-controlled study. *American Journal of Gastroenterology, 85,* 261–265.

Artymowicz, R. J., Childs, A. L., & Paolini, L. (1997). Phenolphthalein-induced toxic epidermal necrolysis. *Annals of Pharmacotherapy, 31*(10), 1157–1159.

Bannister, J. J., Abouzekry, L., & Read, N. (1987). Effect of aging on anorectal function. *Gut, 28,* 353–357.

Barrett, J. A. (1992). Colorectal disorders in elderly people. *British Medical Journal, 305,* 764–766.

Basch, A., & Jensen, L. (1991). Management of fecal incontinence. In D. B. Doughty (Ed.), *Urinary and fecal incontinence: Nursing management* (pp. 235–265). St. Louis, MO: Mosby-Year Book.

Battle, E. H., & Hanna, C. E. (1980). Evaluation of a dietary regimen for chronic constipation. *Journal of Gerontological Nursing, 6,* 527–532.

Behm, R. M. (1985). A special recipe to banish constipation. *Geriatric Nursing, 6,* 216–217.

Bennett, R. G., & Greenough, W. B. (1994). Diarrhea. In W. R. Hazzard, E. L. Bierman, J. P. Blass, et al. (Eds.), *Principles of geriatric medicine and gerontology* (3rd ed., pp. 1275–1284). New York: McGraw-Hill.

Bliss, C. M., & Murray, F. E. (1991). Geriatric constipation: Brief update on a common problem. *Geriatrics, 46*(3), 64–68.

Brocklehurst, J. C. (1992). The large bowel. In J. C. Brocklehurst, R. C. Tallis & H. M. Fillit (Eds.), *Textbook of geriatric medicine and gerontology* (4th ed., pp. 569–591). Edinburgh: Churchill Livingstone.

Burkitt, D. P. (1982). Dietary fiber: Is it really helpful? *Geriatrics, 37*(1), 119–120, 126.

Campbell, A. J., Reinken, J., & McCosh, L. (1985). Incontinence in the elderly: Prevalence and prognosis. *Age and Aging, 14,* 65–70.

Cannon, B. (1981). Bowel function. In N. Martin, N. B. Holt & D. Hicks (Eds.), *Comprehensive rehabilitation nursing* (pp. 223–241). New York: McGraw-Hill.

Castle, S. C. (1989). Constipation: Endemic in the elderly? *Medical Clinics of North America, 73,* 1497–1509.

Castle, S. C., Cantrell, M., & Israel, D. S. (1991). Constipation prevention: Empiric use of stool softeners questioned. *Geriatrics, 46*(11), 84–86.

Cheskin, L. J., & Schuster, M. M. (1994). Constipation. In W. R. Hazzard, E. L. Bierman, J. P. Blass, et al. (Eds.), *Principles of geriatric medicine and gerontology* (3rd ed., pp. 1267–1273). New York: McGraw-Hill.

Davies, G. J., Crowder, M., Reid, B., & Dickerson, J. W. T. (1986). Bowel function measurement of individuals with different eating patterns. *Gut, 27,* 164–169.

Davis, A., Nagelhout, M. J., Hoban, M., & Barnard, B. (1986). Bowel management, a quality assurance approach to upgrading programs. *Journal of Gerontological Nursing, 12,* 13–17.

Devroede, G. (1993). Constipation. In M. H. Sleisenger & J. S. Fordtran (Eds.), *Gastrointestinal disease: Pathophysiology, diagnosis and management, vol. 1* (5th ed., pp. 837–887). Philadelphia: W. B. Saunders.

Donatelle, E. P. (1990). Constipation: Pathophysiology and treatment. *American Family Physician, 42,* 1335–1342.

Dunnick, J. K., & Hailey, J. R. (1996). Phenolphthalein exposure causes multiple carcinogenic effects in experimental model systems. *Cancer Research, 56*(21), 4922–4926.

Fine, K. D., Krejs, G. J., & Fordtran, J. S. (1993). Diarrhea. In M. H. Sleisenger & J. S. Fordtran (Eds.), *Gastrointestinal disease: Pathophysiology, diagnosis, and management, vol. 2* (5th ed., pp. 1043–1072). Philadelphia: W. B. Saunders.

Friedman, L. S., & Isselbacher, K. J. (1994). Diarrhea and constipation. In K. J. Isselbacher, E. Braunwald, J. Wilson, et al. (Eds.), *Harrison's principles of internal medicine* (13th ed., pp. 213–221). New York: McGraw-Hill.

Goldstein, M. K., Brown, E. M., Holt, P., et al. (1989). Fecal incontinence in an elderly man. *Journal of the American Geriatrics Society, 37,* 991–1002.

Halpin, J. E. (1986). Understanding and controlling fecal incontinence. *Ostomy/Wound Management, 13,* 28–36.

Harari, D., Gurwitz, J. H., & Minaker, K. L. (1993). Constipation in the elderly. *Journal of the American Geriatrics Society, 41,* 1130–1140.

Hogstel, M. O., & Nelson, M. (1992). Anticipation and early detection can reduce bowel elimination complications. *Geriatric Nursing, 13,* 28–33.

Isaacs, B., & Walkey, F. A. (1964). A survey on incontinence in elderly hospital patients. *Gerontologia Clinica, 6,* 367–376.

Jensen, L. L. (1997). Fecal incontinence: Evaluation and treatment. *Journal of Wound, Ostomy, and Continence Nursing, 24,* 277–282.

Johanson, J. F., Sonnenberg, A., & Koch, T. R. (1989). Clinical epidemiology of chronic constipation. *Journal of Clinical Gastroenterology, 11,* 525–536.

Kane, R. L., Ouslander, J. G., & Abrass, I. B. (1994). *Essentials of clinical geriatrics* (3rd ed., pp. 145–196). New York: McGraw-Hill.

Koch, T. R. (1995). Part 2: Constipation. In W. S. Haubrich & F. Schaeffer (Eds.) & J. E. Berk (Consult. Ed.), *Bockus' gastroenterology, vol. 1* (5th ed., pp. 87–102). Philadelphia: W. B. Saunders.

Kot, T. V., & Pettit-Young, N. A. (1992). Lactulose in the management of constipation: A current review. *Annals of Pharmacotherapy, 26,* 1277–1282.

Kowlessar, O. D. (1995). Diarrhea. In W. B. Abrams, M. H. Beers & R. Berkow (Eds.), *The Merck manual of geriatrics* (2nd ed., pp. 682–688). Whitehouse Station, NJ: Merck & Co., Inc.

Kubalanza-Sipp, D., & French, E. T. (1990). Procedures to establish and maintain elimination. In E. Carlson, W. P. Grigg & R. B. King (Eds.), *Rehabilitation nursing procedures manual* (pp. 123–178). Rockville, MD: Aspen.

Kumar, D., Bartolo, D. C., Devroede, G., et al. (1992). Symposium on constipation. *International Journal of Colorectal Disease, 7*(2), 47–67.

Lederle, F. A., Busch, D. L., Mattox, K. M., et al. (1990). Cost-effective treatment of constipation in the elderly: A randomized double-blind comparison of sorbitol and lactulose. *American Journal of Medicine, 89,* 597–601.

Leigh, R. J., & Turnberg, L. A. (1982). Faecal incontinence: The unvoiced symptom. *Lancet, 1,* 1349–1351.

Leslie, L. R. (1990). Training for functional independence. In F. J. Kottke & J. F. Lehmann (Eds.), *Krusen's handbook of physical medicine and rehabilitation* (4th ed., pp. 564–570). Philadelphia: W. B. Saunders.

MacLeod, J. H. (1987). Management of anal incontinence by biofeedback. *Gastroenterology, 93,* 291–293.

Madoff, R. D., Williams, J. G., & Caushaj, P. F. (1992). Fecal incontinence. *New England Journal of Medicine, 326,* 1002–1007.

Mager-O'Connor, E. (1984). How to identify and remove fecal impactions. *Geriatric Nursing, 5,* 158–161.

Mahan, L. K., & Escott-Stump, S. (Eds.). (1996). *Krause's food, nutrition, and diet therapy* (9th ed.). Philadelphia: W. B. Saunders.

McCormick, K. A., & Burgio, K. L. (1984). Incontinence: An update on nursing care measures. *Journal of Gerontological Nursing, 10,* 16–23.

McEvoy, G. K. (1998). *Drug information 98.* Bethesda, MD: American Society of Hospital Pharmacists.

Miller, J. (1985). Helping the aged manage bowel function. *Journal of Gerontological Nursing, 11,* 37–41.

Moriarty, K. J., & Irving, M. H. (1992). Constipation. *British Medical Journal, 304,* 1237–1240.

Mowlam, V., North, K., & Myers, C. (1986). Continence: Managing faecal incontinence. *Nursing Times, 82,* 55–59.

Noelker, L. S. (1987). Incontinence in elderly cared for by family. *Gerontologist, 27,* 194–200.

Pattee, J. J., & West, M. S. (1988). Clinical aspects of a fiber supplementation program in a nursing home population. *Current Therapeutic Research, 43,* 1150–1157.

Read, N. W., & Abouzekry, L. (1986). Why do patients with faecal impaction have faecal incontinence? *Gut, 27,* 283–287.

Resnick, B. (1985). Constipation, common but preventable. *Geriatric Nursing, 6,* 213–215.

Robinson, C. H., Lawler, M. R., Chenoweth, W. L., & Garwick, A. E. (1986). *Normal and therapeutic nutrition* (17th ed.). New York: Macmillan.

Rousseau, P. (1988a). Treatment of constipation. *Postgraduate Medicine, 83,* 339–345, 349.

Rousseau, P. (1988b). No soapsuds enemas! *Postgraduate Medicine, 83,* 352–353.

Sandler, R. S., Jordan, M. C., & Shelton, B. J. (1990). Demographic and dietary determinants of constipation in the U.S. population. *American Journal of Public Health, 80,* 185–189.

Sandman, P. O., Adolfsson, R., Hallmans, G., et al. (1983). Treatment of constipation with high-bran bread in the long-term care of severely demented elderly patients. *Journal of the American Geriatrics Society, 31,* 290–293.

Schiller, L. R. (1993). Fecal incontinence. In M. H. Sleisenger & J. S. Fordtran (Eds.), *Gastrointestinal disease: Pathophysiology, diagnosis, and management, vol. I* (5th ed., pp. 934–953). Philadelphia: W. B. Saunders.

Schneeman, B. O., & Tietyen, J. (1994). Dietary fiber. In M. E. Shils, J. A. Olson & M. Shike (Eds.), *Modern nutrition in health and disease* (8th ed., pp. 89–100). Philadelphia: Lea & Febiger.

Shafik, A. (1993). Constipation: Pathogenesis and management. *Drugs, 45,* 528–540.

Smith, R. G., & Lewis, S. (1990). The relationship between digital examination and abdominal radiographs in elderly patients. *Age and Ageing, 19,* 142–143.

Stewart, R. B., Moore, M. T., Marks, R. G., & Hale, W. E. (1992). Correlates of constipation in an ambulatory elderly population. *American Journal of Gastroenterology, 87,* 859–864.

Stryker, R. (1977). *Rehabilitative aspects of acute and chronic nursing care.* Philadelphia: W. B. Saunders.

Talley, N. J., O'Keefe, E. A., Zinsmeister, A. R., & Melton, L. J. (1992). Prevalence of gastrointestinal symptoms and functional bowel disorders in the elderly: A population-based study. *Gastroenterology, 102,* 895–901.

Tedesco, F. J., & DiPiro, J. T. (1985). Laxative use in constipation. *American Journal of Gastroenterology, 80,* 303–309.

Thomas, T. M., Egan, M., Walgrove, A., & Meade, T. W. (1984). The prevalence of faecal and double incontinence. *Community Medicine, 6,* 216–220.

Tobin, G. W., & Brocklehurst, J. C. (1986). Faecal incontinence in residential homes for the elderly. *Age and Ageing, 15,* 41–46.

Towers, A. L., Burgio, K. L., Locher, J. L., et al. (1994). Constipation in the elderly. Influence of dietary, psychological, and physiological factors. *Journal of the American Geriatrics Society, 42,* 701–706.

Turner, A. (1987). Constipation and faecal incontinence. *Professional Nurse, 2,* 256–258.

Wald, A. (1990). Constipation and fecal incontinence in the elderly. *Gastroenterology Clinics of North America, 19,* 405–418.

Wald, A. (1993). Constipation in elderly patients. Pathogenesis and management. *Drugs & Aging, 3,* 220–231.

Wald, A. (1995). Constipation. In W. B. Abrams, M. H. Beers & R. Berkow (Eds.), *The Merck manual of geriatrics* (2nd ed., pp. 674–682). Whitehouse Station, NJ: Merck & Co., Inc.

Whitehead, W. E., Burgio, K. L., & Engel, B. T. (1985). Biofeedback treatment of fecal incontinence in geriatric patients. *Journal of the American Geriatrics Society, 33,* 320–324.

Whitehead, W. E., Drinkwater, D., Cheskin, L. J., et al. (1989). Constipation in the elderly living at home. Definition, prevalence, and relationship to lifestyle and health status. *Journal of the American Geriatrics Society, 37,* 423–429.

Williams, S. G., & DiPalma, J. A. (1990). Constipation in the long-term care facility. *Gastroenterology Nursing, 12,* 179–182.

Williams, S. R. (1992). *Basic nutrition and diet therapy* (9th ed.). St. Louis: Mosby–Year Book.

Winograd, C. H., & Jarvik, L. F. (1986). Physician management of the demented patient. *Journal of the American Geriatrics Society, 34,* 295–308.

Wrenn, K. (1989). Fecal impaction. *New England Journal of Medicine, 321,* 658–662.

Impaired Mobility and Deconditioning

Joyce K. Holohan-Bell
Kenneth Brummel-Smith

The ability to move around under one's own power is one of the most important issues to older people. Mobility is often seen as the final common pathway to independence, a value that many people hold in higher esteem than length of life. Many of the illnesses that afflict older people—most notably, arthritis, neurological diseases, and cardiac conditions—have marked effects on mobility in this population. One of the distinguishing factors in geriatric care is attention to the patient's functional abilities, and mobility is one of the most critical functions.

The term *mobility* is used to describe many different functional activities, including transfers between objects or areas, walking, wheelchair use, and motorized transportation. This chapter discusses transfers, walking, and wheelchair use as well as important associated *geriatric syndromes* such as deconditioning and stroke. (Falls, which constitute another syndrome associated with mobility, are discussed in Chapter 15.)

Large studies of older adults have shown that mobility problems are common in this population. In these studies, the prevalence of mobility deficits was found to vary with the patient's age and living situation as well as the setting in which the problem was identified—community, hospital, or nursing home. In one community-based study, about 15% of the subjects older than 65 years had difficulty with walking; among subjects older than 85 years, 26% of men and 31% of women had these difficulties (Coroni-Huntley et al., 1986). Other studies have shown somewhat lower, although still significant, rates. Approximately 6% were found to have difficulties with bed or chair transfers (Leon & Lair, 1990).

In acute hospitals, as many as 65% of patients older than 70 years have difficulty with walking (Warshaw et al., 1982). Inactivity is promoted during most hospitalizations, often with disastrous results (Lazarus et al., 1991) (Table 12–1). Deficits in bed mobility constitute a recognized risk factor for admission to a nursing home (Kane & Kane, 1987), and 69%

of nursing home residents have difficulty with walking (Brody & Foley, 1987). Although immobility is common in nursing homes, it is infrequently recognized as a problem. In one study, immobility was not identified on the problem list for 85% of immobile residents (Selikson et al., 1988).

Because walking velocity decreases with normal aging (Cohen et al., 1987), even when subjects are not identified as having a "mobility problem," they may experience problems functioning in a society that is oriented to the young and fit. In Sweden a maximum walking speed of 1.4 meters per second is considered a norm for pedestrians at signalized intersections, yet a study of elderly subjects found that none could comfortably achieve this speed (Lundgren-Lindquist et al., 1983). If older patients cannot safely negotiate the streets of the town in which they live, it is likely that other potentially devastating sequelae will develop. Social isolation, depression, poor nutritional intake, and decreased exercise tolerance can all result from immobility.

CAUSES OF IMMOBILITY

The causes of mobility problems are usually myriad and interacting (Fig. 12–1). Arthritis is the most common chronic medical condition of older people, affecting more than 80% of people older than 75 years (Brandt & Slemenda, 1993). Neurological conditions such as stroke, peripheral neuropathy, and Parkinson's disease are also common in old age. The most common cause of death in people older than 65 years is heart disease; however, many patients live long lives while experiencing other consequences of heart disease, such as decreased exercise tolerance or angina occurring with physical activity. Chronic obstructive pulmonary disease also disproportionately affects older populations.

More important than the simple presence of one of these conditions is the fact that many patients have multiple problems that interact to compound their level of disability. For example, the energy cost of walking is generally 30 to 50% higher in people who have survived a stroke than in people with a normal gait. For a younger person, this increased cost is im-

---

T A B L E 1 2 – 1

Provision of Physical Activity in the Hospital

Activity Prescribed	Patients (%)
No activity ordered	13
Never ambulated	24
Activity differed from order	41
Physical therapy ordered	3
Range of motion ordered in best rest patients	0

A restrospective chart review was conducted in five hospitals in Rhode Island (247–719 beds per hospital). A total of 500 patients with a total of 3500 patient days were included. The mean age was 79 years. The medical record was reviewed for any written orders or documentation of the activities indicated in any note in the chart, including those of physicians, nurses, or therapists.

Data from Lazarus et al. (1991).

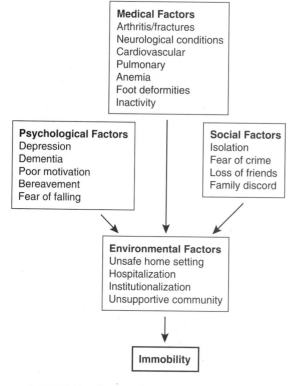

Medical Factors
Arthritis/fractures
Neurological conditions
Cardiovascular
Pulmonary
Anemia
Foot deformities
Inactivity

Psychological Factors
Depression
Dementia
Poor motivation
Bereavement
Fear of falling

Social Factors
Isolation
Fear of crime
Loss of friends
Family discord

Environmental Factors
Unsafe home setting
Hospitalization
Institutionalization
Unsupportive community

Immobility

FIGURE 12–1. Factors contributing to immobility.

portant but rarely a major problem. However, for the older person who may also have underlying cardiac disease or pulmonary insufficiency, it may be enough to precipitate an attack of angina or a myocardial infarction. Similarly, for patients with chronic knee pain from osteoarthritis, learning to walk with a prosthesis following an amputation for peripheral vascular disease may be impossible until the arthritic knee has been treated.

Visual problems are common with old age; these include normal changes such as decreased visual acuity and glare tolerance as well as abnormal conditions such as glaucoma and macular degeneration. For an older person, these problems may interact with an environment that is "stressful" because it has throw rugs, unsafe stairs, or exposed wiring, for example.

Psychological and social conditions may similarly interact with underlying medical con-

ditions to decrease mobility. Patients with depression may be less motivated to be active and thereby decrease their exercise tolerance over time. Patients with dementia may be less attentive to their environment, causing increased risks similar to those seen with decreased vision.

DECONDITIONING

The term *deconditioning* is defined as "the multiple changes in organ system physiology that are induced by inactivity and reversed by activity" (Siebens, 1990). Other terms used frequently to describe this state include *disuse syndrome, immobilization,* and *impaired physical mobility* (Creason, 1990; Thompson et al., 1993). Disuse syndrome, for example, is similarly defined as "deterioration of body systems as the result of prescribed or unavoidable musculoskeletal inactivity" (Thompson et al., 1993).

Several risk factors have been identified that predispose older adults to becoming more readily deconditioned than the young. These include (1) enforced bed rest brought on by acute illness, (2) disability that limits or even temporarily eliminates mobility, (3) chronic disease that causes a gradual decrease in activity, (4) the use of certain medications, and (5) psychosocial factors (Rader & Vaughen, 1994). Normal age-related structural and physiological changes, such as reduced cardiac output and a loss of calcium from bones, also increase the risk of deconditioning in the elderly person (Bortz, 1982). In fact, it is often difficult to identify the specific risk factor(s) that most contributes to inactivity because many may be present in one individual.

Types of Deconditioning

It is helpful to differentiate between *acute* and *chronic* forms of deconditioning, which reflect the risk factors previously noted. Acute deconditioning develops rapidly and is the result of an abrupt cessation of usual activity. An example of acute deconditioning is that caused by enforced bed rest and/or staying in a hospital. Acute immobilization of the body or its parts can also be induced by paralysis; mental health disorders (e.g., catatonia); severe pain; the use of casts, traction, or splints; an altered level of consciousness; and the use of restraints (Dittmer & Teasell, 1993; Thompson et al., 1993). Chronic deconditioning occurs over a prolonged period and may result from psychosocial factors, diseases, or aging effects that, when combined, result in long-term activity limitation. In clinical practice, there may be a blurring of these forms (e.g., acute deconditioning superimposed on underlying chronic inactivity).

ACUTE DECONDITIONING: CAUSES AND CONSEQUENCES

Dating back to the 1800s, resting the body during illness was one of the most frequently prescribed treatments. More recently, however, studies about the effects of immobilization have put an end to the use of bed rest as a therapeutic modality. Despite the evidence from these studies, patients are still assigned a bed on admission to the acute care hospital and often spend the majority of their time either in it or close to it (Harper & Lyles, 1988). This type of severely decreased activity level in the elderly patient can rapidly lead to changes in physiological and psychosocial areas that impair the older person's functional status.

As noted in Table 12–2, bed rest or acute immobilization can have deleterious effects on virtually all major organ systems of the body as well as on several psychosocial functions. Changes in the cardiovascular and musculoskeletal systems can significantly affect an older person's mobility and ability to perform the activities of daily living (ADL); specific aspects of these changes are highlighted in the following section.

The most striking hemodynamic response to lying in bed is the redistribution of approximately 500 mL of blood to the thoracic circulation (Harper & Lyles, 1988). The resulting increase in heart rate, cardiac output, and stroke volume leads to a 20% rise in cardiac workload. This rise almost doubles in the presence of an underlying cardiac disease (Mobily &

TABLE 12-2

Potential Consequences of Immobilization and Strategies for Prevention and Treatment

Consequences	Prevention/Treatment
Cardiovascular	
Thromboembolic phenomena	Intermittent pneumatic compression
Orthostatic hypotension	Prophylactic anticoagulation
Increased cardiac workload	Leg exercises
Decreased aerobic capacity	Reverse Trendelenburg position of bed
	Elastic stockings
	Abdominal binder
	Tilt table
	Elevation of legs
	Leg and abdominal exercises
	Upright position, sitting on side of bed, up in chair
	Isometric exercises
Pulmonary	
Decreased lung volumes	Program of pulmonary hygiene: deep breathing, coughing, postural drainage, vibration
Reduced respiratory muscle strength	Incentive spirometry
Increased ventilation/perfusion mismatching	Frequent position changes
Impaired ciliary function	Adequate hydration
Atelectasis	
Pneumonia	

TABLE 12-2

Potential Consequences of Immobilization and
Strategies for Prevention and Treatment *Continued*

Consequences	Prevention/Treatment
Musculoskeletal	
Joint contracture	Range of motion (active or passive)
Decreased endurance	Regular repositioning of joints
Muscle weakness and atrophy	Neutral positioning of limbs
Bone loss	Resting splints
	Continuous passive motion
	Therapeutic exercises
	Bed mobility training
	Standing or bearing weight
Metabolic/Endocrine	
Negative nitrogen balance	Appropriate diet
Decreased metabolic rate	Increased fluid intake
Glucose intolerance	Isotonic exercises of lower extremities
Increased parathyroid hormone level	
Gastrointestinal	
Anorexia	Small, frequent feedings
Constipation	Regular bowel routine
Fecal impaction	High-fiber diet
	Adequate fluid intake
	Avoid constipating drugs
	Stool softeners or laxatives as needed
Urinary	
Incontinence	Bladder training program
Impaired bladder emptying	Standing or sitting position to urinate
Urinary tract infection	Check for bladder distention
Renal stone formation	Avoid catheterization
	Increased fluid intake
Skin	
Pressure ulcers	Scheduled position changes
	Reduce friction and shear
	Overbed frame and trapeze
	Pressure-relieving devices
	Regular skin inspection
	Control of incontinence
	Adequate nutrition
Neuropsychological	
Sensory deprivation	Adaptive aids (glasses, hearing aids)
Disorientation	Increased sensory stimulation
Dependency	Reality orientation program
Anxiety	Foster self-care and independence
Depression	Psychosocial and physical stimulation
Social isolation	Involvement of family and friends
Intellectual dysfunction	

Data from Coletta & Murphy (1992); Creditor (1993); Dittmer & Teasell (1993); Halar & Bell (1990); Harper & Lyles (1988); Mobily & Kelley (1991); Olson (1967); Rousseau (1993); and Teasell & Dittmer (1993).

Kelley, 1991). These initial cardiac responses are gradually reversed by the action of the atrial baroreceptors, leading to a progressive decrease in stroke volume and cardiac output within 3 to 5 days of bed rest. However, the resting heart rate remains elevated and increases one beat for every 2 days of continued bed rest (Dittmer & Teasell, 1993). Along with cardiovascular deconditioning, maximum oxygen uptake (VO_2 max, a measure of aerobic capacity) markedly diminishes, resulting in an alteration of the usual cardiovascular response to exercise and in diminished exercise tolerance (Halar & Bell, 1990).

The adverse effects of immobility are most obvious in the musculoskeletal system. These effects include joint contractures, osteoporosis caused by disuse, muscle weakness and atrophy, and decreased endurance (Harper & Lyles, 1988). A *contracture* is the lack of a full passive or active range of motion of a joint. Muscle, soft tissue, or joint limitations can lead to the development of contractures, but the most frequent cause is joint immobilization (Halar & Bell, 1993). Bed rest precipitates bone demineralization, probably owing to the increased urinary excretion of calcium and the corresponding increased secretion of parathyroid hormone (Holm & Hedricks, 1989).

The combination of reduced muscle strength, circulation, and metabolic activity leads to decreased endurance. Muscle atrophy also plays a role in muscle strength and endurance changes. With complete bed rest, the loss of muscle strength is estimated to be 10 to 15% per week and is usually greatest in the antigravity muscles of the lower extremities (locomotion muscles) and trunk (postural muscles) (Dittmer & Teasell, 1993; Halar & Bell, 1990). Gogia and colleagues (1988) studied muscle torque in 15 healthy male volunteers from 21 to 54 years of age before and after 5 weeks of strict bed rest and found a significant decrease in muscle strength in all the muscle groups tested except that of the elbow extensors. The largest decreases were noted in the soleus (24%) and gastrocnemius-soleus (26%) of the lower extremities.

The effects of deconditioning on older adults' functional status that are perhaps the least well known, or the least considered and attended to, are the deleterious effects of acute hospitalization and bed rest. These effects are magnified by the fact that many elderly people enter the hospital with preexisting compromised functional status. McVey and associates (1989) found that on admission to a Veterans Affairs hospital, 49 (27%) of 178 patients, mean age 81.5 years, needed help with one to three of the ADL; 39 (22%) needed help with four to six of the ADL; and 21 (12%) were completely dependent in performing all the ADL. After a mean stay of 18.4 days, the overall functional status improved in one third of the patients, remained unchanged in one third, and further declined in one third.

Gillick and colleagues (1982) noted a high rate (40.5%) of functional morbidity in patients older than 70 years admitted to a hospital as opposed to a much lower rate (8.8%) in younger patients. These effects were associated with hospitalization itself and not with the reasons for hospital admission. One study of 279 patients aged 70 years or older found that 50% were confused, 21% had urinary or bowel incontinence, 34% had impaired hearing, 40% had impaired vision, and 25% had speech impairments. More than half of the subjects older than 75 years required assistance with mobility, feeding, and dressing (Warshaw et al., 1982).

In a prospective study, Hirsch and associates (1990) compared the functional status of 71 elderly patients older than 74 years on their second day of hospital admission and the day before discharge. They also collected the same data from patients or caregivers for 2 weeks prior to admission and 1 week after discharge. The patients were admitted for a variety of acute illnesses. There was a statistically significant decline in five of the seven functional domains assessed: mobility, transfer, grooming, feeding, and toileting. Regarding mobility, 40 (65%) of the patients had a decline between admission and the second day of hospitalization, 33 (67%) had not improved at discharge, and 5 (10%) deteriorated further. The investigators concluded that although patients recovered from their acute illnesses during hospitalization, they were left with new and significant functional impairments at discharge.

CHRONIC DECONDITIONING: CAUSES AND CONSEQUENCES

Multiple, interacting components contribute to the development of chronic deconditioning in elderly people. These components can include the biological changes related to normal aging or disease as well as affective, psychological disorders. Finally, the healthcare delivery system itself can contribute to the development and maintenance of chronic disability.

Normal age-related changes have a minimal influence on the development of chronic deconditioning. For example, Bortz (1982) reviewed the presumed normal biological changes associated with aging and noted the striking similarity of these changes to those that occurred with physical inactivity. He suggests that at least some of the changes usually attributed to aging may, in fact, be caused by disuse. Figure 12–2 graphically illustrates the interaction of aging and disuse (Williams, 1984). Although neither author denies the effects of aging on the body systems, it is clear that activity limitation also has a profound influence on organ function. Unfortunately, a sedentary lifestyle appears to be the rule rather than the exception. National surveys of people older than 65 years have revealed that only 2 to 46% participate in physical activity programs, including walking (Fiatarone & Evans, 1990).

Many chronic diseases are associated with old age. The most disabling of these fall into three categories: sensory loss (especially vision and hearing), musculoskeletal diseases (e.g., osteoarthritis, osteoporosis), and neurological diseases (e.g., Parkinson's disease, Alzheimer's disease) (Cassel & Brody, 1990). Some activity limitations caused by chronic illness are found in 41% of people 65 to 74 years of age, in 51% of people 75 to 84 years of age, and in 60% of people 85 or more years of age. The type of activity decrement depends on the specific disease entity. For example, the pain and joint changes of arthritis and the altered movements and posture of parkinsonism result in dissimilar activity deficits.

The affective or emotional state of the elderly can also influence their participation in activities. The presence of depression, with its physical and vegetative signs, can certainly hinder one's motivation to exercise and may also affect stamina, interpersonal relations, and other factors related to activity (Kemp, 1993). Older substance abusers of alcohol often cite physical problems and feeling poorly as excuses for their inactivity (Hopson-Walker, 1990). Both prescription and over-the-counter medications may be intentionally or unintentionally abused by the elderly, leading to decreased vigor (Kemp, 1993). The side effects of drugs frequently prescribed for elderly patients can lead to problems with mobility and ultimately result in reduced activity (Table 12–3).

Health systems may contribute to deconditioning through ageism and overprotectiveness on the part of clinical staff members, which can promote learned helplessness in their patients. *Ageism*, an essentially negative attitude or bias toward older people, can lead to a belief that aged people cannot or should not participate in activities, an attitude that may be shared by staff members and patients alike (Panicucci, 1983). *Learned helplessness* is a loss of independence caused by people's perceived lack of control of themselves and their environment (Slimmer et al., 1987). The responsibility for

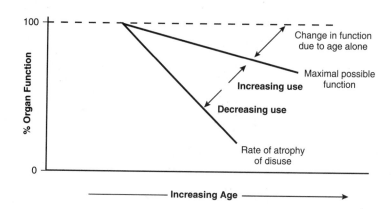

FIGURE 12–2. Interaction of aging and disuse. The upper curve represents the maximal possible performance of a given organ system, whereas the lower curve shows the rate of atrophy when the system is never stressed. Organ function always occurs at some point between the two curves. The slope of the upper curve defines the change in function resulting from aging. (Reproduced from Williams, M. E. [1984]. Clinical implications of aging physiology. *American Journal of Medicine,* 76, 1050. Copyright 1984 by Excerpta Medica Inc.)

TABLE 12-3
Adverse Effects on Mobility from Commonly Used Drugs

Effect on Mobility	Drugs
Impaired alertness	Sedatives (diazepam [Valium], oxazepam [Serax], etc.) Antihistamines (diphenhydramine [Benadryl], etc.) Narcotics (codeine, oxycodone) Alcohol (cough suppressants) Anticonvulsants (phenytoin [Dilantin], carbamazepine [Tegretol], phenobarbital)
Impaired balance	Sedatives Antihypertensives (by orthostatic hypotension) Anticonvulsants
Impaired strength	Diuretics (by hypokalemia) Steroids (by myopathy) Thyroid hormone (by myopathy)
Impaired coordination	Sedatives Narcotics Anticonvulsants
Altered muscle tone	Neuroleptics (haloperidol [Haldol], thioridazine [Mellaril]) Metoclopramide (Reglan)
Impaired sensation	Nitrofurantoin (by peripheral neuropathy) Angiotensin-converting enzyme inhibitors (captopril, etc.) (by peripheral neuropathy) Disulfiram (by peripheral neuropathy) Diphenylhydantoin

From Bottomley, J. M., Blakeney, B., O'Malley, T., et al. (1990). Rehabilitation and mobility of older persons: An interdisciplinary perspective. In S. J. Brody & L. G. Pawlson (Eds.), *Aging and rehabilitation II: The state of practice* (p. 85). New York: Springer. Copyright by Springer Publishing Company, Inc., New York, 10012. Used by permission.

increased functional dependency is frequently shared by both patients who expect staff members to care for them and staff members who provide all aspects of care for their patients (Clark & Siebens, 1993). Avorn and Langer (1982) conducted a trial to explore the concept that disability can be induced by helping. To test performance at various levels of assistance, 72 residents of an intermediate care facility were given a 10-piece jigsaw puzzle and were randomly divided into three groups: helped, encouraged only, and no contact. The investigators found a statistically significant deterioration in both performance and self-confidence in the "helped" group versus the other two groups. They concluded that helping fostered self-induced dependence.

Panicucci (1983) noted that healthcare professionals often fail to allow older people to take risks. For example, in the interest of safety,

nursing staff members often limit patients' mobility and disagree with their choice to return to independent living. She questioned whether in this context caregivers were giving higher priority to their needs than to the patients' needs. She suggested that more trust be placed in the knowledge and experience of the elderly to weigh the risks and benefits of their own actions.

The consequences of chronic inactivity, as with acute immobilization, may be confounded by the changes associated with disease or normal aging (Clark & Siebens, 1993). In many areas of physiological function, the outcomes of both acute and chronic inactivity are similar except that the effects of the latter develop over a more protracted period. The consequences of chronic inactivity are reviewed in Table 12-4 (Siebens, 1990). When viewed from a functional standpoint, chronic deconditioning may

TABLE 12-4

Consequences of Chronic Deconditioning

Impaired balance
Increased reaction time
Decreased maximal oxygen uptake
Prolonged recovery rate of vital signs
Increased resting heart rate
Reduced muscle strength
Accentuation of normal lean body mass and fat changes
Decreased joint flexibility

Data from Siebens (1990).

contribute to falls and injuries (Clark & Siebens, 1993) and to an overall decline in functional abilities and increasing dependence (Vorhies & Riley, 1993).

INTERVENTIONS: ACUTE DECONDITIONING AND IMMOBILIZATION

At the conclusion of her classic article on immobility, Olson (1967) noted that "nursing must not be a partner to disability induced by dependent immobility. It must instead be a catalyst in the prevention of one of the nation's major health problems—immobilization disability" (p. 797). Prevention of the deleterious effects of bed rest remains the cornerstone of treatment. There are, of course, some instances when rest of the body is necessary, such as with extensive trauma or major medical or surgical insults. However, complete bed rest is not indicated for the majority of older patients admitted to the acute care hospital. In fact, uninterrupted activity should be the norm of care.

Geriatric Rehabilitation

Various approaches can be used in preventing and managing the consequences of immobility and bed rest, and one should view all interventions in a rehabilitation context. The primary goal of gerontological nursing is to preserve and restore the greatest degree of independence possible for each elderly person (Butler,

1991; Williams, 1990). This goal is closely intertwined with that of geriatric rehabilitation, which Bottomley (1994) described as "assist[ing] the disabled aged in recovering lost physical, psychological, or social skills so that they may become more independent, live in personally satisfying environments, and maintain meaningful social interactions" (p. 230). The rehabilitative perspective also emphasizes the need for the expertise of various healthcare professionals or an interdisciplinary team to provide holistic, comprehensive care of the elderly.

Prevention and Management

The first step in avoiding or decreasing the consequences of bed rest and hospital-induced deconditioning is to recognize the potential problems that may occur. Nurses should take focused actions that will lead to the prevention and amelioration of these problems. The nursing care plan is based on information from a thorough admission assessment. In addition to identifying patients' medical problems, nurses must also evaluate cognitive and functional status as well as psychosocial and environmental domains.

Specific assessment for acute deconditioning begins with the identification of those older patients most at risk for developing this condition. Siebens (1990) offered several physiological and functional guidelines to use in detecting the presence of deconditioning. These include a resting heart rate above 84 beats per minute and orthostatic hypotension, unless other conditions can account for the change. Another suggestion was to observe the patient's resting heart rate response to undergoing a physical examination. A physical examination includes an evaluation of transfers, ambulation, bed mobility, and manual muscle testing. If it results in an increase of more than 10 to 20 beats per minute, deconditioning is present. Finally, the nurse or therapist can determine physical fitness by observing how patients respond to activities in terms of vital signs, endurance, and symptoms.

The major priority in providing care to acutely ill elderly patients is treating the primary diagnosis(es) that led to hospitalization. At the same time, nurses must be attentive to the potential effects of bed rest or limited activity and should incorporate appropriate interventions into the plan of care. Even in the absence of additional disability from acute illness, reconditioning may take three times as long as it took for deconditioning (Rader & Vaughen, 1994). Table 12–2 lists the consequences of deconditioning and various ways to prevent or minimize these effects. The following discussion focuses mainly on those interventions that are related to acute deconditioning; these include positioning, range of motion (ROM), exercise, general mobilization, self-care activities, and the environment.

Positioning. Although bed rest may be prescribed for patients during the acute stage of illness, there are few instances when movement in bed is not permitted. Ellwood (1990a) suggested using a "positioning prescription" (p. 520), which may include the need for any special equipment (e.g., overbed trapeze or foot board), describe specific positions to be used or avoided, and provide a schedule for repositioning. Turning a patient can improve pulmonary function and decrease the risk of pressure ulcer development (Rousseau, 1993). An upright position in bed also decreases cardiac workload, improves oxygenation, and modifies the orthostasis associated with bed rest (Harper & Lyles, 1988). Varied positioning techniques can be used to prevent joint contractures. For example, the prone position, if tolerated, maintains hip extension and prevents hip flexor contractures (Ellwood, 1990a). The use of pillows, foam wedges, and hand and trochanter rolls helps maintain joints in neutral or functional positions (Silver & Siebens, 1994).

Range of Motion. The importance of ROM exercises in the elderly bedfast patient cannot be overemphasized. These exercises are essential in preventing joint and muscular contractures, promoting joint function, and maintaining an ability to perform ADL. If patients are unable to move their joints, the nurse or therapist must perform passive ROM for them. Family members, too, can be instructed in the proper techniques of ROM. Patients may be able to do all the exercises on their own (active

ROM) or may require assistance with specific joint movements.

The basic components of joint ROM include flexion, extension, abduction, adduction, rotation, supination, and pronation (Earnest, 1993). To prevent muscular contractures, Halar and Bell (1990) recommended 10 to 15 minutes of flexibility exercises three times a week. When mild muscular contractures are present, passive ROM exercises can be performed for 20 to 30 minutes a day with a sustained terminal stretch. A continuous passive mobilization device can be used to provide ROM for joints that are inflamed or infected or have undergone surgery (Kottke, 1990). The presence of severe contractures requires surgical intervention or management by physical and occupational therapists.

Exercise. Kottke (1990) defined therapeutic exercise "as the prescription of bodily movement to correct an impairment, improve musculoskeletal function, or maintain a state of well-being" (p. 436). Specific exercise programs for the elderly during acute hospitalization must be based on each patient's condition and the purpose of such programs. Siebens (1990) noted that the patient's symptoms and vital signs must be monitored in the presence of severe deconditioning. To increase aerobic capacity and maximal oxygen uptake, an exercise should cause an increase of 10 to 20 beats per minute over the patient's resting heart rate, provided the latter is not exceedingly fast (Siebens, 1992). Another guideline is that of perceived exertion on the part of the patient (Siebens, 1992).

Simple bed exercises may be used to attenuate the effects of inactivity on various organ systems. For example, leg and abdominal muscle exercises decrease venous stasis and aid in the prevention of thromboembolic phenomena (Dittmer & Teasell, 1993). Strength in a muscle can be maintained by contracting it for a few seconds a day at 20 to 30% of maximal strength (Halar & Bell, 1990). Isotonic exercise minimizes the effects of body fluid redistribution with bed rest and decreases the severity of orthostatic hypotension when combined with isometric exercises of the lower extremities (Rousseau, 1993). In general, exercise, especially with a nurse, therapist, or family member, may contribute to sensory, psychosocial, and physical stimulation and may thereby foster independence in older people.

General Mobilization. Elderly patients must be mobilized out of bed as soon as their health permits. The first step in mobilization is sitting on the edge of the bed. This strengthens the muscles of the trunk, helps maintain sitting balance, and begins to reverse the loss of postural reflexes (Coletta & Murphy, 1992). The effects of acute deconditioning can be retarded by activities such as the use of a bedside commode or a bathroom (Corcoran, 1991). The use of a commode or toilet also facilitates bladder and bowel elimination. Patients should spend increasing amounts of time sitting in a chair and should ultimately be able to ambulate with assistance as needed. Weight bearing, even for short periods, can reduce the bone demineralization associated with bed rest (Thompson et al., 1993). In short, early mobilization is the primary strategy to prevent the complications of immobility in all organ systems (Coletta & Murphy, 1992).

Self-Care Activities. Elderly patients must be encouraged to participate in ADL as much as they are able. The movements involved in these activities exercise various muscles and joints, maintain muscle strength, and increase self-esteem (Blaylock, 1991; Thompson et al., 1993).

Environment. The environmental factors that influence mobility include physical and architectural characteristics, medical treatments, and staffing (Mobily & Kelley, 1991). These authors cite slippery floors, cluttered rooms, and a lack of assistive devices as additional barriers to mobility that must be addressed. Treatments that limit movement, including intravenous therapy, urinary catheters, and oxygen therapy, should be assessed for their continued need. Adequate numbers of both nursing and therapy staff members are essential for assisting patients in all phases of mobility. Individual patients' goals of care must be mutually set and implemented by all members of the healthcare team, including patients and families (Creditor, 1993).

Discharge Preparation

In general, once the acute illness(es) that required hospitalization has been effectively treated, older patients are discharged. Shine (1983) defined discharge planning as the "process of activities that involve the patient and a team of individuals from various disciplines working together to facilitate the transition of that patient from one environment to another" (p. 403). Shorter hospital stays, which are now common, dictate that discharge planning truly begin at the time of admission. The information obtained on admission and during hospitalization forms the groundwork for decision making, and the early formulation of goals, involving patients, families, and providers, also contributes to the discharge plan. Some hospitals have developed screening criteria that identify the patients at high risk for discharge problems (Fitzig, 1988). The criteria used focus largely on patients' requirements for returning to the desired setting and the type of assistance, if any, that will be available in that setting. At a minimum, a patient returning to independent living, for example, will need to be able to perform ADL safely and effectively. Resources in the community (e.g., home health nursing, homemakers, the Meals on Wheels program) may be used to assist with instrumental ADL and other needs.

If caregivers are available to care for the patient at home, their age, physical abilities, and willingness to help should be determined (Silver & Siebens, 1994). To provide the necessary care, they should be included in all teaching sessions with nurses and therapists. When possible, the home setting should be evaluated to identify accessibility, safety issues, and equipment needs. A wide range of rehabilitative services are available for continued care in the home, and an individualized therapeutic program that is consistent with patient and family goals and abilities can be designed and carried out there (Council on Scientific Affairs, 1990). Rehabilitative services may also be offered in outpatient clinics and adult daycare centers.

For elderly patients who cannot return to independent living at the time of discharge, multiple options are available on a temporary or permanent basis. The choice of settings is dependent on the patient's unresolved impairments or disabilities (Silver & Siebens, 1994). A patient dependent in most ADL may require continued care in a skilled or intermediate long-term care facility. An adult foster home, assisted living facility, or retirement care center may be sufficient for those people who require some assistance or supervision.

INTERVENTIONS: CHRONIC DECONDITIONING

Older adults who are chronically deconditioned can be assessed in much the same way as for acute deconditioning (Siebens, 1990). Much information can be gained from observing patients perform various functional activities. When watching a patient ambulate, for example, clinicians can also assess the patient's endurance (Hoenig & Rubenstein, 1991). They can also observe how a patient gets in and out of a car, as difficulty in this task may be caused by quadriceps weakness (Clark & Siebens, 1993).

A reconditioning program to restore fitness in older adults consists of flexibility and strength training as well as cardiovascular endurance exercises (Kligman & Pepin, 1992). Before beginning any exercise program, patients must be evaluated by their medical care provider and be given precise guidelines and instructions to ensure their safety (Benison & Hogstel, 1986). Several authors provide guidelines and precautions for prescribing exercise for elderly people (Gillett et al., 1993; Larson & Bruce, 1987; Shephard, 1990). Others have reviewed the benefits of exercise in the chronically ill (Hogue et al., 1993) and have researched and reported the specific outcomes of various programs of exercise (Fiatarone et al., 1990). In some patients, simply being encouraged to walk may be sufficient incentive to achieve some improvement in fitness and function (Siebens, 1990).

Functional Levels of Mobility

The concept of mobility has been reviewed by several authors (Creason et al., 1985; Mehmert & Delaney, 1991; Ouellett & Rush, 1992). Rush and Ouellet (1993) described mobility as multidimensional and, based on a literature review, defined four common attributes of mobility: (1) having free and independent movement involving all aspects of life; (2) being goal-directed and purposeful; (3) knowing self in relation to one's environment; and (4) having an ability to adapt and adjust to both the environment and instability. These attributes are significant in that they focus on the person-environment components involved in mobility. Problems with movement are clustered under the umbrella term *impaired physical mobility*, which Creason (1990) defined as a "limitation or absence of person-controlled movement within the physical environment" (p. 55).

Various ways exist of evaluating the mobility of older people, including comprehensive neurological and musculoskeletal examinations. But as Tinetti and Ginter (1988) found in their study of 336 community-dwelling people older than 75 years, neuromuscular findings on examination often did not detect the mobility problems of the subjects. The following discussion focuses on the assessment of various mobility tasks as patients perform them. A functional approach to mobility can help identify both personal and environmental needs. The movements discussed include bed mobility, transfers, wheelchair mobility, and walking and stair climbing.

Bed Mobility

The ability to move in bed is the most fundamental mobility skill. It should be assessed with and without aids such as side rails, electric controls on a bed, and an overbed trapeze. The patient should be asked to perform various activities, which can include turning from side to side, rolling over from a supine to a prone position, moving up in bed and to the side of the bed, shifting weight, sitting up in bed, and bridging or elevating the hips off the bed while in a supine position (McCourt, 1993; Vorhies & Riley, 1993). An inability to perform these tasks may be due to pain, disease, or profound deconditioning. Clinicians should assist patients with these movements as needed while addressing the treatment of the underlying problems. Therapy should begin as soon as possible and, if necessary, family members should be taught the correct techniques of helping with bed mobility. As previously noted, the use of adaptive aids may enhance the patient's ability to move in bed.

Transfers

A *transfer* is a group of movements that enables people to move from one surface to another (Ellwood, 1990b). Transfers may be performed in a sitting or a standing position and with or without assistance. They are believed to be the most important ability for maintaining physical independence (Cooney, 1993). A prerequisite skill in performing a transfer is the ability to achieve a static and dynamic sitting balance (Stolov & Hays, 1990). Patients may not be able to do the necessary movements involved in a transfer because of pain or a lack of strength, flexibility, and coordination. Clinicians can identify these problems while observing the patient attempt to complete a transfer. Other conditions that may contribute to the inability to move from a sitting to a standing position include osteoarthritis of the hip, myopathies and neuropathies of the lower extremities, hip flexor contractures from prolonged sitting, and sciatic nerve impairment. Arthritis of the knee and quadriceps atrophy are conditions that mainly interfere with the knee extension necessary to perform a transfer from sitting to standing (Cooney, 1993). Patients and, if indicated, families need to be taught the correct and safe techniques of transfers, such as the step-by-step procedures, the proper position of the surface and their position in relation to it, and specific precautions.

Various devices can be used to facilitate transfers, including a transfer or sliding board and a disk. The former is used when patients are unable to stand, and the latter when they are unable to pivot on their own. A gait or transfer belt may be used by staff members to assist in transfers; it is thought to reduce the likelihood of injuries to both staff members and patients (Heeschen, 1989). Other equipment that facilitates transfers includes grab-bars and raised toilet seats. A mechanical lifting device should be used by nursing staff members if the patient is heavy and completely unable to safely assist in transfers (Galarneau, 1993).

Wheelchair Mobility

Wheelchairs may be the only mode of mobility for some patients, and in other patients they may be used as an adjunct to walking (e.g., to go longer distances or conserve energy) (McCourt, 1993). Many types of wheelchairs are available, and prescribing a specific chair for an individual patient should be a team process that addresses not only medical and physical concerns but also optimal positioning, cosmetic factors, the type of propulsion, and needs for assistance, comfort, and rest (Currie et al., 1993). Wheelchairs prescribed for stroke patients with hemiplegia, for example, should be of a height that enables them to propel the wheelchair with their unaffected foot.

Wheelchair skills may be measured as the distance traveled before resting, the time it takes to go a certain distance, or the ability to navigate in a variety of environments (Erickson & McPhee, 1993). Clinicians should observe how safely patients transfer in and out of wheelchairs (e.g., by locking the brakes or moving foot rests and leg supports out of the way). Because self-propelling a wheelchair can require considerable strength and cardiovascular endurance, patients should initially be monitored during this activity for excessive stress and exertion (Vorhies & Riley, 1993).

Nurses should provide input into the final choice of a wheelchair for a specific patient. They are in a position to closely observe how the patient uses the wheelchair and to discuss any concerns and suggestions they may have based on their observations. To use a wheelchair safely, patients must have functional hearing and vision and an ability to control its movement, especially if they are using an electric cart or scooter-type device. Nurses can assess patients for deficits in these areas and report their findings to the team. If patients cannot propel or independently transfer to and from the wheelchair, their family members must work with nurses and therapists to learn the necessary skills.

Walking and Stair Climbing

Ambulation is the highest level of mobility and most frequently refers to walking, although people who are confined to wheelchairs and able to move about easily are also referred to as *ambulators*. The act of walking requires adequate strength, balance, coordination, and an ability to bear weight (Vorhies & Riley, 1993). These authors suggest that one way to evaluate these characteristics is to have patients, when appropriate, walk on uneven surfaces, up stairs, on ramps, and over curbs. Other measurements of ambulation include the distance walked, the number of rest periods needed, and the scope of the environment (i.e., whether the patient is limited to mobility in the home or is able to go outside the home to walk, shop, use public transportation) (Erickson & McPhee, 1993).

Tinetti (1986) suggested that walking be assessed by observing various maneuvers of both gait and balance. Her evaluation tool includes seven components of gait and nine of balance and enables care providers to cite specific areas of dysfunction (see Chapter 15).

Several types of assistive devices may significantly improve patients' ability to ambulate; these include canes, crutches, and walkers. Selection of the most appropriate device must be tailored to each patient's needs and abilities, and the device should be adjusted for proper and safe use. A cane can improve stability during walking and can support approximately 25% of the body's weight, thus relieving the strain on one leg (Redford, 1992). It should be used on the side opposite the limited extremity, and the top should just reach the wrist while the patient is standing erect (Wasson et al., 1990). The four-legged, or quad, cane provides more stability than the standard cane and is often prescribed for hemiplegics (Redford, 1992). However, it is unsafe to use outdoors because of the uneven terrain often encountered.

Crutches allow ambulation with minimal or no weight bearing on one leg. The use of both axillary and forearm crutches requires excellent balance and upper extremity strength and thus may be inappropriate for older adults (Cooney, 1993). However, crutches are able to support twice as much body weight as a cane (Wasson et al., 1990).

Because the base of a walker provides maximum support for walking, elderly people with balance deficits and functional arms and hands may benefit from using this device (Wasson et al., 1990). Several types of walkers are available. A *pick-up walker* requires good balance and the strength to pick it up and move it forward (Cooney, 1993). It can be used outdoors and is useful when weight-bearing restrictions are needed, for example, when only touch-down weight bearing of a lower extremity is allowed. However, this type of walker fosters an abnormal gait pattern and is unsafe for retropulsive patients. A wide-based, standalone *hemiwalker* is most often used for patients with dense hemiparesis (Fig. 12–3). It helps by distributing and balancing weight. The *front-wheeled walker* promotes a normal gait pattern, requires less strength to use than the pick-up walker, and can be used by people with a retropulsive gait. It is difficult to use outdoors and over thick carpets and thresholds (Wasson et al., 1990). The newer *four-wheeled walker* is good on all surfaces, promotes a good gait pattern, and often has a seat to enable the patient to rest and a basket for carrying objects. Patients need to be able to set the brakes and control momentum for safety.

Patients must be taught the correct use and ambulation techniques specific to the assistive device prescribed. If they require supervision or assistance with the device, the caregiver must be instructed about the specific aid required as well as safe techniques for use. The living environment should also be assessed and if necessary changed to accommodate the assistive device.

Stair climbing is another aspect of ambulation. It requires a combination of good balance, strength, and hip and knee function (Cooney, 1993). Ascending stairs is especially dependent on hip flexion and knee extension, and descending stairs is especially dependent on knee flexion. Therefore, an assessment of a patient's ability to climb stairs should focus on the hip and knee joints. An assessment should also include the number of steps a patient can climb and will need to climb in his or her own living setting. A handrail on both sides of the stair-

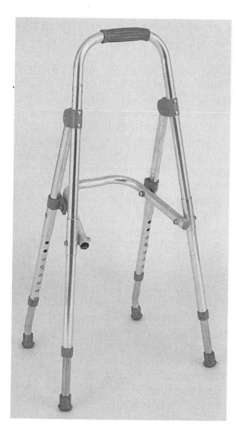

FIGURE 12–3. Hemiwalker. This type of walker allows the patient to lean more weight on the device than a standard four-point cane. Unlike the usual walker, it requires the use of only one arm.

well, good lighting, and strips of color to mark the border of each step will increase the patient's safety while using the stairs.

IMPAIRED MOBILITY DUE TO A STROKE

Epidemiology

Strokes are the third leading cause of death among older people. Approximately 500,000 strokes occur each year, and about 2.5 million community-dwelling people have survived a stroke (Goldstein & Matchar, 1994). Stroke is the classic geriatric disease. Its peak incidence is in the 75 to 84 years of age group, and it

has no cure; working with the effects of the disabling results is the thrust of treatment.

The majority of strokes are caused by infarction (thrombosis is more common than embolism), and in these patients there is a 20 to 40% 30-day mortality rate (Bladin & Chambers, 1994). About 12% of strokes are caused by hemorrhages, which have a much higher mortality rate (50–80%). Regardless of the cause, most patients are left with some form of disability. Only 10% of survivors return to full functional independence. About 40% have minimal amounts of functional problems but can live independently. Another 40% have more significant disability and may require some assistance with daily activities for the rest of their life. As few as 10% of survivors need total assistance.

Virtually all patients who survive a stroke require retraining and rehabilitation for a wide range of functional deficits. Although sensory and perceptual problems, speech difficulties, and psychosocial complications are extremely common and important in the care of older stroke survivors, a full discussion of these topics is beyond the scope of this chapter. The reader is referred to an excellent review of these topics (Kelly, 1990). The following section addresses the enhancement of mobility in stroke survivors.

Neurological and Musculoskeletal Components of Mobility in Stroke

All aspects of movement require a complex integration of (1) neurological control, (2) musculoskeletal responsiveness, and (3) cardiopulmonary capacity to provide the energy for that movement. Following a stroke, it is common for the first two of these components to be affected, and geriatric patients often have underlying problems with the third. A comprehensive approach to mobility problems necessarily involves attention to all these areas.

Most of the functional return is dependent on chance. Patients who regain some return of motor function usually start to do so within the first week, and most of the return of motor function is seen during the first month. However, some improvements may be seen as late as 6 months after the stroke. Sensory deficits or swallowing problems may improve more slowly and may continue up to 2 years after the stroke.

Despite these endogenous improvements, the use of rehabilitation efforts following a stroke has been shown to lead to higher functional levels and is also cost effective (Lehman & Wieland, 1975). A recent metaanalysis of rehabilitation research demonstrated that the average person receiving rehabilitative treatment functioned better than 66% of those who did not receive rehabilitation, with ADL performance and visual-perceptual function showing the most improvement. Younger patients generally fared better than older ones, but gains were also seen among the oldest subjects (Ottenbacher & Jannell, 1993). Age, in itself, does not affect rehabilitation outcome (Falconer et al., 1994). The Agency for Health Care Policy and Research's clinical practice guideline on poststroke rehabilitation provides an excellent summary of rehabilitation studies (Gresham et al., 1995).

The patient usually has flail limbs immediately after a stroke. When motor function returns, the patient will be more functional if his or her arm has been positioned properly to prevent subluxation of the shoulder. Reflex sympathetic dystrophy (the *hand-shoulder syndrome*) can also be prevented by ROM exercises, attention to proper bed positioning, and protecting the shoulder when moving the patient (Braus et al., 1994). Proper body positioning also prevents nerve palsies from occurring. Footboards are sometimes used to prevent plantar flexion contractures of the ankle; however, this technique is controversial and should not be used as a substitute for active ranging of the patient's ankles.

Intensive rehabilitation usually begins once the patient's condition is "stable." True stability is elusive in the older person, and risks of an intervention must be weighed against risks of continued bed rest and deconditioning. The nurse's role in enhancing function is crucial, as interventions left only to physical therapists may be inadequate and delayed. The best outcomes are achieved through a close working relationship between the therapist, who assesses and trains the patient in the gym setting,

and the nurse, who promotes a fuller understanding and facility with these newly learned techniques.

Motor return usually occurs in a fairly predictable sequence; however, not all patients go through this exact sequence and some never achieve all steps. Initially, the limbs are flaccid and there are hyperactive reflexes. This is followed by mass flexor synergism, in which the limb flexes at multiple joints when movement is attempted. Flexor synergism interferes with, but does not completely prevent, learning to reuse the upper extremities; however, the patient cannot learn to walk if every time he or she tries to stand up his or her leg goes into flexion. Extensor synergism usually follows. Once the patient has an extensor synergy pattern, even with poor control, ambulation may be possible, although a brace and adequate physical training are typically needed. If the patient is fortunate to have continued motor return, selective flexion of individual joints may develop, followed by selective extension with decreased flexor tone.

Unfortunately, the return of sensory function is far less predictable. In comparison to motor return, sensory return more significantly affects upper extremity function and the ability to accomplish ADL. There are many ways to adapt to weak muscles. However, if a patient is unaware of his or her deficit owing to perceptual neglect, learning new techniques for independence is much more difficult.

Enhancing Mobility

Mobility enhancement training begins at the bedside as soon as the patient can tolerate sitting up. Even older patients who have been in bed for only a few days should have their blood pressure checked because of the risk of hypotension. A drop of more than 20 mm Hg indicates orthostatic hypotension and may require treatment. Strokes, dehydration, medications, and deconditioning can affect blood pressure regulation. Hypotension should be avoided during the poststroke period, as it may adversely affect outcomes (VanOuwenaller et al., 1986).

The patient should first learn basic bed mobility skills, such as moving from a supine to a seated position and maintaining balance while sitting on the bed. Once his or her sitting balance is stable, the patient should begin practicing transfers. The patient should be taught to move from the bed to a chair or wheelchair, from a chair to the wheelchair, and from the wheelchair to a toilet. An important technique he or she must master is the *stand-pivot transfer*, which consists of movements that are usually practiced in the physical therapy gym, where the therapist can more easily support the patient on an exercise mat. As the patient regains strength and control in the lower extremity, he or she should practice standing in a *standing frame*, which supports an upright position. When the lower extremities have "good strength" (i.e., 4/5—"full range of motion against gravity, some resistance"; Seidel et al., 1995, p. 665) and the patient can balance on the uninvolved side, gait training can be initiated. The patient should progress to walking in parallel bars with the therapist close at hand for safety.

Once the patient can ambulate safely in the parallel bars, he or she should be advanced to using a walker and eventually a cane in many cases. When significant arm weakness or balance problems are present, the patient must use a hemiwalker (see Fig. 12–3). If the patient needs less support than is provided by a hemiwalker, a cane may be used. However, because a single-point cane provides insufficient support for most stroke patients, a four-point cane (platform cane) is often used. Such canes must be used with care when walking out of doors, as a flat surface is required for safe placement of all four points of the cane. Most patients also require a properly fitted wheelchair when traveling long distances. The standard sling seat and back wheelchair seen on most hospital units is inappropriate for long-term use. For the hemiplegic patient, the seat should be lowered to facilitate directional control with the uninvolved leg, and a special cushion may be required if the patient spends a significant amount of time in the chair. A brake handle extension should also be provided so the patient can reach across with the uninvolved arm to set the brake. All these modifications highlight the importance of having a physical therapist evaluate and prescribe the correct equipment.

Facilitating Muscle Tone and Inhibiting Spasticity

A variety of techniques can be used to facilitate muscle tone. Good muscle tone promotes function and inhibits muscle spasticity, which can interfere with independence. Tone and spasticity are not inherently good or bad; rather, the functional effect of these muscle changes should be determined. In many instances, a mild to moderate degree of extensor spasticity can facilitate ambulation. On the other hand, if a patient uses a wheelchair, even mild problems with extensor back muscle tone may make it impossible to control the chair or sit comfortably.

Stretching, ROM exercises, modalities such as heat or massage, and different body positioning techniques are all used to control tone and spasticity. If a patient has weak dorsiflexors of the foot (causing a foot drop) and little spasticity, he or she may benefit from the use of a polyethylene ankle-foot orthosis (AFO) (Fig. 12–4). Patients with less ankle control or more significant spasticity will probably require a metal AFO (Fig. 12–5). Older patients tend to prefer the plastic type, as it is lighter, easier to don, and more cosmetically acceptable. However, the patient's stability and safety are the primary reasons for using an AFO, so the choice is best based on a measurement of functional improvement. The final decision is, of course, the patient's, and there is no use in prescribing a device that the patient is sure to reject once he or she is at home.

Strengthening

An important component in the enhancement of mobility is strengthening. Before they have a stroke, many older people are already chronically deconditioned and have little muscle power in reserve. Performing physical activities is more taxing to the cardiovascular system when one is weak; as a result, it is not uncommon to see deconditioned older people become easily fatigued or even develop angina with minimal exertion. Recent research, however,

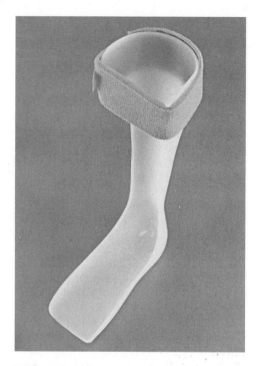

FIGURE 12–4. Polyethylene ankle-foot-orthosis, which is used when there is reasonable stability of the ankle and minimal spasticity.

has shown that 90-year-old nursing home patients are capable of and respond positively to high-intensity strength training (Fiatarone et al., 1990). Following a stroke, the patient's unaffected arm, leg, and trunk muscles need strength training to accept the additional burden of walking with a hemiparetic gait. The patient should attempt to stand (with assistance if necessary) when being tested for strength, because supine testing may give falsely weak results. Close attention must be paid to the patient's cardiopulmonary function, as transfers, walking, and using a wheelchair are very energy consuming.

Home Modifications

Most stroke survivors will need to have handrails installed if there are any steps in the house or will need a ramp built if they use a wheelchair. Ramps require 12 inches of length for

every inch of rise. The doorways in the home will also need to be measured to ensure that they allow the passage of a walker or wheelchair; many doorways in manufactured homes are not wide enough. The bathroom may need modifications such as arm attachments for the toilet, a raised toilet seat, and grab-bars in the tub or near the toilet. If the patient has a bathtub, a tub bench is usually necessary, as tub seats are often unstable. In either case, a hand-held shower hose is necessary.

SUMMARY

The prevention of deconditioning and mobility problems is the foundation of good nursing

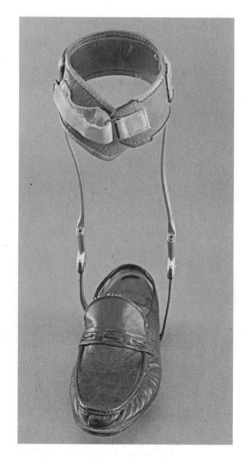

FIGURE 12–5. Rigid metal ankle-foot-orthosis, which is often used by stroke survivors who have excessive spasticity. It can be adjusted for variable degrees of flexion.

care of the elderly patient. Opportunities exist in all care settings to enhance the older person's mobility skills. Functional mobility improves well-being, enhances quality of life, often prevents nursing home placement, and promotes independence (Blocker, 1992). These are worthwhile goals all healthcare providers can work toward during their patients' later stages of life.

REFERENCES

Avorn, J., & Langer, E. (1982). Induced disability in nursing home patients. *Journal of the American Geriatrics Society, 30*, 397–400.

Benison, B., & Hogstel, M. O. (1986). Aging and movement therapy: Essential interventions for the immobile elderly. *Journal of Gerontological Nursing, 12*(12), 8–16.

Bladin, C. F., & Chambers, B. A. (1994). Frequency and pathogenesis of hemodynamic stroke. *Stroke, 25*(11), 2179–2182.

Blaylock, B. (1991). Mobility and ambulation. *Advancing Clinical Care, 6*(6), 20–21, 41.

Blocker, W. P. (1992). Maintaining functional independence by mobilizing the aged. *Geriatrics, 47*(1), 42, 48–50, 53–56.

Bortz, W. M. (1982). Disuse and aging. *Journal of the American Medical Association, 248*, 1203–1208.

Bottomley, J. M. (1994). Principles and practice in geriatric rehabilitation. In D. G. Satin (Ed.), *The clinical care of the aged person: An interdisciplinary perspective* (pp. 230–280). New York: Oxford University Press.

Brandt, K. D., & Slemenda, C. W. (1993). Osteoarthritis: Epidemiology, pathology, and pathogenesis. In H. R. Schumacher (Ed.), *Primer on rheumatic diseases* (pp. 184–190). Atlanta, GA: Arthritis Foundation.

Braus, D. F., Krauss, J. K., & Strobel, J. (1994). The shoulder-hand syndrome after stroke: A prospective clinical trial. *Annals of Neurology, 36*, 728–733.

Brody, J. A., & Foley, D. J. (1987). Epidemiologic considerations. In E. J. Schneider (Ed.), *The teaching nursing home* (pp. 23–41). New York: Raven Press.

Butler, M. (1991). Geriatric rehabilitation nursing. *Rehabilitation Nursing, 16*, 318–321.

Cassel, C. K., & Brody, J. A. (1990). Demography, epidemiology, and aging. In C. K. Cassel, D. E. Riesenberg, L. B. Sorensen & J. R. Walsh (Eds.), *Geriatric medicine* (2nd ed., pp. 16–27). New York: Springer-Verlag.

Clark, G. S., & Siebens, H. C. (1993). Rehabilitation of the geriatric patient. In J. A. DeLisa & B. M. Gans (Eds.), *Rehabilitation medicine: Principles and practice* (2nd ed., pp. 642–665). Philadelphia: J. B. Lippincott.

Cohen, J. J., Sveen, J. D., Walker, J. M., & Brummel-Smith, K. (1987). Establishing criteria for community ambulation. *Topics in Geriatric Rehabilitation, 3*, 71–77.

Coletta, E. M., & Murphy, J. B. (1992). The complications of immobility in the elderly stroke patient. *Journal of the American Board of Family Practice, 5*, 389–397.

Cooney, L. M. (1993). Assessment of immobility in the elderly. *Connecticut Medicine, 57*, 281–286.

Corcoran, P. J. (1991). Use it or lose it—hazards of bedrest and inactivity. *Western Journal of Medicine, 154*, 536–538.

Coroni-Huntley, J., Brock, D. B., Ostfeld, A. M., et al. (1986). *Established populations for epidemiological studies of the elderly. Resource data book.* NIH Publication No. 86-2443 (pp. 1–443). Hyattsville, MD: Department of Health and Human Services, Public Health Service.

Council on Scientific Affairs (1990). Home care in the 1990s. *Journal of the American Medical Association, 263*, 1241–1244.

Creason, N. S. (1990). Mobility: Current bases for practice. In S. G. Funk, E. M. Tornquist, M. T. Champagne, et al. (Eds.), *Key aspects of recovery: Improving nutrition, rest, and mobility* (pp. 55–73). New York: Springer.

Creason, N. S., Pogue, N. J., Nelson, A. A., & Hoyt, C. A. (1985). Validating the nursing diagnosis of impaired physical mobility. *Nursing Clinics of North America, 20*, 669–683.

Creditor, M. C. (1993). Hazards of hospitalization of the elderly. *Annals of Internal Medicine, 118*, 219–223.

Currie, D. M., Hardwick, K., Marburger, R. A., & Britell, C. W. (1993). Wheelchair prescription and adaptive seating. In J. A. DeLisa & B. M. Gans (Eds.), *Rehabilitation medicine: Principles and practice* (2nd ed., pp. 563–585). Philadelphia: J. B. Lippincott.

Dittmer, D. K., & Teasell, R. (1993). Complications of immobilization and bed rest. Part 1: Musculoskeletal and cardiovascular complications. *Canadian Family Physician, 39*, 1428–1437.

Earnest, V. V. (1993). *Clinical skills in nursing practice* (2nd ed.). Philadelphia: J. B. Lippincott.

Ellwood, P. M., Jr. (1990a). Bed positioning. In F. J. Kottke & J. F. Lehmann (Eds.), *Krusen's handbook of physical medicine and rehabilitation* (4th ed., pp. 520–528). Philadelphia: W. B. Saunders.

Ellwood, P. M., Jr. (1990b). Transfers—method, equipment, and preparation. In F. J. Kottke & J. F. Lehmann (Eds.), *Krusen's handbook of physical medicine and rehabilitation* (4th ed., pp. 529–547). Philadelphia: W. B. Saunders.

Erickson, R. P., & McPhee, M. C. (1993). Clinical evaluation. In J. A. DeLisa & B. M. Gans (Eds.), *Rehabilitation medicine: Principles and practice* (2nd ed., pp. 51–95). Philadelphia: J. B. Lippincott.

Falconer, J. A., Naughton, B. J., Strasser, D. C., & Sinacore, J. M. (1994). Stroke inpatient rehabilitation: A comparison across age groups. *Journal of the American Geriatrics Society, 42*, 39–44.

Fiatarone, M. A., & Evans, W. J. (1990). Exercise in the oldest old. *Topics in Geriatric Rehabilitation, 5*(2), 63–77.

Fiatarone, M. A., Marks, E. C., Ryan, N. D., et al. (1990). High-intensity strength training in nonagenarians. *Journal of the American Medical Association, 263*, 3029–3034.

Fitzig, C. (1988). Discharge planning: Nursing focus. In P. J. Volland (Ed.), *Discharge planning: An interdisciplinary approach to continuity of care* (pp. 93–117). Owings Mills, MD: National Health Publishing.

Galarneau, L. (1993). An interdisciplinary approach to mobility and safety education for caregivers and stroke patients. *Rehabilitation Nursing, 18*, 395–399.

Gillett, P. A., Johnson, M., Juretich, M., et al. (1993). The nurse as exercise leader. *Geriatric Nursing, 14*, 133–137.

Gillick, M. R., Serrell, N. A., & Gillick, L. S. (1982). Adverse consequences of hospitalization in the elderly. *Social Science and Medicine, 16*, 1033–1038.

Gogia, P. P., Schneider, V. S., LeBlanc, A. D., et al. (1988). Bed rest effect on extremity muscle torque in healthy men. *Archives of Physical Medicine and Rehabilitation, 69,* 1030–1032.

Goldstein, L. B., & Matchar, B. D. B. (1994). Clinical assessment of stroke. *Journal of the American Medical Association, 271,* 1114–1120.

Gresham, G. E., Duncan, P. W., Stason, W. B., et al. (1995). *Post-stroke rehabilitation.* Clinical Practice Guideline, No. 16. Agency for Health Care Policy and Research Publication No. 95-0662. Rockville, MD: U.S. Department of Health and Human Services, Public Health Service, Agency for Health Care Policy and Research.

Halar, E. M., & Bell, K. R. (1990). Rehabilitation's relationship to inactivity. In F. J. Kottke & J. F. Lehmann (Eds.), *Krusen's handbook of physical medicine and rehabilitation* (4th ed., pp. 1113–1133). Philadelphia: W. B. Saunders.

Halar, E. M., & Bell, K. R. (1993). Contracture and other deleterious effects of immobility. In J. A. DeLisa & B. M. Gans (Eds.), *Rehabilitation medicine: Principles and practice* (2nd ed., pp. 681–699). Philadelphia: J. B. Lippincott.

Harper, C. M., & Lyles, Y. M. (1988). Physiology and complications of bed rest. *Journal of the American Geriatrics Society, 36,* 1047–1054.

Heeschen, S. J. (1989). Getting a handle on patient mobility. *Geriatric Nursing, 10,* 124–125.

Hirsch, C. H., Sommers, L., Olsen, A., et al. (1990). The natural history of functional morbidity in hospitalized older patients. *Journal of the American Geriatrics Society, 38,* 1296–1303.

Hoenig, H. M., & Rubenstein, L. Z. (1991). Hospital-associated deconditioning and dysfunction. *Journal of the American Geriatrics Society, 39,* 220–222.

Hogue, C. C., Cullinan, S., & McConnell, E. (1993). Exercise interventions for the chronically ill: Review and prospects. In S. G. Funk, E. M. Tornquist, M. T. Champagne & R. A. Wiese (Eds.), *Key aspects of caring for the chronically ill: Hospital and home* (pp. 59–79). New York: Springer.

Holm, K., & Hedricks, C. (1989). Immobility and bone loss in the aging adult. *Critical Care Nursing Quarterly, 12*(1), 46–51.

Hopson-Walker, S. D. (1990). Substance abuse in older persons with disability: Assessment and treatment. In B. Kemp, K. Brummel-Smith & J. W. Ramsdell (Eds.), *Geriatric rehabilitation* (pp. 279–293). Boston: Little, Brown, and Co.

Kane, R. A., & Kane, R. L. (1987). *Long-term care* (pp. 31–42). New York: Springer.

Kelly, J. F. (1990). Stroke rehabilitation for elderly patients. In B. Kemp, K. Brummel-Smith & J. W. Ramsdell (Eds.), *Geriatric rehabilitation* (pp. 61–89). Austin, TX: Pro-Ed Press.

Kemp, B. J. (1993). Psychologic care of the older rehabilitation patient. *Clinics in Geriatric Medicine, 9,* 841–857.

Kligman, E. W., & Pepin, E. (1992). Prescribing physical activity for older patients. *Geriatrics, 47*(8), 33–34, 37–44, 47.

Kottke, F. J. (1990). Therapeutic exercise to maintain mobility. In F. J. Kottke & J. F. Lehmann (Eds.), *Krusen's handbook of physical medicine and rehabilitation* (4th ed., pp. 436–451). Philadelphia: W. B. Saunders.

Larson, E. B., & Bruce, R. A. (1987). Health benefits of exercise in an aging society. *Archives of Internal Medicine, 147,* 353–356.

Lazarus, B. A., Murphy, J. B., Coletta, E. M., et al. (1991). The provision of physical activity to hospitalized elderly patients. *Archives of Internal Medicine, 151,* 2452–2456.

Lehman, J. F., & Wieland, G. D. (1975). Stroke: Does rehabilitation affect outcome? *Archives of Physical Medicine and Rehabilitation, 56,* 375–382.

Leon, J., & Lair, T. (1990). *Functional status of noninstitutionalized elderly: Estimates of ADL and IADL difficulties.* Department of Health & Human Services Publication No. PHS90-3462. Rockville, MD: Agency for Health Care Policy and Research.

Lundgren-Lindquist, B., Aniansson, A., & Rundgren, A. (1983). Functional studies in 79-year-olds. III. Walking performance and climbing capacity. *Scandanavian Journal of Rehabilitation Medicine, 15,* 125–131.

McCourt, A. E. (Ed.) (1993). *The specialty practice of rehabilitation nursing: A core curriculum* (3rd ed.). Skokie, IL: Rehabilitation Nursing Foundation.

McVey, L. J., Becker, P. M., Saltz, C. C., et al. (1989). Effect of a geriatric consultation team on functional status of elderly hospitalized patients. *Annals of Internal Medicine, 110,* 79–84.

Mehmert, P. A., & Delaney, C. C. (1991). Validating impaired physical mobility. *Nursing Diagnosis, 2,* 143–154.

Mobily, P. R., & Kelley, L. S. (1991). Iatrogenesis in the elderly: Factors of immobility. *Journal of Gerontological Nursing, 17*(9), 5–11.

Olson, E. V. (1967). The hazards of immobility. *American Journal of Nursing, 67*(4), 780–797.

Ottenbacher, K. J., & Jannell, S. (1993). The results of clinical trials in stroke rehabilitation research. *Archives in Neurology, 50,* 37–44.

Ouellet, L. L., & Rush, K. L. (1992). A synthesis of selected literature on mobility: A basis for studying impaired mobility. *Nursing Diagnosis, 3,* 72–80.

Panicucci, C. L. (1983). Functional assessment of the older adult in the acute care setting. *Nursing Clinics of North America, 18,* 355–363.

Rader, M. C., & Vaughen, J. L. (1994). Management of the frail and deconditioned patient. *Southern Medical Journal, 87,* S61–S65.

Redford, J. B. (1992). Assistive devices for the elderly. In E. Calkins, A. B. Ford & P. R. Katz (Eds.), *Practice of geriatrics* (2nd ed., pp. 185–196). Philadelphia: W. B. Saunders.

Rousseau, P. (1993). Immobility in the aged. *Archives of Family Medicine, 2,* 169–177.

Rush, K. L., & Ouellet, L. L. (1993). Mobility: A concept analysis. *Journal of Advanced Nursing, 18,* 486–492.

Seidel, H. M., Ball, J. W., Dains, J. E., & Benedict, G. W. (1995). *Mosby's guide to physical examination* (3rd ed.). St. Louis: Mosby.

Selikson, S., Damus, K., & Hamerman, D. (1988). Risk factors associated with immobility. *Journal of the American Geriatrics Society, 36,* 707–712.

Shephard, R. J. (1990). The scientific basis of exercise prescribing for the very old. *Journal of the American Geriatrics Society, 38,* 62–70.

Shine, M. S. (1983). Discharge planning for the elderly patient in the acute care setting. *Nursing Clinics of North America, 18,* 403–410.

Siebens, H. (1990). Deconditioning. In B. Kemp, K. Brummel-Smith & J. W. Ramsdell (Eds.), *Geriatric rehabilitation* (pp. 177–191). Boston: Little, Brown, and Co.

Siebens, H. (1992). Practical issues in physical medicine, rehabilitation, and pain management. In E. Calkins, A. B. Ford & P. R. Katz (Eds.), *Practice of geriatrics* (2nd ed., pp. 171–184). Philadelphia: W. B. Saunders.

Silver, K. H. C., & Siebens, A. (1994). Rehabilitation medicine. *Surgical Clinics of North America, 74,* 465–488.

Slimmer, L. W., Lopez, M., LeSage, J., & Ellor, J. (1987). Perceptions of learned helplessness. *Journal of Gerontological Nursing, 13*(5), 33–37.

Stolov, W. C., & Hays, R. M. (1990). Evaluation of the patient. In F. J. Kottke & J. F. Lehmann (Eds.), *Krusen's handbook of physical medicine and rehabilitation* (4th ed., pp. 1–19). Philadelphia: W. B. Saunders.

Teasell, R., & Dittmer, D. K. (1993). Complicatons of immobilization and bed rest. Part 2: Other complications. *Canadian Family Physician, 39,* 1440–1446.

Thompson, J. M., McFarland, G. K., Hirsch, J. E., & Tucker, S. M. (1993). *Mosby's clinical nursing* (3rd ed.). St. Louis: Mosby.

Tinetti, M. E. (1986). Performance-oriented assessment of mobility problems in elderly patients. *Journal of the American Geriatrics Society, 34,* 119–126.

Tinetti, M. E., & Ginter, S. F. (1988). Identifying mobility dysfunctions in elderly patients. *Journal of the American Medical Association, 259,* 1190–1193.

VanOuwenaller, C., Laplace, P. M., & Chantraine, A. (1986). Painful shoulder in hemiplegia. *Archives of Physical Medicine & Rehabilitation, 67*(1), 23–26.

Vorhies, D., & Riley, B. E. (1993). Deconditioning. *Clinics in Geriatric Medicine, 9,* 745–763.

Warshaw, G. A., Moore, J. T., Friedman, W., et al. (1982). Functional disability in the hospitalized elderly. *Journal of the American Medical Association, 248,* 847–850.

Wasson, J. H., Gall, V., McDonald, R., & Liang, M. H. (1990). The prescription of assistive devices for the elderly: Practical considerations. *Journal of General Internal Medicine, 5,* 46–54.

Williams, M. E. (1984). Clinical implications of aging physiology. *American Journal of Medicine, 76,* 1049–1054.

Williams, T. F. (1990). Introduction to rehabilitation and aging. In S. J. Brody & L. G. Pawlson (Eds.), *Aging and rehabilitation II: The state of the practice* (pp. 3–8). New York: Springer.

CHAPTER | 13 |

Pressure Sores

Barbara J. Braden
Janet Cuddigan

Pressure sores are tissue injuries that occur as a result of excessive pressure and cause significant mortality. These lesions are debilitating and frequently painful and can greatly increase the cost of care (Alterescu, 1989; Frantz, 1989; Krouskop et al., 1983).

ETIOLOGICAL FACTORS IN PRESSURE SORE FORMATION

Multiple factors contribute to pressure sore formation in varying degrees by increasing the intensity and duration of pressure exposure or by decreasing tissue tolerance for pressure (Fig. 13–1). Early investigators (e.g., Husain, 1953; Kosiak, 1959) demonstrated that lower pressures of longer duration could produce the same tissue injury as intense pressures of short duration. Daniel and colleagues (1981) also demonstrated that muscle is more susceptible to pressure injury than is normothermic skin.

Because they are more likely to be exposed to pressure of high intensity and long duration, people with conditions that compromise mobility, activity, or sensory perception have a higher risk of developing pressure sores than do people who can independently move in bed, ambulate, and respond purposefully to the painful pressure sensations (Allman et al., 1986; Barbenel et al., 1977; Ek & Boman, 1982; Manley, 1978; Moolten, 1972). Nevertheless, the intensity and duration of pressure does not explain every pressure lesion. Two studies in which the sitting patterns of spinal cord–injured patients were continuously monitored found multihour exposure to high sitting pressures and wide variability among subjects without subsequent pressure sore formation (Merbitz et al., 1985; Patterson & Fisher, 1986). This variability has prompted scientists to consider other factors that interact with pressure to increase or decrease susceptibility to skin injury.

Factors affecting tissue tolerance for pressure can be classified as either *extrinsic* or *intrinsic*. Extrinsic factors are physical factors that weaken the outer layers of the skin, making it more susceptible to the effects of pressure. Intrinsic factors influence either the supporting structures of the skin or physiological processes in such a way that tissue injury occurs at lower external pressures.

Extrinsic Factors

Extrinsic factors affecting tissue tolerance include friction, shear, and exposure to moisture. Friction affects the superficial layers of the skin and may be a problem in patients who cannot lift or be lifted sufficiently during a position change to avoid dragging the skin over the bed linens. It also may be a problem with patients who are agitated or spastic or who use orthopedic devices that become sources of friction. In experiments using swine to investigate the effects of friction, Dinsdale (1974) compared the amount of pressure required to produce ulceration between hips that had been treated with friction and untreated hips. He found that in the absence of friction a pressure of 290 mm Hg was required to produce ulceration, whereas a pressure of only 45 mm Hg would produce ulceration in skin pretreated with friction.

Shear forces, which refer to tangential rather than perpendicular pressure, also diminish tissue tolerance. Shearing injuries most com-

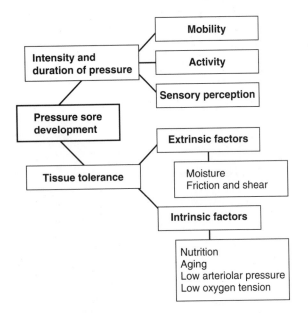

FIGURE 13–1. Conceptual schema for etiological factors in pressure sore development.

monly occur when the head of the bed is elevated and the patient slides downward, causing shear to develop in the sacral area. This results in deformation and destruction of the vascular bed (Newell et al., 1970; Reichel, 1958). In a study examining shearing in normal, geriatric, and paraplegic subjects, investigators found that geriatric and paraplegic subjects developed substantially greater shearing forces (accompanied by decrements in pulsatile blood flow) than did healthy, young subjects (Bennett et al., 1984). These findings support clinical studies demonstrating a higher incidence of pressure sores among geriatric and spinal cord–injured patients (Ek & Boman, 1982; Richardson & Meyer, 1981).

Exposure of the skin to moisture is frequently mentioned as a risk factor. Sources of moisture most frequently implicated are urine and feces, although perspiration may be a significant source in certain patients. Flam (1987) found that as many as 200 g of moisture are transmitted through the skin of the supine patient. Not unexpectedly, fecal incontinence is most strongly associated with pressure sore formation. In one study, however, urinary catheterization was more strongly associated with pressure sore formation than was urinary incontinence.

Intrinsic Factors

Certain intrinsic factors can change the skin architecture or the oxygen delivery capabilities of the blood and vascular bed to such an extent that the external mechanical load required to cause ischemia is decreased. Examples of these factors include undernutrition, aging, low arteriolar pressure, and elevations in body temperature.

The nutritional deficiencies most frequently related to pressure sores are protein-calorie, iron (Bergstrom & Braden, 1992; Moolten, 1972; Vasile & Chaitin, 1972), ascorbic acid (Hunter & Rajan, 1971), and trace mineral deficiencies (Prasad, 1982). All of these deficiencies can contribute to a decrease in the quality and integrity of the components of soft tissue, particularly collagen. Protein nutriture, as reflected by serum albumin and hemoglobin concentra-

tions, has been related to the presence of pressure sores (Allman et al., 1986; Artigue & Hyman, 1979; Bennett et al., 1984; Moolten, 1972; Ryan, 1979). In a prospective study of at-risk patients, Bergstrom and Braden (1992) found that patients who did not develop pressure sores consumed a higher average amount of protein (mean = 118.5% recommended daily allowance [RDA]) than those who developed pressure sores (mean = 88.8% RDA).

Hypocholesterolemia has been associated with pressure sore formation. Trumbore and associates (1990) examined 40 patients on low-fat, low-cholesterol, tube-fed diets and found that low cholesterol was a better predictor of pressure sores than was serum albumin. There is also some evidence that fatty acid deficiencies affect skin integrity. Linoleic acid, for example, contributes to the waterproof barrier with the stratum corneum (Roe, 1986).

Ascorbic acid deficiency can impair wound healing in animals and humans (Irwin & Hutchins, 1976; Ringsdorf & Cheraskin, 1982), probably as a result of problems in the formation and maintenance of collagen. Vitamin C supplementation (1000 mg/day) has been shown to increase the rate at which pressure sores heal (Taylor et al., 1974) and may have a role in the prevention of pressure sores (Irwin & Hutchins, 1976; Taylor et al., 1974). Certain trace minerals such as zinc and copper have also been related to improved quality of collagen and hypothetically decreased pressure sore formation (Prasad, 1982). No direct evidence of this link exists, however, although zinc supplementation has been shown to increase wound healing (Haeger et al., 1974; Hallbook & Lanner, 1972; Prasad, 1982).

With aging, certain changes occur in the skin and its supporting structures (Kenney, 1982). Elastin fibers become more rigid, allowing for a greater degree of mechanical load to be transferred from externally applied pressure to the underlying vasculature, thereby leading to ischemia (Krouskop, 1983). One study showed that when sitting on an instrumented seat, elderly subjects have median blood flow rates roughly one third of those of younger subjects (Bennett et al., 1984). Several studies have suggested that older people are more susceptible to pressure sore formation (Andersen & Kvorning, 1982; Bergstrom & Braden, 1992; Ek & Boman, 1982; Manley, 1978).

Low blood pressure diminishes tissue tolerance for pressure by decreasing the pressure that is required to effect vascular closure (Seiler & Stahelin, 1979). Larsen and colleagues (1979) found that hypertensive subjects could withstand higher external pressures before vascular occlusion occurred than could normotensive subjects. In a retrospective study, more than 20% of the subjects with pressure sores had a systolic blood pressure below 100 mm Hg (Moolten, 1972); in another prospective study, subjects with a diastolic blood pressure below 60 mm Hg were found to be predisposed to developing pressure sores (Bergstrom & Braden, 1992).

Pressure sore development has also been related to psychological factors, including those that influence patients' motivation and emotional energy to deal with their self-care needs (Anderson & Andberg, 1979). A relationship between stress and pressure sore formation has been hypothesized based on the effect of cortisol on mechanical properties of the skin. In a study of nursing home residents, Braden (1990) found significantly higher levels of serum cortisol in those residents who developed pressure sores.

Cigarette smoking has been reported to have a significant positive correlation with pressure sores in a group of spinal cord–injured patients, and the incidence and severity of existing sores were greater in those patients with higher pack-year histories (Lamid & El Ghatit, 1983). Smoking's effect on wound healing also is supported in animal model studies (Mosely et al., 1978).

Several investigators have demonstrated an association between disease states and pressure sore formation (Allman et al., 1986; Berlowitz & Wilking, 1989; Hassard, 1975). With the exception of diabetes and vascular disease, the disease states identified in these studies lead to immobility and probably do not represent independent risk factors.

STAGING

Histological studies of pressure sores have demonstrated consistent patterns of tissue in-

flammation, ischemia, injury, and necrosis (Shea, 1975; Witkowski & Parish, 1982). Shea's work is used as the basis for the most commonly used pressure sore classification system. The following adaptation of Shea's classification is recommended by the pressure ulcer panels sponsored by the Agency for Health Care Policy and Research (AHCPR) (Bergstrom et al., 1994; Panel for the Prediction and Prevention of Pressure Ulcers in Adults, 1992), the National Pressure Ulcer Advisory Panel (National Pressure Ulcer Advisory Panel, 1989), and the Wound, Ostomy, and Continence Nurses Society (International Association for Enterostomal Therapy, 1991). According to this system, pressure sores can be staged as follows (Fig. 13–2):

Stage I: Nonblanchable erythema of intact skin, the heralding lesion of skin ulceration. In individuals with darker skin, discoloration of the skin, warmth, edema, induration, or hardness may also be indicators.

Stage II: Partial-thickness skin loss involving epidermis and/or dermis. The ulcer is superficial and presents clinically as an abrasion, blister, or shallow crater.

Stage III: Full-thickness skin loss involving damage to or necrosis of subcutaneous tissue that may extend down to, but not through, underlying fascia. The ulcer presents clinically as a deep crater, with or without undermining the adjacent tissue.

Stage IV: Full-thickness skin loss, with extensive destruction, tissue necrosis, or damage to muscle, bone, or supporting structures (e.g., tendon or joint capsule). Undermining and sinus tracts may also be associated with stage IV pressure ulcers.

Extra vigilance is required when applying these criteria to dark-skinned individuals (see stage I) and patients with casts or other orthopedic devices. Clinicians should check under the edges of casts for pressure sores and be alert to the need to revise casts that are too tight or painful (Panel for the Prediction and Prevention of Pressure Ulcers in Adults, 1992).

Although this classification system is highly practical in clinical settings in which staff

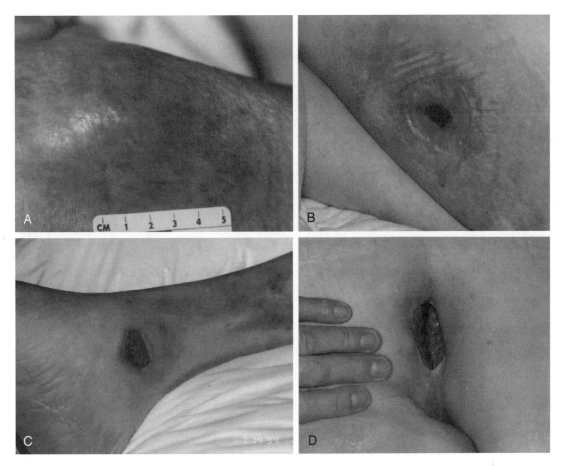

FIGURE 13–2. Examples of pressure sore stages. *A*, Stage I pressure sore. *B*, Stage II pressure sore. *C*, Stage III pressure sore. *D*, Stage IV pressure sore.

members vary in educational level and expertise, it has many limitations. This four-stage system provides only a gross assessment of the severity of a pressure sore. It reveals nothing related to wound size, severity, or the potential for healing. As a result, it does little to assist the advanced practice nurse (APN) in making decisions concerning treatment or monitoring the efficacy of that treatment.

A wound assessment tool that does assist in detailing the severity and status of a pressure sore is the Pressure Sore Status Tool (PSST) developed by Barbara Bates-Jensen (Fig. 13–3) (Bates-Jensen, 1990). It is composed of 13 subscales, each rated from 1 to 5 and representing a physical attribute of pressure sores that clini-

cians consider when evaluating wound status. Scores range from 13 to 65. Lower scores indicate lesser severity and greater healing potential, and higher scores indicate greater severity and lesser healing potential. These scores can also be used to monitor treatment. Scores that trend downward over time indicate progress toward healing, and scores that trend upward indicate degeneration of the wound (Bates-Jensen et al., 1992). The PSST has demonstrated good reliability and validity and can be a valuable asset to the APN who treats chronic wounds and pressure sores (Bates-Jensen et al., 1992).

The Pressure Ulcer Scale for Healing (PUSH) was recently developed by the National Pres-

PRESSURE SORE STATUS TOOL   NAME_____

Complete the rating sheet to assess pressure sore status. Evaluate each item by picking the response that best describes the wound and entering the score in the item score column for the appropriate date.

Location: Anatomic site. Circle, identify right (**R**) or left (**L**) and use "**X**" to mark site on body diagrams:

_____	Sacrum & coccyx	_____	Lateral ankle
_____	Trochanter	_____	Medial ankle
_____	Ischial tuberosity	_____	Heel Other Site _____

Shape: Overall wound pattern; assess by observing perimeter and depth.
Circle and <u>date</u> appropriate description:

_____	Irregular	_____	Linear or elongated
_____	Round/oval	_____	Bowl/boat
_____	Square/rectangle	_____	Butterfly Other Shape _____

Item	Assessment	Date	Date	Date
		Score	Score	Score
1. Size	1 = Length x width < 4 sq cm 2 = Length x width 4 -16 sq cm 3 = Length x width 16.1 - 36 sq cm 4 = Length x width 36.1 - 80 sq cm 5 = Length x width > 80 sq cm			
2. Depth	1 = Non-blanchable erythema on intact skin 2 = Partial thickness skin loss involving epidermis &/or dermis 3 = Full thickness skin loss involving damage or necrosis of subcutaneous tissue; may extend down to but not through underlying fascia; &/or mixed partial & full thickness &/or tissue layers obscured by granulation tissue 4 = Obscured by necrosis 5 = Full thickness skin loss with extensive destruction, tissue necrosis or damage to muscle, bone or supporting structures			
3. Edges	1 = Indistinct, diffuse, none clearly visible 2 = Distinct, outline clearly visible, attached, even with wound base 3 = Well-defined, not attached to wound base 4 = Well-defined, not attached to base, rolled under, thickened 5 = Well-defined, fibrotic, scarred or hyperkeratotic			
4. Under-mining	1 = Undermining < 2 cm in any area 2 = Undermining 2-4 cm involving < 50% wound margins 3 = Undermining 2-4 cm involving > 50% wound margins 4 = Undermining > 4 cm in any area 5 = Tunneling &/or sinus tract formation			
5. Necrotic Tissue Type	1 = None visible 2 = White/grey non-viable tissue &/or non-adherent yellow slough 3 = Loosely adherent yellow slough 4 = Adherent, soft, black eschar 5 = Firmly adherent, hard, black eschar			
6. Necrotic Tissue Amount	1 = None visible 2 = < 25% of wound bed covered 3 = 25% to 50% of wound covered 4 = > 50% and < 75% of wound covered 5 = 75% to 100% of wound covered			

FIGURE 13–3 *See legend on opposite page*

Item	Assessment	Date	Date	Date
		Score	Score	Score
7. Exudate Type	1 = None or bloody 2 = Serosanguineous: thin, watery, pale red/pink 3 = Serous: thin, watery, clear 4 = Purulent: thin or thick, opaque, tan/yellow 5 = Foul purulent: thick, opaque, yellow/green with odor			
8. Exudate Amount	1 = None 2 = Scant 3 = Small 4 = Moderate 5 = Large			
9. Skin color Surrounding Wound	1 = Pink or normal for ethnic group 2 = Bright red &/or blanches to touch 3 = White or grey pallor or hypopigmented 4 = Dark red or purple &/or non-blanchable 5 = Black or hyperpigmented			
10. Peripheral Tissue Edema	1 = Minimal swelling around wound 2 = Non-pitting edema extends < 4 cm around wound 3 = Non-pitting edema extends $\geq$ 4 cm around wound 4 = Pitting edema extends < 4 cm around wound 5 = Crepitus &/or pitting edema extends $\geq$ 4 cm			
11. Peripheral Tissue Induration	1 = Minimal firmness around wound 2 = Induration < 2 cm around wound 3 = Induration 2-4 cm extending < 50% around wound 4 = Induration 2-4 cm extending $\geq$ 50% around wound 5 = Induration > 4 cm in any area			
12. Granulation Tissue	1 = Skin intact or partial thickness wound 2 = Bright, beefy red; 75% to 100% of wound filled &/or tissue overgrowth 3 = Bright, beefy red; < 75% & > 25% of wound filled 4 = Pink, &/or dull, dusky red &/or fills $\leq$ 25% of wound 5 = No granulation tissue present			
13. Epithelialization	1 = 100% wound covered, surface intact 2 = 75% to <100% wound covered &/or epithelial tissue extends >0.5cm into wound bed 3 = 50% to <75% wound covered &/or epithelial tissue extends to <0.5cm into wound bed 4 = 25% to < 50% wound covered 5 = < 25% wound covered			
TOTAL SCORE				
SIGNATURE				

PRESSURE SORE STATUS CONTINUUM

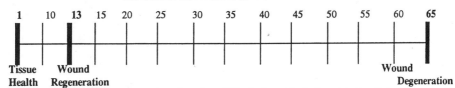

Plot the total score on the Pressure Sore Status Continuum by putting an "X" on the line and the date beneath the line. Plot multiple scores with their dates to see-at-a-glance regeneration or degeneration of the wound.

FIGURE 13–3. Pressure sore status tool. (Copyright 1990 by B. Bates-Jensen: New pressure ulcer status tool.)

sure Ulcer Advisory Panel. This tool focuses on three critical parameters (i.e., surface area, exudate amount, and predominant tissue type) to provide a simple and reliable tool to monitor pressure ulcer healing (or deterioration) (Thomas et al., 1997). The tool was developed using research data and has been validated in a multisite, retrospective study.

PREVENTION OF PRESSURE SORES

Risk Assessment

Over the years, an assortment of screening tools have been used or proposed to determine if a patient is at risk for pressure sore development. These tools vary from simple (e.g., rating scales, serum albumin, serum transferrin) to complex (e.g., thermography, laser Doppler flowmetry, ultrasound) and also vary in terms of cost, invasiveness, clinical utility, reliability, and predictive validity. Fortunately, the tools with the highest predictive validity and acceptable reliability are also the least costly, least invasive, and most utilitarian. These tools are the rating scales that have emerged from nursing practice and research.

The two rating scales that have been recommended by the AHCPR panel in the Pressure Ulcer Prevention Guidelines are the Norton Scale (Norton et al., 1962) and the Braden Scale (Bergstrom et al., 1987). These tools were judged by the panel to have undergone sufficient testing to justify their use in making clinical judgments. A brief description of each of these tools and their reliability and validity may be helpful in selecting one or the other for clinical implementation.

The Norton Scale consists of five parameters: physical condition, mental state, activity, mobility, and incontinence, each rated from 1 to 4 (Fig. 13–4). It has good sensitivity (ability to identify true positives while minimizing false negatives) but low to moderate specificity (ability to identify true negatives while minimizing false positives) (Goldstone & Goldstone, 1982; Goldstone & Roberts, 1980). No tests of interrater reliability have been reported.

The Braden Scale (Bergstrom et al., 1987; Braden & Bergstrom, 1989, 1992, 1994) is composed of six subscales reflecting sensory perception, skin moisture, activity, mobility, nutritional intake, and friction and shear (Fig. 13–5). Subscales are rated from 1 to 3 or 1 to 4, and each rating is accompanied by criteria for rating. Potential scores range from 4 to 23. The Braden Scale has demonstrated excellent sensitivity and good specificity in hospital and nursing home settings as well as excellent interrater reliability when used by registered nurses (RNs) (Bergstrom et al., 1987, in press; Braden & Bergstrom, 1994).

These risk assessments measure broad categories of factors that put patients at risk but do not measure all factors. Other factors that have been found to predict risk for developing pressure sores are advanced age, low diastolic blood pressure, elevated body temperature, and inadequate current intake of protein (Allman et al., 1986). Clinicians should keep in mind that the risk assessment tools are intended to supplement nursing judgment but not replace it. They should consider these additional factors when they are assessing risk for pressure sore development.

Using Risk Assessment in Prevention Programs

Patients at risk for pressure sores should be identified on admission to healthcare facilities and homecare services. The activity subscales of these risk assessment tools can be used as an initial screen, and all patients who are bedfast or chairfast should be further assessed. Following the initial assessment, reassessment should be conducted at periodic intervals depending on the rapidity with which the condition changes and whenever a major change in condition occurs. The APN should be aware that the first 2 weeks following admission are the time of highest risk for pressure sore development. In one prospective study of nursing home residents, investigators followed the cases of new admissions for 3 months and found that 80% of those individuals who developed a pressure sore did so within 2 weeks of admission and that 96% did so within 3

Norton Scale

		Physical condition		Mental condition		Activity		Mobility		Incontinent		
		Good	4	Alert	4	Ambulant	4	Full	4	Not	4	Total
		Fair	3	Apathetic	3	Walk/help	3	Slightly limited	3	Occasional	3	score
		Poor	2	Confused	2	Chairbound	2	Very limited	2	Usually/urine	2	
		Very bad	1	Stupor	1	Stupor	1	Immobile	1	Doubly	1	
Name	Date											

FIGURE 13–4. Norton Scale. (From Norton, D., McLaren, R., & Exton-Smith, A. N. ([1962], *An investigation of geriatric nursing problems in hospitals.* London: National Corporation for the Care of Old People [now the Centre for Policy on Ageing]).

weeks of admission (Allman et al., 1986). Thus, an appropriate schedule for reassessing pressure sore risk in nursing homes might be every week for 4 weeks with routine quarterly assessments thereafter. Intervals for reassessment have not been studied in other settings. In hospitals that have implemented risk assessment, protocols have typically called for reassessments to be performed daily in the intensive care unit and every other day in general medical-surgical units. In homecare, it is thought that screening should be done with every RN visit, as these visits are generally correlated with the severity of illness of the patient.

Preventive Protocols Based on the Level of Risk

If a risk assessment tool is being used, preventive interventions should become more intense as risk increases. Although Norton did much of the seminal work on pressure sore prevention, she made no recommendations concerning appropriate protocols based on level of risk. Most of the subsequent discussion focuses on the use of the Braden Scale, since Braden and Bergstrom (1992) did make such recommendations. However, the following protocols should also be helpful to those clinicians using the Norton Scale.

The prevention of pressure sores is based on the elimination of those risk factors that are amenable to intervention. Because exposure to intense and prolonged pressure is the primary risk factor, at any level of risk the initial nursing intervention is to reduce pressure. Pressure reduction may be achieved in a variety of ways. The patient can be frequently repositioned using pillows, foam wedges, or other protective devices that assist in special positioning problems or protect specific bony prominences; in addition, pressure reduction surfaces can be used on the bed or chair.

Mild Risk. This level of risk is indicated by Braden Scale scores of 15 to 18. (If major risk factors not measured by the Braden Scale are present, the nurse should advance to interventions appropriate at the next level of risk.) The patient should use a pressure reduction surface and should be moved according to a turning schedule. If narcotics or sedatives are being used, particularly at night, extra attention should be paid to turning during those times of heavy sedation. Any potential that the patient has for remobilization should be optimized. Problems related to moisture, nutrition, friction, and shear should be managed.

Moderate Risk. Braden Scale scores of 12 to 14 indicate moderate risk. Close attention should be paid to an individualized turning schedule that accounts for periods when the patient must be on his or her back, such as during meals and morning care. Sample turning schedules are presented in Figure 13–6, and these should be further altered to meet

Braden Scale for Predicting Pressure Sore Risk

Patient's Name _____ Evaluator's Name _____ Date of Assessment

SENSORY PERCEPTION ability to respond meaningfully to pressure-related discomfort	**1. Completely limited:** Unresponsive (does not moan, flinch, or grasp) to painful stimuli, due to diminished level of consciousness or sedation OR limited ability to feel pain over most of body surface.	**2. Very limited:** Responds only to painful stimuli. Cannot communicate discomfort except by moaning or restlessness OR has a sensory impairment which limits the ability to feel pain or discomfort over 1/2 of body.	**3. Slightly limited:** Responds to verbal commands, but cannot always communicate discomfort or need to be turned. OR has some sensory impairment which limits ability to feel pain or discomfort in 1 or 2 extremities.	**4. No impairment:** Responds to verbal commands. Has no sensory deficit which would limit ability to feel or voice pain or discomfort.			
MOISTURE degree to which skin is exposed to moisture	**1. Consistently moist:** Skin is kept moist almost constantly by perspiration, urine, etc. Dampness is detected every time patient is moved or turned.	**2. Very moist:** Skin is often but not always moist. Linen must be changed at least once a shift.	**3. Occasionally moist:** Skin is occasionally moist, requiring an extra linen change approximately once a day.	**4. Rarely moist:** Skin is usually dry; linen requires changing only at routine intervals.			
ACTIVITY degree of physical activity	**1. Bedfast:** Confined to bed.	**2. Chairfast:** Ability to walk severely limited or non-existent. Cannot bear own weight and/or must be assisted into chair or wheelchair.	**3. Walks occasionally:** Walks occasionally during day, but for very short distances, with or without assistance. Spends majority of each shift in bed or chair.	**4. Walks frequently:** walks outside the room at least twice a day and inside room at least once every 2 hours during waking hours.			
MOBILITY ability to change and control body position	**1. Completely immobile:** Does not make even slight changes in body or extremity position without assistance.	**2. Very limited:** Makes occasional slight changes in body or extremity position but unable to make frequent or significant changes independently.	**3. Slightly limited:** Makes frequent though slight changes in body or extremity position independently.	**4. No limitations:** Makes major and frequent changes in position without assistance.			

	1. Very poor:	2. Probably inadequate:	3. Adequate:	4. Excellent:	
NUTRITION *usual* food intake pattern	Never eats a complete meal. Rarely eats more than ⅓ of any food offered. Eats 2 servings or less of protein (meat or dairy products) per day. Takes fluids poorly. Does not take a liquid dietary supplement OR is NPO and/or maintained on clear liquids or IVs for more than 5 days	Rarely eats a complete meal and generally eats only about ½ of any food offered. Protein intake includes only 3 servings of meat or dairy products per day. Occasionally will take a dietary supplement OR receives less than optimum amount of liquid diet or tube feeding.	Eats over half of most meals. Eats a total of 4 servings of protein (meat, dairy products) each day. Occasionally will refuse a meal, but will usually take a supplement if offered. OR is on a tube feeding or TPN regimen which probably meets most of nutritional needs.	Eats most of every meal. Never refuses a meal. Usually eats a total of 4 or more servings of meat and dairy products. Occasionally eats between meals. Does not require supplementation.	
	1. Problem:	2. Potential problem:	3. No apparent problem:		
FRICTION AND SHEAR	Requires moderate to maximum assistance in moving. Complete lifting without sliding against sheets is impossible. Frequently sliding against sheets is impossible. Frequently slides down in bed or chair, requiring frequent repositioning with maximum assistance. Spasticity, contractures or agitation leads to almost constant friction	Moves feebly or requires minimum assistance. During a move skin probably slides to some extent against sheets, chair, restraints, or other devices. Maintains relatively good position in chair or bed most of the time but occasionally slides down.	Moves in bed and in chair independently and has sufficient muscle strength to lift up completely during move. Maintains good position in bed or chair at all times.		

Total Score

FIGURE 13–5. Braden Scale. (Copyright 1988 by B. J. Braden & N. Bergstrom: The Braden Scale for predicting pressure sore risk.)

Turning Schedules

These turning schedules may be used to organize care on nursing units with large numbers of patients who are at risk for pressure sores. Patients on a team or unit can be assigned to one of three schedules in a balanced manner (e.g., if six patients are at risk, two would be assigned to each of the three schedules). These schedules may have to be adjusted to each day, depending on other components of the patients schedule.

Direction of Turn	Schedule 1	Schedule 2	Schedule 3
1. Back **(breakfast & bath)**	7:00–9:00	7:30–9:30	8:00–10:00
2. Right side	9:00–11:00	9:30–11:30	10:00–12:00
3. Back **(lunch)**	11:00–1:00	11:30–1:30	12:00–2:00
4. Right side	1:00–3:00	1:30–3:30	2:00–4:00
5. Left side	3:00–5:00	3:30–5:30	4:00–6:00
6. Back **(dinner)**	5:00–7:00	5:30–7:30	6:00–8:00
7. Left side	7:00–9:00	7:30–9:30	8:00–10:00
8. Right side	9:00–11:00	9:30–11:30	10:00–12:00
9. Left side	11:00–1:00	11:30–1:30	12:00–2:00
10. Back	1:00–3:00	1:30–3:30	2:00–4:00
11. Right side	3:00–5:00	3:30–5:30	4:00–6:00
12. Left side	5:00–7:00	5:30–7:30	6:00–8:00

FIGURE 13–6. Sample turning schedules.

individual patient needs. The patient should be repositioned with assistance and attention to good body mechanics, using pillows and pads to protect bony prominences. To avoid pressure on the trochanter, lateral positioning should not exceed 30 degrees (Seiler & Stahelin, 1985). Legs should be supported on pillows with the heels off the mattress when lying recumbent.

High Risk. Braden Scale scores of less than 12 indicate high risk. Turning schedules for these patients should include either increased frequency of turns or assisted frequent, small shifts in body weight. Lateral turns should not exceed 30 degrees, and if at all possible the head of the bed should not be elevated beyond 30 degrees. Foam wedges are helpful in lateral positioning and can be used to increase the frequency of repositioning by being pulled out slightly every 30 minutes to 1 hour. When patients can tolerate the prone position, it should be added to the turning schedule, as it allows the most common sites of pressure sore formation (e.g., sacrum, trochanters, heels) to be totally relieved of pressure while also preventing flexion contractures of the hips. Impeccable

padding and positioning are required if the prone position is to be employed. If supporting the legs on pillows fails to protect the heels while the patient is supine, consult physical therapy or occupational therapy to construct devices that adequately protect the heels from excessive pressure.

If the Braden Score is below 9 or the patient has intractable or severe pain exacerbated by turning, use of a low–air loss bed may be indicated. It is important to remember that low pressures of long duration are capable of causing pressure sores, and that turning is still necessary to prevent pressure sores and other complications of immobility. However, the nurse must be clear about the goal of care for these patients. If the patient is terminally ill and the goal of care is the provision of comfort, a rigorous schedule of turning may not be appropriate.

Interventions for Specific Problems

Risk assessment allows the APN to identify not only the level of risk but also specific problems or factors that contribute to that level of risk. In some instances the problems identified are amenable to intervention, whereas at other times they are not. It may be possible, for example, to restore mobility to the person who has fractured a hip, but it is not possible to restore mobility to a person whose spinal cord has been transected at the cervical level. In instances in which mobility, activity, or sensory perception cannot be restored, the potential consequences (exposure to prolonged, intense pressure) can usually be mitigated.

Reducing the Exposure to Pressure

Remobilization of the Immobile. When a patient is found to have deficits in activity or mobility, the nurse should always be alert to the patient's potential to become remobilized. During an episode of illness, it is very easy for an elderly person to be less active than is warranted and to enter into a spiral of deconditioning and gradual decline. This leads to a myriad of complications as well as increased pressure sore risk. A physical therapy consultation may be helpful in determining the degree to which remobilization is possible and to begin the process of remobilization. The physical therapist, the nurse, and, if possible, the patient should collaborate in developing a plan that is clear about the responsibilities that each person holds in the process of remobilization.

In instances in which the return to full mobility is not possible, the patient can be taught to make small shifts in body position. This can be achieved by moving the legs and shifting weight from one buttock to another. Wheelchair-bound people need to be taught to lift their buttocks off the seating surface every 20 minutes. It may be helpful to teach the person to use some external cue (such as television commercials) to remember to "lift-off." If the patient is incapable of performing lift-offs or making shifts in his or her seating position, the nurse or caregiver should implement an hourly schedule for repositioning (Panel for the Prediction and Prevention of Pressure Ulcers in Adults, 1992).

Use of Special Surfaces. If the patient is bedbound or chairbound, use of a special support surface for the bed or wheelchair is advised to decrease interface pressure over bony prominences (Panel for the Prediction and Prevention of Pressure Ulcers in Adults, 1992). These surfaces include overlays (mattress or wheelchair seating), mattress replacements, and specialty beds. Mattress overlays and replacements may be classified as either static (i.e., foam, gels) or dynamic (i.e., alternating pressure surfaces). Specialty beds are classified as either low air loss or air fluidized.

The comparative effectiveness of mattress overlays, mattress replacements, and specialty beds is difficult to evaluate, but findings converge on the following results:

1. Almost every surface tested reduces interface pressure below that of a standard hospital mattress (Bliss et al., 1967; Goldstone et al., 1982; Jacobs, 1989)
2. Foam overlays that are 2 to 3 inches thick do not compare favorably with other pressure-reduction surfaces (Stapleton, 1986), including thicker foam surfaces (Krouskop, 1986)
3. Gel-filled overlays and mattresses reduce pressure better than most foam overlays (Berjian et al., 1983; Krouskop, 1986)
4. Solid foam overlays and foam mattress replacements that are 4 or more inches thick are more effective in preventing pressure sores than are convoluted foam overlays (Kemp et al., 1993; Vyhlidal et al., 1997).
5. Air-fluidized beds and low–air loss beds result in substantial pressure reduction and appear to be beneficial in healing pressure sores, although results are not always dramatic (Allman et al., 1987; Bennett et al., 1989; Ferrell et al., 1993; Jackson et al., 1988)

Ferguson-Pell identified several characteristics of a pressure reduction surface that must be considered: moisture accumulation and resistance, heat accumulation or loss, stability during care procedures, frictional properties, flammability, safety, durability, and maintenance (Ferguson-Pell, 1990). These factors may be used to make purchasing decisions or to prescribe surfaces for specific patients. For example, although gel pads or gel mattresses are effective, they are difficult to handle and contribute to heat loss. Heat loss is a disadvantage for a thin, elderly person but might be advantageous for a younger, heavier person.

It also is important to know whether the product requires special linens; is easy to clean, disinfect, or deodorize; is designed for single or multiple use; or has special problems or costs related to disposal. The practicality of special care procedures, such as reinflation and hand checks for "bottoming out" (placing the hand underneath the surface to see if the buttocks can be felt), should be considered. The life of these products must be weighed against their cost, and if the weight a surface can support is limited, other products should be used for heavier patients. Krouskop and Garber (1987) recommended that foam products have a base height of 3 to 4 inches (thicker for a mattress replacement), a density of 1.3 to 1.6 lb per cubic foot, a 25% indentation load deflection (ILD) of around 30 lb, and a 60% ILD to 25% ILD ratio of two and a half or greater. Agencies considering new support surfaces should try several products and obtain feedback from the nursing staff on care and handling problems. Special attention should be given to comments from patients regarding acceptability and comfort.

Addressing Problems that Reduce Tissue Tolerance

Moisture. Exposure of the skin to excessive moisture from any source can cause skin maceration. One of the most common causes of this exposure is incontinence. A variety of interventions are aimed at reducing or eliminating incontinent episodes in elderly patients, including the use of bladder training, prompted voiding, or other behavioral methods (see Chapter 10). When incontinence is unavoidable, the nurse should use a very mild soap to cleanse the skin gently but thoroughly, pat the skin dry, and apply a commercial moisture barrier. Absorbent underpads or briefs should be used, checked frequently, and changed as needed.

Diarrhea is very caustic to the skin and can lead quickly to skin breakdown. An attempt should be made to determine the cause of diarrhea and to eliminate that cause (see Chapter 11). If this does not bring quick results, a fecal incontinence bag should be used while further attempts at control are made.

Perspiration can also be problematic, especially with neurological injuries that are accompanied by autonomic instability. Absorbent materials should be used beneath the patient's body and next to the patient's skin. The use of absorbent powders is generally not advisable, as they may collect in skinfolds and become a source of injury. If perspiration occurs on a nonbreathing support surface, an alternative surface should be sought.

Friction and Shear. Several options are available to prevent or ameliorate exposure of the skin to friction and shear. The use of a trapeze or turning sheet for assisting movement in bed can be effective in preventing friction and shear. Ankle and heel protectors, which do nothing to relieve pressure, may nevertheless be helpful in protecting these areas from friction. In some instances, hydrocolloid dressings may be used over a particular prominence that is being exposed to friction. The nurse should understand that shearing and excessive sacral pressure begin to develop when the head of the bed is elevated more than 30 degrees and that this position should be avoided.

Nutritional Repletion. Although long-term problems with nutrition make patients more prone to pressure sore development, it appears that immediate nutritional repletion, particularly for protein intake, can provide some protection. If the patient has good liver and renal function, it may be helpful to increase protein intake above 100% of the RDA. It is also important to encourage adequate caloric intake, as protein is used for energy if caloric intake is inadequate. Although there is no evidence that vitamin deficiencies increase the risk for developing pressure sores, certain vitamins and minerals are known to be important in building new tissue and healing injured tissue. A vitamin supplement containing vitamin C, vitamin A, and zinc may be helpful.

If there are problems with assessing or meeting the patient's nutritional needs, a consultation with a registered dietitian should be considered. This is particularly important for patients who are fed enterally to ensure that the formula meets their nutritional needs. It is not unusual for the patient on tube feedings to develop some diarrhea, but this problem can and should be addressed immediately. A change to a feeding with a lower osmolality, higher fiber content, or lack of artificial coloring may be sufficient to take care of the diarrhea. Bacterial contamination from the feeding equipment is also a potential problem. Antidiarrheal medication may occasionally be necessary. Whatever the situation, this problem needs aggressive intervention.

MANAGEMENT OF PRESSURE SORES

Treatment of pressure sores is more expensive than their prevention, in terms of both emotional and economic costs. Oot-Giromini and colleagues (1989) estimated that the economic cost of pressure sore treatment is two and a half times greater than that of prevention. Unfortunately, despite our best efforts at prevention, pressure sores do develop in very–high-risk patients and often require weeks (or months) of diligent care to heal.

Brandeis and colleagues (1990) monitored healing rates of 377 individuals developing pressure sores after admission to 51 nursing homes. After 3 months, 51.2% of stage II sores, 25.9% of stage III sores, and only 18% of stage IV sores healed. Rather than accept these figures as "norms," APNs should try to improve treatment for the patients under their care.

No data are currently available to determine the time required for healing under optimal conditions. However, a clean pressure sore with adequate innervation and blood supply should show some progress toward healing within 2 to 4 weeks (Robson, Phillips, Thomason, et al., 1992a, 1992b; van Rijswijk, 1993). If some sign of healing (e.g., decreased size, less exudate, granulation tissue, or epithelialization) is not evident during this time, the plan of care should be reevaluated.

Pressure sores should be assessed at least weekly. Any deterioration in the pressure sore or the patient's general condition makes immediate reevaluation of the treatment plan man-

datory (Bergstrom et al., 1994). Effective pressure sore management can be accomplished by creating a wound environment that has the following characteristics:

- Is free of pressure
- Is free of nonviable tissue
- Is free of clinical infection
- Is free of dead space
- Supports tissue growth
- Contains adequate substrate for tissue repair

Creating a Pressure-Free Wound Environment

Pressure of sufficient intensity and duration to cause tissue ischemia also delays or prevents healing. Positioning techniques and support surfaces should be used to (1) keep all pressure off the pressure sore and (2) prevent new pressure sores in patients who remain at risk.

The selection of positioning techniques and support surfaces to achieve these goals depends on available research, clinical judgment, and the unique needs of the patient. Only one randomized controlled clinical trial has explored the role of pressure-reducing beds to facilitate pressure sore healing in long-term care patients. Ferrell and colleagues (1993) randomly assigned 84 nursing home residents having stage II, III, or IV pressure sores to use either a low–air loss bed or a 4-inch corrugated foam mattress overlay. Residents on the low–air loss beds were two and a half times more likely to heal than those on foam mattresses (P = .004). Of course, not all patients require low–air loss beds.

A panel sponsored by the AHCPR developed recommendations for the treatment of pressure sores based on a comprehensive review of the research literature (Bergstrom et al., 1994). Their suggestions regarding the selection of support surfaces are summarized in Table 13–1.

Creating a Wound Environment Free of Nonviable Tissue

The presence of nonviable tissue promotes the growth of pathogens and impairs healing.

TABLE 13-1
Considerations When Selecting a Support Surface for Pressure Sore Treatment

Category	Examples	Indications for Use
Static support surface	Convoluted foam overlay or mattress replacement Static flotation device (air or water filled)	The individual can assume a variety of positions without bearing weight on the pressure sore and without "bottoming out."*
Dynamic support surface	Alternating-air overlay	The individual (1) cannot assume a variety of positions without bearing weight on a pressure sore or (2) fully compresses the static support surface OR the pressure sore does not show evidence of healing on a static support surface.
Specialty beds	Low-airloss bed Air-fluidized bed	The individual (1) has large Stage III or IV sores on multiple turning surfaces or (2) bottoms out or fails to heal on a dynamic support surface. The airflow provided by these beds may be helpful in controlling excess moisture.

*To check for bottoming out, the caregiver should place an outstretched hand (palm up) under the overlay, below the pressure sore. If the overlay is compressed to less than 1 inch, the individual has bottomed out.

Débridement, followed by routine wound cleansing, creates an environment conducive to healing. Accepted methods include sharp, autolytic, enzymatic, and mechanical débridement. The method (or combination of methods) used should be consistent with the patient's condition and the goals of care. Every effort should be made to prevent or manage débridement-induced pain.

Sharp débridement involves the use of sharp instruments (e.g., scalpels, scissors) or lasers to remove dead tissue. When faced with serious infectious complications such as advancing cellulitis and sepsis, rapid débridement of necrotic tissue is critical, and sharp débridement is the method of choice (Bergstrom et al., 1994). Anyone performing sharp débridement should meet local licensing requirements and demonstrate the necessary skills to safely débride the sore and manage complications such as bleeding, infection, and pain (Bergstrom et al., 1994).

Glenchur and colleagues (1981) documented transient bacteremia following sharp débridement. Although this is usually a self-limiting process, patients should be monitored for signs of sepsis (e.g., fever, tachycardia, hypotension, confusion) following sharp débridement. Antibiotic coverage is not necessary in most situations but should be considered if (1) the pressure sores are large and deep, (2) the patient is immunosuppressed, or (3) the patient has conditions warranting subacute bacterial endocarditis prophylaxis (Allman, 1989).

For routine débridement in severely debilitated patients, less aggressive methods of débridement are often chosen. Autolytic débridement is an appropriate choice for patients with a low risk of infection and a poor tolerance for sharp débridement. Occlusive or semiocclusive dressings are placed over the pressure sore, allowing the natural enzymes in wound fluid to digest necrotic tissue (Maklebust & Sieggreen, 1996). The liquefied necrotic tissue is then irrigated from the wound. Clinical research supporting this technique is limited to an uncontrolled clinical trial (Carr & Lalagos, 1990). This method is contraindicated in infected sores.

Enzymatic débridement, in which a topical enzyme preparation is applied to digest necrotic tissue, is another option for the débridement of noninfected sores. Manufacturer instructions should be followed carefully because some preparations are pH dependent and others may be inactivated by wound care products. Collagenase is the most thoroughly researched product and demonstrates débridement within an average of 3 days and growth of granulation tissue within 30 days (Barrett & Klibanski, 1973).

Mechanical débridement includes the use of wet-to-dry dressings, irrigation, a whirlpool, and dextranomers. The wet-to-dry (or wet-to-moist) dressing technique involves applying a wet saline dressing to the wound, allowing the dressing to dry, then pulling adherent eschar off with the dry (or moist) dressing. Irrigation and the use of a whirlpool are effective cleansing methods and are also useful in softening and mechanically removing necrotic tissue and debris. Dextranomer beads and dressings absorb exudate and necrotic debris but do not appreciably decrease healing time (Shand & McClemont, 1979) and may obstruct sinus tracts in wounds (Freeman et al., 1981).

All mechanical débridement techniques are nonselective, in that they remove both viable and nonviable tissue. The mechanical force used with these methods may damage granulation tissue and new epithelial tissue (Alvarez et al., 1983). Wet-to-dry dressings may desiccate the wound bed and thus impede healing. These methods may also be painful. Despite these limitations, mechanical débridement can be effective if (1) pain is managed, (2) minimal necessary mechanical force is used, and (3) débridement is discontinued when the wound bed is clean and granulation tissue appears.

Pressure sores should be cleansed initially and with each dressing change (Bergstrom et al., 1994). Skin cleansers and antiseptic agents are cytotoxic to healing tissue and should not be used for wound cleansing (Burkey et al., 1993; Foresman et al., 1993). Although nontoxic commercial wound cleansers can be used, nor-

mal saline irrigation safely and effectively cleanses most pressure sores.

Irrigation pressures should be between 4 and 15 lb per square inch (psi) (Bergstrom et al., 1994). Higher pressures may damage granulation tissue and drive bacteria into the wound (Wheeler et al., 1976), and lower pressures are ineffective (Hamer et al., 1975). Bulb syringes deliver saline at approximately 2 psi and are not recommended for cleansing pressure sores. A 35–mL syringe with a 19-gauge needle or angiocatheter delivers saline at 8 psi and is more effective in removing bacteria than a bulb syringe (Stevenson et al., 1976).

A whirlpool may be particularly beneficial for treating multiple, extensive, necrotic pressure sores (Braden et al., 1993). To avoid damaging granulation tissue, stop whirlpool treatments when the sore is clean and do not position the sore too close to the high-pressure water jets (Feedar & Kloth, 1990). Disinfect whirlpool equipment between patients to prevent cross-contamination (Rutala, 1990).

Creating a Wound Environment Free of Clinical Infection

There is a direct correlation between high levels of bacteria (i.e., $>10^5$ organisms/g tissue) and the failure of pressure sores to heal (Bendy et al., 1964; Sapico et al., 1986). Additionally, local pressure sore infections may lead to serious complications such as cellulitis, osteomyelitis, and sepsis. Prevention, early detection, and aggressive treatment of clinical infection are critical. Usually, local infection can be prevented with effective wound cleansing, débridement, and avoidance of fecal contamination (Bergstrom et al., 1994).

Preventing the spread of pathogens among patients is essential. Nurses should adopt and rigorously follow body substance isolation (BSI) precautions or an equivalent infection-control system (Bergstrom et al., 1994). The BSI system emphasizes handwashing and barrier precautions to control potentially infectious body substances (Lynch et al., 1987).

Sterile instruments should be used for sharp débridement (Bergstrom et al., 1994). Because pressure sores are already colonized with some bacteria, some institutions have elected to use clean rather than sterile dressings. In a small pilot study ($N = 30$), Stotts and associates (1994) found no difference in the rate of wound healing for surgical patients treated with clean versus sterile dressing techniques. Additional research is needed, however. Anyone considering the use of clean dressings in an institutional setting should ensure that the dressings remain clean and that BSI precautions are consistently observed. Clean dressing techniques may not be appropriate for severely immunosuppressed patients or in institutions in which nosocomial infections are not adequately controlled.

Once the skin's protective covering has been lost, pressure sores become colonized with low levels of bacteria. Colonization can usually be controlled with cleansing and débridement. Infection occurs when the number of microorganisms increases to a level that damages tissue or impairs healing (i.e., $\geq 10^5$ organisms per gram of tissue). Clinical signs of local pressure sore infection include localized erythema, warmth, tenderness, edema, pain, and purulent drainage. A foul odor is frequently detectable when anaerobic organisms are present (Sapico et al., 1986). Unfortunately, these signs may be absent in immunosuppressed patients, and infection may go undetected.

Swab cultures often detect surface contaminants that may or may not be the organisms causing tissue infection (Rousseau, 1989). The Centers for Disease Control and Prevention recommend the use of quantitative bacterial cultures from fluid obtained by needle aspiration or biopsy of pressure sore tissue (Garner et al., 1988). When needle aspiration and tissue biopsy techniques are not feasible, quantitative swab cultures (obtained using specific protocols) provide reasonably accurate results (Stotts, 1995).

Localized pressure sore infections can usually be treated with more vigilant cleansing and débridement. There is no evidence that topical antiseptics decrease bacterial counts in the deeper tissues; further, these agents harm healing cells (Bergstrom et al., 1994). Some clinicians advocate the use of broad-spectrum topical antibiotics when cleansing and débridement fail to resolve local infections. Two clinical trials showed reductions in bacterial levels

and improvements in wound appearance when treated with topical silver sulfadiazine and gentamicin (Bendy et al., 1964; Kucan et al., 1981); however, adverse reactions and the growth of resistant organisms are continuing concerns.

Systemic antibiotics should be reserved for the treatment of systemic infections such as cellulitis, osteomyelitis, and sepsis. Cellulitis is an invasive infection of the tissue surrounding the pressure sore. The erythema accompanying cellulitis is more intense than normal periwound inflammation and tends to spread or advance if left untreated. The clinician can mark the edges of the erythema on the skin's surface and check for advancing erythema 24 hours later.

Osteomyelitis is more difficult to diagnose. Pathological examination of bone tissue is the gold standard for diagnosing this condition, yet bone biopsy can be very stressful for a debilitated patient. Lewis and colleagues (1988) compared bone biopsy examination with a combination of three less invasive techniques (white blood cell count $> 15,000$ mm^3; erythrocyte sedimentation rate > 120 mm/hour; and positive plain x-ray). They concluded that these tests accurately exclude osteomyelitis 96% of the time when all tests are negative and accurately diagnoses osteomyelitis 69% of the time when all tests are positive.

Patients with pressure sores who develop bacteremia have a mortality rate of 55% (Bryan et al., 1983). Symptoms of sepsis (e.g., fever, leukocytosis, tachycardia, hypotension, change in mental status) require immediate evaluation and treatment, including blood cultures and sharp débridement of pressure sores that may be a source of infection. Pending blood culture results, antibiotics should be initiated to combat the organisms most commonly associated with pressure sore–related sepsis (i.e., *Bacteroides fragilis, Proteus mirabilis, Staphylococcus aureus,* and *Escherichia coli*) (Bryan et al., 1983; Chow et al., 1977; Galpin et al., 1976).

Several systemic antibiotics are effective against pressure sore–related infections. Clindamycin and aminoglycosides (e.g., gentamicin, amikacin) effectively penetrate necrotic tissue; however, cefazolin, cephalothin, and penicillin do not (Berger et al., 1978, 1981;

Chow et al., 1977; Segal et al., 1990). Aminoglycosides are preferred when *Proteus, Pseudomonas,* or *Bacteroides* are cultured, whereas vancomycin is often recommended with *Staphylococcus* and *Enterococcus* species (Braden et al., 1993).

The duration of systemic antibiotic therapy varies with the nature and severity of the infectious complication. Seven to 10 days are usually sufficient for localized soft tissue infections, but 14 to 21 days may be required with sepsis or the involvement of muscle or deep fascia (Braden et al., 1993). Continuing osteomyelitis and joint infections may require 6 weeks of intravenous antibiotics and surgical excision of infected tissue (Lewis et al., 1988).

Creating a Wound Environment Free of Dead Space

Dead space exists in wounds with undermining or sinus tracts. Left untreated, dead space can lead to abscess formation. Nurses should identify dead space by examining the edges and the base of the wound with a sterile cotton applicator and should then loosely fill the space with dressing material. Overpacking can increase the pressure within the wound and damage the tissue further (Maklebust & Sieggreen, 1996).

Creating a Wound Environment that Supports Tissue Growth

Tissue growth is best supported by an environment that keeps the wound moist yet the surrounding tissue dry (Maklebust & Sieggreen, 1996). Research clearly shows the advantages of a moist wound environment in supporting significantly faster rates of collagen synthesis and reepithelialization (Alvarez et al., 1983).

Various types of occlusive dressings help retain moisture in the wound bed. These include polyurethane films, hydrocolloids, hydrogels, and foams. The unique characteristics, indications, and contraindications of these dressings have been described by other authors (Bolton & van Rijswijk, 1991; Braden & Bryant, 1990). Occlusive dressings should never be left

on infected pressure ulcers for several days at a time. Infected sores require frequent cleansing and débridement to prevent systemic infectious complications.

Although occlusive dressings are generally effective and convenient, five controlled trials have demonstrated no significant differences in wound healing when comparing continuously moist saline gauze with a variety of moisture-retaining dressings (Alm et al., 1989; Colwell et al., 1992; Neill et al., 1989; Oleske et al., 1986; Xakellis & Chrischilles, 1992). The initial cost of gauze is less than film or hydrocolloid dressings; however, gauze dressings take more time to change and remoisten every 6 to 8 hours (Colwell et al., 1992; Xakellis et al., 1992).

Ultimately, the choice of dressings is a matter of clinical judgment based on the condition of the wound. Table 13–2 provides recommendations for dressing selection based on the amount of wound exudate.

Creating a Wound Environment with Adequate Substrate for Tissue Repair

Pressure sores require an oxygenated blood supply and essential nutrients for healing. There is no evidence that hyperbaric oxygen improves pressure sore healing. However, other interventions can improve the supply of

---

TABLE 13-2

Dressing Selection Based on the Amount of Wound Exudate

Amount of Exudate	Dressing Choice
Excess exudate	Calcium alginates Hydrophilic beads Gauze (dry or moistened with saline) Hydrophilic foam Wound pouch
Normal exudate	Hydrocolloids Polyurethane Moist saline gauze
Minimal exudate or dry wound	Hydrogels Gels Continuously moist saline gauze

oxygenated blood to affected areas. These include (1) treating peripheral vascular disease, (2) keeping affected areas warm to prevent vasoconstriction, and (3) positioning patients to maximize arterial flow and venous return.

The provision of adequate nutrients is essential for pressure sore healing. Patients who develop a pressure sore should be immediately assessed for their current nutritional status and future nutritional needs. Nutritional support should place and keep the patient in positive nitrogen balance. This usually requires 30 to 35 calories and 1.25 to 1.50 g protein per kg per day (Chernoff et al., 1990; Kaminski, 1976). Breslow and colleagues (1993) conducted a nonrandomized nutritional intervention study involving 28 malnourished nursing home patients with pressure sores. They found that a reduction in pressure sore size was significantly correlated with higher protein ($P < .01$) and caloric ($P < .03$) intake. Vitamin and mineral supplements should also be provided if deficiencies are confirmed or suspected (Bergstrom et al., 1994).

Plans for nutritional support, whether they include assisted feeding, oral supplements, tube feedings, or hyperalimentation, should always be consistent with the needs and desires of the patient. Reevaluate nutritional status at least weekly and modify the nutritional plan as needed. Caloric count, weekly weight, body mass index, serial serum albumin, and total lymphocyte count are useful indices of nutritional status.

Treatments of the Future

Electrical stimulation shows promise as an adjunctive therapy for the treatment of pressure sores that do not respond to more conventional therapies (Baker et al., 1996; Carley & Wainapel, 1985; Feedar et al., 1991; Gentzkow et al., 1991; Griffin et al., 1991; Itoh et al., 1991; Kloth & Feedar, 1988; Salzberg et al., 1995). Because this is a new therapy in pressure sore treatment, clinicians should ensure that trained personnel use proper equipment and follow research-based protocols (Bergstrom et al., 1994).

A few controlled clinical trials have tested the effects of growth factors on pressure sore healing. Although encouraging results have been documented with the use of recombinant platelet-derived growth factor BB and basic fibroblast growth factor, there is insufficient evidence to approve these agents for general clinical use (Mustoe et al., 1994; Pierce et al., 1994; Robson, Phillips, Lawrence, et al., 1992; Robson, Phillips, Thomason, et al., 1992a, 1992b; Vande-Berg et al., 1995).

Education for Self-Care

Addressing the psychosocial and educational needs of the patient is critical to any effective pressure sore prevention or treatment program. Patients should receive a psychosocial assessment to evaluate their ability and motivation to comprehend and adhere to the treatment program (Bergstrom et al., 1994). Nurses should design and implement psychosocial interventions and educational strategies to support the restoration of an optimal level of self-care for the patient.

SUMMARY

This chapter summarized the research base for the prevention and treatment of pressure sores. A review of the research related to risk factors and risk assessment was used to construct detailed protocols for prevention. In addition, specific criteria were provided for selecting support surfaces that are appropriate for preventing or treating pressure sores in a variety of situations. Issues involved in the local care of pressure sores and appropriate clinical responses to optimize healing were examined, and problems that must be addressed with systemic interventions were reviewed. The clinical recommendations for both prevention and treatment are consistent with the guidelines published by the AHCPR but also provide the research and specificity necessary for advanced practice.

REFERENCES

Allman, R. M. (1989). Epidemiology of pressure sores in different populations. *Decubitus, 2*(2), 30–33.

Allman, R. M., Laprade, C. A., Noel, L. B., et al. (1986). Pressure sores among hospitalized patients. *Annals of Internal Medicine, 105*(3), 337–342.

Allman, R. M., Walker, J. M., Hart, M. K., et al. (1987). Air-fluidized beds or conventional therapy for pressure sores. A randomized trial. *Annals of Internal Medicine, 107*(5), 641–648.

Alm, A., Hornmark, A. M., Fall, P. A., et al. (1989). Care of pressure sores: A controlled study of the use of a hydrocolloid dressing compared with wet saline gauze compresses. *Acta Dermato-Venereologica, 149*(suppl.), 1–10.

Alterescu, V. (1989). The financial costs of inpatient pressure ulcers to an acute care facility. *Decubitus, 2*(3), 14–23.

Alvarez, O. M., Mertz, P. M., & Eaglstein, W. H. (1983). The effect of occlusive dressings on collagen synthesis and re-epithelialization in superficial wounds. *Journal of Surgical Research, 35*(2), 142–148.

Andersen, K. E., & Kvorning, S. A. (1982). Medical aspects of the decubitus ulcer. *International Journal of Dermatology, 21*(5), 265–270.

Anderson, T. P., & Andberg, M. M. (1979). Psychosocial factors associated with pressure sores. *Archives of Physical Medicine and Rehabilitation, 60,* 341–346.

Artigue, R. S., & Hyman, W. A. (1979). The effect of myoglobin on the oxygen concentration in skeletal muscle subjected to ischemia. *Annals of Biomedical Engineering, 4,* 128–137.

Baker, L. L., Rubayi, S., Villar, F., & Demuth, S. K. (1996). Effect of electrical stimulation waveform on healing of ulcers in human beings with spinal cord injury. *Wound Repair and Regeneration 4*(1), 21–28.

Barbenel, J. C., Jordan, M. M., Nicol, S. M., & Clark, M. O. (1977). Incidence of pressure sores in the Greater Glasgow Health Board area. *Lancet, 2*(8037), 548–550.

Barrett, D., Jr., & Klibanski, A. (1973). Collagenase debridement. *American Journal of Nursing, 73*(5), 849–851.

Bates-Jensen, B. (1990). New pressure ulcer status tool. *Decubitus, 3*(3), 14–15.

Bates-Jensen, B., Vredevoe, D., & Brecht, M. (1992). Validity and reliability of the Pressure Sore Status Tool. *Decubitus, 5*(6), 20–28.

Bendy, R. H., Jr., Nuccio, P. A., Wolfe, E., et al. (1964). Relationship of quantitative wound bacterial counts to healing of decubiti: Effect of topical gentamicin. *Antimicrobial Agents and Chemotherapy, 4,* 147–155.

Bennett, L., Kavner, D., Lee, B. Y., et al. (1984). Skin stress and blood flow in sitting paraplegic patients. *Archives of Physical Medicine and Rehabilitation, 65,* 186–190.

Bennett, R. G., Bellantoni, M. F., & Ouslander, J. G. (1989). Air-fluidized bed treatment of nursing home patients with pressure sores. *Journal of the American Geriatrics Society, 37*(3), 235–242.

Berger, S. A., Barza, M., Haher, J., et al. (1978). Penetration of clindamycin into decubitus ulcers. *Antimicrobial Agents and Chemotherapy, 14*(3), 498–499.

Berger, S. A., Barza, M., Haher, J., et al. (1981). Penetration of antibiotics into decubitus ulcers. *Journal of Antimicrobial Chemotherapy, 7*(2), 193–195.

Bergstrom, N., Bennett, M. A., Carlson, C. E., et al. (1994, December). *Treatment of Pressure Ulcers.* Clinical Practice Guideline No. 15. Agency for Health Care Policy and Research Publication No. 95-0652. Rockville, MD: U.S. Department of Health and Human Services, Public Health Service, Agency for Health Care Policy and Research.

Bergstrom, N., & Braden, B. A. (1992). Prospective study of pressure sore risk among institutionalized elderly. *Journal of the American Geriatrics Society, 40,* 747–758.

Bergstrom, N., Braden, B., Kemp, M., & Champagne, M. (in press). Reliability and validity of the Braden Scale: A multi-site study. *Nursing Research.*

Bergstrom, N., Braden, B. J., Laguzza, A., & Holman, V. (1987). The Braden Scale for predicting pressure sore risk. *Nursing Research, 36*(4), 205–210.

Berjian, R. A., Douglass, H. O., Jr., Holyoke, E. D., et al. (1983). Skin pressure measurements on various mattress surfaces in cancer patients. *American Journal of Physical Medicine, 62*(5), 217–226.

Berlowitz, D. R., & Wilking, S. V. (1989). Risk factors for pressure sores. A comparison of cross-sectional and cohort-derived data. *Journal of the American Geriatrics Society, 37*(11), 1043–1050.

Bliss, M. R., McLaren, R., & Exton-Smith, A. N. (1967). Preventing pressure sores in hospital: Controlled trial of a large-celled ripple mattress. *British Medical Journal, 1*(537), 394–397.

Bolton, L., & van Rijswijk, L. (1991). Wound dressings: Meeting clinical and biological needs. *Dermatology Nursing, 3*(3), 146–161.

Braden, B. J. (1990). Emotional stress and pressure sore formation among the elderly recently relocated to a nursing home. In S. G. Funk, E. M. Tornquist, M. T. Champagne, et al. (Eds.), *Key aspects of recovery: Improving mobility, rest, and nutrition* (pp. 188–196). New York: Springer.

Braden, B. J., & Bergstrom, N. (1989). Clinical utility of the Braden Scale for predicting pressure sore risk. *Decubitus, 2*(3), 44–51.

Braden, B. J., & Bergstrom, N. (1992). Pressure reduction. In G. M. Bulechek & J. C. McCloskey (Eds.), *Nursing interventions, essential nursing treatments* (2nd ed., pp. 94–108). Philadelphia: W. B. Saunders.

Braden, B. J., & Bergstrom, N. (1994). Predictive validity of the Braden Scale for Pressure Sore Risk in a nursing home population. *Research in Nursing and Health, 17,* 459–470.

Braden, B. J., & Bryant, R. (1990). Innovations to prevent and treat pressure ulcers. *Geriatric Nurse, 11*(4), 182–186.

Braden, B. J., Kemp, M. G., Overton, M. H., et al. (1993). The etiology, prevention and treatment of pressure sores. In P. R. Katz, R. L. Kane, & M. D. Mezey (Eds.), *Advances in long-term care, vol. 2* (pp. 72–97). New York: Springer.

Brandeis, G. H., Morris, J. N., Nash, D. J., & Lipsitz, L. A. (1990). The epidemiology and natural history of pressure ulcers in elderly nursing home residents. *Journal of the American Medical Association, 264*(22), 2905–2909.

Breslow, B. A., Hallfrisch, J., Guy, D. G., et al. (1993). The importance of dietary protein in healing pressure ulcers. *Journal of the American Geriatrics Society, 41*(4), 357–362.

Bryan, C. S., Dew, C. E., & Reynolds, K. L. (1983). Bacteremia associated with decubitus ulcers. *Archives of Physical Medicine and Rehabilitation, 143*(11), 2093–2095.

Burkey, J. L., Weinberg, C., & Brenden, R. A. (1993). Differential methodologies for the evaluation of skin and wound cleansers. *Wounds, 5*(6), 284–291.

Carley, P. J., & Wainapel, S. G. (1985). Electrotherapy for acceleration of wound healing: Low intensity direct current. *Archives of Physical Medicine and Rehabilitation, 66*(7), 443–446.

Carr, R. D., & Lalagos, D. E. (1990). Clinical evaluation of a polymeric membrane dressing in the treatment of pressure ulcers. *Decubitus 3*(3), 38–42.

Chernoff, R., Milton, K., & Lipschitz, D. (1990). The effect of a very high-protein liquid formula (Replete®) on decubitus ulcer healing in long-term tube-fed institutionalized patients [abstract]. *Journal of the American Dietetic Association, 90*(9), A-130.

Chow, A. W., Galpin, J. E., & Guze, L. B. (1977). Clindamycin for treatment of sepsis caused by decubitus ulcers. *Journal of Infectious Diseases, 135*(suppl.), S65–S68.

Colwell, J. C., Foreman, M. D., & Trotter, J. P. (1992). A comparison of the efficacy and cost-effectiveness of two methods of managing pressure ulcers. *Decubitus, 6*(4), 28–36.

Daniel, R. K., Priest, D. L., Wheatley, D. C., & Eng, B. (1981). Etiologic factors in pressure sores: An experimental model. *Archives of Physical Medicine and Rehabilitation, 62*, 492–498.

Dinsdale, S. M. (1974). Decubitus ulcers: Role of pressure and friction in causation. *Archives of Physical Medicine and Rehabilitation, 55*(4), 147–152.

Ek, A. C., & Boman, G. A. (1982). Descriptive study of pressure sores: The prevalence of pressure sores and the characteristics of patients. *Journal of Advanced Nursing, 7*(1), 51–57.

Feedar, J. A., & Kloth, L. C. (1990). Conservative management of chronic wounds. In L. C. Kloth, J. M. McCulloch & J. A. Feedar (Eds.), *Wound healing: Alternatives in management* (pp. 32–40). Philadelphia: F. A. Davis.

Feedar, J. A., Kloth, L. C., & Gentzkow, G. D. (1991). Chronic dermal ulcer healing enhanced with monophasic pulsed electrical stimulation. *Physical Therapy, 71*(9), 639–649.

Ferguson-Pell, M. W. (1990). Seat cushion selection: Technical considerations. *Journal of Rehabilitation Research and Development Clinical Supplement 2*, 49–73.

Ferrell, B. A., Osterweil, D., & Christenson, P. (1993). A randomized trial of low-air-loss beds for treatment of pressure ulcers. *Journal of the American Medical Association, 269*(4), 494–497.

Flam, E. (1987). Optimum skin aeration in pressure sore management. *Proceedings of the Annual Conference of Engineering in Medicine and Biology Abstracts, 29*, 84.

Foresman, P. A., Payne, D. S., Becker, D., et al. (1993). A relative toxicity index for wound cleansers. *Wounds, 5*(5), 226–231.

Frantz, R. A. (1989). Pressure ulcer costs in long-term care. *Decubitus, 2*(3), 56–57.

Freeman, B. G., Carwell, G. R., & McCraw, J. B. (1981). The quantitative study of the use of dextranomer in the management of infected wounds. *Surgery, Gynecology and Obstetrics, 153*, 81–86.

Galpin, J. E., Chow, A. W., Bayer, A. S., & Guze, L. B. (1976). Sepsis associated with decubitus ulcers. *American Journal of Medicine, 61*(3), 346–350.

Garner, J. S., Jarvis, W. R., Emori, T. G., et al. (1988). CDC definitions for nosocomial infections. *American Journal of Infection Control, 16*(3), 128–140 [published erratum appears in *American Journal of Infection Control, 16*(4), 177].

Gentzkow, G. D., Pollack, S. V., Kloth, L. C., & Stubbs, H. A. (1991). Improved healing of pressure ulcers using dermapulse, a new electrical stimulation device. *Wounds, 3*(5), 158–170.

Glenchur, H., Patel, B. S., & Pathmarajah, C. (1981). Transient bacteremia associated with debridement of decubitus ulcers. *Military Medicine, 146*(6), 432–433.

Goldstone, L. A., & Goldstone, J. (1982). The Norton score: An early warning of pressure sores? *Journal of Advanced Nursing, 7*(5), 419–426.

Goldstone, L. A., Norris, M., O'Reilly, M., & White, J. (1982). A clinical trial of a bead bed system for the prevention of pressure sores in elderly orthopaedic patients. *Journal of Advanced Nursing, 7*(6), 545–548.

Goldstone, L. A., & Roberts, B. V. (1980). A preliminary discriminant function analysis of elderly orthopaedic patients who will or will not contract a pressure sore. *International Journal of Nursing Studies, 17*(1), 17–23.

Griffin, J. W., Tooms, R. E., Mendius, R. A., et al. (1991). Efficacy of high voltage pulsed current for healing of pressure ulcers in patients with spinal cord injury. *Physical Therapy, 71*(6), 433–442.

Haeger, K., Lanner, E., & Magnusson, P. (1974). Oral zinc sulphate in the treatment of venous leg ulcers. *Vasa, 1*, 62–69.

Hallbook, T., & Lanner, E. (1972). Serum zinc and healing of venous leg ulcers. *Lancet, 14*(2), 780–782.

Hamer, M. L., Robson, M. C., Krizek, T. J., & Southwick, W. O. (1975). Quantitative bacterial analysis of comparative wound irrigations. *Annals of Surgery, 181*(6), 819–822.

Hassard, G. H. (1975). Heterotopic bone formation about the hip and unilateral decubitus ulcers in spinal cord injury. *Archives of Physical Medicine and Rehabilitation, 56*(8), 355–358.

Hunter, T., & Rajan, K. T. (1971). The role of ascorbic acid in the pathogenesis and treatment of pressure sores. *Paraplegia, 8*(4), 211–216.

Husain, T. (1953). An experimental study of some pressure effects on tissues, with reference to the bed-sore problem. *Journal of Pathology and Bacteriology, 66*, 347–358.

International Association for Enterostomal Therapy (1991). *Standards of care for dermal wounds: Pressure ulcers* (rev. ed.). Irvine, CA: International Association for Enterostomal Therapy.

Irwin, M. I., & Hutchins, B. K. (1976). A conspectus of research on vitamin C requirements in man. *Journal of Nutrition, 106*, 823–879.

Itoh, M., Montemayor, J. S., Jr., Matsumoto, E., et al. (1991). Accelerated wound healing of pressure ulcers by pulsed high peak power electromagnetic energy (Diapulse). *Decubitus, 4*(1), 24–25, 29–34.

Jackson, B. S., Chagares, R., Nee, N., & Freeman, K. (1988). The effects of a therapeutic bed on pressure ulcers: An experimental study. *Journal of Enterostomal Therapy, 15*(6), 220–226.

Jacobs, M. A. (1989). Comparison of capillary blood flow using a regular hospital bed mattress, ROHO mattress, and Mediscus bed. *Rehabilitation Nursing, 14*(5), 270–272.

Kaminski, M. V., Jr. (1976). Enteral hyperalimentation. *Surgery, Gynecology and Obstetrics, 143*(1), 12–16.

Kemp, M. G., Kopanke, D., Todecilla, L., et al. (1993). The role of support surfaces and patient attributes in preventing pressure ulcers in elderly patients. *Research in Nursing and Health, 16*(2), 89–96.

Kenney, R. A. (1982). *Physiology of aging: A synopsis.* Chicago: Year Book Medical Publishers.

Kloth, L. C., & Feedar, J. A. (1988). Acceleration of wound healing with high voltage, monophasic, pulsed current. *Physical Therapy, 68*(4), 503–508 [published erratum appears in *Physical Therapy, 69*(8), 702].

Kosiak, M. (1959). Etiology and pathophysiology of ischemic ulcers. *Archives of Physical Medicine and Rehabilitation, 40*(2), 62–69.

Krouskop, T. A. (1983). A synthesis of the factors that contribute to pressure sore formation. *Medical Hypotheses, 11*(2), 255–267.

Krouskop, T. A. (1986). The effect of surface geometry on interface pressures generated by polyurethane foam mattress overlays. *Reports by the Rehabilitation Engineering Center at the Institute for Rehabilitation & Research.* Houston, TX: The Rehabilitation Engineering Center at the Institute for Rehabilitation & Research.

Krouskop, T. A., & Garber, S. L. (1987). The role of technology in the prevention of pressure sores. *Ostomy Wound Management, 16,* 44–45, 48–49, 52–54.

Krouskop, T. A., Noble, P. C., Garber, S. L., & Spencer, W. A. (1983). The effectiveness of preventive management in reducing the occurrence of pressure sores. *Journal of Rehabilitation Research and Development, 20*(1), 74–83.

Kucan, J. O., Robson, M. C., Heggers, J. P., & Ko, F. (1981). Comparison of silver sulfadiazine, povidone-iodine and physiologic saline in the treatment of chronic pressure ulcers. *Journal of the American Geriatrics Society, 29*(5), 232–235.

Lamid, S., & El Ghatit, A. Z. (1983). Smoking, spasticity and pressure sores in spinal cord–injured patients. *American Journal of Physical Medicine, 62*(6), 300–306.

Larsen, B., Holstein, P., & Lassen, N. A. (1979). On the pathogenesis of bedsores. Skin blood flow cessation by external pressure on the back. *Scandinavian Journal of Plastic and Reconstructive Surgery, 13*(2), 347–350.

Lewis, V. L., Jr., Bailey, M. H., Pulawski, G., et al. (1988). The diagnosis of osteomyelitis in patients with pressure sores. *Plastic and Reconstructive Surgery, 81*(2), 229–232.

Lynch, P., Jackson, M. M., Cummings, M. J., & Stamm, W. E. (1987). Rethinking the role of isolation practices in the prevention of nosocomial infections. *Annals of Internal Medicine, 107*(2), 243–246.

Maklebust, J., & Sieggreen, M. (1996). *Pressure ulcers: Guidelines for prevention and nursing management* (2nd ed.). Springhouse, PA: Springhouse Corporation.

Manley, M. T. (1978). Incidence, contributory factors and costs of pressure sores. *South African Medical Journal, 53*(6), 217–222.

Merbitz, C. T., King, R. B., Bleiberg, J., & Grip, J. C. (1985). Wheelchair push-ups: Measuring pressure relief frequency. *Archives of Physical Medicine and Rehabilitation, 66*(7), 433–438.

Moolten, S. E. (1972). Bedsores in the chronically ill patient. *Archives of Physical Medicine and Rehabilitation, 53*(9), 430–438.

Mosely, L. H., Finseth, F., & Goody, M. (1978). Nicotine and its effects on wound healing. *Plastic and Reconstructive Surgery, 61*(4), 570–575.

Mustoe, T. A., Cutler, N. R., Allman, R. M., et al. (1994). A phase II study to evaluate recombinant platelet-derived growth factor-BB in the treatment of stage 3 and 4 pressure ulcers. *Archives of Surgery, 129*(2), 213–219.

National Pressure Ulcer Advisory Panel (1989). Pressure ulcer prevalence, cost and risk assessment: Consensus development conference statement. *Decubitus, 2*(2), 24–28.

Neill, K. M., Conforti, C., Kedas, A., & Burris, J. F. (1989). Pressure sore response to a new hydrocolloid dressing. *Wounds, 1*(3), 173–185.

Newell, P. H., Thornburgh, J. D., & Fleming, W. C. (1970). The management of pressure and other external factors in the prevention of ischemic ulcers. *Journal of Basic Engineering, 92,* 590–596.

Norton, D., McLaren, R., & Exton-Smith, A. N. (1962). *An investigation of geriatric nursing problems in hospitals.* London: National Corporation for the Care of Old People.

Oleske, D. M., Smith, X. P., White, P., et al. (1986). A randomized clinical trial of two dressing methods for the treatment of low-grade pressure ulcers. *Journal of Enterostomal Therapy, 13*(3), 90–98.

Oot-Giromini, B., Bidwell, F. C., Heller, N. B., et al. (1989). Pressure ulcer prevention versus treatment, comparative product cost study. *Decubitus, 2*(3), 52–54.

Panel for the Prediction and Prevention of Pressure Ulcers in Adults (1992). *Pressure ulcers in adults: Prediction and prevention.* Clinical Practice Guideline No. 3. Agency for Health Care Policy and Research Publication No. 92-0047. Rockville, MD: U.S. Department of Health and Human Services, Public Health Service, Agency for Health Care Policy and Research.

Patterson, R. P., & Fisher, S. V. (1986). Sitting pressure-time patterns in patients with quadriplegia. *Archives of Physical Medicine and Rehabilitation, 67*(11), 812–814.

Pierce, G. F., Tarpley, J. E., Allman, R. M., et al. (1994). Tissue repair processes in healing chronic pressure ulcers treated with recombinant platelet-derived growth factor BB. *American Journal of Pathology, 145*(6), 1399–1410.

Prasad, A. S. (1982). *Clinical, biochemical, and nutritional aspects of trace elements.* New York: Alan R. Liss.

Reichel, S. M. (1958). Shearing force as a factor in decubitus ulcers in paraplegics. *Journal of the American Medical Association, 166*(7), 762–763.

Richardson, R. R., & Meyer, P. R., Jr. (1981). Prevalence and incidence of pressure sores in acute spinal cord injuries. *Paraplegia, 19*(4), 235–247.

Ringsdorf, W. M., Jr., & Cheraskin, E. (1982). Vitamin C and human wound healing. *Oral Surgery, Oral Medicine, Oral Pathology, 53*(3), 231–236.

Robson, M. C., Phillips, L. G., Lawrence, W. T., et al. (1992). The safety and effect of topically applied recombinant basic fibroblast growth factor on the healing of chronic pressure sores. *Annals of Surgery, 216*(4), 401–408.

Robson, M. C., Phillips, L. G., Thomason, A., et al. (1992a). Recombinant human platelet-derived growth factor BB for the treatment of chronic pressure ulcers. *Annals of Plastic Surgery, 29,* 193–201.

Robson, M. C., Phillips, L. G., Thomason, A., et al. (1992b).

Platelet-derived factor BB for treatment of chronic pressure ulcers. *Lancet, 339,* 23–25.

Roe, D. A. (Ed.). (1986). Nutrition and the skin. *Contemporary issues in clinical nutrition, vol. 10* (entire issue). New York: Alan R. Liss.

Rousseau, P. (1989). Pressure ulcers in an aging society. *Wounds, 1*(2), 135–141.

Rutala, W. A. (1990). APIC guideline for selection and use of disinfectants. *American Journal of Infection Control, 18*(2), 99–117.

Ryan, T. J. (1979). Blood supply and decubitus ulcers. *International Journal of Dermatology, 18*(2), 123–124.

Salzberg, C. A., Cooper-Vastola, S. A., Perez, F. J., et al. (1995). The effects of non-thermal pulsed electromagnetic energy (Diapulse®) on wound healing of pressure ulcers in spinal cord–injured patients: A randomized, double-blind study. *Wounds, 7*(1), 11–16.

Sapico, F. L., Ginunas, V. J., Thornhill-Joynes, M., et al. (1986). Quantitative microbiology of pressure sores in different stages of healing. *Diagnostic Microbiology and Infectious Disease, 5*(1), 31–38.

Segal, J. L., Brunnemann, S. R., & Eltorai, I. M. (1990). Pharmacokinetics of amikacin in serum and in tissue contiguous with pressure sores in humans with spinal cord injury. *Antimicrobial Agents and Chemotherapy, 34*(7), 1422–1428.

Seiler, W. O., & Stahelin, H. B. (1979). Skin oxygen tension as a function of imposed skin pressure: Implication for decubitus ulcer formation. *Journal of the American Geriatrics Society, 27*(7), 298–301.

Seiler, W. O., & Stahelin, H. B. (1985). Decubitus ulcers: Preventive techniques for the elderly patient. *Geriatrics, 40*(7), 53–58, 60.

Shand, J. E., & McClemont, E. (1979). Recent advances in the treatment of pressure sores. *Paraplegia, 17*(4), 400–408.

Shea, J. D. (1975). Pressure sores: Classification and management. *Clinical Orthopaedics and Related Research, 112,* 89–100.

Stapleton, M. (1986). Preventing pressure sores—an evaluation of three products. *Geriatric Nursing (London), 6*(2), 23–25.

Stevenson, T. R., Thacker, J. G., Rodeheaver, G. T., et al. (1976). Cleansing the traumatic wound by high pressure syringe irrigation. *Journal of the American College of Emergency Physicians, 5*(1), 17–21.

Stotts, N. A. (1995). Determination of bacterial burden in wounds. *Advances in Wound Care, 8*(suppl.), 46–52.

Stotts, N. A., Barbour, S., Griggs, K., et al. (1994). Sterile vs. clean technique in wound care of patients with open surgical wounds in the post-op period: A pilot study [abstract]. *Proceedings of the Ninth Annual Clinical Symposium on Pressure Ulcer and Wound Management* (p. 72). Nashville, TN: Springhouse.

Taylor, T. V., Rimmer, S., Day, B., et al. (1974). Ascorbic acid supplementation in the treatment of pressure-sores. *Lancet, 2*(7880), 544–546.

Thomas, D. R., Rodeheaver, G. T., Bartolucci, A. A., et al. (1997). Pressure Ulcer Scale for Healing: Derivation and validation of the PUSH tool. *Advances in Wound Care, 10*(5), 96–101.

Trumbore, L. S., Miles, T. P., Henderson, C. T., et al. (1990). Hypocholesterolemia and pressure sore risk with chronic tube feeding [abstract]. *Clinical Research, 38*(2), 76OA.

Vande-Berg, J. S., Robson, M. C., & Mikhail, R. J. (1995). Extension of the life span of pressure ulcer fibroblasts with recombinant human interleukin-1 beta. *American Journal of Pathology, 146*(5), 1273–1282.

van Rijswijk, L. (1993). Full-thickness pressure ulcers: Patient and wound healing characteristics. *Decubitus, 6*(1), 16–21.

Vasile, J., & Chaitin, H. (1972). Prognostic factors in decubitus ulcers of the aged. *Geriatrics, 27*(4), 126–129.

Vyhlidal, S. K., Moxness, D., Bosak, K. S., et al. (1997). Mattress replacement or foam overlay? A prospective study on the incidence of pressure ulcers. *Applied Nursing Research, 10*(3), 111–120.

Wheeler, C. B., Rodeheaver, G. T., Thacker, J. G., et al. (1976). Side-effects of high pressure irrigation. *Surgery, Gynecology and Obstetrics, 143*(5), 775–778.

Witkowski, J. A., & Parish, L. C. (1982). Histopathology of the decubitus ulcer. *American Academy of Dermatology, 6*(6), 1014–1021.

Xakellis, G. C., & Chrischilles, E. A. (1992). Hydrocolloid versus saline gauze dressings in treating pressure ulcers: A cost-effectiveness analysis. *Archives of Physical Medicine and Rehabilitation, 73*(5), 463–469.

Failure to Thrive

Helen Lamberta
Jean F. Wyman

Historical Perspective

Frailty

Definition of Failure to Thrive

Clinical Features

Predisposing Factors

Management of Failure to Thrive
Assessment
Intervention

Role of the Advanced Practice Nurse

Summary

Frailty in the elderly population is often mistakenly attributed to old age and senility, thus overlooking the range of diagnostic possibilities that contribute to impaired physical and psychological health (Hodkinson, 1973). As one ages, the interactions among physical, psychological, social, and economic factors become increasingly important in maintaining health status. A growing number of older adults are presenting with deterioration in their functional abilities that cannot be directly attributed to an active disease process. This deterioration, sometimes referred to as *failure to thrive*, may be rapid or may occur over a period of several months. It can appear intractable to nursing and medical intervention and eventually lead to death if a reversible cause is not properly diagnosed and treated. Older patients

may show a lack of response to initial interventions and continue in a downward trajectory; as a result, healthcare teams who are caring for these individuals can experience disappointment and frustration, resulting in a failure to search for treatable causes.

The exact prevalence of failure to thrive is unknown. Estimates of the prevalence of failure to thrive range from 5 to 35% in community-dwelling elders, 25 to 40% among nursing home residents, to 50 to 60% of hospitalized veterans (Verdery, 1997b). Individuals who present with this syndrome are usually in acute care or long-term care institutions. Because the signs of failure to thrive are subtle and gradual, this syndrome is usually not detected in outpatient settings until significant functional decline has occurred, necessitating hospitalization or nursing home placement. Failure to thrive in the elderly has a high morbidity and mortality rate and incurs significant costs.

The authors thank Laura Finch, MS, RN, CS, GNP, for her review and helpful suggestions.

313

Physical consequences of failure to thrive include dependency, falls with associated injuries, pressure sores, and altered immune functioning with subsequent infections. Mortality rates are 12 to 16% during acute care hospitalization (Berkman et al., 1989; Hildebrand et al., 1997; Osato et al., 1993) and 35% during the first 6 months posthospitalization (Osato et al., 1993). Caregiver burden and stress may occur, increasing the risk of mistreatment. Acute care costs are high, with the length of hospital stays averaging 19.8 days (Berkman et al., 1989). Hospital recidivism rates are also high (Osato et al., 1993). The majority of patients with failure to thrive are discharged from acute care to long-term care settings (Berkman et al., 1989; Osato et al., 1993); the cost of long-term institutional care can be substantial.

The geriatric syndrome of failure to thrive is becoming more widely accepted as a diagnostic entity. This chapter discusses the concept of failure to thrive and its application to older adults. Predisposing factors are identified and serve as a basis for the assessment and management of patients who present with failure to thrive. The role of the advanced practice nurse in the prevention, early detection, and treatment of failure to thrive is described.

HISTORICAL PERSPECTIVE

Failure to thrive was originally used in the pediatric literature to characterize malnourished infants. In 1894, Holt described *marasamus*, a condition in breast-fed babies similar to failure to thrive. These infants initially thrived, but after weaning they ceased to grow, lost weight and strength, and were eventually brought to the hospital in a wasted, debilitated state from which they could not recover. In 1915, Chapin (as cited in Newbern & Krowchuk, 1994) used *failure to thrive* to describe the rapid weight loss, listlessness, and subsequent death he observed in institutionalized infants.

The term *failure to thrive* was first attributed to a group of elderly patients when diagnostic-related groupings (DRGs) were being developed at Yale University in 1970. Certain older patients did not readily fit within a specific diagnosis; rather, these patients shared a non-

specific set of symptoms that developed insidiously and were described as failure to thrive. Since then, failure to thrive has been used as an admission diagnosis in acute care hospitals.

Failure to thrive involves similar components in pediatric and geriatric populations. Comparable characteristics include undernutrition, impaired physical and cognitive function, and subsequent death (Braun et al., 1988). *Undernutrition* refers to inadequate caloric intake and a failure to gain and maintain weight. These symptoms are classic in infant failure to thrive, and studies have also shown this to be evident in older patients with failure to thrive. In geriatric failure to thrive, caloric consumption is inadequate, even for patients with a sedentary lifestyle. Although impaired physical and cognitive functioning can lead to poor nutritional intake, the reverse is also true: Poor nutrition can inadvertently result in physical and mental dysfunction, making the elderly more at risk for undernutrition.

In pediatric and geriatric populations, depression can lead to surrendering and wasting away. This "giving up" can precipitate death. Giving up is seen in both children and older adults who have experienced substantial loss. However, whereas infants have not developed the ability for self-care, the elderly lose their ability to perform the usual activities of daily living (ADL).

In older adults, failure to thrive can be viewed as a broad symptom complex involving a variety of physiological, psychological, and social characteristics with clinical symptoms analogous to infant failure to thrive. Although similarities exist between pediatric and geriatric failure to thrive at the time of diagnosis, the conditions ultimately differ. In children, there is failure to grow and develop, leading to physical, psychological, and social deficits. In older adults, there is regression or failure to maintain weight, with losses of functional abilities and social skills (Egbert, 1993b).

Unlike pediatric failure to thrive, geriatric failure to thrive is not well established in the literature or as a diagnostic category. In a study conducted at two Department of Veterans Affairs Medical Centers, Osato and colleagues (1993) found a lack of specificity in the diagnosis and treatment of failure to thrive in the geriatric population. This diagnosis was instead used to describe the general deterioration seen in patients with chronic or incurable illnesses.

Caution should be exercised in using failure to thrive as a diagnostic label, because the term may reinforce the stereotype of older people as demented and decrepit and may also halt the diagnostic workup for potentially treatable diseases (Berkman et al., 1989). It is unclear whether failure to thrive is a primary diagnosis with an obscure cause or a secondary diagnosis attributable to treatable diseases; some studies suggest that it occurs both ways (Verdery, 1996). Additional research is needed to determine the applicability of the diagnostic category of failure to thrive in the elderly, with specific reference to the reversibility of the diagnosis.

Early research on patients with failure to thrive used cross-sectional evaluations of the characteristics of people who died. This led to the concept of *predeath* as a condition that included one or more problems with cognition, continence, weight loss, or chronic disease (Issacs et al., 1971). More recent studies have focused on physiological abnormalities of nursing home patients and the risk factors for death. Risk factors include low weight, low muscle mass, decreased physical function, weakness, low albumin and cholesterol levels, anergy, and other signs of immunodeficiency (Adler & Nagel, 1981; Rudman et al., 1989; Ryan et al., 1995; Verdery & Goldberg, 1991). Further research is needed to examine the risk factors of failure to thrive and to clarify the processes of moving from a state of good health to a state of frailty and from frailty to frank cachexia (Verdery, 1994, 1996, 1997b).

FRAILTY

The frail elderly are the most physically and socially vulnerable population and are at the greatest risk for developing failure to thrive. Between 10 and 20% of older adults 65 years and older are estimated to be "frail," and the proportion increases dramatically with age (Fried, 1994). Although the terms *frail* and *frailty* are used often in gerontology and geriat-

rics, these words have been poorly defined. Most definitions agree that frail older adults are vulnerable and have the highest risk of adverse health outcomes. These definitions commonly equate frailty with functional dependence in performing ADL (National Institute on Aging, 1991; Woodhouse et al., 1988); the presence of multiple chronic diseases (MacAdam et al., 1989; Pawlson, 1988); common geriatric syndromes of confusion, falls, immobility, incontinence, and extreme old age (Winograd et al., 1991); and reduced daily activities, feelings about social relationships, and mental health (Strawbridge et al., 1998).

Aging is associated with almost universal changes in organs and metabolism, leading to a reduced homeostatic reserve. In a comprehensive review, Buchner and Wagner (1992) defined frailty as "losses of physical reserve" that serve as a "precursor state" to disability and dependence on others for ADL. They suggested three important components of the precursor state: (1) impaired neurological control (a decreased ability to perform complex tasks), (2) decreased mechanical performance (diminished strength), and (3) impaired energy metabolism (e.g., decreased aerobic status due to cardiac or pulmonary disease).

As a clinical syndrome, frailty reflects underlying physiological changes of aging that are not disease specific. Frailty has a constellation of symptoms such as weakness, fatigue, poor appetite, undernutrition, dehydration, and weight loss. These symptoms lead to the adverse outcomes of falls, injuries, acute illnesses, hospitalizations, disability, dependency, institutionalization, and death (Fried, 1994).

If frailty is a state or an outcome occurring on a continuum, then risk factors can be identified to predict functional dependence. Based on Brocklehurst's work (1985), Rockwood and colleagues (1994) presented a dynamic model of frailty in older adults that recognized the complex interaction of assets and deficits, both medical and social, that maintain or threaten independence (Fig. 14–1). On one side of the scale are the assets that help a person maintain his or her independence in the community: health, attitudes toward health and health practices, resources, and caregiver availability. On the other side of the scale are deficits that

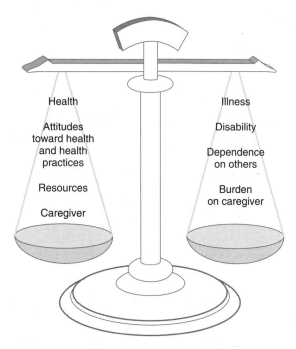

FIGURE 14–1. Dynamic model of frailty in elderly people. (Redrawn from Rockwood, K., Fox, R. A., Stolee, P., et al. [1994]. *Canadian Medical Association Journal, 150*[4], 490.)

threaten independence: ill health (especially chronic disease), disability, dependence on others, and caregiver burden. In well older adults, the scale is heavily weighted toward the assets. Frail older adults, however, are in a precarious balance in which the scale can be easily tipped toward one side or the other as a result of any of the variables, such as the loss of a caregiver. As the scale tips toward dependence, the individual develops risk for failure to thrive.

DEFINITION OF FAILURE TO THRIVE

Failure to thrive can be defined as a syndrome related to classical nutritional abnormalities (Verdery, 1997b). It is the progressive loss of physical and psychological function that occurs in frail people, leading to cachexia and eventually death. The process is marked by the loss of weight, strength, and ability to perform daily activities (Verdery, 1994). Failure to thrive in

older adults has also been referred to as "the dwindles," failure to maintain, physical and psychosocial atrophy, and biopsychosocial failure (Egbert, 1993b).

In addition to deterioration in physical and psychological functioning, failure to thrive presents with problems in social relatedness. These problems are demonstrated by disconnectedness and an inability to give of oneself, find meaning in life, and attach to others (Newbern & Krowchuk, 1994). Problems in social relatedness may be a consequence of significant physical, social, environmental, economic, and other losses as well as feelings of exclusion, shame, helplessness, worthlessness, loneliness, and dependency.

A conceptual distinction can be made among the following conditions: (1) frailty, the condition of being at risk for deterioration; (2) failure to thrive, the process of deterioration; and (3) the various frail states that occur after failure to thrive begins, which have been called *pre-death* or *cachexia* (Verdery, 1994). Verdery (1994) proposed a "trigger" model to explain why failure to thrive occurs in some older adults (Fig. 14–2). In this model, failure to thrive is related to a decline in a measured function, such as walking, muscle strength, cognition, cardiac output, forced expiratory volume (FEV) greater than what would be expected with normal aging, chronic disease, or a combination of both. At some point, the individual who is already frail begins to decline at a rate greater than is typical for his or her age and condition. Usually this increased rate of decline occurs as a result of a trigger event such as a hip fracture, the death of a spouse, or a serious illness.

Failure to thrive is listed in the International Classification of Diseases (ICD code 783.4) as a diagnostic category for use with infants and children (Bernard, 1996). Although an ICD code has not yet been developed for use with adult patients, the diagnosis of failure to thrive is increasingly being used for patients admitted to tertiary care settings with chronic or incurable illnesses (Osato et al., 1993). It is a syndrome that can be defined as "a paradigm of the frail elderly with unexplained decline in physical and/or cognitive function" (Palmer, 1990, p. 47). Typically, the person with this syndrome has seriously deteriorated; has expe-

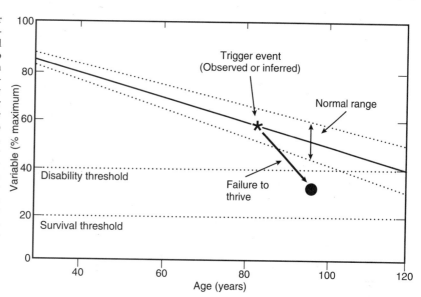

FIGURE 14–2. Trigger model for failure to thrive in elderly persons. In the context of normal changes in function, failure to thrive is defined as decline at a rate greater than expected, leading to a level of function below the age-adjusted norm. A trigger event such as a hip fracture or severe illness is often observed to occur prior to failure to thrive, but in many instances such a trigger event must be inferred. (Redrawn from Verdery, R. B. [1994]. Failure to thrive. In W. R. Hazzard, E. L. Bierman, J. P. Blass, et al. [Eds.], *Principles of geriatric medicine and gerontology* [3rd ed., p. 1206]. New York: McGraw-Hill. Copyright 1994 by McGraw-Hill. Reproduced with permission of The McGraw-Hill Companies.)

rienced multiple hospitalizations, chronic illnesses, and many coping problems; has poor social and financial resources; has experienced no significant improvement with initial interventions; and is not responding to medical treatment. This type of patient is at high risk for further functional deterioration, long-term care institutionalization, and death (Berkman et al., 1989; Hildebrand et al., 1997; Osato et al., 1993).

Failure to thrive is neither an aspect of normal aging nor a synonym for dementia. It is not synonymous with predeath or the end stage of a terminal illness (Egbert, 1993b; Verdery, 1994). Although many patients in a predeath stage with terminal illness, organ failure, or systemic infection have failure to thrive, their decline in function is not reversible. In failure to thrive patients without these diagnoses, the decline may be reversible if it is caused by functional or psychosocial problems that result in poor food intake (Verdery, 1994, 1997b).

CLINICAL FEATURES

Failure to thrive is multifactorial, with multiple causes and precipitating factors. It eventually involves multiple organ systems. Symptoms are vague and insidious. Key diagnostic elements include (1) a decline or deterioration in physical, psychological, and social functioning; (2) weight loss or evidence of malnutrition; and (3) the lack of a readily explained cause such as a known terminal disease (Egbert, 1993b). Initially, the older adult may exhibit weight loss, a gradual decline in physical and/or cognitive function, and a decreased interest and involvement in social activities (Braun et al., 1988). The slow, downward trajectory may go unnoticed or may be attributed to other conditions such as dementia. As the failure to thrive progresses without appropriate intervention, the clinical course can be visualized as a downward spiral (Fig. 14–3). Anorexia can cause weight loss and malnutrition, which then spiral to depression. The resulting cognitive dysfunction contributes to social withdrawal and isolation, leading to giving up and ultimately death.

PREDISPOSING FACTORS

Age-related and sociodemographic factors predispose older adults to failure to thrive (Palmer, 1990). The 11 "D's" of the dwindles as described by Egbert (1993b) reflect the biopsychosocial failure common in the condition.

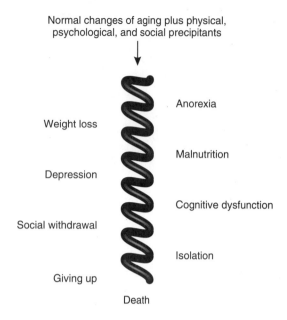

Normal changes of aging plus physical, psychological, and social precipitants

Weight loss

Anorexia

Depression

Malnutrition

Social withdrawal

Cognitive dysfunction

Isolation

Giving up

Death

FIGURE 14–3. Downward spiral of geriatric failure to thrive. (Redrawn from Egbert, A. [1993]. "The dwindles." Failure to thrive in older patients. *Postgraduate Medicine, 94*[5], 201.)

A more comprehensive list of the predisposing factors includes a 12th "D" for functional dependency (Table 14–1). Alone, each precipitant may not be significant, but when combined with malnutrition and the normal physiologi-

---

TABLE 14-1

The 12 D's of the Dwindles: Predisposing Factors of Geriatric Failure to Thrive

Diseases
Dementia
Delirium
Dependency
Drinking alcohol or abusing other substances
Drugs
Dysphagia
Deafness, blindness, or other sensory deficits
Depression
Desertion by family and/or friends (social isolation)
Destitution (poverty)
Despair (giving up)

Adapted from Egbert, A. (1993). "The dwindles." Failure to thrive in older patients. *Postgraduate Medicine, 94*(5), 204.

cal changes of aging, each precipitant can lead to failure to thrive.

Diseases. The most common diseases contributing to failure to thrive are chronic lung diseases, congestive heart failure, cancer (particularly of the pancreas and gastrointestinal tract), infections (particularly endocarditis, tuberculosis, pneumonia, and urinary tract infection), thyroid disease, and disease processes that produce prolonged immobility such as stroke and hip fractures (Fox et al., 1996; Palmer, 1990; Verdery, 1997a).

Dementia. Dementia is the most common cause of failure to thrive, in which the patient's functional capacity for independent ADL or instrumental activities of daily living (IADL) deteriorates. Dementia interferes with nutritional status by making it difficult for people to obtain and prepare food and feed themselves. Anorexia and weight loss are associated with the later stages of dementia. Berkman and colleagues' study of hospitalized elderly patients (1989) found that 40% of those patients diagnosed with failure to thrive had dementia. Reversible (delirium) and nonreversible dementias should be differentiated (see Chapter 18).

Delirium. Delirium is often mistaken for dementia but can usually be differentiated by its acute onset, greater fluctuations in symptoms, and shorter course. It is also associated with acute febrile illness, dehydration, drug reactions or interactions, severe anemia, myocardial infarction, stroke, and toxic metabolic disorders. It is usually reversible when its cause is identified and corrected (see Chapter 18).

Dependency. Functional decline is both a precursor and an outcome of failure to thrive. Frail older people with preexisting functional impairments are the most vulnerable to continued deterioration. Dependency can result from other predisposing factors, such as chronic disease, dementia, delirium, depression, sensory impairments, and drug reactions.

Drinking Alcohol. Older people have a lower tolerance for alcohol and thus require less alcohol to get intoxicated or addicted. Excessive drinking or substance abuse is often missed in this age group because older adults tend to live alone, are retired or unemployed, and do not drive (see Chapter 23).

Drugs. Drug-induced failure to thrive can

result from side effects, adverse reactions, and drug interactions of both prescribed and over-the-counter medications. Nausea and vomiting caused by adverse drug reactions can lead to dehydration and malnutrition and can initiate the downward spiral of failure to thrive. Anorexia, with resulting weight loss, is a possible side effect of the long-term use of antibiotics, digoxin, or acetazolamide (Diamox) (Haken, 1996). Depression is associated with several drug classes used to treat chronic diseases (see Tables 17–3 and 26–5).

Dysphagia. Swallowing difficulties as well as choking and drooling can lead to social embarrassment and decreased food intake. These problems are associated with diseases more prevalent in the elderly (e.g., Parkinson's disease or stroke) or may have a functional cause (e.g., having ill-fitting dentures).

Sensory Deficits. Hearing and visual impairments can induce failure to thrive by affecting communication skills, increasing isolation, and causing social withdrawal (see Chapter 22). Sensory deficits are linked to injurious falls, which can trigger the failure to thrive syndrome.

Depression. Depressed older patients may show symptoms of irritability or memory problems rather than mood alterations. Depression usually results in a poor appetite, which reduces food intake and can lead to failure to thrive. Clinicians should keep a high index of suspicion for drug-induced depression associated with the use of antihypertensives, cardiovascular agents, corticosteroids, narcotic and nonsteroidal antiinflammatory analgesics, antihistamines (e.g., cimetidine), antiparkinsonian agents, antimicrobials (especially sulfonamides and isoniazid), psychotropic drugs (including sedatives, hypnotics, and antipsychotics), estrogen, and chemotherapeutic agents (Kane et al., 1994).

Desertion. A high percentage of geriatric failure to thrive is caused by social isolation resulting from the loss of friends and family through death, travel, or moving as well as patient or family indifference. Isolation leads to loneliness, anxiety, depression, denial, apathy, or suicidal ideation and may also cause alterations in eating behaviors (White, 1994).

For example, older adults who live alone tend to consume fewer calories (Davis et al., 1990).

Destitution. Poverty results in an inability to afford food, medication, travel, or recreational activities. It therefore contributes to social isolation and malnutrition as well as noncompliance with drug regimens. Many older individuals or families who are eligible for economic assistance never receive this aid. Fewer than 8% of elderly low-income households receive Supplemental Security Income, and fewer than 6% receive food stamps (Schwenk, as cited in White, 1994).

Despair. The loss of the will to live, or *giving up,* is lethal in old age. Giving up occurs when the individual determines that his or her life is not worth continuing. It is usually seen in patients who are experiencing a combination of social or environmental losses, a chronic debilitating illness, and a poor response to treatment or rehabilitation. These patients then withdraw from goal-directed activities such as making meals, eating, and drinking. This withdrawal can subsequently lead to death (Egbert, 1993b). Other terms synonymous with giving up are *passive suicide* and *psychogenic mortality.* These terms are used to describe conditions in which older patients turn their heads to the wall and lose their will to live (Newbern & Krowchuk, 1994).

MANAGEMENT OF FAILURE TO THRIVE

All frail elderly patients should have a comprehensive geriatric assessment as described in Chapters 5 and 6. To halt the downward trajectory, the risk of failure to thrive should be detected early and intervention directed toward the predisposing causes. The following principles adapted from Egbert (1993b) serve to guide the management of failure to thrive:

- Identify all precipitating factors
- Use a multidisciplinary approach, including an advanced practice gerontological nurse, geriatrician, dietician, social worker, physical therapist, occupational therapist, and psychologist; other disciplines may also be included as appropriate, such as a

speech pathologist, pastoral counselors, and art and music therapists
- Treat early before failure to thrive becomes irreversible
- Correct deficits that can be easily treated, such as visual and sensory impairments
- Interview family members and caregivers
- Obtain laboratory and diagnostic studies as indicated

Assessment

Failure to thrive results from multiple and interacting medical, psychological, social, and functional causes. Signs and symptoms of failure to thrive are often subtle and can reflect disorders in multiple body systems. Any patient who presents with unexplained weight loss, a gradual decline in functional status, or a discontinuation of usual or favorite hobbies and activities is considered at risk for failure to thrive and should receive a detailed assessment (Table 14–2). This evaluation is focused

TABLE 14-2
Assessment of Failure to Thrive

History and physical examination
Psychosocial assessment
  Mental status screening
  Depression screening
  Social history
Functional assessment
  Activities of daily living
  Instrumental activities of daily living
Nutritional assessment
  Height and weight (body mass index)
  Dietary history
  Food diary
  Anthropometric measures
Caregiver assessment
  Collateral history
  Caregiver burden
  Risk of elder mistreatment
Laboratory and diagnostic tests
  Initial: complete blood count, fasting chemistry panel, erythrocyte sedimentation rate, thyroid panel, urinalysis, purified protein derivative (PPD) skin test, chest x-ray
  Additional: Other blood studies, urine culture, other x-rays, diagnostic imaging as indicated
Values history

TABLE 14-3
Differential Diagnoses in Failure to Thrive

Alcoholism
Acquired immune deficiency syndrome
Anemia (folate or vitamin B_{12} deficiencies)
Cancer (especially gastrointestinal, colorectal, pancreatic)
Cerebrovascular accident
Chronic lung disease
Congestive heart failure
Coronary artery disease
Delirium
Dementia
Dental problems
Depression
Diabetes mellitus
Drug reactions
End-stage organ failure (heart, kidney, lung, or liver)
Hyperthyroidism or hypothyroidism
Infections (especially pneumonia, urinary tract infections, bacterial endocarditis, tuberculosis)
Malabsorption or maldigestive syndromes
Primary hyperparathyroidism with hypercalcemia

on the identification of predisposing factors that might be treatable and reversible. In addition, the patient's values should be clarified to help determine the most appropriate treatment plan.

HISTORY AND PHYSICAL EXAMINATION

A thorough history and physical examination should be performed to detect any of the conditions or diseases commonly associated with failure to thrive (Table 14–3). Attention should be given to screening for high-risk conditions that affect cardiac output, exercise tolerance, strength, mobility, functional independence, and nutritional status. These conditions include organ failure, delirium, depression, stroke, cancer, anemia, and gastrointestinal disorders. The patient may have an acute illness superimposed on multiple chronic diseases, which confounds a diagnosis of the precipitating cause(s).

Current medications, including prescription and over-the-counter preparations, should be reviewed to assess for drug misuse (overuse or underuse) as well as for adverse effects (see Chapter 26). The use of three or more medications is linked to nutritional deficiencies (Lipschitz, 1994; Nutrition Screening Initiative, 1992). Some drugs have potentially harmful effects on nutritional status and may cause depression, which contributes to anorexia (see Table 17–3). Some drugs such as digoxin and antibiotics may cause anorexia or nausea, which then leads to weight loss. Medications with anticholinergic effects, such as the anticholinergics, antihistamines, antipsychotics, and antidepressants, may cause a dry mouth, which interferes with the pleasure of eating. They can also cause delirium even at normal adult doses. Other delirium-inducing drugs are the benzodiazepines, centrally acting antihypertensive agents, digoxin, cimetidine, and nonsteroidal antiinflammatory agents. Overuse of over-the-counter drugs such as laxatives, antacids, antihistamines, and nonsteroidal antiinflammatory agents (e.g., ibuprofen) may cause symptoms that adversely affect appetite and nutrient absorption or may cause a drug-induced anemia.

The use of tobacco, alcohol, and other recreational drugs should be included in the patient's medication history. If possible, the clinician should determine who is supplying the drug. Alcoholism is a common disease in older adults, affecting as many as 10% of those living at home and as many as 40% of those living in nursing homes (Egbert 1993a). Alcohol use greatly increases the risk of drug-induced nutritional deficiency (Roe, 1994). Symptoms of alcoholism tend to be nonspecific and may include failure to thrive, depression, insomnia, diarrhea, and dementia (Egbert, 1993a) (see Chapter 23).

The physical examination includes an assessment of height and weight, with an emphasis on evaluating the special senses (vision, hearing, taste, smell), oral health, and cardiovascular, pulmonary, musculoskeletal, gastrointestinal, and neurological systems (see Chapter 6). Clinicians should keep a high index of suspicion whenever there is involuntary weight loss exceeding 10 pounds or 10% of body weight in 6 months; 7.5% in 3 months; 5% in 1 month; or a body weight below 80% of desirable weight (Nutrition Screening Initiative, 1992; Lipschitz, 1994; Silver, 1993). Low body weight

is highly predictive of increased morbidity and mortality (Andres, 1994; Ryan et al., 1995).

PSYCHOSOCIAL ASSESSMENT

A hallmark of failure to thrive is the lack of interest in usual activities. Thus, a careful assessment of mental and affective status is essential. A variety of standardized instruments can be used to screen for depression and dementia (see Chapters 7, 17, and 18). Patients with severe depressive symptoms or who fail an antidepressant trial should be referred for psychological evaluation.

A social history as described in Chapters 8 and 9 is also important to identify familial attachments and support systems. Frequently, patients with failure to thrive have few or no family or friends. The social history should include cultural and religious affiliations; the loss of significant others, including pets; and other losses, such as those of homes, jobs, or finances and relocations of the patient or his or her family members.

FUNCTIONAL ASSESSMENT

Difficulty in managing self-care activities is one of the first signs of failure to thrive. A functional assessment including ADL and IADL should be conducted. The patient's baseline level of functioning should be determined early so that it can be compared with any later changes as recognized by the patient, family member, or staff member. The most common causes of decreased self-care are activity intolerance, decreased endurance, and cognitive and psychological impairment. Standardized instruments that are useful in assessing physical functioning (e.g., the Katz Index and the Functional Independence Measure) are described in Chapter 9.

NUTRITIONAL ASSESSMENT

Anorexia, decreased food intake, and weight loss are cardinal features of failure to thrive. Unexplained weight loss occurs in 13% of outpatients (Wallace et al., 1995), in 35 to 50% of general medical-surgical patients (Bistrian et al., 1974, 1976), and in 45% of nursing home patients (Keller, 1991). Although cancer is a leading cause, weight loss can occur for a variety of other reasons, including poor dentition, a lack of financial resources to purchase food, problems in preparing food, dysphagia, depression, dementia, diarrhea, and chronic diseases (Robbins, 1989).

Early detection of nutritional problems is essential to prevent complications from malnutrition. A slightly nutritionally compromised older adult rapidly becomes malnourished if his or her metabolic needs rise, whether from infection or tissue loss (Hamm, 1994). Patients with multiple chronic illnesses or severe disability or who are residing in long-term care institutions are at high risk for malnutrition. Table 14–4 lists other risk factors for malnutrition in the elderly.

Nutritional status should be carefully assessed using a dietary history; a food diary; height, weight, and anthropometric measurements; and selected laboratory data. Key indicators of nutritional problems are listed in Table 14–5. It may be beneficial to consult with a dietitian who can assist in nutritional assessment and management.

The nutritional history should include information in the following areas (Table 14–6):

- Finances
- Physical activity
- Sociocultural influences
- Eating and diet patterns
- Appetite, including smell and taste perception
- Attitudes toward food and eating
- Food allergies, intolerances or avoidances, including fad diets
- Dental and oral health
- Gastrointestinal problems
- Acute and chronic illnesses and any treatment requiring dietary modification prescribed by a primary care provider
- Medication and dietary supplement use
- Recent weight history
- Patient perceptions

A 3-day food diary is helpful in assessing for adequate intake of calories, protein, carbohydrates, fat, vitamins, and minerals. At the end of the 3 days, nutrient intake is calculated, averaged, and compared with the recom-

---

TABLE 14-4

Risk Factors for Malnutrition in Older Adults

Age-related changes
  Loss of subcutaneous fat or muscle mass
  Hypodipsia
  Diminished palatability
  Altered neuropeptide control of feeding

Disease
  Acquired immune deficiency syndrome
  Alcoholism
  Cancer
  Cardiomyopathy or congestive heart failure
  Cerebrovascular disease
  Chronic renal insufficiency
  Chronic lung disease
  Diabetes mellitus
  Malabsorption syndromes
  Parkinson's disease
  Poorly healing wounds
  Tuberculosis

Psychiatric disorders
  Depression
  Dementia
  Distorted body image

Environment
  Isolation
  Limited income

Drugs
  Adverse drug effects
  Polypharmacy
  Drug-nutrient interactions
  Drug-drug interactions

Laboratory measures
  Low cholesterol (<160 mg/dL)
  High cholesterol (>240 mg/dL)
  Low albumin (<3.5 g/dL)
  Prealbumin (10–15 mg/dL)
  Anemia
  Weight loss greater than 10% in 6 months

Other
  Poor oral or dental hygiene
  Constipation
  Dependency or disability

Data from DeHoog (1996); Nutrition Screening Initiative (1992); and Silver (1993).

---

mended daily allowances (RDA) (Table 14–7) or food pyramid guidelines. If a food diary cannot be obtained, a food frequency review or a 24-hour recall can be used. This review or recall should focus on the period during which failure to thrive was first detected as well as the period before it occurred. A food frequency

TABLE 14-5

Key Indicators in the Assessment of Undernutrition

Height and weight
Percentage of desirable body weight
Body mass index (weight/height in kg^2;
  should be 22–27)
Weight loss within 6 months
Clinical features
  Difficulty chewing or swallowing
  Digestive problems
  Problems with mouth, teeth, or gums
  Skin changes, which suggest
    malnutrition
  Angular stomatitis
  Glossitis
  History of bone pain
  Bone fractures
Living environment
  Income (<$6,000/yr/person)
  Lives alone
  Concerned about home security
  Inadequate heating or cooling
  No stove or refrigerator
  Unable or prefers not to spend money
    on food
Functional status
  Needs assistance with activities of daily
    living and instrumental activities of
    daily living
Mental or affective status
  Mini-Mental State Examination (<26)
  Geriatric Depression Scale (>5) or Beck
    Depression Inventory (<15)

Drug use
  More than three prescription drugs
  More than three nonprescription drugs
  Vitamin and mineral supplements
Dietary data
  Insufficient food intake each day
  Number of days per month without any food
  Poor appetite
  Usually eats alone
  Special dietary needs
    Self-defined
    Prescribed
    Problems with compliance or meeting special
      needs
  Multiple diet prescriptions
  Other unusual dietary practices
Usual daily food intake
  Fewer than two servings of milk or dairy products
  Fewer than two servings of meat, protein, fish, or
    eggs
  Fewer than three servings of fruit or juice
  Fewer than three servings of vegetables
  Fewer than six servings of bread, cereal, or grains
  More than 2 ounces of alcohol for men or 1 ounce
    of alcohol for women
Laboratory and anthropometric data
  Serum albumin (<3.5 g/dL)
  Serum cholesterol (<160 mg/dL or <240 mg/dL)
  Prealbumin (10–15 mg dL)
  Triceps skinfold thickness (<10th percentile)
  Mid-arm circumference (<10th percentile)

Data from DeHoog (1996); Lipschitz (1994); and Nutrition Screening Initiative (1992).

---

determination provides a retrospective review of dietary intake over the past day, week, or month and organizes food into groups that have common nutrients (Appendix 14–1). A 24-hour recall asks the person to list specific foods consumed during the past 24 hours (Appendix 14–2). The recall method can be problematic because of short-term memory difficulties, an atypical intake on the day being recalled, and the tendency to overreport or underreport intake. Using both questionnaires provides a cross-check of the accuracy of estimated intake (DeHoog, 1996).

Whenever possible, observe the patient eating, noting problems with handling, chewing, and swallowing food. If chewing is a problem because of the lack of teeth or poorly fitting dentures, the patient should be referred for dental care. If choking or swallowing problems are present, the patient should be referred to a speech pathologist for an evaluation of dysphagia.

The body mass index (BMI) should be determined, as it is an important indicator of nutritional status. A nomogram for calculating BMI is illustrated in Figure 14–4. Desirable BMI ranges between 22 and 27 (Nutrition Screening Initiative, 1992). Anthropometric measurements using the midarm muscle circumference and triceps skinfold are also recommended in assessing nutritional status. Because measurement error can occur, clinicians should be trained by an individual skilled in performing anthropometric assessments. A triceps skinfold that is less than the 10th percentile indicates poor nutritional status (Nutrition Screening

TABLE 14-6
Dietary History

Finances

Income
Amount of money for food each week or month and
   individual's perception of its adequacy for meeting
   food needs
Eligibility for food stamps

Physical Activity and Rest

Mobility impairment
Daily activity
Exercise—type, amount, frequency
Sleep—hours/day, including naps
Manual dexterity and strength to open containers, set up
   meals, hold utensils
Fatigue while eating or self feeding

Sociocultural Influences

Education
Ethnic and religious background
Cultural influences on diet
Recent loss of spouse
Depression

Eating Pattern

When and where individual eats
Whether individual eats alone or with people; recent
   changes in eating companion
Time of day
Environmental influences that affect eating (e.g., noisy
   dining room, disruptive eating companions)
Snacks
Ability to shop and prepare food
Person who does shopping (if applicable)
Person who does cooking (if applicable)
Food storage and cooking facilities (stove, refrigerator)
Vision problems impairing shopping, food preparation, or
   eating
Transportation difficulties impairing shopping

Appetite

Good, poor; any changes
Taste and smell perception and any changes

Attitudes Toward Food and Eating

Disinterested in food
Irrational ideas about food, eating, and body weight
Changes in food preferences

Diet Pattern

Typical day's eating pattern
Food preferences
Foods avoided and reason
Food allergies and intolerances (describe)
Fluid intake and types
Special diet order by primary care provider
Compliance with diet order
Self-prescribed special diet (describe)

Dental and Oral Health

Dentures (wear with eating?)
Dental caries and missing teeth
Sore mouth
Bleeding gums
Problems with chewing
Problems with swallowing, salivation, food sticking

Gastrointestinal

Problems with heartburn, bloating, gas, diarrhea, vomiting,
   constipation, distention
Changes in bowel habits
Use of home remedies
Use of antacid, laxative, or other drug use
Chronic gastrointestinal disease
Surgery on gastrointestinal tract

Illness

Acute infection or illness
Chronic diseases and their treatment
Acute or chronic confusion
Length of time of treatment

Medication History

Current medications—type, dosage, frequency, and time of
   medication (both prescribed and over-the-counter drugs)
Vitamins and mineral supplements—type, dosage, and
   frequency
Alcohol intake
History of alcohol abuse

Recent Weight Change

Loss or gain; over what time period
Rapid or slow change
Intentional or involuntary

Dietary or Nutritional Problems (as perceived by patient)

Data from DeHoog (1966); and Rajcevich & Wakefield (1991).

Initiative, 1992). Table 14–8 lists norms for arm
circumference and triceps skinfold for older
men and women.

CAREGIVER ASSESSMENT

Separate interviews should be conducted with
family members and other caregivers who can
provide valuable information regarding the
cause and progression of the failure to thrive.
An assessment of the caregiver's burden, coping abilities, and strengths should also be conducted. Caregiver stress and burden may be a
contributing factor in the development of failure to thrive, and when there is high caregiver

TABLE 14-7

Recommended Dietary Allowances for People Older Than 50 Years

	Men	Women
Energy (kcal)	2300.0	1900.0
Protein (g)	63.0	50.0
Vitamin A (μg RE)	1000.0	800.0
Vitamin D (μg)	5.0	5.0
Vitamin E (mg a-TE)	10.0	8.0
Vitamin K (μg)	80.0	65.0
Thiamin (mg)	1.2	1.0
Riboflavin (mg)	1.4	1.2
Niacin (mg NE)	15.0	13.0
Vitamin B_6 (mg)	2.0	1.6
Folate (μg)	200.0	180.0
Vitamin B_{12} (μg)	2.0	2.0
Calcium (mg)	800.0	800.0
Phosphorus (mg)	800.0	800.0
Magnesium (mg)	350.0	280.0
Iron (mg)	10.0	10.0
Zinc (mg)	15.0	12.0
Iodine (μg)	150.0	150.0
Selenium (μg)	70.0	55.0

Adapted from National Academy of Sciences (1989). *Recommended dietary allowances* (10th ed.). Philadelphia: National Academy of Sciences. Reprinted with permission from *Recommended dietary allowances: 10th edition.* Copyright 1989 by the National Academy of Sciences. Courtesy of the National Academy Press, Washington, D.C.

stress, the risk of elder mistreatment should be evaluated (see Chapter 29).

LABORATORY AND OTHER TESTS

Based on the findings from the history and physical examination, relevant diagnostic tests should be ordered. Initial tests should include a complete blood count with differential, fasting chemistry panel, prealbumin level, erythrocyte sedimentation rate, thyroid panel, urinalysis, two-step purified protein derivative (PPD), and chest x-ray. Depending on the differential diagnoses, additional tests may be ordered. For suspected anemia, total iron binding capacity as well as the levels of folate, vitamin B_{12}, transferrin, and ferritin should be measured. If a dipstick urinalysis is positive for urinary tract infection, a follow-up urine culture should be obtained. For suspected cardiovascular disease, an electrocardiogram, echocardiogram, and ra-

dionucleotide scans may be indicated. If endocarditis is suspected, blood cultures should be ordered. For suspected pulmonary disease, pulmonary function tests and sputum for cytology and acid-fast bacilli may be indicated. If cancer is suspected, chest and other x-rays, a mammogram, Papanicolaou (Pap) smear, and prostatic specific antigen (PSA) test may be ordered. Diagnostic imaging such as computed tomography or magnetic resonance imaging may also be indicated. However, these expensive studies are rarely needed, because most of the causes of failure to thrive can usually be diagnosed through a comprehensive geriatric assessment as described in Chapter 5.

VALUES CLARIFICATION

A *values history* is aimed at determining whether the length or quality of life is more important to the patient (Doukas & McCullough, 1991). If the patient values quality of life over longevity, questions should be aimed at defining issues of quality of life that are specific to the patient. Appendix 14–3 includes an example of a values history used in establishing advance directives.

Intervention

Advanced practice nurses have an important role in managing patients with failure to thrive. Scientific knowledge, ethical decision making, and humanistic concern should be integrated into the development of the patient's plan of care. The goals of treatment are to (1) treat underlying conditions that may be contributing to the failure to thrive, (2) maintain or improve nutritional status, (3) maintain or improve functional status, and (4) maintain comfort and dignity.

When reversing the failure to thrive is no longer a therapeutic goal, care should focus on managing the symptoms and preventing complications (Osato et al., 1993). The ultimate goal is to improve the quality of life for whatever quantity of life remains. Religious and cultural preferences are important considerations when developing the care plan, especially as individuals approach death and dying.

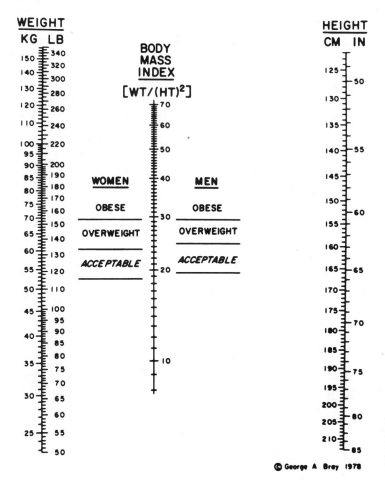

FIGURE 14–4. Nomogram for body mass index. (Copyright 1978 by George A. Bray, M.D., Executive Director, Pennington Biomedical Research Center, Louisiana State University, Baton Rouge, LA.)

Interventions in failure to thrive depend on the underlying causes; they can include health promotion and education, nutritional counseling and/or supplementation, exercise prescription, family counseling, and referral to appropriate community resources. All precipitants of failure to thrive should be identified and treated, if feasible. Table 14–9 presents a summary of potential interventions based on the predisposing causes of failure to thrive.

Undernutrition may be both a cause and an effect of failure to thrive. However, unlike some of the other predisposing factors, it can usually be treated. Medications that have an adverse effect on nutritional status (e.g., anorexia, nausea, dry mouth, depression) should be identified and changed if possible. Patients with a dry mouth from anticholinergic medications should be encouraged to drink water and other fluids and to eat foods with sauces or that require a lot of chewing. Snacking on sugarless hard candies is also beneficial (Nutrition Screening Initiative, 1992).

A critical intervention in failure to thrive is nutritional supplementation (Verdery, 1997b). Food intake should be planned using a calculation of daily calorie, protein, carbohydrate, and fat requirements based on ideal body weight. Table 14–10 presents age-adjusted weight norms for older adults. Protein intake is essential in correcting protein-energy malnutrition. In this situation, protein intake of 1.5 g per kg of body weight is recommended (Silver, 1993); otherwise, 1 g per kg of body weight is recom-

TABLE 14-8

Norms for Arm Circumference and Triceps Skinfold

Percentile	Men		Women	
	55–65 yr	65–75 yr	55–65 yr	65–75 yr
Arm Circumference (cm)				
10th	27.3	26.3	25.7	25.2
50th	31.7	30.7	30.3	29.9
95th	36.9	35.5	38.5	27.9
Arm Muscle Circumference (cm)				
10th	24.5	23.5	19.6	19.5
50th	27.8	26.8	22.5	22.5
95th	32.0	30.6	28.0	27.9
Triceps Skinfold (mm)				
10th	6	6	16	14
50th	11	11	25	24
95th	22	22	38	36

From Frisancho, A. R. (1981). New norms of upper limb fat and muscle areas for assessment of nutritional status. *American Journal of Clinical Nutrition, 34*, 2540–2545.

mended for those older adults with chronic illness (Barrocas et al., 1994). If there has been significant weight loss, the goal is to optimize caloric intake to 35 kcal per kg (Morley et al., 1986). Daily fluid intake of at least 1500 mL of water or other fluids should be encouraged. Commercial sports drinks that are high in calories and fortified with vitamins and electrolytes can be used. Vitamin and mineral supplements should be instituted.

Meals should be planned according to daily requirements as well as the patient's food preferences. Food and fluids of choice should be available in frequent, small meals and snacks throughout the day rather than in only regularly scheduled meals. The use of oral nutritional supplements should be considered if protein and calorie counts cannot be increased sufficiently with normal food intake or because of special dietary considerations.

Patients who lack teeth or who have ill-fitting dentures or dental caries that is severe enough to impair eating should be referred to a dentist to improve oral health. For those with chewing difficulty, food should be chopped, ground, pureed, or blended. Patients with choking difficulties may benefit from the use of cold, thick foods and sauces and chopped, ground, or pureed meals. All patients should be encouraged to exercise, which helps promote appetite and improve mood (Silver, 1993). Wheelchair-bound patients can participate in sitting exercises, and ambulatory patients should be advised to begin walking as much as tolerated.

When making the nutritional plan, clinicians should consider the importance of the social nature of eating. Providing meal times with other people either through social groupings within an institutional setting or in congregate meal site programs may improve dietary adequacy (Walker & Beauchene, 1991).

The effectiveness of nutritional intervention should be evaluated. Improvements in a patient's nutritional status can be determined by observing food intake; performing periodic daily calorie counts of protein, calories, and micronutrients; and monitoring weekly or monthly weights. If oral intake is poor or if the individual has difficulty with swallowing and choking, nasogastric, nasoenteric, or percutaneous tube feeding may be indicated. This type of feeding may be temporary until the patient can learn to swallow again. Prior to initiating enteral nutrition, the clinician should discuss wishes and preferences regarding feeding deci-

TABLE 14-9

Management of Predisposing Factors (The 12 D's) of Failure to Thrive

Predisposing Factors	Interventions
Diseases	
Anemias	Correct underlying deficiency or condition causing anemia
Cancer	Refer to oncologist for evaluation and treatment; optimize nutritional status; provide symptom management as needed
Congestive heart failure	Correct any reversible cause; moderately restrict sodium in diet; use diuretic therapy in combination with cardiac drugs; monitor weights
Chronic lung disease	Stop smoking; avoid airway irritants and allergens; use bronchodilator therapy, antibiotic therapy if airway infection is present, chest physiotherapy, cough and pursed lip training, abdominal breathing, supplemental oxygen in severe cases, and energy conservation techniques; refer to occupational therapy
Infections	Use appropriate antibiotic therapy; maintain adequate fluid intake
Thyroid disease	Correct hypothyroidism; refer hyperthyroidism to specialist
Dementia	Treat comorbidity; use validation, stimulation, and touch therapy; provide caregiver education and support groups; refer to community resources as indicated
Delirium	Treat underlying cause; modify environment for safety
Depression	Assess for suicide risk; refer for detailed psychological evaluation; provide antidepressant therapy; encourage development of social networks
Drinking alcohol	Provide patient education and alcohol detoxification followed by alcohol treatment program if indicated
Drugs	Carefully review drugs; remove all unnecessary drugs; consider drug holiday (trial off drug or drugs); change drug class or group to one that has fewer side effects
Dysphagia	Refer to speech pathology for evaluation; ensure proper fit of dentures; encourage patient to eat thick, cold foods and sauces, add thickening agent to foods, and to chop, grind, or puree foods
Sensory deficits	Refer for audiology evaluation and hearing aids if indicated; refer for ophthalmology evaluation, cataract removal if indicated, and appropriate corrective lenses; provide good illumination, magnifying glasses or other optical aids as needed; encourage the use of herbs and spices to increase taste perception
Functional dependency	Refer to physical therapist to increase muscle strength and endurance; refer to occupational therapist if indicated; prescribe assistive devices as needed; refer for appropriate community resources (e.g., in-home personal care aide or health aide, home-delivered meals, caregiver support programs, adult day care)
Desertion	Identify social network; contact family and friends to encourage visits; help establish new social contacts
Destitution	Refer to social worker or local Area Agency on Aging and local welfare office to assist in determining eligibility and application for food stamps, Social Security, supplemental security income, Medicare, Medicaid, housing assistance, veterans' benefits, energy assistance, meal programs
Despair	Refer for spiritual counseling; encourage family participation and visits; provide caregiver education and counseling; maintain nursing contact

TABLE 14-10
Height/Weight Tables for Ages 65 to 94 Years

Height (in)	Age (yrs)					
	65–69	70–74	75–79	80–84	85–89	90–94
			Men			
61*	128–156	125–153	123–151	122–148		
62	130–158	127–155	125–153	122–148		
63	131–161	129–157	127–155	122–150	120–146	
64	134–164	131–161	129–157	124–152	122–148	
65	136–166	134–164	130–160	127–155	125–153	117–143
66	139–169	137–167	133–163	130–158	128–156	120–146
67	140–172	140–170	136–166	132–162	130–160	122–150
68	143–175	142–174	139–169	135–165	133–163	126–154
69	147–179	146–178	142–174	139–169	137–167	130–158
70	150–184	148–182	146–178	143–175	140–172	134–164
71	155–189	152–186	149–183	148–180	144–176	139–169
72	159–195	156–190	154–188	153–187	148–182	
73	164–200	160–196	158–192			
			Women			
58	120–146	112–138	111–135			
59	121–147	114–140	112–136	100–122	99–121	
60	122–148	116–142	113–139	106–130	102–124	
61	123–151	118–144	115–141	109–133	104–128	
62	125–153	121–147	118–144	112–136	108–132	107–131
63	127–155	123–151	121–147	115–141	112–136	107–131
64	130–158	126–154	123–151	119–145	115–141	108–132
65	132–162	130–158	126–154	122–150	120–146	112–136
66	136–166	132–162	128–157	126–154	124–152	116–142
67	140–170	136–166	131–161	130–161	128–156	
68	143–175	140–170				
69	148–180	144–176				

*Formula for calculating stature from knee height (from Chumlea, W. [1984]. *Nutritional assessment of the elderly through anthropometry* [p. 10]. Columbus, OH: Ross Laboratories):

Stature for men = 64.19 − (0.04 × age) + (2.02 × knee height)

Stature for women = 84.88 − (0.24 × age) + (1.83 × knee height)

Adapted from Master, A. M., Laser R. P., Beckman, G. (1960). Tables of average weight and height of Americans age 65–94. *Journal of the American Medical Association, 172*, 658–662. Copyright 1960 by the American Medical Association.

sions with the patient and/or family members. If the patient's wishes are to have enteral nutrition, consultation with an interdisciplinary nutritional support team composed of a physician, dietitian, nurse, and pharmacist may help determine the most appropriate enteral and parenteral route and the nutritional products that should be used.

Functional status may be improved through physical and occupational therapy. Exercise programs have been shown to be effective in improving physical function and strength in frail, very old nursing home residents (Fiatarone et al., 1990). The use of assistive devices may be necessary to compensate for functional deficits in these patients. Interventions to improve the safety of the environment may help in preventing injuries from falls. To increase residents' functional independence and self-esteem, caregivers should use patience and should encourage the residents to complete their own ADL. Nonprofessional staff and family members should be educated regarding the importance of the patient participating in his or her own care to the fullest extent possible, even if considerable time is required to prevent excess disability (see Chapter 16).

Depression, a major component underlying undernutrition and functional dependence, should be addressed, as the risk of passive and active suicide is high among older adults. Any individual exhibiting suicidal ideation or behavior should be referred for psychological evaluation. A trial of antidepressant medication such as sertaline (Zoloft) or nortriptyline (Pamelor) may be effective in improving mood as well as appetite and motivation. Modifying the social environment with the depressed individual is also important. Providing more frequent nursing visits to decrease the feelings of isolation is frequently beneficial. Visits by family members and friends should be encouraged. Long-distance relatives can stay connected with each other by making telephone calls or by sending audiocassette or videocassette recordings to the patient. Chapter 17 discusses additional interventions for the depressed individual.

Discharge planning should be initiated early in the hospitalization process. Patients should be given referrals to home healthcare and other appropriate community resources to support optimal functioning in the home environment. Patient and family education are required to maintain progress in weight gain or stabilization, improve muscle strength and physical functioning, and prevent falls and injuries. The primary care provider and a home health nurse should provide follow-up every 1 to 2 weeks until the patient has stabilized.

If failure to thrive cannot be reversed, symptoms should be treated so that the patient can be made more comfortable. Advance directives should be discussed if they have not been determined previously. Patient and family counseling should be provided as a means of support through the dying trajectory. Referral for pastoral counseling may be beneficial for individuals who desire this intervention.

ROLE OF THE ADVANCED PRACTICE NURSE

Across all practice settings, advanced practice nurses have a crucial role in the early detection of patients at risk for failure to thrive. Important components of the advanced practice role include health screening, health education and promotion, counseling, and patient advocacy. By working within a broad interdisciplinary team (composed of physicians, psychologists, psychiatrists, dieticians, ethicists, chaplains, social workers, and occupational, physical, and recreational therapists), nurses can help establish protocols for the assessment and management of patients with failure to thrive and can develop guidelines for supporting patients, families, and staff members when the situation is not reversible. The advanced practice nurse should act as an advocate for the elderly to ensure that they receive full informed consent and to help them develop advanced directives such as a living will and a durable power of attorney. This may help decrease the risk of an ethical dilemma occurring before a critical health situation arises. Decision making is more effective while patients are competent and are not experiencing an acute illness or crisis (see Chapters 3 and 4).

SUMMARY

Failure to thrive is a clinical syndrome that is being increasingly recognized in frail older patients who show weight loss and functional deterioration not directly attributable to a disease process. Prompt treatment of all potentially correctable precipitating causes is necessary to halt or reverse failure to thrive. If left untreated, failure to thrive eventually results in death.

The advanced practice nurse has a key role in the prevention, early detection, assessment, and management of failure to thrive. As part of a multidisciplinary or interdisciplinary team, the nurse can help develop protocols to evaluate and treat failure to thrive; to educate patients, families, and staff members about its causes and management; and to serve as an advocate to ensure the highest quality of remaining life for patients.

REFERENCES

Adler, W. H., & Nagel, J. E. (1981). Studies of immune function in a human publication. In D. Serge & L. Smith (Eds.), *Immunological aspects of aging* (pp. 296–311). New York: Dekker.

Andres, R. (1994). Mortality and obesity: The rationale for age-specific height-weight tables. In W. R. Hazzard, E. L. Bierman, J. P. Blass, et al. (Eds.), *Principles of geriatric medicine and gerontology* (3rd ed, pp. 847–853). New York: McGraw-Hill.

Barrocas, A., Craig, L. D., & Foltz, M. B. (1994). Nutrition support, supplementation, and replacement. *Primary Care, 21*, 149–173.

Berkman, B., Foster, L. W. S., & Campion, E. (1989). Failure to thrive: Paradigm for the frail elderly. *Gerontologist, 29*, 654–659.

Bernard, S. (1996). *1997 Standard ICD-9: 2 volumes in 1.* Salt Lake City, UT: Medicode, Inc.

Bistrian, B. R., Blackburn, G. L., Hollowell, E., et al. (1974). Protein status of general surgical patients. *Journal of the American Medical Association, 230*, 858–860.

Bistrian, B. R., Blackburn, G. L., Vitale, J., et al. (1976). Prevalence of malnutrition in general medical patients. *Journal of the American Medical Association, 235*, 1567–1570.

Braun, J., Wykle, M., & Cowling, W. R. (1988). Failure to thrive in older persons: A concept derived. *Gerontologist, 28*, 809–812.

Brocklehurst, J. C. (Ed.). (1985). The day hospital. *Textbook of geriatric medicine and gerontology* (3rd ed., pp. 982–995). London: Churchill Livingstone.

Buchner, D. M., & Wagner, E. H. (1992). Preventing frail health. *Clinics in Geriatric Medicine, 8*, 1–17.

Davis, L., Murphy, S. P., Neuhaus, J. M., et al. (1990). Living arrangements and dietary quality of older U.S. adults. *Journal of the American Dietetic Association, 90*, 1167–1672.

DeHoog, S. (1996). The assessment of nutritional status. In L. K. Mahan & S. Escott-Stump (Eds.), *Krause's food, nutrition, and diet therapy* (9th ed., pp. 361–386). Philadelphia: W. B. Saunders.

Doukas, D. J., & McCullough, L. B. (1991). The values history: The evaluation of the patient's values and advance directives. *Journal of Family Practice, 32*, 145–153.

Egbert, A. (1993a). The older alcoholic: Recognizing the subtle clinical cues. *Geriatrics, 48*(7), 63–69.

Egbert, A. (1993b). "The dwindles." Failure to thrive in older patients. *Postgraduate Medicine, 94*(5), 199–212.

Fiatarone, M. A., Marks, E. C., Ryan, N. D., et al. (1990). High intensity strength training in octogenarians. Effects on skeletal muscle. *Journal of the American Medical Association, 263*, 3029–3034.

Fox, K. M., Hawkes, W. G., Magaziner, J., et al. (1996). Markers of failure to thrive among older hip fracture patients. *Journal of the American Geriatrics Society, 44*, 371–376.

Fried, L. (1994). Frailty. In W. R. Hazzard, E. L. Bierman, J. P. Blass, et al. (Eds.), *Principles of geriatric medicine and gerontology* (3rd ed., pp. 1149–1156). New York: McGraw-Hill.

Haken, V. (1996). Interactions between drugs and nutrients. In L. K. Mahan & S. Escott-Stump (Eds.), *Krause's food, nutrition, and diet therapy* (9th ed., pp. 387–402). Philadelphia: W. B. Saunders.

Hamm, R. J. (1994). The signs and symptoms of poor nutritional status. *Primary Care, 21*, 33–53.

Hildebrand, J. K., Joos, S. K., & Lee, M. A. (1997). Use of the diagnosis "Failure to thrive" in older veterans. *Journal of the American Geriatrics Society, 45*, 1113–1117.

Hodkinson, H. M. (1973). Non-specific presentation of illness. *British Medical Journal, 4*, 94–96.

Issacs, B., Gunn, J., McKechan A., et al. (1971). The concept of predeath. *Lancet, 1*, 1115–1118.

Kane, R. L., Ouslander, J. G., & Abrass, I. B. (1994). Diagnosis and management of depression. *Essentials of clinical geriatrics* (3rd ed., pp. 115–143). New York: McGraw Hill.

Keller, H. H. (1991). Malnutrition in institutionalized elderly: How and why? *Journal of the American Geriatrics Society, 41*, 1212–1218.

Lipschitz, D. A. (1994). Screening for nutritional status in the elderly. *Primary Care, 21*, 55–67.

MacAdam, M., Capitman, J., Yee, D., et al. (1989). Case management for frail elders: The Robert Wood Johnson Foundation's program for hospital initiatives in long-term care. *Gerontologist, 29*, 737–744.

Morley, J. E., Silver, A. J., Fiatarone, M., et al. (1986). UCLA Geriatric Grand Rounds: Nutrition and the elderly. *Journal of the American Geriatrics Society, 34*, 823–832.

National Institute on Aging (1991). *Physical frailty: A reducible barrier to independence for older Americans.* Report to the U.S. House of Representatives Committee on Appropriations. Bethesda, MD: U.S. Department of Health and Human Services, Public Health Service, Agency for Health Care Policy and Research.

Newbern, V. B., & Krowchuk, H. V. (1994). Failure to thrive in elderly people: A conceptual analysis. *Journal of Advanced Nursing, 19*, 840–849.

Nutrition Screening Initiative (1992). *Nutrition interventions manual for professionals caring for older Americans.* Washington, D.C.: Nutrition Screening Initiative.

Osato, E. E., Stone, J. T., Phillips, S. L., & Winne, D. M. (1993). Clinical manifestations: Failure to thrive in the elderly. *Journal of Gerontological Nursing, 19*(8), 28–34.

Palmer, R. M. (1990). 'Failure to thrive' in the elderly: Diagnosis and management. *Geriatrics, 45*(9), 47–55.

Pawlson, L. G. (1988). Hospital length of stay of frail elderly patients: Primary care by general internists versus geriatricians. *Journal of the American Geriatrics Society, 36*, 202–208.

Rajcevich, K., & Wakefield, B. (1991). Altered nutrition: Less than body requirements. In M. Maas, K. C. Buckwalter & M. Hardy (Eds.), *Nursing diagnoses and interventions for the elderly* (pp. 97–101). Redwood City, CA: Addison-Wesley Nursing.

Robbins, L. J. (1989). Evaluation of weight loss in the elderly. *Geriatrics, 44*(4), 31–37.

Rockwood, K., Fox, R. A., Stolee, P., et al. (1994). Frailty in elderly people: An evolving concept. *Canadian Medical Association Journal, 150*, 489–495.

Roe, D. A. (1994). Medications and nutrition in the elderly. *Primary Care, 21*, 135–142.

Rudman, D., Mattson, D. E., Feller, A. G., et al. (1989). A mortality risk index for men in a Veterans Administration extended care facility. *Journal of Parenteral and Enteral Nutrition, 13*, 189–195.

Ryan, C., Bryant, E., Eleazer, P., et al. (1995). Unintentional weight loss in long-term care: Predictor of mortality in the elderly. *Southern Medical Journal, 88*, 721–724.

Silver, A. J. (1993). The malnourished older patient: When and how to intervene. *Geriatrics, 48*(7), 70–74.

Strawbridge, W. J., Shema, S. J., Balfour, J. L., et al. (1998). Antecedents of frailty over three decades in an older cohort. *Journal of Gerontology: Social Sciences, 53B*, S9–S16.

Verdery, R. B. (1994). Failure to thrive. In W. R. Hazzard, E. L. Bierman, J. P. Blass, et al. (Eds.), *Principles of geriatric medicine and gerontology* (3rd ed., pp. 1205–1211). New York: McGraw-Hill.

Verdery, R. B. (1996). Failure to thrive in older people [Editorial]. *Journal of the American Geriatrics Society, 44*, 467–469.

Verdery, R. B. (1997a). Clinical evaluation of failure to thrive in older people. *Clinics in Geriatric Medicine, 13*, 769–778.

Verdery, R. B. (1997b). Failure to thrive in old age: Follow-up on a workshop. *Journal of Gerontology: Medical Sciences, 52A*, M333–M336.

Verdery, R. B., & Goldberg, A. P. (1991). Hypocholesterolemia as a predictor of death. A prospective study of 224 nursing home residents. *Journal of Gerontology: Medical Sciences, 46*, M84–M90.

Walker, D., & Beauchene, R. E. (1991). The relationship of loneliness, social isolation, and physical health to dietary adequacy of independent living elderly. *Journal of the American Dietetic Association, 91*, 300–304.

Wallace, J. I., Schwartz, R. S., LaCroix, A. Z., et al. (1995). Involuntary weight loss in older outpatients: Incidence and clinical significance. *Journal of the American Geriatrics Society, 43*, 329–337.

White, J. V. (1994). Risk factors for poor nutritional status. *Primary Care, 21*, 17–31.

Winograd, C. H., Gerety, M. B., Chung, M., et al. (1991). Screening for frailty: Criteria and predictors of outcomes. *Journal of the American Geriatrics Society, 39*, 778–784.

Woodhouse, K., Wynne, H., Baillie, S., et al. (1988). Who are the frail elderly? *Quarterly Journal of Medicine, 28*, 505–506.

APPENDIX │ **14-1**

Food Frequency Questionnaire

For the frequency of food use, the following pattern of questions may be useful. However, questions may have to be modified after learning some information from the 24-hour recall. For instance, if the patient has said he or she had a glass of milk yesterday, you wouldn't ask "Do you drink milk?" but rather "How much milk do you drink?" Record answers as 1/day, 1/wk, 3/mo, for example, or as accurately as possible. It may have to be noted just as "occasionally" or "rarely."

1. Do you drink milk? If so, how much?   What kind? whole   low-fat   skim

2. Do you use fat? If so, what kind?   How much?

3. How many times do you eat meat?   eggs   cheese   beans

4. Do you eat snack foods? If so, which ones?   How often?   How much?

5. What vegetables do you eat? (in each group) How often?

    a. Broccoli   green peppers   cooked greens   carrots   sweet potato

    b. Tomatoes   raw cabbage

    c. Asparagus   beets   cauliflower   corn   cooked cabbage

       celery   peas   lettuce

6. What fruits and how often?

    a. Apples or applesauce   apricots   bananas   berries   cherries

       grapes or grape juice   peaches   pears   pineapple   plums   prunes

       raisins

    b. Oranges   orange juice   grapefruit   grapefruit juice

7. Bread and cereal products

    a. How much bread do you usually eat with each meal?   Between meals?

    b. Do you eat cereal (daily, weekly) cooked?   Dry?

    c. How often do you eat foods such as macaroni, spaghetti, noodles, etc.?

    d. Do you eat whole grain breads and cereals?   How often?

8. Do you use salt?   Do you salt your food before tasting it?
   Do you cook with salt?   Do you "crave" salt or salty foods?

9. How many tsp of sugar do you use per day (1 packet = 1 tsp)?
(Be sure to ask patient about sugar on cereal, fruit, toast and in coffee, tea, etc.)

10. Do you eat desserts?   If so, how often?

11. Do you drink sugar-containing beverages such as soda pop?   How often?

12. How often do you eat candy or cookies?

13. Do you drink water?   How often during the day?
How much each time?   How much would you say you drink each day?

14. Do you use sugar substitutes in packet form or in drinks?
What is your use?   How often?

15. Do you drink alcohol?
Beer, wine, liquor?   How often?   How much?

16. Do you drink caffeinated beverages?   How often?   How much per day?

17. Do you drink pop?   How often?   How much?

From DeHoog, S. (1996). The assessment of nutritional status. In L. K. Mahan & S. Escott-Stump (Eds.), *Krause's food, nutrition, and diet therapy* (9th ed., p. 373). Philadelphia: W. B. Saunders.

24-Hour Recall Form and Food Group Evaluation

Food and Fluid Intake from Time of Awakening Until the Next Morning

TIME	Food and Drink Consumed		Number of Servings from Each Food Group*				
	NAME AND TYPE AMOUNT	MILK GROUP	MEAT GROUP	FRUITS AND VEGETABLES	BREADS AND CEREALS	FATS, SWEETS, AND ALCOHOLIC BEVERAGES
	Totals					

Recommended Number of Servings Daily (Adults)

	MILK GROUP	MEAT GROUP	FRUITS AND VEGETABLES	BREADS AND CEREALS	FATS, SWEETS, AND ALCOHOLIC BEVERAGES
	2–3	2–3	5–9	6–11	Avoid too many
*Evaluation					

* Evaluation: L = low, A = adequate, and E = excessive.

Adapted from DeHoog, S. (1996). The assessment of nutritional status. In L. K. Mahan & S. Escott-Stump (Eds.), *Krause's food, nutrition, and diet therapy* (9th ed., p. 375). Philadelphia: W. B. Saunders.

Values History

Patient Name _____

This values history serves as a set of my specific value-based directives for various medical interventions. It is to be used in healthcare circumstances when I may be unable to voice my preferences. These directives shall be made a part of the medical record and used as supplementary to my living will.

VALUES

There are several values important in decisions about terminal treatment and care. This section of the values history invites you to identify your most important values.

Basic Life Values

Perhaps the most basic values in this context concern length of life versus quality of life. Which of the following two statements is the most important to you?

___ 1. I want to live as long as possible, regardless of the quality of life that I experience.
___ 2. I want to preserve a good quality of life, even if this means that I may not live as long.

Quality of Life Values

Many values help to define the quality of life that we want to live. The following list contains some that appear to be the most common. Review this list (and feel free to either elaborate on it or add to it) and circle those values that are important to your definition of quality of life.

1. I want to maintain my capacity to think clearly.
2. I want to feel safe and secure.
3. I want to avoid unnecessary pain and suffering.
4. I want to be treated with respect.
5. I want to be treated with dignity when I can no longer speak for myself.
6. I do not want to be an unnecessary burden on my family.
7. I want to be able to make my own decisions.
8. I want to experience a comfortable dying process.
9. I want to be with my loved ones before I die.
10. I want to leave good memories of me to my loved ones.
11. I want to be treated in accord with my religious beliefs and traditions.
12. I want respect shown for my body after I die.
13. I want to help others by making a contribution to medical education and research.
14. Other values or clarification of values above:

RANKING VALUES

Of the above values, which are the three that are the most important to you? _____ _____ _____

DIRECTIVES

Some directives involve simple yes/no decisions. Others provide for the choice of trial of intervention.

Initials/Date

_____ 1. I want to undergo cardiopulmonary resuscitation.
___ Yes
___ No
Why?

_____ 2. I want to be placed on a ventilator.
___ Yes
___ TRIAL for the period of _____
___ TRIAL to determine effectiveness using reasonable medical judgment.
___ No
Why?

_____ 3. I want to have an endotracheal tube used in order to perform items 1 and 2.
___ Yes
___ TRIAL for the period of _____
___ TRIAL to determine effectiveness using reasonable medical judgment.
___ No
___Why?

_____ 4. I want to have total parenteral nutrition administered for my nutrition.
___ Yes
___ TRIAL for the period of _____
___ TRIAL to determine effectiveness using reasonable medical judgment.
___ No
Why?

_____ 5. I want to have intravenous medication and hydration administered; regardless of my decision, I understand the intravenous medication and hydration to alleviate discomfort or pain will not be withheld from me if I so request them.
___ Yes
___ TRIAL for the period of _____
___ TRIAL to determine effectiveness using reasonable medical judgment.
___ No
Why?

_____ 6. I want to have all medications used for the treatment of my illness continued; regardless of my decision, I understand that pain medication will continue to be administered, including narcotic medications.

___ Yes
___ TRIAL for the period of _____
___ TRIAL to determine effectiveness using reasonable medical judgment.
___ No
Why?

_____ 7. I want to have nasogastric, gastrostomy, or other enteral feeding tubes introduced and administered for my nutrition.

___ Yes
___ TRIAL for the period of _____
___ TRIAL to determine effectiveness using reasonable medical judgment.
___ No
Why?

_____ 8. I want to be placed on a dialysis machine.

___ Yes
___ TRIAL for the period of _____
___ TRIAL to determine effectiveness using reasonable medical judgment.
___ No
Why?

_____ 9. I want to have an autopsy done to determine the cause(s) of my death.

___ Yes
___ No
Why?

_____ 10. I want to be admitted to the Intensive Care Unit.

___ Yes
___ No
Why?

_____ 11. [For patients in long-term care facilities who experience a life-threatening change in health status] I want 911 called in case of medical emergency.

___ Yes
___ No
Why?

_____ 12. Other directives: I consent to these directives after receiving honest disclosure of their implications, risks, and benefits by my physician, free from constraints and being of sound mind.

_____	_____
Signature	Date
_____	_____
Witness	Date
_____	_____
Witness	Date

_____ 13. Proxy negation: I request that the following persons *not* be allowed to make decisions on my behalf in the event of my disability or incapacity.

_____	_____	_____
	Signature	Date
_____	_____	_____
	Witness	Date
_____	_____	_____
	Witness	Date

_____ 14. Organ donation [Specific state version inserted here]

_____ 15. Durable power of attorney [Specific state version inserted here]

_____

Adapted from Doukas, D. J., & McCullough, L. B. (1991). The values history: The evaluation of the patient's values and advance directives. *Journal of Family Practice, 32*, 145–153. Reprinted by permission of Appleton & Lange, Inc.

Falls

Joyce Takano Stone
Jean F. Wyman

Falls and their sequelae pose a serious threat to the health, functioning, and independence of older adults. Unintentional injury is the seventh leading cause of death in the elderly, with falls accounting for a majority of these deaths (National Safety Council, 1995).

This chapter reviews the epidemiology of falls and their consequences. Risk factors associated with falls and with injurious falls in community-dwelling and institutionalized elderly populations are described. Strategies for the prevention of falls across different care settings are also presented.

EPIDEMIOLOGY

Prevalence

A fall has been defined as "an event which results in a person coming to rest inadvertently on the ground or other lower level and other than as a consequence of sustaining a violent blow, loss of consciousness, sudden onset of paralysis, as in a stroke, or an epileptic seizure" (Kellogg International Work Group on the Prevention of Falls in the Elderly, 1987, p. 4). The exact prevalence of falls is unknown because of under-reporting by the community-dwelling elderly due to either forgetting (Cummings et al., 1988) or denying a fall has occurred because of embarrassment or the fear of losing one's independence. Falls in institutional settings frequently are not witnessed or go unreported by staff for a variety of reasons, including how a fall event is defined and the nursing staff's lack of time for completing incident reports.

Falls occur in approximately 25 to 33% of community-dwelling older adults (Nevitt et al., 1989; Tinetti, Speechley, & Ginter, 1988), 50 to 67% of nursing home residents (Downton,

1992; Robin, 1995), and in between these two rates for the hospitalized older patients (Robin, 1995). Falls are the most frequently reported incident in hospitals (Maciorowski et al., 1988) and in nursing homes (Gurwitz et al., 1994). The higher prevalence rate of falls in institutional settings is attributed to the greater degree of frailty and dependency of the patients and to more accurate reporting of falls (Robin, 1995; Tinetti, 1994a).

The rate of falls increases with advancing age in both women and men. Research on gender differences is inconsistent (Tinetti, 1994b), although a majority of studies find that women have higher fall rates than men at most ages (Sattin, 1992). Racial differences in fall rates are unclear. In both community-dwelling and institutionalized elderly populations, the number of falls increases as the number of disabilities and other risk factors increase (Rubenstein et al., 1994; Tinetti, 1994a).

Consequences of Falls

Falls can have physical, psychosocial, and economic consequences. Although the majority of older people who fall are not injured or suffer only minor injury, falls have the potential to negatively affect an older person's health and quality of life. The severity of fall consequences increases with advancing age (Rubenstein et al., 1991; Tinetti, Doucette, Claus, & Marottoli, 1995).

PHYSICAL CONSEQUENCES

Falls can result in physical injuries, disability, and death. Approximately 30 to 55% of people who fall suffer minor injury, 4 to 6% sustain fractures, 2 to 20% have injuries severe enough to require hospitalization, and 2.2% die as a result of a fall-related injury (Nevitt et al., 1991; O'Loughlin et al., 1993; Sattin, 1992; Tinetti, 1997). The risk of major injury is greatest with falls associated with loss of consciousness, as compared with nonsyncopal falls (Nevitt et al., 1991).

Hip fractures constitute one of the most serious injuries resulting from falls. Annually, more than 233,000 hip fractures occur in older people, with more than 13,000 deaths (Sattin, 1992). The incidence of hip fracture increases exponentially by age, doubling every 5 years after the age of 50 years (Grisso & Kaplan, 1994). Hip fracture rates vary markedly by gender and racial groups. The majority of hip fractures (75%) occur in women. Whites have age-adjusted hip fracture rates that are twice as high as rates for people of all other races (Sattin, 1992).

Mortality during hospitalization for hip fracture is 5% (Fisher et al., 1991), and the overall 1-year mortality rate is 12 to 67% (Robin, 1995; Sattin, 1992). For those who survive hip fracture, significant disability and dependency occur. Half of those individuals who were ambulatory prior to a hip fracture cannot walk afterwards, and half are no longer able to live independently. Less than 30% regain their prefracture levels of physical functioning (Mossey et al., 1989).

Nearly 50% of community-dwelling elderly people who fall are unable to get up without assistance, and 10% of these individuals remain on the floor or ground for more than 1 hour (Tinetti, Liu, & Claus, 1993). The "long lie" after a fall may result in dehydration, pneumonia, hypothermia, pressure ulcers, and a fear of falling. Characteristics associated with a person who has fallen and is unable to get up include the following: older age (over 80 years), physical frailty, decreased strength, poor balance and gait, arthritis, and functional decline. This person is likely to have more frequent hospitalization and be at higher risk for death (Tinetti, Liu, & Claus, 1993).

Ten to 25% of falls in long-term care settings result in minor and major injuries. In comparison with the community-dwelling elderly person, nursing home residents have a higher incidence of hip fractures, especially those who fall frequently, and a higher mortality rate after hip fracture. Annually, about 1800 nursing home residents die after a fall (Luukinen et al., 1995; Rhymes & Jaeger, 1998; Rubenstein et al., 1996).

A clustering of falls over a short period is a marker for general physical decline. The risk of long-term institutionalization and death is high for older adults who have multiple falls or are hospitalized for injurious falls (Alexander et al., 1992; Dunn et al., 1992; Kiel et al., 1991; Wolinsky et al., 1992). The rate of death due to falls rises rapidly with increasing age for all race and sex groups aged 75 years and older. Men have a higher death rate in the 65 to 74 age group, whereas women have a higher rate in the 75 and over age group (National Safety Council, 1995).

PSYCHOSOCIAL CONSEQUENCES

Psychosocial reactions to falls may be even more debilitating than physical injuries. Falls can result in fear of falling, depression, anxiety, loss of confidence, social withdrawal, dependency, and institutionalization (Arfken et al., 1994; Brummel-Smith, 1989; Downton, 1992; Nevitt et al., 1991). Fear of falling occurs in older people who fall as well as those who have never fallen. Studies indicate that 40 to 73% of people who have fallen and 20 to 60% of those who have never fallen fear falling (Maki et al., 1991; Nevitt et al., 1989; Tinetti et al., 1988). Fear of falling increases with age and is greater in women and people with gait and balance disorders (Arfken et al., 1994).

Approximately 27 to 50% of community-dwelling elderly people who are fearful of falling restrict or eliminate social and physical activities because of their fear (Downton & Andrews, 1990; Kosorok et al., 1992; Lachman et al., 1998; Nevitt et al., 1991; Tinetti et al., 1988). This occurs in people who have fallen as well as in those who have never fallen. The restriction of mobility following a fall has been called the *postfall syndrome.*

Brummel-Smith (1989) described how the fear of falling leads to a vicious cycle in which the older person who has fallen begins to avoid previously performed activities, thus becoming deconditioned, which then leads to losses in strength, flexibility, joint mobility, and righting reflexes. These losses can potentiate the risk of a more serious fall in the future (Fig. 15–1). To protect the older person from a future fall, family and nursing staff may impose unnecessary activity restrictions or the use of restraints, which further compounds the problem.

ECONOMIC CONSEQUENCES

High health service use occurs with falls (Kiel et al., 1991; Wolinsky et al., 1992). Falls injuries

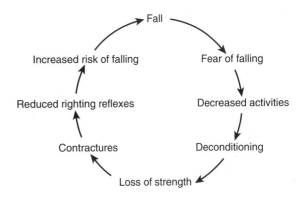

FIGURE 15–1. Vicious cycle of fear of falling. (Redrawn from Brummel-Smith, K. [1989]. Falls in the aged. *Primary Care, 16,* 377–393.)

result in utilization costs that have been estimated at nearly $10 billion of the $158 billion lifetime economic costs of all injuries (Rice et al., 1989). Falls in older people account for nearly 70% of emergency room visits and for the highest rate of acute care hospitalizations for injuries. The average length of hospital stay is 11.6 days, which is higher than for most other diagnostic-related groups (DRGs) (Robin, 1995; Sattin, 1992). Falls are a contributory factor in 30 to 40% of admissions to nursing homes (King & Tinetti, 1995).

•CLASSIFICATION OF FALLS

Several schemes have been used to classify falls so that differences in types of falls by age, gender, and other factors can be determined (Lach et al., 1991; Rubenstein et al., 1994; Wild et al., 1981). Falls are grouped by cause or by contributing circumstances. However, no classification scheme has received widespread acceptance. Generally, these schemes fail to consider the interactions of multiple risk factors (King & Tinetti, 1995).

One method of classifying falls is to identify predisposing and situational risk factors (Fig. 15–2). Predisposing or intrinsic factors are those related to the individual's physiological functioning, such as normal age-related changes, acute and chronic disease, and medication use. Situational or extrinsic factors are

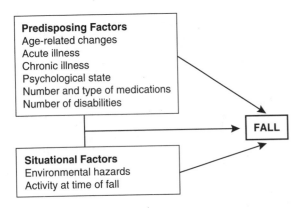

FIGURE 15–2. Etiology of falls.

those related to environmental hazards or the individual's activity at the time of the fall. It is often difficult to pinpoint the single cause of a fall. Usually, a complex interaction of predisposing and situational factors results in falling. For example, an individual with several predisposing risk factors might not fall until he or she walks across a slippery surface or becomes preoccupied by a stressful life event and misses a step when descending stairs.

RISK FACTORS

The multitude of comorbid conditions and contributing factors associated with falls is similar among community-dwelling and institutionalized elderly persons (Table 15–1). The rate, circumstances, and outcome of falls may vary, however.

In community-dwelling adults younger than 75 years of age, environmental factors play a significant role; in those older than 75 years, intrinsic factors have a more substantial role (Lach et al., 1991; Rubenstein et al., 1994). Risk factors associated with falls in community-dwelling elderly people identified in prospective studies include older age; white race; cognitive impairment; palmomental reflex; medication use; specific chronic diseases, including arthritis, lung disease, diabetes, and stroke; foot problems; impairments in muscle strength, balance, and gait; and dizziness

TABLE 15-1

Causes of Falls in Nursing Home and Community Populations: Comparison of Studies that Conducted Post-Fall Evaluations

Cause of Falls	Nursing Home, % (range)*	Community, % (range)†
Gait or balance disorder or weakness	26 (20–39)‡	13 (2–29)
Dizziness or vertigo	25 (0–30)	8 (0–19)
"Accident" or environment-related	16 (6–27)	41 (23–53)
Confusion	10 (0–14)	2 (0–7)
Visual disorder	4 (0–5)	0.8 (0–4)
Postural hypotension	2 (0–16)	1 (0–6)
Drop attack	0.3 (0–3)	13 (0–25)
Syncope	0.2 (0–3)	0.4 (0–3)
Other specified causes§	12 (10–34)	17 (2–39)
Unknown	4 (0–34)	6 (0–16)

*Four studies and 1076 falls.
†Seven studies and 2312 falls.
‡Mean percentage calculated from the total number of falls in the studies reviewed. Ranges indicate the percentage reported in each of the studies. Percentages do not total 100% because some studies reported more than one cause per fall.
§This category includes arthritis, acute illness, drugs, alcohol, pain, epilepsy, and falling from bed.
From Rubenstein, L. Z., Josephson, K. R., & Robbins, A. S. (1994). Falls in the nursing home. *Annals of Internal Medicine, 121,* 442–451. Copyright 1994 by the American College of Physicians. Adapted with permission.

(Campbell et al., 1989; Nevitt et al., 1989; O'Loughlin et al., 1993; Tinetti et al., 1988). Risk factors may vary between men and women (Campbell et al., 1989). The recurrent faller may be more predictable than the individual who will experience a single fall (Nevitt et al., 1989).

The likelihood of falling increases with the number of predisposing risk factors present (King & Tinetti, 1995). Fall rates in two prospective studies for individuals with no risk factors ranged from 8 to 10%, whereas for those individuals with four to seven risk factors the fall rates were 68 to 73% (Nevitt et al., 1989; Tinetti et al., 1988). These studies also indicate, however, that a significant number of older adults fall despite having no or few risk factors for falls.

In the institutionalized population, predisposing factors are more significant than environmental factors as the cause of falls (Luukinen et al., 1994; Rubenstein et al., 1994; Tinetti, 1997). Sixteen percent of the falls in nursing homes are attributed to environmental factors (Tinetti, 1997). In hospitalized elderly people, key risk factors include history of previous falls, change in mental status, sensory deficits, weakness, debilitated physical status with impaired mobility, use of multiple medications, and postural hypotension (Janken et al., 1986; Spellbring, 1992). In elderly nursing home residents, risk factors include weakness, gait or balance disorders, dizziness, dementia, depression, musculoskeletal and neurological disorders, use of multiple medications, functional status impairment, vision and hearing deficits, and postural hypotension (Lipsitz et al., 1991; Rubenstein et al., 1994; Sattin, 1992; Tinetti et al., 1986).

Predisposing Factors

Walking can be considered controlled falling. One "throws" oneself forward, and then "catches" oneself before falling. The maintenance of an upright position or postural stability depends on the constant integration of sensory, nervous, and motor input. Age-related changes in the sensory, musculoskeletal, and central and peripheral nervous systems can predispose an older person to fall (Table 15–2). Superimposed acute and chronic illness can significantly impair the functioning of body systems, thereby raising the risk of falling (Table 15–3). In the elderly person, acute illness may present atypically, with falls being an early sign of underlying illness (Downton, 1992; Miceli et al., 1994). Medications can cause iatrogenic complications leading to balance and gait disturbances and postural hypotension (Table 15–4). Disability, particularly multiple disabilities, arising from age-related changes and disease also contributes in a cumulative fashion to the risk of falling (Tinetti et al., 1986).

Situational Factors

Environmental hazards in combination with the individual's activity or movements create a

TABLE 15-2
Age-Related Changes Predisposing to Falls

Visual Function

Decreased accommodation
Decreased acuity
Decreased dark adaptation
Decreased depth perception
Decreased peripheral vision
Decreased glare tolerance
Decreased contrast sensitivity

Neurological Function (Including Balance)

Slower reaction time
Decreased position sense
Decreased vibratory sense
Increased postural sway
Impaired righting reflexes
Decreased proprioception
Altered gait
    Shorter steps
    Decreased toe-floor clearance
    Limited extension and swing through
    Slower gait speed

Musculoskeletal Function

Decreased muscle strength
Decreased joint flexibility

Data from Kane et al. (1994); Robin (1995); and Tinetti & Ginter (1988).

TABLE 15-3

Medical Risk Factors Associated with Falls

Sensory

Vision loss
Cataracts
Glaucoma
Macular degeneration
Vestibular disorders (e.g., acute labyrinthitis, Meniere's disease, benign positional vertigo, vertebrobasilar ischemia and infarction, drug toxicity)

Neurological

Balance and gait disorders
Cerebellar disorders
Cervical spondylosis
Delirium
Dementia
Myelopathy
Normal pressure hydrocephalus
Parkinson's disease
Peripheral neuropathy
Seizure disorder
Stroke
Transient ischemic attack

Musculoskeletal

Arthritis
Inflammatory joint disorders
Muscle weakness
Myopathy
Podiatric problems

Cardiovascular

Aortic stenosis
Arrhythmia
Carotid sinus sensitivity
Conduction disorders
Myocardial infarction
Postural hypotension
Syncope
Vertebrobasilar insufficiency
Volume depletion

Respiratory

Pneumonia
Hypoxemia

Gastrointestinal

Diarrhea
Defecation syncope
Postprandial syncope

Metabolic

Anemia
Dehydration
Diabetes
Hypokalemia
Hypomagnesemia
Hyponatremia
Hypothyroidism

Genitourinary

Incontinence
Micturition syncope
Nocturia
Urgency and frequency

Psychological

Anxiety
Depression
Stress
Fear of falling
Impaired judgment
Impulsiveness

Data from Baloh (1992); Duthie (1989); Gross et al. (1990); Gulya (1995); Kane et al. (1994); Lord et al. (1991); Resnick (1996); Stewart et al. (1992); Vlahov (1990); Wolfson (1992); Wolfson et al. (1995).

unique situation that can precipitate falls independently or in association with predisposing factors. The degree to which the environment poses a threat depends on the vulnerability of the person. Environmental hazards that can be tripped over or slipped on are thought to be responsible for 44 to 55% of falls in community-dwelling older adults (Tinetti et al., 1988; Lach et al., 1991; Luukinen et al., 1994). Hazards that can cause falls include poor lighting, slippery surfaces, objects in the walking path, scatter rugs, patterned carpets and rugs, frayed carpeting, electrical cords, uneven or cracked walking surfaces, stairs, unstable furniture, low furniture and toilets, and pets. The majority of falls (54–70%) occur at home, especially in the bathroom and bedroom (Campbell et al., 1990; DeVito et al., 1988). Approximately 10% of falls occur on stairs, with descending stairs being

more hazardous than ascending (Tinetti et al., 1988). Falls on stairs are associated with an increased risk of serious injuries (Tinetti, Doucette & Claus, 1995). Men tend to fall more outside, whereas women fall more inside the home (Campbell et al., 1990; Luukinen et al., 1994).

Most falls occur during only mildly or moderately displacing activities such as walking, stepping up or down, performing a basic activity of daily living, getting up or sitting down, or bending over or reaching (Tinetti et al., 1988). Falls by men are more likely to occur at the highest level of activity, such as gardening, than are those by women (Campbell et al., 1990). Falls occur mostly during the day during periods of activity (Luukinen et al., 1994).

There are fewer environmental related falls in the hospital and nursing home than in the

TABLE 15-4
Drugs Associated with Falls

Increased risk for falls associated with
 Number of medications
  Taking four or more medications
 New medication
 Increase in dosage of a current medication
 Type of drug
  Alcohol
  Antihypertensives
  Barbiturates
  Benzodiazepines
  Diuretics
  Narcotics
  Nonmiotic topical eye medications
  Phenothiazines
  Tricyclic antidepressants
  Oral hypoglycemics
  Cardiac medications

Data from Glynn et al. (1991); Lipsitz et al. (1991); Liu et al. (1995); Malmivaara et al. (1993); Miceli et al. (1994); Monane & Avorn (1996); Myers et al. (1991); Tinetti, Doucette & Claus (1995); Vernon (1995).

community. Environmental hazards account for approximately 16 to 19% of the falls in nursing homes (Luukinen et al., 1994). This low rate is attributed to several factors. Institutions are often designed to accommodate frail elderly residents or the acutely ill older person. The institutionalized or ill elderly person is less likely to be engaged in hazardous activities. The environment of the nursing home and hospital is usually monitored closely for hazards, and prompt attention is paid to any potential safety problems (Tinetti, 1994b). Nevertheless, the design and activities of the hospital and nursing home may pose hazardous situations. Mobility aids (canes, walkers, and wheelchairs) and toileting equipment, such as urinals and commodes, at the bedside increase the risk for falls. Inadequate lighting and inaccessible call lights may lead to falls, as may restraints and siderails. One study found that the design for privacy contributed to a higher incidence of falls because it decreased staff's ability to observe and monitor the patients. Equipment, such as wheelchairs and commodes, was involved in fall-related injuries of nonambulatory residents (Thapa et al., 1996).

The most common location for falls is in the patient's room, with most falls occurring during bed, chair, or wheelchair transfers. Another location for falls is the bathroom, also during transfers (Rubenstein et al., 1991; Tideiksaar, 1988).

The stress of relocation to a new setting and unfamiliarity with the environment places the older patient at risk for falls (Friedman et al., 1995). Most falls in acute care settings occur during the first week of hospitalization (Janken et al., 1986; Uden, 1985), the first 45 days in the nursing home (Miceli et al., 1994), and the first 60 days in a rehabilitation hospital (Vlahov et al., 1990). The risk for falls increases as a patient feels better and becomes more independent and active, thereby increasing the opportunity to fall.

Studies on staffing patterns and activity level found that most falls occurred during periods of high activity or when the staffing level was poor (Robin, 1995; Rubenstein & Robbins, 1989; Whedon & Shedd, 1989). In their study on frequent fallers, Wright and associates (1990) found that people who fell did not ask for assistance because they perceived resentment from the staff when assistance was requested. Organizational and attitudinal factors, such as head nurse leadership, group work cohesion, staff job expectations, and positive attitude of the staff, were found to have some effect on patient falls (Harris, 1989).

Trauma Risk Factors

The likelihood of suffering a serious fall injury depends on a number of factors (Table 15–5).

TABLE 15-5
Factors Associated with Trauma

Velocity of the fall
Energy absorbing capacity of the landing surface
Protective responses of the faller
Injury threshold of the tissue
Direction and location of impact
Number and frequency of falls

Data from Melton & Rigg (1985); Myers et al. (1991); Nevitt et al. (1991); O'Loughlin et al. (1993); Tinetti, Doucette, Claus & Marottoli (1995).

There is a relationship between the height of the fall, the position of the person, the velocity of the fall, and an increased risk for injury. Fewer injuries were noted in people who fell at standing height or lower, such as while transferring, stooping, bending, or standing still (Melton & Riggs, 1985; Nevitt et al., 1991). Falling while turning, rather than falling while walking in one direction, was associated with increased risk for hip fracture (Cumming & Kleinberg, 1994).

The ability to quickly respond and protect oneself in the event of a fall determines whether an injury will occur. Neuromuscular and cognitive dysfunction results in delayed reaction time, slowed motor speed, poor coordination, and upper extremity weakness and impairs a person's ability to prevent or break a fall (Nevitt et al., 1991).

The risk for injurious falls depends on the injury threshold of bone and tissues. While it is known that osteoporosis results in decreased bone resistance to mechanical energy, there is controversy over the role of osteoporosis in the cause of hip fractures. The average force needed to fracture the neck of the femur has been shown to be about 1/20 to 1/10 of the force available in a typical fall (Cumming & Kleinberg, 1994; Sattin, 1992). Other determinants, such as the velocity of the fall, the position and location of the impact, or the concentration and absorption of energy, may be more critical than bone strength in determining the risk of fractures (Lotz & Hayes, 1990; Sattin, 1992). Older adults with low body mass are at higher risk for injury. Low body mass reflects loss of the cushioning effect of soft tissue and lower bone-mineral density (Tinetti, Doucette, Claus & Marottoli, 1995).

The energy-absorbing capacity of the landing surface is another factor that determines the likelihood of an injury. The older person who falls on a rug-covered floor in the home, as compared with a person who falls on a tile floor or the ground, has a lower risk for injury because of the energy-absorbing capacity of the rug. If the person were then unable to get up for some time after a fall on a rug, the serious consequences of the fall would be less than if the person fell on a hard surface (Nevitt et al., 1991).

People who suffer an injury in a fall, in comparison with those who do not suffer an injury, are also more likely to have had a recent fall. The cumulative risk of injury is proportional to the number of falls (Cumming & Kleinberg, 1994; Tinetti, 1987).

MANAGEMENT OF FALLS

Assessment

Falls have a multifactorial etiology and may be a sign of underlying disease. The key to preventing falls or reducing the seriousness of fall consequences is early detection of risk factors that may be amenable to intervention (Rubenstein et al., 1996; Tinetti, Doucette & Claus, 1995). This should occur during annual health examinations or following a fall event. Older adults who report a fall that is clearly not due to an accidental trip or slip should be carefully evaluated. A thorough fall assessment consists of a focused history, physical examination, mobility evaluation, environmental assessment, and, in certain cases, selected diagnostic tests (Table 15–6). An interdisciplinary approach to fall assessment and intervention is recommended for the person who has had multiple falls.

HISTORY

A targeted history focused on prior falls and identification of key risk factors is critical in the prevention of falls. Many older adults fail to report a history of falling when asked during routine health examinations for several reasons. They may have forgotten noninjurious falls, be embarrassed, minimized the significance of a fall by attributing it to carelessness, or be fearful of losing their independence. The advanced practice nurse may want to initiate a discussion about falls by saying, "It's common for people to fall as they get older. Tell me about the falls you have had this year." Because the definition of a fall event varies among individuals, the advanced practice nurse may need to define a fall by asking "Have you had any experiences in which you accidentally came to rest on the floor or ground this past year?"

If the older adult indicates that a fall occurred, then a fall history should be taken. Tideiksaar (1996) coined the mnemonic device SPLATT to help recall the components of the fall history (Table 15–7). These include the symptoms at the time of the fall, history of previous falls, location and activity prior to the fall, the time of the fall and the time on the ground, and any trauma or injury that occurred. The symptoms that occurred immediately prior to the fall or with the fall help indicate the presence of new or exacerbated

---

TABLE 15-6
Fall Assessment

History

Fall history: SPLATT (see Table 15–7)
Risk factor assessment
    Predisposing factors
    Environmental factors

Physical Examination

Postural blood pressure
    Postural hypotension
Sensory examination
    Visual acuity, fields, cataracts, glaucoma, macular
        degeneration, hearing loss
Cardiovascular examination
    Arrhythmias, valvular disorders, heart failure, carotid
        bruits
Neurological examination
    Mental status (delirium, dementia)
    Mood and behavior (depression, anxiety, stress,
        agitation)
    Focal deficits, peripheral neuropathy, myelopathy,
        tumor
    Parkinson's disease, cerebellar disease
    Balance and gait disorders
Musculoskeletal examination
    Muscle weakness
    Limited range of motion
    Severe arthritis
    Foot abnormalities
    Type and condition of footwear

Mobility Evaluation

Balance
Gait
Transfers (wheelchair patients)

Environmental Assessment

Diagnostic Tests (in selected cases)

TABLE 15-7
Evaluation of a Fall Episode: SPLATT

Symptoms
    Lightheadedness, dizziness, or vertigo
    Palpitations, chest pain, or shortness of breath
    Sudden focal neurological symptoms (e.g., weakness,
        sensory disturbance, dysarthria, ataxia, confusion,
        aphasia)
    Aura
    Loss of consciousness
    Urinary or bowel incontinence
Previous falls (during past year)
Location
Activity at time of fall
Time of fall and time on ground
Trauma or injury with fall

Data from Tideiksaar (1996).

---

underlying illness. Falls resulting from syncope should be evaluated for underlying central nervous system, cardiovascular, and metabolic disease.

Each fall episode should be carefully evaluated because several causes can coexist and precipitate falling by different mechanisms. Recurrent falls may follow a similar pattern that helps reveal the etiology. For example, falls that occur consistently after getting up and are associated with the complaint of lightheadedness may be due to postural hypotension. Many older adults will not be able to give any details about a fall. If the individual is unable to recall the circumstances surrounding his or her falls or had a loss of consciousness with the fall, question family, friends, or other caregivers who may have witnessed the event.

The fall history should also include an assessment of the individual's fear of falling while performing specific daily activities (i.e., taking a bath or shower, getting dressed, walking outdoors) and identify what activities the individual is now avoiding or limiting because of his or her fear of falling (Myers et al., 1996). Several standardized instruments are available to measure fear of falling, such as the Fall Efficacy Scale (FES) (Tinetti et al., 1990), the Activities-Specific Balance Confidence Scale (ABC) (Powell & Myers, 1995), and the Falls Handicap Inventory (FHI) (Rai et al., 1995).

In addition to the fall history, a targeted assessment on risk factors associated with falling should be conducted. Tables 15–3 and 15–4 summarize the medical problems and medications that can precipitate falls. As the number of chronic medical conditions increases, so does the risk of falling. Medications have been highly associated with an increased risk of falls and fall-related injuries in both community and institutionalized populations. Thus, a drug history is especially important, with careful review of the risks and benefits of each medication (Monane & Avorn, 1996). The focus should be on new or recently increased drugs, key drugs that have been associated with falls, as well as on the number and combination of drugs that could be causing iatrogenic complications. Community-dwelling adults should be asked to bring all their prescription and over-the-counter drugs to their annual health examination.

PHYSICAL EXAMINATION

The physical examination is important in helping to confirm or detect the presence of selected risk factors. Emphasis in the examination is placed on the sensory, cardiovascular, musculoskeletal, and neurological systems. Near and far visual acuity and visual fields should be checked. Visual acuity of 20/70 or worse reduces the ability to detect environmental hazards and to perform normal activities of daily living safely. Reduced visual fields may indicate glaucoma. Nystagmus is a sign of vestibular dysfunction. Evidence of macular degeneration and cataracts should be noted.

Postural hypotension should be assessed by having the individual rest in a supine position for at least 5 minutes. Blood pressure should be checked initially in the supine position, and then rechecked 1 and 3 minutes after the individual comes to either a sitting or a standing position. A systolic drop in pressure of 20 mm Hg or a diastolic drop in pressure of 10 mm Hg is diagnostic for postural hypotension. Postural hypotension may appear in healthy, asymptomatic older adults as well as in those who have venous insufficiency. It can also be the result of a drug side effect, dehydration, or acute blood loss from gastrointestinal bleeding. The cardiac evaluation should assess for ar-

rhythmias, valvular disorders, heart failure, and carotid bruits.

The musculoskeletal examination should assess for deformities, range-of-motion limitations in the lower extremities, active inflammatory processes, arthritis, foot abnormalities, and the type and condition of footwear. Lower extremity weakness can easily be assessed during the mobility evaluation by observing ability to rise from a chair. If a mobility aid is used, such as a cane or walker, proper sizing as well as safety features (rubber tips, tightness of any joints, functioning of any wheels) should also be checked.

The neurological examination should screen for focal deficits, myelopathy, peripheral neuropathy (loss of vibratory and position sense), tumors, cerebellar disease (abnormal heel to shin testing), and Parkinson's disease (resting tremor, muscle rigidity, weakness, cogwheeling, bradykinesia; see Chapter 19). Mental status testing using a standardized instrument such as the Mini-Mental State Examination (see Chapter 7) should be conducted to rule out dementia, delirium, or depression. If depression is suspected, a standardized mood assessment instrument such as the Geriatric Depression Scale (see Chapter 17) can be helpful.

MOBILITY ASSESSMENT

Gait and balance impairments are strong predictors of fall risk. Assessment of mobility, that is, the ability to walk and transfer safely and independently within the individual's environment, is especially important. Careful observation of the individual through simple gait and balance maneuvers will provide critical data for determining fall risk and appropriate interventions to improve safety. Common abnormal gait patterns are described in Table 15–8. Patients who are wheelchair bound should be observed performing bed, chair, and toilet transfers.

A simple mobility test that provides valuable information on gait, balance, muscle strength, and functional performance is the Get Up & Go Test (Mathias et al., 1986) (see Chapter 6). The examiner should walk along side the patient for safety. For frail or large patients, a

TABLE 15-8
Common Abnormal Gait Patterns

Gait	Cause	Characteristic
Circumduction	Stroke or hemiparesis	Lower extremity assumes triple extension of hip, knee, and ankle; leg swings in an outward arc to ensure ground clearance
Scissoring	Bilateral upper motor neuron disease	Bilateral circumduction gait
Festinating	Parkinson's disease	Symmetric shuffling of feet; poor ground clearance, especially at beginning and end; turning en bloc; forward flexed posture; easy displacement backward or forward; walking at running pace
Cerebellar, ataxic	Chronic alcoholism, spinocerebellar atrophy, progressive supranuclear palsy, multiple sclerosis, cerebellar tumor, acute onset vascular event	Broad-based, irregular steps; veering side to side, backward, or forward
Frontal lobe apraxia	Normal pressure hydrocephalus	Slowed initiation of movement; mild broad-based gait; short, slow, shuffling steps; forward-flexed posture; normal strength
Senile gait	Arterial degeneration	Flexed posture, shuffling steps prominent on turns, retropulsion on turning (falling backward)
Sensory ataxia	Vitamin B_{12} deficiency, cervical spondylosis, spinocerebellar degeneration	Broad-based, foot stamping; patient looking at feet; inability to stand with eyes closed (positive Romberg)
Waddling gait	Severe degenerative disease of hips, severe proximal muscle weakness (e.g., myositis or polymyalgia rheumatica)	Wide-based waddling, swaying gait
Asymmetric gait (hopping gait)	Painful disorders of weight-bearing joint; osteoarthritis of hip or knee	Shortened stance phase on affected side
Discontinuous gait	Painful forefoot disease (e.g., hallux rigidus)	No toe-off on affected side

From Hough, J. C. (1992). Falls and falling. In R. J. Ham & P. D. Sloane (Eds.), *Primary care geriatrics: A case-based approach* (2nd ed., pp. 362–380). St. Louis: Mosby–Year Book.

safety belt can be placed around the patient's waist that can quickly be grasped should the patient lose his or her balance. Hip extensor weakness will present as an inability to arise from the chair without assistance from the hands. Patients with muscle weakness may rock forward a few times before standing.

A more detailed test is Tinetti's Performance-Oriented Mobility Test (1986) (Table 15–9). Balance maneuvers most associated with falls include sitting down, turning, sternal nudge, and standing on one leg (Tinetti & Ginter, 1988). Abnormal gait changes that are highly linked to falls in the community-dwelling elderly include increased trunk sway, an inability to increase walking pace, and increased path devia-tion (Tinetti & Ginter, 1988). In one study, scores on this test were the best single predictor of recurrent falls in nursing home residents (Tinetti et al., 1986).

ENVIRONMENTAL ASSESSMENT

Ideally, an environmental assessment should be conducted for all patients, both community-dwelling and institutionalized. Key features to evaluate in a home environmental assessment can be found in Chapter 5. Environmental hazards in institutional settings that should be assessed are listed in Table 15–10.

TABLE 15-9

Performance-Oriented Mobility Test

Balance

Instructions: The subject begins this assessment seated in a backless or (straight-backed), armless, firm chair. A walking aid is defined as a cane or walker. Circle the appropriate score.

1. **Sitting balance**

Leans or slides down in chair	=0
Steady, stable, safe	=1

2. **Rising from chair**

Unable without human assistance	=0
Able but uses arms (on chair or walking aid) to pull or push up	=1
Able to rise in a single movement without using arms on chair or walking aid (Note: use of arms on subject's own thighs scores a 2)	=2

3. **Attempts to arise**

Unable without human assistance	=0
Able but requires multiple attempts	=1
Able to rise with one attempt	=2

4. **Immediate standing balance** (first 3–5 seconds)

Any sign of unsteadiness (defined as grabbing at objects for support, staggering, moving feet, or more than minimal trunk sway	=0
Steady but uses walking aid or grabs other object for support	=1
Steady without holding onto walking aid or other object for support	=2

5. **Standing balance**

Any sign of unsteadiness regardless of stance, or holds onto object	=0
Steady but wide stance (medial heels more than 4 inches apart) or uses walking aid or other support	=1
Steady with narrow stance (medial heels less than 4 inches apart) and without holding onto any object for support	=2

6. **Nudge on sternum** (with subject standing with feet as close together as possible, examiner pushes with light even pressure over sternum three times)

Begins to fall or examiner has to help to maintain balance	=0
Needs to move feet but able to maintain balance (e.g., staggers, grabs, but catches self)	=1
Steady, able to withstand pressure	=2

7. **Balance with eyes closed for 5 seconds** (with subject standing with feet as close together as possible with arms at side)

Any sign of unsteadiness or needs to hold onto an object	=0
Steady without holding onto any object with feet close together	=1

8. **Turning balance (360 degrees)** (Have subject turn around in a complete circle from a standing still position; demonstrate this first and give the subject one time to practice)

Steps are discontinuous (subject puts one foot completely on the floor before raising the other foot)	=0
Steps are continuous (turn is a flowing movement)	=1
Any sign of unsteadiness or holds onto an object	=0
Steady without holding onto any object	=1

9. **Sitting down**

Unsafe (falls into chair, misjudges distances, lands off-center)	=0
Needs to use arms to guide self into chair or not a smooth movement	=1
Able to sit down in one safe, smooth motion	=2

Balance Score _____/16

TABLE 15-9
Performance-Oriented Mobility Test (Continued)

Gait

Instructions: The subject stands with the examiner. They walk down the hallway or across a room (preferably) when there are few people or obstacles. The subject should be told to walk at his or her "usual" pace using his or her usual walking aid. Circle the appropriate score.

10. **Initiation of gait** (subject is asked to begin walking down the hallway immediately after being told to "go")

Any hesitancy, multiple attempts to start, or initiation of gait not a smooth motion = 0
Subject begins walking immediately without observable hesitation and initiation of gait in a single, smooth motion = 1

11. **Step length and height** (observe distance between toe of stance foot and heel of swing foot; observe from the side; do not judge first few or last few steps; observe one foot at a time)

Right swing foot does *not* pass left stance foot with each step = 0
Right swing foot passes left stance foot with each step = 1

Right swing foot does *not* clear floor completely with each step (may hear scraping) or is raised markedly high (e.g., due to drop foot) = 0
Right foot completely clears floor but is not markedly high = 1

Left swing foot does *not* pass left stance foot with each step = 0
Left swing foot passes left stance foot with each step = 1

Left swing foot does *not* clear floor completely with each step (may hear scraping) or is raised markedly high (e.g., due to drop foot) = 0
Left foot completely clears floor but is not markedly high = 1

12. **Step symmetry** (observe distance between toe of each stance foot and heel of each swing foot; observe from the side; do not judge first few or last few steps)

Step length varies between sides or subject advances with same foot with every step = 0
Step length same or nearly same on both sides for most step cycles = 1

13. **Step continuity**

Steps are *discontinuous* (subject places entire foot, heel and toe, on floor before beginning to raise other foot) or subject stops completely between steps = 0
Steps are *continuous* (subject begins raising heel of one foot as heel of other foot touches the floor) and there are no breaks or stops in the subject's stride = 1

14. **Path deviation** (observe in relation to floor tiles or a line on the floor; observe one foot over several strides—about 10 feet of path length; observe from behind; difficult to assess if subject uses a walking aid)

Marked deviation of foot from side-to-side or toward one direction = 0
Mild/moderate deviation, or subject uses a walking aid = 1
Foot follows close to a straight line as subject advances = 2

15. **Trunk stability** (observe from behind)

Marked side-to-side trunk sway, or subject uses a walking aid = 0
No side-to-side trunk sway, but subject flexes knees or back or subject spreads arms out while walking = 1
Trunk does not sway, knees and back are not flexed, arms are not abducted in an effort to maintain stability = 2

16. **Walk stance** (observe from behind)

Feet apart with stepping = 0
Feet should almost touch as one foot passes the other = 1

Gait score _____ /12

TOTAL SCORE _____ /28

Reprinted with permission from M. Tinetti.

TABLE 15-10

Environmental Hazards in Institutional Settings

Lighting:	Dark, too dim, glare, shadows
Walking surface:	Wet and slippery from spills, patterned floor
Hallways:	Cluttered, people traffic
Stairs:	Inadequate handrails, edges not clearly defined, poor step design
Furniture:	Too low, too high, too soft, tips easily, on wheels
Bathroom:	Slippery tub or shower, lack of grab bars for toilet or tub
Shoes/slippers:	Too loose, badly worn heels, soles too slick
Clothing:	Too long, loose, and flowing
Equipment:	Worn out or broken, improper use of equipment, use of restraints, full length siderails
Staff:	Too busy, inadequate number, attitude

DIAGNOSTIC TESTS

The routine use of diagnostic tests in fall assessment is generally not recommended unless the history and physical examination suggest that a specific clinical condition may exist or if the individual has had repeated falls. If acute illness is suspected, appropriate laboratory studies should be ordered, such as a complete blood count, blood chemistries, chest x-ray, and electrocardiogram. If a heart block or transient arrhythmia is suspected, ambulatory electrocardiographic monitoring is indicated. Electrocardiography should be considered in patients with histories suggestive of aortic stenosis and a grade 2 systolic heart murmur. If the history suggests anterior circulation transient ischemic attack, noninvasive vascular studies should be considered to rule out treatable vascular lesions. If a seizure disorder is suspected, an electroencephalogram should be ordered. When there is high suspicion for an intracranial lesion, a computed tomographic scan should be considered (Kane et al., 1994).

Prevention

The overall goal of fall prevention is to reduce falls and fall-related injuries. Specific objectives include the following: (1) modify or eliminate predisposing and environmental risk factors, (2) improve or maintain physical function and mobility, (3) reduce fear of falling, and (4) maintain patient autonomy to the fullest extent possible. Balancing interventions to ensure safety while at the same time encouraging independence may be difficult. Tables 15–11 and 15–12 provide a summary of selected medical, environmental, psychological, and rehabilitative interventions associated with fall risk factors.

GENERAL FALL PREVENTION STRATEGIES

Fall prevention in community-dwelling and institutionalized elderly people follows similar strategies. The first strategy is to conduct a targeted assessment to determine individuals at high risk for falling. Identified fall risk factors should be modified or corrected to the fullest extent possible. All underlying medical problems should be appropriately treated. Medications should be carefully selected based on a cost-benefit analysis and judiciously used. The use of long-acting sedatives and tranquilizers should be avoided. The axiom of "start low, and go slow" with drug dosing is critical in the elderly, especially in frail adults. Drug effects should be closely monitored for adverse reactions and iatrogenic complications.

Because a significant number of community-dwelling people who fall may have no identified risk factors for falls, all older adults and their families should be given fall prevention education. In institutionalized settings, patients, their families, and staff (e.g., nursing, dietary, housekeeping) that work within patient care areas should also be instructed in fall prevention. A greater awareness of risk factors and safety issues may help alter individuals' behavior.

The environment should be modified for optimal safety (see Tables 15–11 and 15–12). Attention should be given to areas where falls are most likely to occur, such as bathrooms, bedrooms, and stairs. Fall alarm systems should be considered for the person who has had multiple falls or is at high risk for falling, who lives alone at home, or who is institution-

TABLE 15-11

Interventions for Predisposing Risk Factors

Risk Factor	Intervention
Sensory	
Vision changes	Appropriate refraction, proper placement of bifocal or trifocal lenses; clean glasses; good lighting especially at steps and entranceways; cataract surgery if indicated; glaucoma treatment; allow time for eyes to adjust when going from light to dark room and vice versa
Hearing loss	Cerumen removal; referral for audiologic evaluation; hearing aids
Vestibular dysfunction	Avoidance of toxic drugs; balance retraining; surgery if indicated
Dizziness	Treat underlying cause
Proprioceptive changes	Treatment of underlying disease, e.g., vitamin B_{12}; use of assistive device if indicated; educate patient to use extra caution when climbing stairs, crossing streets, walking on uneven surfaces; appropriate footwear
Neuromuscular	
Balance problems	Consider use of assistive device; balance retraining; water exercises; good lighting; appropriate footwear; use of adaptive devices, e.g., reachers, grab bars, bath stools; educate patient to sit when putting on underwear, slacks, and footwear and to avoid sudden movement
Gait disorders	Referral for physical therapy evaluation; consider use of assistive device
Muscle weakness	Strengthening exercises; use high, firm chair with arms; consider use of ejection chairs; use of grab bars, reachers
Joint inflexibility	Flexibility exercises
Arthritis	Use of nonsteroidal anti-inflammatory agents; low-intensity exercise; water exercise
Osteoporosis (fracture risk)	Hormone replacement therapy in women if not contraindicated; consideration of alendronate or calcitonin if estrogen contraindicated; calcium and vitamin D supplementation; walking program; protective hip pads
Foot problems	Referral to podiatrist for painful foot abnormalities; keep toe nails and calluses well-trimmed; appropriate footwear
Cognitive/Affective	
Delirium	Treat underlying cause; monitor closely for safety
Dementia	Supervised environment; judicious use of anticholinergic and centrally acting drugs
Depression	Careful consideration of risk/benefit of antidepressant medication; social support; for severe depression, consider referral for psychological evaluation
Fear of falling	Discuss fears with patient; desensitization program for severe fear
Cardiovascular	
Postural hypotension	Educate patient about arising slowly (count to 30 before changing position); adequate hydration; lowest effective dose of necessary medications; elevate head of bed 8–12 inches, TED stockings; reconditioning exercises
Postprandial hypotension	Small, frequent meals; rest period after meals; give antihypertensive medication after meals; reduced dosage of antihypertensive drug
Cardiac causes (e.g., arrhythmias, conduction disorders)	Treat underlying disease
Metabolic	
Metabolic diseases (e.g., diabetes, hypothyroidism)	Treat underlying disease; educate patient about signs and symptoms of hypoglycemia and need to carry concentrated sugar
Fluid and electrolyte disturbances	Correct underlying problem
Urinary	
Urinary urgency, nocturia, incontinence	Two-hour timed voiding; urinal/bedside commode at bedside; accessible call light and quick response to call
Medications	Discontinue all unnecessary medications; use lowest effective dose of necessary medications; avoid long-acting sedatives and tranquilizers; monitor drugs closely, especially new medications or increased dosages
Environment	Eliminate obstacles; modify environment for optimal safety (see Tables 15–12 and 15–14); consider use of fall alarm system or telephone reassurance program; cellular phone or telephones in several rooms

TABLE 15-12
Environmental Interventions for Falls in the Home

Hazards	Modifications
Lighting Problems	
Poor access to switches or lamps	Provide ample lighting in rooms and hallways, with switches located at room entrances
Low lighting	Provide extra lighting along path from bedroom to bathroom, by one- and two-step elevations, and by top and bottom of stairway landings
	Use 100 to 200 watt bulbs and three-way light bulbs to increase lighting levels
Lack of night lights	Use night lights; keep flashlight in bedside table in case of power failures
Increased lighting glare	Eliminate glare from exposed light bulbs by using translucent light shades or frosted light bulbs
Floors and Hallway Problems	
Clutter	Arrange furnishings so that pathways are not obstructed
Low-lying objects	Remove low-lying objects
Limited walking space	Provide stable furnishings along pathways for balance support
Waxed/wet floors	Provide nonskid rugs and carpet runners on slippery floors; use nonskid floor wax; wipe up spills immediately
Sliding throw rugs	Replace sliding area rugs with nonskid rugs or place nonskid tape or pads underneath existing rugs
Worn carpets	Repair or replace worn, loose, wrinkled, or torn carpets
Upended or curled carpet edges	Tape down all carpet edges prone to buckling or curling
Raised door sills	Remove or place carpeting over threshold to create smooth transition between rooms
Patterned carpet or floor coverings	Avoid floor coverings with complex patterns
Bathroom Problems	
Low toilet seat	Use elevated toilet seat or install toilet safety frame
Inaccessible tub or shower stall	Install wall-mounted or tub-attached grab bar or shower chair or tub transfer bench
Slippery floor tile	Apply nonskid strips or decals to bathroom tiled floors
Slippery tub or shower floor	Apply nonskid rubber mat on tub floor
Unstable towel or shower rods	Replace with grab rails that can be bolted to wall studs
Lack of telephone or alarm device	Take cellular phone into bathroom when bathing or using toilet; avoid locking bathroom door
Stairway Problems	
Lack of handrails	Install well-anchored cylindrical handrails on both sides (for hand grasp)
Slippery steps	Apply nonskid treads to steps
Steps in poor repair	Repair worn carpet on steps; repair outdoors steps
Lack of step visibility	Apply color-contrasted nonskid tape for visibility
Furniture Problems	
Low chair seats	Replace low chairs with those that are easy to get up from and sit down in or add a seat cushion to raise seat height
Armless chairs	Provide chairs with armrest support
Low or high bed	Replace existing mattress with one that is thinner (to lower bed height) or thicker (to raise)
Unstable table	Remove pedestal tables; obtain table that can support weight of person leaning on table edges
Storage Problems	
Shelves too low or high	Keep frequently used objects at waist level; use reacher device to obtain objects
Unstable chairs or step stools	Replace chairs; obtain stable step stool with a handrail
Lack of adequate storage space	Install shelves and cupboards at accessible height

Adapted with permission from Tideiksaar, R. (1996). Preventing falls: How to identify factors, reduce complications. *Geriatrics*, 51(2), 43–50. Copyright by Advanstar Communications Inc.

alized either in an acute or long-term care setting.

Chemical and physical restraints should be avoided if at all possible because of the increased fall risk associated with their use. Alternatives to restraint use are identified in Table 15–13 and discussed in greater detail in Chapter 25.

Attention should also be given to clothing that might cause accidents. Individuals should be instructed to avoid wearing long nightgowns, long robes, or other clothing that can easily be tripped on or get caught on furniture and doorknobs.

Good nutrition with adequate protein and calories should be maintained to prevent weakness, particularly in frail older adults. Unless there is a contraindication, all older women should be on hormone replacement therapy, with calcium and vitamin D supplementation to counteract bone loss and reduce the risk of fracture with falls. For postmenopausal women who are unable or unwilling to use estrogen

and have confirmed low bone density or history of osteoporotic fractures, use of alendronate (Fosamax) or calcitonin salmon (Miacalcin) may also reduce the fracture risk associated with falls. Women who use alendronate should be instructed to take their medication at least 30 minutes prior to having any fluid or food in the morning for optimal absorption. However, they should be cautioned not to return to bed after taking the medication because of the risk of esophageal and gastric irritation. Miacalcin, a nasal spray, may be a suitable alternative to the use of alendronate. At the present time, the Food and Drug Administration (FDA) is studying whether to add an indication to use these drugs for the prevention of osteoporosis without having an established diagnosis.

Attention to foot care and proper foot wear is essential. Individuals with painful calluses, bunions, and toe abnormalities should be referred for podiatric care. Toe nails should be kept well trimmed. Well-fitting, low-heeled

---

TABLE 15-13
Alternatives to Restraints to Prevent Falls

Environment

Wheelchair adaptions, e.g. antitipper
Wedge seat
Alternative seating
   High-backed stationary chairs
   Recliner chairs
   Rocking chairs
   Modular couches
Removal of wheels from overbed table
Body props
Alarm devices
Improve lighting
Bed
   Lowest position
   Half-length siderails
   Position next to wall

Nursing

Assess patients for risk of falling
Anticipate patient's needs, individualize care
   Ambulation
   Toileting
   Activity/rest
   Discomfort/pain
   Positioning

Nursing *Continued*

Review medications
Increase observation and monitoring
   Locate near nurses' station
   Make frequent rounds
Frequent reminders to avoid certain behaviors and to encourage other behaviors (e.g., not to get up without asking for assistance)
Encourage family to participate in rehabilitative and safety activities
Psychosocial
   Provide structured, meaningful activity
   Monitor environmental stimuli
   Distract, redirect

Organization

Permit risk of falling
Ensure adequate staffing

Education

Assessment of fall risk
Consequences of restraint use
Alternative strategies to restraints use

Data from Brower (1991); Cutchins (1991); Masters & Marks (1990); Strumpf et al. (1991); and Werner et al. (1994).

shoes and slippers with a nonskid surface should be worn to prevent slips and trips.

Regular exercise should be encouraged for all older adults with normal gait and balance. For patients with gait and balance disorders, referral for physical therapy is important. The Frailty and Injuries Cooperative Studies of Intervention Techniques (FICSIT) trials, a set of independent, randomized, controlled clinical trials in community and long-term institutionalized elderly populations, demonstrated that even the oldest, most frail nursing home patients can benefit from exercise interventions in reducing frailty and falls (Province et al., 1995).

PREVENTING FALLS IN THE COMMUNITY

Interventions for preventing falls in the community-dwelling elderly include risk factor modification (see Tables 15–11 and 15–12), education, and exercise. Results from randomized controlled trials of different low-intensity interventions have shown mixed results in reducing falls and fall-related injuries (Hornbrook et al., 1994; Lord et al., 1995; Reinsch et al., 1992; Tinetti et al., 1994; Vetter et al., 1992; Wagner et al., 1994). Although the prevention of all falls is probably not a realistic goal, the reduction of predisposing risk factors along with environmental alterations may help decrease some falls and reduce the risk of injurious falls.

Risk Factor Modification

Research has suggested that identifying and treating predisposing and environmental risk factors in community-dwelling elderly people may reduce falls and possibly injurious falls (Tinetti et al., 1994; Wagner et al., 1994; Wolf-Klein et al., 1988). One of the FICSIT trials that studied the effect of a multidisciplinary risk abatement program in 301 community-dwelling adults aged 70 years and over who had at least one fall risk factor found a 31% reduction of falls in the follow-up year (Tinetti et al., 1994). The intervention group received an environmental assessment, medication review with a focus on reducing the use of multiple drugs as well as selected drugs, treatment of postural hypotension, or physical therapy to improve

upper and lower extremity strength, range of motion, and balance and gait impairments, or a combination of these. The risk of falling was reduced by 11% for each decrease of one risk factor. In addition, researchers noted that the total mean annual healthcare cost in the intervention group was approximately $2000 less than the comparison group (Rizzo et al., 1996).

Education

Education will also be beneficial in fall prevention; however, education alone will probably not be sufficient to achieve significant reductions in falls and fall-related injuries. Research investigating educational approaches to fall prevention have had mixed results. In the Study of Accidental Falls in the Elderly (SAFE), elderly members of health maintenance organizations (HMO) attended group meetings to improve awareness of environmental hazards and medical and behavioral risk factors for falls and to learn a low-intensity exercise program. The intervention group reduced the odds of falling during the 23-month study by 0.85, but it reduced the number of falls among those who fell by only 7% and did not decrease the number of falls requiring medical treatment (Hornbrook et al., 1994). Another study investigating exercise and a cognitive-behavioral intervention that included discussion of fall prevention, recommendations for exercise, and relaxation training failed to find a significant benefit on fall and fall-injury reduction, fear of falling, or perceived health in senior center participants (Reinsch et al., 1992). A third study of elderly HMO enrollees found that the provision of a brief nursing visit to seniors with targeted risk factors resulted in less disability and fewer falls over a 1-year period but that these differences disappeared by 2 years (Wagner et al., 1994).

The educational program should include information on the types and circumstances surrounding falls; environmental hazards, key medical and behavioral risk factors and how to modify them; strategies to empower individuals to better manage their own health care; and what to do if a fall occurs. Appendix 15–1 lists resources for patient education materials.

It is beneficial to provide anticipatory guidance for managing a fall event and how to get up from the floor after a fall if no one is available to help. Many older adults report feeling surprised and stunned when they have fallen, which affects their ability to think clearly about what they should do. Having an opportunity to rehearse what they might do in a fall situation, and practicing how to get up from the floor, may help reduce anxiety if an actual fall should occur. Individuals should be instructed to remain still for a few minutes after a fall and then to check themselves to see if they are injured. In the case of an injury, they should crawl to the nearest phone to call the rescue squad to help them get up. If they are not injured, they should try to get themselves back to an upright position. To get up from the floor without physical assistance, the individual should be instructed to turn from a supine position to the prone position, and then try to arise to a kneeling position with hands still held on the floor. If a chair or table is nearby, the person should crawl over to it and pull himself or herself up holding on to the furniture. If there is no sturdy piece of furniture available to pull oneself up with, the person can attempt to get up without help by flexing one knee, keeping the foot flat on the floor. The person's hand should be placed on the flexed knee, and he or she should push down on the knee until he or she arises to a standing position.

Exercise

One of the more promising approaches to reducing falls is exercise interventions designed to improve balance, strength, flexibility, coordination, and endurance. However, the type, intensity, and duration of the exercise program need further explication. Four of the FICSIT sites investigating the effects of short-term exercise programs in community-dwelling older adults used approaches such as tai chi, balance retraining, flexibility and resistance exercises, and endurance training. A meta-analysis of individual patient data from seven of the eight FICSIT sites (includes two nursing homes) suggests that subjects assigned to exercise interventions are less likely to fall in the follow-up period, and those whose interventions were

designed to improve balance had even a lower incidence of falls (Province et al., 1995). Unfortunately, the sample size of the clinical trials was not large enough to detect an effect on reduction of fall injuries.

Based on the findings of the FICSIT trial as well as the recent recommendations from the Surgeon General's Report on Physical Activity and Health (U.S. Department of Health and Human Services [USDHHS], 1996), older adults should be encouraged to engage in moderate physical activity for 30 minutes, 5 days a week. A 5- to 10-minute warm-up and cool-down period is recommended. Low-intensity exercise has been shown to improve joint flexibility and reduce pain in elders with arthritis (Ettinger & Afable, 1994). Sedentary elderly people should follow a graduated exercise program, beginning with 5 or 10 minutes per day and adding 5 minutes per week until 30 minutes is achieved. Walking is an excellent exercise that not only increases overall physical fitness but also helps with maintenance of bone mineral density. Low-intensity exercise designed to improve balance, such as tai chi and water exercises, can be safely and easily performed by most older adults (Simmons & Hansen, 1996; Wolf et al., 1993).

PREVENTING FALLS IN NURSING HOMES AND HOSPITALS

A multidimensional approach with interdisciplinary involvement is necessary to reduce the risk of falls in healthcare institutions. Many management strategies are known but their success rates vary. A systemic approach to the prevention of falls includes a careful admission assessment to identify the patient at high risk for falls (Rhymes & Jaeger, 1988; Tinetti & Speechley, 1989). Assessments are made throughout the period of hospitalization and nursing home stay because the patient's condition changes over time. An individualized plan of care is developed with the focus on elimination or modification of predisposing and situational risk factors to the extent possible (Table 15–14 and see Table 15–11).

Risk Factor Modification

Physical and Psychological Factors. The most modifiable of the known fall risk factors

TABLE 15-14
Fall-Prevention Strategies Used in Hospitals and Nursing Homes

PATIENT	ENVIRONMENT *(Continued)*
Restraints and Devices Reduce or eliminate use of restraints Use electronic alarm devices, such as Ambularm, Bed-Check, Wander Guard	Lock wheels on all furniture, equipment Keep equipment on one side of hallway Maintain equipment in good repair Night lights in rooms Safety (grab) bars in bathroom and corridors Chairs with various seat height and raised toilet seats Use of bedside commodes Remove wheels from bedside commodes Safety posters in room to encourage asking for help
Medications Note hypnotic and sedative drugs given at night, especially to elderly, postoperative patients Note diuretics and laxatives given at night	
	PATIENT EDUCATION
Activities of Daily Living Assist patient to void every 4 hours Check for properly fitting clothes Check for proper slippers or footwear (nonskid footwear) Keep patient's belongings close to the bed Provide rehabilitation training to improve functional ability	Hand out safety brochure to patient and family on admission Teach patient about safety and equipment Encourage patient to request assistance Encourage use of bathroom and corridor handrails Teach safe transfer from bed to chair
ENVIRONMENT	NURSING
Relocation of patient with high fall risk to room close to nurses' station or in hallway Nurse call light system in place, e.g. pinned to pillow, within reach Teach patient and family how to use the call light system and bed controls; show location of bathroom; point out movable furniture Half to three-quarter length siderails Bed in low position Room light on, adequate intensity TV controls within reach Clutter-free room and hallways Carpet all hard surfaces Nonskid wax Clean up spills	Perform assessment at admission and throughout hospital stay Assign safety risk Note subtle changes in health status Provide closer observations shortly after admission, transfer, during acute illness, after a fall Frequent rounds/checks/observations Move slowly around unsteady ambulatory patients
	ORGANIZATION
	Monitor falls, watch for trends, and conduct in-service when trend emerges Adequate staffing

Data from Brower (1991); Kellogg International Work Group (1987); Rubenstein et al. (1994); Tinetti (1994a, 1994b); Whedon & Shedd (1989).

are weakness and impairment of balance (Tinetti, 1994b). A mobility exercise program helps maintain mobility and reduces the likelihood of falling and the seriousness of the consequences. The optimal intensity of exercise programs has yet to be determined (Tinetti, 1997). Exercise programs for the very frail nursing home resident have shown limited and modest benefits. In one study, a physical therapy program for the very frail nursing home resident resulted in modest mobility benefits and no significant improvement in other areas of physical performance, self-perceived func-

tion, and activities of daily living (Mulrow et al., 1994). A study on the effects of a walking program for very frail ambulatory nursing home residents showed that 12 weeks of daily walking produced significant improvement in walk endurance capacity but did not effect significant changes in physical activity level, mobility, or quality of life. Improvement was not noted when the program was extended to 22 weeks (MacRae et al., 1996). The deconditioning of hospitalized elderly patients can be prevented by initiating a gradual, progressive exercise program (Hoenig & Rubenstein, 1991).

To prevent postprandial hypotension, walking after a meal to restore normal circulation was recently proposed. The older person should be closely observed or accompanied during the walk (Lipsitz, 1995).

The older person who has a fear of falling can be assisted to increase his or her self-efficacy or level of confidence. Mobility and transfer skills may be improved with consultation from a physical therapist. The older person's self-confidence can be increased by setting attainable short-term goals toward independence (Tinetti & Powell, 1993).

Protective hip pads have been used to prevent or diminish the impact and the seriousness of an injury during a fall. The pads have been found to reduce hip fracture rates in a nursing home (Lauretizen et al., 1993).

Environment. A safe, supportive, enabling environment is one that meets the special needs of the older person with diminished competence and a decreased ability to adapt. A bed height of about 18 inches from the floor to the top of the mattress is the ideal height for safe transfer. Chair height should be at a level where the person's feet are firmly on the floor when sitting with the knees flexed at 90 degrees. Armrests that extend beyond the edge of the seat provide leverage when moving in and out of the chair.

Restraints have been the focus of many studies. Although restraints are used primarily to prevent falls and injury, the study results indicate that alternatives to restraints were not sufficiently taken into consideration and that restraint use was associated with continued falls and serious injuries (Gross et al., 1990; MacPherson et al., 1990; Tinetti et al., 1992). Reducing the use of restraints resulted in an increase in nonserious falls, but no increase in serious, injurious falls (Ejaz et al., 1994). A number of care alternatives to restraints are available (see Table 15–13). Restraint use can be eliminated with the implementation of an individualized approach to care (see Chapter 25).

Effective interventions to prevent falls that minimize work on the part of patients and also the staff include various types of fall-monitoring devices (Llewellyn et al., 1988; Morse, 1993; Morton, 1989; Ross, 1991). Alarm devices such as Bed Check and Ambularm (Fig. 15–3) will

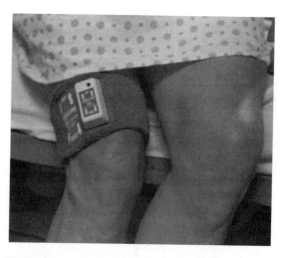

FIGURE 15–3. The Ambularm is worn just above the knee. The alarm is activated when the patient moves this leg to a vertical position. (Used with permission from AlertCare, Mill Valley, California.)

sound a warning that the person is trying to leave the bed or chair. The appropriate device to use depends on the situation and the patient. Some devices can be taken off by patients.

Fall Prevention Program

Fall prevention programs have been established in many nursing homes and hospitals. In an effort to prevent falls, the fall prevention programs present a comprehensive, systematic approach to the problem. Patients are assessed for fall risk on admission. Assessment forms have been developed to determine a patient's risk and to formalize staff awareness and assessment skills. Common factors included in fall assessment instruments are fall history, mental status, sensory deficits, physical disabilities, postoperative condition, admission or transfer to a hospital or unit in a hospital, drug and alcohol use, gait disturbances, incontinence, attitude, and mood state. Patients should be assessed on an ongoing basis throughout their stay.

Once a patient is determined to be at risk, all staff should be alerted. The use of an orange adhesive sticker or other eye-catching device on the patient's chart, name band, Kardex, door, or bedside is a popular method to indicate that a patient is at risk for falls (Fife et al., 1984; Spellbring et al., 1988). Figure 15–4 shows one hospital's fall alert design.

Once risk factors have been identified, efforts are directed to modify the factors. Fall prevention strategies commonly used in hospitals and nursing homes are presented in Table 15–14. Comprehensive review articles by Maciorowski and associates (1988), Morse (1993), Rawsky (1998), and Whedon and Shedd (1989) are helpful in developing prevention strategies.

After an extensive review of the literature on falls, Whedon and Shedd (1989) concluded that staff nurses know the basic interventions necessary to prevent patient falls. Instead of focusing on the actions to prevent falls, Whedon and Shedd suggest that efforts should be focused on raising staff awareness in relation to falls.

Providing staff members with statistical data on falls, providing inservice education on risk factors and preventive measures, and involving the staff in designing a fall prevention program have been shown to increase staff aware-

ness and use of fall prevention measures. A standardized care plan should be developed with the interventions focusing on high risk factors. Periodic review and revision of the plan are essential (Spellbring, 1992).

It is recommended that a focused fall risk assessment be included in the periodic physical examination of nursing home residents. The purpose of the focused assessment should be to identify potentially correctable problems. This assessment should include postural blood pressure measurement, visual acuity testing, manual muscle testing of lower extremities, balance and gait evaluation, functional status and mental status evaluation, and a review of medications and dosing (Rubenstein et al., 1991; Tinetti, 1994b).

SUMMARY

Falls are a common problem among older people. They represent an important clinical syndrome in terms of their frequency, morbidity, threat to the quality and length of life of the older person, and the increased use of healthcare services. Falls are caused by a multitude of factors that include the personal characteristics of the person who falls, the environment, and the interaction between the two. The incidence, circumstances, and outcomes of falls differ between community dwelling elderly persons and the elderly who are in healthcare institutions. The advanced practice nurse has a crucial role in the early detection of fall risk factors, in monitoring fall events, and in the development of fall prevention programs for community and institutional settings.

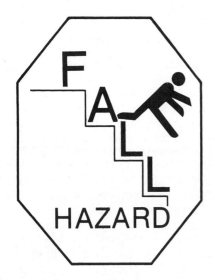

FIGURE 15–4. Safety alert sticker. The safety alert sticker is designed to signal all staff that this patient is at high risk for falling. It can be placed on the patient's chart or care plan or affixed at the patient's bedside. (Redrawn from Spellbring, A. M., Gannon, M. E., Kleckner, T., & Conway, K. [1988]. Improving safety for hospitalized elderly. *Journal of Gerontological Nursing, 14,* 31–37.)

REFERENCES

Alexander, B. H., Rivara, F. P., & Wolf, M. E. (1992). The cost and frequency of hospitalization for fall-related injuries in older adults. *American Journal of Public Health, 82,* 1020–1023.

Arfken, C. L., Lach, H. W., Birge, S. J., & Miller, J. P. (1994). The prevalence and correlates of fear of falling in elderly persons living in the community. *American Journal of Public Health, 84,* 565–570.

Baloh, R. W. (1992). Dizziness in older people. *Journal of the American Geriatrics Society, 40,* 713–721.

Brower, H. T. (1991). The alternatives to restraints. *Journal of Gerontological Nursing, 17*(2), 18–22.

Brummel-Smith, K. (1989). Falls in the aged. *Primary Care, 16*, 377–393.

Campbell, A. J., Borrie, M. J., & Spears, G. F. (1989). Risk factors for falls in a community-based prospective study of people 70 years and older. *Journal of Gerontology: Medical Sciences, 44*, M112–M117.

Campbell, A. J., Borrie, M. J., Spears, G. F., et al. (1990). Circumstances and consequences of falls experienced by community population 70 years and over during a prospective study. *Age and Aging, 19*, 136–141.

Cutchins, C. H. (1991). Blueprint for restraint-free care. *American Journal of Nursing, 91*(7), 36–42.

Cumming, R. G., & Klineberg, R. J. (1994). Fall frequency and characteristics and the risk of hip fractures. *Journal of the American Geriatrics Society, 42*, 774–778.

Cummings, S. R., Nevitt, M. C., & Kidd, S. (1988). Forgetting falls: The limited accuracy of recall of falls in the elderly. *Journal of the American Geriatrics Society, 36*, 613–616.

DeVito, C. A., Lambert, D. A., Sattin, R. W., et al. (1988). Fall injuries among the elderly. Community-based surveillance. *Journal of the American Geriatrics Society, 36*, 1029–1035.

Downton, J. (1992). Falls in the elderly. In J. C. Brocklehurst, R. C. Tallis & H. M. Fillit (Eds.), *Textbook of geriatric medicine and gerontology* (4th ed., pp. 317–325). Edinburgh: Churchill Livingstone.

Downton, J. H., & Andrews, K. (1990). Postural disturbance and psychological symptoms amongst elderly people living at home. *International Journal of Geriatric Psychology, 5*, 93–98.

Dunn, J. E., Rudberg, M. A., Turner, S. E., & Cassel, C. K. (1992). Mortality, disability, and falls in older persons: The role of underlying disease and disability. *American Journal of Public Health, 82*, 395–400.

Duthie, E. H. (1989). Falls. *Medical Clinics of North America, 73*, 1321–1336.

Ejaz, F. K., Jones, J. A., & Rose, M. S. (1994). Falls among nursing home residents: An examination of incident reports before and after restraints reduction programs. *Journal of the American Geriatrics Society, 42*, 960–964.

Ettinger, W. H. Jr., & Afable, R. F. (1994). Physical disability from knee osteoarthritis: The role of exercise as an intervention. *Medical Science, Sports, and Exercise, 26*, 1435–1440.

Fife, D. P., Solomon, P., & Stanton, M. (1984). A risk/falls program: Code orange for success. *Nursing Management, 15*, 50–53.

Fisher, E. S., Baron, J. A., Malenka, D. J., et al. (1991). Hip fracture incidence and mortality in New England. *Epidemiology, 2*, 116–122.

Friedman, S. M., Williamson, J. D., Lee, B. H., et al. (1995). Increased fall rates in nursing home residents after relocation to a new facility. *Journal of the American Geriatrics Society, 43*, 1237–1242.

Glynn, R. J., Seddon, J. M., Krug, J. H., et al. (1991). Falls in elderly patients with glaucoma. *Archives of Ophthalmology, 109*, 205–210.

Grisso, J. A., & Kaplan, F. (1994). Hip fractures. In W. R. Hazzard, E. L. Bierman, J. P. Blass, et al. (Eds.), *Principles of geriatric medicine and gerontology* (3rd ed., pp. 1321–1328). New York: McGraw-Hill.

Gross, Y. T., Shimamoto, Y., Rose, C. L., & Frank, B. (1990). Why do they fall? Monitoring risk factors in nursing homes. *Journal of Gerontological Nursing, 16*(6), 20–25.

Gulya, A. J. (1995). Dizziness and vertigo. In W. B. Abrams, M. H. Beers & R. Berkow (Eds.). *The Merck manual of geriatrics* (2nd ed., pp. 1331–1337). Whitehouse Station, NJ: Merck & Co., Inc.

Gurwitz, J. H., Sanchez-Cross, M. T., Echler, M. A., & Matulis, J. (1994). The epidemiology of adverse and unexpected events in the long-term care setting. *Journal of the American Geriatrics Society, 42*, 33–38.

Harris, P. B. (1989). Organizational and staff attitudinal determinants of falls in nursing home residents. *Medical Care, 27*, 739–749.

Hoenig, H. M., & Rubenstein, L. Z. (1991). Hospital-associated deconditioning and dysfunction. *Journal of the American Geriatrics Society, 39*, 220–222.

Hornbrook, M. C., Stevens, V. J., Wingfield, D. J., et al. (1994). Preventing falls among community-dwelling older persons: Results from a randomized trial. *Gerontologist, 34*, 16–23.

Hough, J. C. (1992). Falls and falling. In R. J. Ham & P. D. Sloane (Eds.), *Primary care geriatrics. A case-based approach* (2nd ed., pp. 362–380). St. Louis: Mosby–Year Book.

Janken, J. K., Reyonds, B. A., & Sweich, K. (1986). Patient falls in the acute care setting: Identifying risk factors. *Nursing Research, 35*, 215–219.

Kane, R., Ouslander, J. G., & Abrass, I. B. (Eds.). (1994). Instability and falls. *Essentials of clinical geriatrics* (3rd ed., pp. 197–220). New York: McGraw-Hill.

Kellogg International Work Group on the Prevention of Fall in the Elderly (1987). The prevention of falls in late life. *Danish Medical Bulletin, 34*(suppl. 4), 1–24.

Kiel, D. P., O'Sullivan, P., Teno, J. M., & Mor, V. (1991). Health care utilization and functional status in the aged following a fall. *Medical Care, 29*, 221–228.

King, M. B., & Tinetti, M. E. (1995). Falls in community-dwelling older persons. *Journal of the American Geriatrics Society, 43*, 1146–1154.

Kosorok, M. R., Omenn, G. S., Diehr, P., et al. (1992). Restricted activity days among older adults. *American Journal of Public Health, 82*, 1263–1267.

Lach, H. W., Reed, A. T., Arfken, C. L., et al. (1991). Falls in the elderly: Reliability of a classification system. *Journal of the American Geriatrics Society, 39*, 197–202.

Lachman, M. E., Howland, J., Tennstedt, S., et al. (1998). Fear of falling and activity restriction: The survey of activities and fear of falling in the elderly (SAFE). *Journal of Gerontology: Psychological Sciences, 53B*, P43–P50.

Lauritzen, J. B., Petersen, M. M., & Lund, B. (1993). Effect of external hip protectors on hip fractures. *Lancet, 341*, 11–13.

Lipsitz, L. A. (1995). Syncope. In W. B. Abrams, M. H. Beers & R. Berkow (Eds.). *The Merck manual of geriatrics* (2nd ed., pp. 58–65). Whitehouse Station, NJ: Merck & Co., Inc.

Lipsitz, L. A., Jonsson, P. V., Kelley, M. M., & Koestner, J. S. (1991). Causes and correlates of recurrent falls in ambulatory frail elderly. *Journal of Gerontology: Medical Sciences, 46*, M114–M122.

Liu, B. A., Topper, A. K., Reeves, R. A., et al. (1995). Falls among older people: Relationship to medication use and orthostatic hypotension. *Journal of the American Geriatrics Society, 43,* 1141–1145.

Llewellyn, J., Martin, B., Shekleton, M., & Firlit, S. (1988). Analysis of falls in the acute surgical and cardiovascular surgical patients. *Applied Nursing Research, 1,* 116–121.

Lord, S. R., Clark, R. D., & Webster, I. W. (1991). Physiological factors associated with falls in an elderly population. *Journal of the American Geriatrics Society, 39,* 1194–1200.

Lord, S. R., Ward, J. A., Williams, P., et al. (1995). The effect of a 12-month exercise trail on balance, strength, and falls in older women: A randomized controlled trial. *Journal of the American Geriatrics Society, 43,* 1198–1206.

Lotz, J. C., & Hayes, W. C. (1990). The use of quantitative computed tomography to estimate the risk of fracture of the hip from falls. *Journal of Bone and Joint Surgery, 72A,* 689–700.

Luukinen, H., Koski, K., Hiltunen, L., & Kivela, S. (1994). Incidence rate of falls in an aged population in northern Finland. *Journal of Clinical Epidemiology, 47,* 843–850.

Luukinen, H., Koski, K., Honkanen, R., & Kivela, S. (1995). Incidence of injury-causing falls among older adults by place of residence: A population-based study. *Journal of the American Geriatrics Society, 43,* 871–876.

Maciorowski, L. F., Munro, B. H., Dietrick-Gallagher, M., et al. (1988). A review of the patient fall literature. *Journal of Nursing Quality Assurance, 3*(1), 18–27.

MacPherson, D. S., Lofgren, R. P., Granieri, R., & Myllenbeck, S. (1990). Deciding to restrain medical patients. *Journal of the American Geriatrics Society, 78,* 516–520.

MacRae, P., Asplund, L. A., Schnelle, J. F., et al. (1996). A walking program for nursing home residents: Effects on walk endurance, physical activity, mobility, and quality of life. *Journal of the American Geriatrics Society, 44,* 178–180.

Malmivaara, A., Helioovaara, M., Knekt, P., et al. (1993). Risk factors for injurious falls leading to hospitalization or death in a cohort of 19,500 adults. *American Journal of Epidemiology, 138,* 384–394.

Maki, B. E., Holliday, P. J., & Topper, A. K. (1991). Fear of falling and postural performance in the elderly. *Journal of Gerontology: Medical Sciences, 46,* M123–M131.

Masters, R., & Marks, S. F. (1990). The use of restraints. *Rehabilitation Nursing, 15,* 22–25.

Mathias, S., Nayak, U. S. L., & Isaacs, B. (1986). Balance in elderly patients: The "get-up and go" test. *Archives in Physical Medicine and Rehabilitation, 67,* 387–389.

Melton, L. J., & Riggs, B. L. (1985). Risk factors for injury after a fall. *Clinics in Geriatric Medicine, 1,* 525–539.

Miceli, D. L. G., Waxman, H., Cavalieri, T., & Lage, S. (1994). Prodromal falls among older nursing home residents. *Applied Nursing Research, 7,* 18–27.

Monane, M., & Avorn, J. (1996). Medication and falls. *Clinics in Geriatric Medicine, 12,* 847–858.

Morse, J. M. (1993). Nursing research on patient falls in health care institutions. In J. J. Fitzpatrick & J. S. Stevenson (Eds.), *Annual review of nursing research, vol. 2* (pp. 299–316). New York: Springer.

Morton, D. (1989). Five years of few falls. *American Journal of Nursing, 89,* 204–205.

Mossey, J. M., Mutram, E., Knott, K., & Craik, R. (1989). Determinants of recovery 12 months after hip fracture: The importance of psychosocial factors. *American Journal of Public Health, 79,* 279–286.

Mulrow, C. D., Gerety, M. B., Kanten, D., et al. (1994). A randomized trial of physical rehabilitation for very frail nursing home residents. *Journal of the American Medical Association, 271,* 519–524.

Myers, A. H., Baker, S. P., Van Natta, M. L., et al. (1991). Fall factors associated with falling and injuries among elderly institutionalized persons. *American Journal of Epidemiology, 133,* 1179–1190.

Myers, A. M., Powell, L. E., Maki, B. E., et al. (1996). Psychological indicators of balance confidence: Relationship to actual and perceived abilities. *Journal of Gerontology: Medical Sciences, 51A,* M37–M43.

National Safety Council (1995). *Accident facts.* Chicago: National Safety Council.

Nevitt, M. C., Cummings, S. R., & Hudes, E. S. (1991). Risk factors for injurious falls: A prospective study. *Journal of Gerontology: Medical Sciences, 46,* M164–M170.

Nevitt, M. C., Cummings, S. R., Kidd, S., & Black, D. (1989). Risk factors for recurrent nonsyncopal falls. *Journal of the American Medical Association, 261,* 2663–2668.

O'Loughlin, J. L., Robitaille, Y., Boivin, J., & Suissa, S. (1993). Incidence of and risk factors for falls and injurious falls among the community-dwelling elderly. *American Journal of Epidemiology, 137,* 342–354.

Powell, L. E., & Myers, A. M. (1995). The Activities-Specific Balance Confidence Scale. *Journal of Gerontology: Medical Sciences, 50A,* M28–M34.

Province, M. A., Hadley, E. C., Hornbrook, M. C., et al. (1995). The effects of exercise on falls in elderly patients. A preplanned meta-analysis of the FICSIT Trials. *Journal of the American Medical Association, 272,* 1341–1347.

Rai, G. S., Kiniorns, M., & Wientjes, H. (1995). Falls Handicap Inventory (FHI)—An instrument to measure handicaps associated with repeated falls. *Journal of the American Geriatrics Society, 43,* 723–724.

Rawsky, E. (1998). Review of the literature on falls among the elderly. *Image: Journal of Nursing Scholarship, 30,* 47–52.

Reinsch, S., MacRae, P., Lachenbruch, P. A., & Tobis, J. S. (1992). Attempts to prevent falls and injury: A prospective community study. *Gerontologist, 32,* 450–456.

Resnick, N. M. (1996). Geriatric medicine. In L. M. Tierney Jr., S. J. McPhee & M. A. Papadakis (Eds.), *Current medical diagnosis and treatment* (35th ed., pp. 36–55). Stamford, CT: Appleton & Lange.

Rhymes, J., & Jaeger, R. (1988). Falls: Prevention and management in the institutional setting. *Clinics in Geriatric Medicine, 4,* 613–622.

Rice, D. P., MacKenzie, E. J., Jones, A. S., et al. (1989). *Cost of injury in the United States. A report to Congress.* San Francisco: Institute for Health and Aging, University of California, San Francisco; and Baltimore: Injury Prevention Center, the Johns Hopkins University.

Rizzo, J. A., Baker, D. I., McAvay, G., & Tinetti, M. E. (1996). Cost-effectiveness of the multi-factorial targeted prevention program for falls among community elderly persons. *Medical Care, 34,* 954–969.

Robin, D. W. (1995). Falls and gait disorders. In W. B. Abrams, M. H. Beers & R. Berkow (Eds.). *The Merck manual of geriatrics* (2nd ed., pp. 65–78). Whitehouse Station, NJ: Merck & Co., Inc.

Ross, J. E. R. (1991). Iatrogenesis in the elderly: Contributors to falls. *Journal of Gerontological Nursing, 17*(9), 19–23.

Rubenstein, L. Z., Josephson, K. R., & Osterweil, D. (1996). Falls and fall prevention in the nursing home. *Clinics in Geriatric Medicine, 4,* 881–902.

Rubenstein, L. Z., Josephson, K. R., & Robbins, A. S. (1994). Falls in the nursing home. *Annals of Internal Medicine, 121,* 442–451.

Rubenstein, L. Z., & Robbins, A. S. (1989). Falling syndromes in elderly persons. *Comprehensive Therapy, 15*(6), 13–18.

Rubenstein, L. Z., Robbins, A. S., & Josephson, K. R. (1991). Falls in the nursing-home setting: Causes and preventive approaches. In P. R. Katz, R. L. Kane & M. D. Mezey (Eds.), *Advances in Long-Term Care, vol. 1* (pp. 28–42). New York: Springer.

Sattin, R. W. (1992). Falls among older persons: A public health perspective. *Annual Review of Public Health, 13,* 489–508.

Simmons, V., & Hansen, P. D. (1996). Effectiveness of water exercise on postural mobility in the well elderly: An experimental study on balance enhancement. *Journal of Gerontology: Medical Sciences, 51A,* M233–M238.

Spellbring, A. M. (1992). Assessing elderly patients at high risk for falls: A reliability study. *Journal of Nursing Care Quality, 6*(3), 30–35.

Spellbring, A. M., Gannon, M. E., Kleckner, T., & Conway, K. (1988). Improving safety for hospitalized elderly. *Journal of Gerontological Nursing, 14,* 31–37.

Stewart, R. B., Moore, M. T., May, F. E., et al. (1992). Nocturia: A risk factor for falls in the elderly. *Journal of the American Geriatrics Society, 40,* 1217–1220.

Strumpf, N. E., Evans, L. K., & Schwartz, D. (1991). Physical restraint of the elderly. In W. C. Chenitz, J. Takano Stone & S. A. Salisbury (Eds.), *Clinical gerontological nursing. A guide to advanced practice* (pp. 329–344). Philadelphia: W. B. Saunders Company.

Thapa, P. B., Brockman, K. G., Gideon, P., et al. (1996). Injurious falls in nonambulatory nursing home residents: A comparative study of circumstances, incidences, and risk factors. *Journal of the American Geriatrics Society, 44,* 272–278.

Tideiksaar, R. (1988). Falls in the elderly. *Bulletin of the New York Academy of Medicine, 64,* 145–163.

Tideiksaar, R. (1996). Preventing falls: How to identify risk factors, reduce complications. *Geriatrics, 51*(2), 43–46, 49–53.

Tinetti, M. E. (1986). The performance-oriented assessment of mobility problems in elderly patients. *Journal of the American Geriatrics Society, 34,* 119–126.

Tinetti, M. E. (1987). Factors associated with serious injury during falls by ambulatory nursing home residents. *Journal of the American Geriatrics Society, 36,* 644–648.

Tinetti, M. E. (1994a). Falls. In W. R. Hazzard, E. L. Bierman, J. P. Blass, et al. (Eds.), *Principles of geriatric medicine and gerontology* (3rd ed., pp. 1313–1320). New York: McGraw-Hill.

Tinetti, M. E. (1994b). Prevention of falls and fall injuries in elderly persons: A research agenda. *Preventive Medicine, 23,* 756–762.

Tinetti, M. E. (1997). Falls. In C. K. Cassel, H. J. Cohen, E. B. Larson, et al. (Eds.), *Textbook of geriatric medicine* (3rd ed., pp. 787–799). New York: Springer-Verlag.

Tinetti, M. E., Baker, J. J., McAvay, G., et al. (1994). A multifactorial intervention to reduce the risk of falling among elderly people living in the community. *New England Journal of Medicine, 331,* 821–827.

Tinetti, M. E., Doucette, J. T., & Claus, E. B. (1995). The contribution of predisposing and situational risk factors to serious fall injuries. *Journal of the American Geriatrics Society, 43,* 1207–1213.

Tinetti, M. E., Doucette, J., Claus, E., & Marottoli, R. (1995). Risk factors for serious injury during falls by older persons in the community. *Journal of the American Geriatrics Society, 43,* 1214–1221.

Tinetti, M. E., & Ginter, S. F. (1988). Identifying mobility dysfunction in elderly patients. *Journal of the American Medical Association, 259,* 1190–1193.

Tinetti, M. E., Liu, A. L., & Claus, E. (1993). Predictors and prognosis of inability to get up after falls among elderly persons. *Journal of the American Medical Association, 265,* 269–270.

Tinetti, M. E., Liu, W. L., & Ginter, S. F. (1992). Mechanical restraint use and fall-related injuries among residents of skilled nursing facilities. *Annals of Internal Medicine, 116,* 369–374.

Tinetti, M. E., & Powell, L. (1993). Fear of falling and low self-efficacy: A cause of dependence in elderly persons. *Journal of Gerontology, 48* (special issue), 35–38.

Tinetti, M. E., Richman, D., & Powell, L. (1990). Falls efficacy as a measure of fear of falling. *Journal of Gerontology, 45,* 239–243.

Tinetti, M. E., & Speechley, M. (1989). Prevention of falls among the elderly. *New England Journal of Medicine, 320,* 1055–1059.

Tinetti, M. E., Speechley, M., & Ginter, S. F. (1988). Risk factors for falls among elderly persons living in the community. *New England Journal of Medicine, 319,* 1701–1707.

Tinetti, M. W., Williams, T. F., & Mayewski, R. (1986). Fall risk index for elderly patients based on number of chronic disabilities. *American Journal of Medicine, 80,* 429–434.

Uden, G. (1985). Inpatient accidents in hospitals. *Journal of the American Geriatrics Society, 33,* 833–841.

U.S. Department of Health and Human Services (1996). *Physical activity and health: A report of the Surgeon General.* Atlanta, GA: U.S. Department of Health and Human Services, Centers for Disease Control and Prevention, National Center for Chronic Disease Prevention and Health Promotion.

Vernon, M. S. (1995). Accidents in the elderly population. In W. Reichel (Ed.), *Care of the elderly. Clinical aspects of aging* (4th ed., pp. 547–555). Baltimore: Williams & Wilkins.

Vetter, N. J., Lewis, P. A., & Ford, D. (1992). Can health visitors prevent fractures in elderly people? *British Medical Journal, 304,* 888–890.

Vlahov, D., Myers, A. H., & Al-Ibrahim, M. S. (1990). Epidemiology of falls among patients in a rehabilitation hospital. *Archives of Physical Medicine and Rehabilitation, 71,* 8–12.

Wagner, E. H., LaCroix, A. Z., Grothaus, L., et al. (1994). Preventing disability and falls in older adults: A population-based randomized trial. *American Journal of Public Health, 84,* 1800–1806.

Werner, P., Koroknay, V., Braun, J., & Cohen-Mansfield, J. (1994). Individualized care alternatives used in the process of removing physical restraints in the nursing home. *Journal of the American Geriatrics Society, 43,* 321–325.

Whedon, M. B., & Shedd, P. (1989). Prediction and prevention of patient falls. *Image: Journal of Nursing Scholarship, 21,* 108–114.

Wild, D., Nayak, U. S. L., & Isaacs, B. (1981). Description, classification, and prevention of falls in old people at home. *Rheumatology and Rehabilitation, 20,* 153–159.

Wolf, S., Kutner, N., Green, R., & McNeeley, E. (1993). The Atlanta FICSIT study: Two exercise interventions to reduce fraility in elders. *Journal of the American Geriatrics Society, 41,* 329–332.

Wolf-Klein, G. P., Silverstone, F. A., Basavaraju, N., et al.

(1988). Prevention of falls in the elderly population. *Archives of Physical Medicine and Rehabilitation, 69,* 589–691.

Wolfson, L. (1992). Falls and gait. In R. Katzman & J. W. Rowe (Eds.), *Principles of geriatric neurology* (pp. 281–299). Philadelphia: F. A. Davis.

Wolfson, L., Judge, J., Whipple, R., & King, M. (1995). Strength is a major factor in balance, gait, and the occurrence of falls. *Journal of Gerontology, Series A, 50A* (special issue), pp. 64–67.

Wolinsky, F. D., Johnson, R. J., & Fitzgerald, J. F. (1992). Falling, health status, and the use of health services by older adults. *Medical Care, 30,* 587–597.

Wright, B. A., Aizenstein, S., Vogler, G., et al. (1990). Frequent fallers. Leading groups to identify psychological factors. *Journal of Gerontological Nursing, 16*(4), 15–19.

Resources

American Association of Retired Persons
Consumer Affairs Section
601 E. Street, N.W.
Washington, DC 20049
Telephone (202) 434-2277
(Publishes patient education materials on creating a safe home environment)

National Safety Council
Central Region Office
1121 Spring Lake Drive
Itasca, IL 60143-3201
Telephone (708) 285-1121
(Catalog of brochures, posters, and other safety training materials)

U. S. Consumer Safety Commission
Washington, D. C. 20207
(Provides information on consumer safety and offers a home safety checklist pamphlet)

Walker, Bonnie L.
Injury Prevention in the Elderly
Aspen Publishers
Rockville, MD
Telephone (301) 417-7500
(Publishes 10 modules on safety, including fall prevention; includes workbook and video for use in caregiver education)

Iatrogenesis

Joyce Takano Stone
Catherine Steinbach

Iatrogenesis refers to the unintended, harmful incidents or conditions that result from diagnostic, prophylactic, or therapeutic interventions or omissions (Lefevre et al., 1992; Rubins & Moskowitz, 1990). It occurs frequently in the elderly because of their increased exposure to the healthcare system (Gorbien et al., 1992). Its incidence in this population is the consequence of age; the number and severity of illnesses (Schiff, 1993); healthcare providers' attitudes, beliefs, skills, and knowledge; and system-related factors such as the environment of care settings, high technology, or a lack of services (Gorbien et al., 1992). This chapter describes the nature and extent of iatrogenesis in the elderly and addresses common iatrogenic occurrences and conditions in this age group.

Age has been implicated as a major risk factor for iatrogenic conditions. In the Harvard Medical Practice Study, researchers found that adverse events occurred in 3.7% of hospitalizations and that the rate of adverse events rose with age (Brennan et al., 1991; Leape et al., 1991). In another study, Lefevre and associates (1992) determined that 58% of patients older than 65 years suffered at least one iatrogenic complication and that 36% of these complications were considered potentially preventable. The most common complications occurring in this study population were infections and respiratory and vascular complications. The authors found that complications could have been prevented if greater emphasis had been placed on the initial assessment, including documentation of the older patient's functional status; in doing so, clinicians could have more appropriately targeted the interventions. Low functional status was found to be a significant predictor of experiencing subsequent iatrogenic complications (Lefevre et al., 1992; Potts et al., 1993).

Gurwitz and associates (1994) concluded that falls, nonrelated fall injuries, medication-related events, and wandering episodes are the most frequently reported incidents in the long-term care setting. The investigators identified the need for systematic examination of adverse events in this setting to identify patterns and trends as well as specific areas of care requiring further attention. They also noted that an adverse outcome such as a fall may represent an acceptable outcome in the context of maintaining a restraint-free environment.

The iatrogenesis seen in elderly patients commonly has multiple causes—a cascade of mishaps or trigger events that leads, directly or indirectly, to the final undesired outcome (Potts et al., 1993). Usually, there is not a single, linear, cause-and-effect explanation for most events. Many high-risk interventions are accepted as usual and customary care, and there is a heavy reliance on biomedical technology. In addition, an unfavorable outcome is often not preventable or predictable. An analysis of iatrogenic events must include more than the outcome: It requires an analysis of the relationship and interaction among the patient; the illness; the complicated, highly technical healthcare system (with its diverse group of healthcare providers and support personnel); and the numerous healthcare industries that provide equipment, drugs, and supplies (Leape et al., 1991; Schiff, 1993).

IATROGENIC INFECTIONS

The incidence and severity of infections is greatest in the elderly. Older patients account for 38% of hospital patient days, yet they acquire 54% of nosocomial infections (Emori et al., 1991). Infections in nursing homes are a significant problem, with 5 to 10% of the residents acquiring an infection during a given month (Smith, 1988). The elderly are more susceptible to infections; although the mechanisms underlying this increased susceptibility are not known, multiple factors appear to be involved.

Predisposing Factors

Age. With aging, alterations in the structure and function of many tissues and organs diminish the older person's ability to respond to stressors such as infection. The immune system, skin, mucosa, and respiratory, gastrointestinal, and urinary tracts all change in ways that may predispose the elderly to infections.

Age-related changes in the immune system result in a decreased ability to resist bacterial, fungal, and viral infections and an increased risk of reactivating latent infections. In addition, the classic signs and symptoms of infection are frequently absent in the elderly. Often there is no fever or only a low-grade fever and little pain, and the presenting signs and symptoms are not specific enough to localize the site of infection (Crome & Bruce-Jones, 1992).

With age, specific antibody responses to foreign antigens are significantly impaired. The response to vaccines, for example, is diminished in older populations (Fagiolo et al., 1993; Powers, 1992). Studies of healthy older people show that host defenses appear the same or slightly diminished in comparison to younger people. Decreased immune response frequently accompanies chronic illness or malnutrition (Bradley, 1992).

The susceptibility to infections is increased as a result of age-related changes in the skin, which functions as an important barrier to microorganisms. Increased vulnerability to trauma and a slower rate of healing result from the thinning of the epidermis, a slowing of cell replacement in the stratum corneum, a loss of subcutaneous fat, and a diminished blood supply (Cerimele et al., 1990; Terpenning & Bradley, 1991). The susceptibility of older people to bacterial infections may also result from altered mucosal defense barriers. The mucosal surfaces may be more vulnerable to attachment and colonization by bacterial pathogens (Arranz et al., 1992).

Changes in the respiratory and gastrointestinal systems may predispose the elderly to infections. Elderly people have decreased ciliary action in the respiratory tree and a diminished cough reflex (Tockman, 1995). In the gastrointestinal tract, the stomach secretes less acid, motility slows (Altman, 1990), and the amount of immunoglobulin and antibody in the mucosal cells may be altered (Arranz et al., 1992).

Disease States. Disease states frequently seen in the elderly, such as diabetes, malignancies, and respiratory diseases, are associated with a high incidence of infections. An enlarged prostate is common in older men and predisposes them to urinary retention, treatment with genitourinary instrumentation, and urinary tract infection (UTI) (Krough et al., 1993). Immobility, incontinence, and dementia have been linked to increased rates of infection in elderly men and women (Jones, 1990).

Deficiencies in certain vitamins—notably, cyanabalamin, folate, and pyridoxine—have produced a decline in immunological responses (Ek et al., 1990). Other nutritional deficiencies, such as insufficient zinc, may also contribute to a diminished immunological response (Prasad et al., 1993).

Types of Infection

The hospitalized elderly frequently acquire the most devastating types of infections. The incidence of urinary tract infection, pneumonia, surgical wound infection, and bacteremia increases with age (Gingrich, 1990). Surveys have indicated that elderly people living in nursing homes have more urinary tract, respiratory tract, skin, and gastrointestinal tract infections than do their community-dwelling counterparts (Beck-Sague et al., 1993; Jones, 1990). Factors contributing to the problem of nosocomial infections include high staff turnover rates, high numbers of nonprofessional staff members, understaffing, minimal education of personnel in infection control, substandard practices, and inadequate facilities for isolation and handwashing.

Urinary Tract Infection. The urinary tract is the most common site of infection in the elderly, both in the community and in the hospital (Hooten, 1990). Nosocomial UTI occurs in 2 to 3% of hospitalized patients, and 80% of these infections are secondary to urinary catheterization (Griffith & Schell, 1987). UTI is the most common cause of bacteremia in hospitalized elderly patients, accounting for up to 50% of such infections (Cools, 1994). Other predisposing factors for UTI in the elderly are poor hygiene, urine stasis, bacterial growth, and decreased immune competence (Gleckman, 1992).

Pneumonia. Pneumonia is a major source of morbidity and mortality for the elderly. The clinical features of pneumonia are insidious, often leading to a delayed diagnosis of this illness in the elderly. Instead of the expected fever, cough, and pleuritic chest pain, pneumonia in the elderly presents as confusion or delirium, anorexia, lethargy, and deterioration of preexisting medical conditions such as congestive heart failure (Niederman, 1993). Breath sounds are diminished, and rales may be difficult to auscultate (Jones, 1990; Raju & Khan, 1988).

The most common cause of nosocomial pneumonia is the aspiration of bacteria-laden secretions from the oropharynx into the lungs. The causative organisms are most often enteric, gram-negative aerobic bacteria (Bates et al., 1992). These organisms colonize the oropharynx in frail elderly people who have diminished cough and glottic reflexes (Gingrich, 1990). Patients who are at the greatest risk for nosocomial pneumonia include those with incontinence; immobility; neurological impairments; debilitation from malignant, cardiac, and respiratory disease; and deteriorating or preterminal states (Beck-Sague et al., 1993).

Aspiration pneumonia occurs when drugs, anesthesia, or neurological conditions interfere with normal swallowing and protective mechanisms. It can also be caused by improper positioning during mealtimes or nasogastric feeding. Other factors contributing to pneumonia include poor technique during procedures such as tracheal intubation and suction, inadequate provision of fluids to thin bronchial secretions, prolonged bedrest, and neglect of deep-breathing exercises.

Methicillin-Resistant Staphylococcus aureus. Infections caused by methicillin-resistant *Staphylococcus aureus* (MRSA) have become a significant problem in hospitals and nursing homes. These organisms cause UTI, pneumonia, wound infections, and bacteremia and are difficult to treat because of a diminished response to almost all antibiotics. MRSA colonizes the skin and mucus membranes of affected hospitalized patients and is found in secretions from these areas. Patients colonized with MRSA are often bedridden with poor functional status, have feeding tubes or urinary catheters, and have pressure sores (Bradley, 1992). Only 3% of colonized patients become infected with the organism; patients with the highest risk of infection are diabetics and those who have received treatment with antibiotics (Inamatsu et al., 1992). MRSA is spread by person-to-person contact, usually on the hands of healthcare workers (MRSA Interagency Advisory Panel, 1993).

Vancomycin-Resistant Enterococcus. Another resistant organism that has recently emerged is the vancomycin-resistant *Enterococcus* (VRE) (Bartlett & Froggatt, 1995; Flournoy, 1994). This organism is multidrug resistant and may reflect selection of these organisms in the hospital environment by antibiotic use (Bates et al., 1994). Because VRE is most often cultured from the stool of infected patients, researchers believe that the intestinal tract harbors the VRE, which overgrows when normal intestinal flora are diminished by the antibiotics (Montecalvo et al., 1994). VRE most often causes bacteremia, UTIs, and wound infections (Frainow et al., 1994; Moreno et al., 1994; Swartz, 1994).

Risk factors for developing VRE infections are prolonged hospitalization, neutropenia, central line placement, staying in an intensive care unit, and treatment with broad-spectrum antibiotics (Gray et al., 1994; Spera & Farber, 1994; Swartz, 1994). VRE has been isolated from the hands of healthcare workers and from overbed trays, used linens, bedside stands, and bed rails in the rooms of infected patients (Yamaguchi et al., 1994).

Prevention

The prevention of infections is critical. In elderly patients, pneumonia may be prevented with an annual influenza vaccine as well as a one-time pneumococcal vaccine for patients at risk for respiratory infection (Govaert et al., 1994; Henschke, 1993; Quick et al., 1993). Adhering to infection-control principles—especially handwashing, universal precautions, and aseptic techniques—is important in preventing and controlling iatrogenic infections (Gingrich, 1990). The incidence of infection can be significantly reduced by identifying potential sources of infection, such as indwelling urinary catheters and prolonged immobility, and eliminating these practices whenever possible. Understanding the atypical presentation of infectious conditions in the elderly allows for their early recognition and prompt and appropriate treatment. Presentations in the elderly can include vague, nonspecific symptoms and changes in mental status, as opposed to more typical symptoms of fever, chills, and leukocytosis. Antibiotic therapy should be based on culture and sensitivity tests, and the overuse of antibiotics should be avoided. Although these suggested interventions are considered fundamental, they are all important in preventing infections.

IATROGENIC MALNUTRITION

Factors Leading to Iatrogenic Malnutrition

Malnutrition is a common complication seen in the elderly as a result of illness, hospitalization, or entry into the nursing home. Mion and colleagues (1994) estimated that 20 to 60% of hospitalized elderly patients and as many as 85% of nursing home patients have significant nutritional deficits. Other researchers have also found high levels of malnutrition in these populations (Cederholm & Hellstrom, 1992; Constans et al., 1992; Keller, 1993). Older people are especially at risk because they are often admitted in a compromised nutritional state (McWhirter & Pennington, 1994). Nutritional problems may result from multiple chronic conditions, limited mobility, loneliness, poor dentition, or poverty (Lehmann, 1989). Elderly patients who are marginally malnourished can quickly become deficient when physiologically stressed during illness or hospitalization. Malnutrition in hospitalized geriatric patients is associated with increased mortality rates for these patients (Lipschitz, 1997; Volkert et al., 1992).

During hospitalization, many factors can contribute to weight loss (Table 16–1). These include underlying physical or mental conditions, medical treatment, institutional policies, and environmental factors. Elderly patients often have many medical conditions in addition to their reason for hospitalization.

The treatment of medical conditions may lead to nutritional deficits. Medications can cause nausea and vomiting, dryness of mouth, or taste changes (Bell et al., 1993; Schiffman, 1993; Wujick, 1992). Polypharmacy is common in the elderly, and drugs may interfere or interact with nutrients or cause constipation, diarrhea, anorexia, or toxic reactions (Roe, 1994; Varma, 1994). Restricted diets, which are sometimes prescribed to treat diseases, can increase the risk of drug-induced side effects or can decrease appetite, as the patient cannot eat his or her favorite foods (Roe, 1994). Patients are frequently kept on nothing by mouth (NPO) treatment for days following surgery, receiving only saline or glucose intravenous solution. Often the increased metabolic needs of sick or injured patients are not recognized (Shikora & Blackburn, 1991), and care providers may fail to initiate early nutritional supplementation for those patients at risk for undernutrition (Roebothan & Chandra, 1994).

Dietary intake may decrease after admission to a hospital or nursing home because of poor food palatability; dietary restrictions; and a loss of control over food choices, mealtimes, and meal frequency (Buckler et al., 1994; Lipschitz, 1997). The food may not meet the cultural preferences of the older person. One study found that nursing home residents who became mal-

TABLE 16-1
Factors Leading to Iatrogenic Malnutrition

Medical conditions
  Stroke
  Cancer
  Infections
  Chronic airflow limitation (e.g., emphysema)
  Peptic ulcer disease
  Colitis
  Kidney and liver disease
  Mental impairment (e.g., Alzheimer's disease)

Illness-related factors
  Polypharmacy
  Pain
  Decreased mobility and activity
  Dysphagia
  Anorexia
  Dietary modifications and restrictions
  Poorly fitting dentures

Hospital or nursing home conditions
  Insufficient staff and time to provide needed assistance at mealtimes
  Unmet cultural or personal preferences in diet
  Change in usual mealtimes
  Absence of family members
  Packaging of food and utensils
  Unpleasant environment
  Lack of adaptive devices
  Lack of opportunity for oral hygiene, handwashing
  Lack of dentures, glasses, hearing aid
  Use of restraints
  Multiple activities resulting in fatigue
  Prolonged use of glucose and saline intravenous fluids
  Fasting for diagnostic tests and procedures
  Failure to recognize increased metabolic needs with illness or injury

Data from Buckler et al. (1994); Collinsworth (1991); Lipschitz (1997); Lugger (1994); Shikora & Blackburn (1991); and Zahler et al. (1993).

nourished consumed significantly smaller amounts of their meals than those who did not become malnourished (Thomas et al., 1991). Poor planning and scheduling of activities such as physical therapy and treatments may interfere with mealtimes or cause the older patient to be too tired to eat. Patients who are having diagnostic procedures may be kept NPO or miss meals because they are away from their rooms during mealtimes (Patterson, 1986).

Environmental factors that may affect food intake include serving food in containers that are difficult to open; the absence of family members to share mealtimes; and unpleasant sights, sounds, and odors in the institution. In addition, a lack of staff members to provide the necessary assistance with meals and insufficient time can contribute to malnutrition. This staffing problem especially applies to total care patients who may require 30 to 45 minutes of nursing time for feeding (Keller, 1993). Malnourished patients may require more help with eating than other patients and may become even more malnourished when they do not receive the necessary assistance (Thomas et al., 1991).

Prevention

The key to preventing malnutrition is recognizing those elderly who are at risk for nutritional problems during hospitalization (Volkert et al., 1992). Nurses working in collaboration with the dietitian and healthcare team have an important role in screening patients for these problems. They should conduct a careful assessment for prior nutritional problems and obtain a previous weight history. During hospitalization, accurate measurements of height, weight, and food and fluid intake are also important. An intake record should be obtained over a 3-day period to provide the most accurate information about dietary intake. An early identification of nutritional deficit or weight loss will allow early intervention.

If aged people are admitted to the hospital or nursing home in a malnourished state, they may benefit from supplementation initiated at the beginning of their hospital stay (Larsson et al., 1990). Those elderly patients who lose weight during hospitalization may benefit from supplements when the problem is noted. Patients who are experiencing medication side effects that may contribute to malnutrition should receive treatment to prevent these side effects or should be switched to a medication that is better tolerated (Kotzmann & Gisslinger, 1992).

Patients who need assistance with meals should be identified on admission so this assistance will be provided. A consultation from the occupational therapist may be necessary to provide the appropriate assistive devices, and

a dietary consultation may be requested to discuss food preferences and possible meal modifications. Mealtime assistance includes opening hard-to-open containers; cutting up food as needed; offering patients an opportunity to wash hands before meals; making sure that patients have their glasses, hearing aids, or dentures if needed; and allowing enough time for the meal to be consumed before the tray is taken away. Inservices to educate the staff about mealtime practices should be offered frequently.

Nurses can help patients by monitoring the schedule of diagnostic tests or procedures so as to minimize interference with mealtimes; offering snacks between meals to increase intake; and encouraging family members to be present at mealtimes to improve intake through socialization. Preventing and treating malnutrition in elderly patients who are hospitalized or in nursing homes is critical in preventing excess morbidity and mortality in this vulnerable population.

IATROGENIC INCONTINENCE

Causes

Incontinence may be attributed to the physical design of a hospital or other healthcare building and to the multiple practices carried out in these settings (Table 16–2). The building may have been poorly designed, with toilets shared by several patients, no toilet in areas of high activity, or inadequate or difficult-to-read signs for locating the toilets. Transportation from one test or appointment to another may not include

TABLE 16–2
Causes of Iatrogenic Incontinence

Unable to locate bathroom
Shared bathroom; bathroom not available when needed
Inaccessible urinal or commode
Delayed response to call light
No bathroom stop between tests, procedures, etc.
Restraints
Medications
Prolonged bedrest and inactivity

a bathroom stop. Restraints and tubing for oxygen and intravenous therapy are major barriers to getting to a bathroom. Other situations that may result in incontinence include a delayed response to patients using a call light to request assistance to the bathroom and a failure to provide urinals or commodes for older people with decreased mobility. In the home, hospital, or other setting, prescribed medications such as diuretics and laxatives may precipitate incontinence. If these medications are administered without consideration of the time of peak action, problems may occur during the night. Hypnotics or sedatives may make the older person too drowsy to be aware of toileting needs. Prolonged bed rest or inactivity and weakness from illness may prevent an older person from getting to the bathroom in time, and clothing that is difficult to remove may also contribute to incontinence.

Prevention

Incontinence caused by iatrogenic factors can be prevented or greatly reduced by recognizing the possible iatrogenic factors of incontinence and by taking measures to avoid poor practices. Orienting the patient to toilet facilities and assisting them promptly when called may reduce incontinence. Urinals and bedpans should be placed within reach of bedbound patients, and commode chairs should be made available to those who need them. Diuretics or laxatives should be given with consideration of when peak effect occurs so that patients can be near the bathroom and receive assistance if needed. Lastly, episodes of incontinence in the nursing home and hospital setting may be reduced by toileting patients with incontinence problems either according to their usual pattern, before and after mealtimes, or every 2 to 4 hours.

IATROGENIC ACCIDENTS AND INJURIES

Factors Contributing to Accidents and Injuries

The hospital or nursing home environment presents potential safety hazards for older peo-

ple, especially if they are more vulnerable to these hazards because of the effects of illness and treatment, including sedation, restricted mobility, and pain. Special attention to the environment can prevent or reduce iatrogenic accidents and possible injuries. Potential hazards for hospitalized older people are listed in Table 16–3.

Initially, an unfamiliar environment poses special problems. The first week of hospitalization has been identified as a time of high accident frequency for elderly hospitalized patients (Catchen, 1983). Things are not in their usual places, and maneuvering around a

TABLE 16-3
Potential Hazards

Floor

Slippery due to wax or spills

Light

Inadequate lighting
Glare

Corridors

Cluttered corridors
Human traffic

Equipment

Wheels not locked on wheelchairs, commode, bedside stand and table, and bed
Bed not in low position
Objects and obstacles
  Siderails
  Trapeze bar
  Tubing (nasogastric, oxygen, catheter, or intravenous)
  Cords
  Doors and dresser drawers left open
  Needles and instruments not disposed in proper containers
  Special equipment (e.g., intravenous poles)
Defective or broken equipment

Patient

Clothing
  Poorly fitting clothes or hospital gowns/robes
  Poorly fitting shoes or slippers
  Shoes or slippers not placed under bed, bedside stand, or in closet
Medications
  Sedatives and hypnotics
  Diuretics
  Antihypertensive agents

strange hospital environment may prove awkward, difficult, and hazardous. Elderly patients with musculoskeletal or cognitive impairments are particularly at risk for accidents. Medications such as sedatives, hypnotics, analgesics, and antihypertensive agents may cause sedation, orthostatic hypotension, decreased coordination, and instability in the elderly.

Prevention

Older patients at risk for accidents and possible injuries can be identified through a careful and systematic assessment that includes a consideration of causative factors, such as a history of falls, incontinence, and weakness. Providing a clean, safe environment requires the awareness and cooperation of all personnel to identify potentially dangerous situations and to intervene before an incident occurs. Patients should be oriented to their new surroundings and educated about equipment and special precautions necessitated by illness and treatment.

IATROGENIC DISTURBANCES OF THE SLEEP-WAKE CYCLE

The sleep-wake cycle is a complex process consisting of wakefulness, rapid eye movement (REM) sleep, and non–REM sleep (Bootzin et al., 1994; Feinsilver & Hertz, 1993). The cycle should be viewed on a 24-hour continuum in which the quality of sleep influences daytime functioning and vice versa. A consideration of this 24-hour continuum should be used in assessing and managing any problems related to the sleep-wake pattern (Ancoli-Israel & Kripke, 1991).

Factors Contributing to Alterations in the Sleep-Wake Pattern

Disturbances in sleep pattern and complaints related to sleep increase with age (Ancoli-Israel & Kripke, 1991; Pressman & Fry, 1988; Prinz et al., 1990). However, chronological age per se often does not correlate with the higher prevalence of sleep disturbances. The majority of healthy elderly people express satisfaction with their sleep (Evans & Rogers, 1994; Wauquier et al., 1992). In this population, evidence points to disease, late-life issues, and environmental factors as causes for the deterioration in sleep (Table 16–4). These conditions include nocturia, asthma, menopause, rheumatoid arthritis, cardiovascular symptoms, gastrointestinal illness, sleep apnea, nocturnal myoclonus (periodic leg movements in sleep), anxiety, dementia, depression, and fear of death in sleep (Ancoli-Israel & Kripke, 1991; Bliwise, 1993; Prinz et al., 1990; Satlin, 1994). The elderly are more sensitive than younger people to environmental stimuli such as noise, light, and temperature extremes. Recent studies have suggested that the timing and intensity of environmental light affect sleep. A lack of exposure to bright light during the day predisposes people to poor sleep (Ancoli-Israel et al., 1991; Bliwise,

---

TABLE 16-4

Causes of Disturbances in Sleep Patterns

Sleep pattern
   Disruption in usual sleep pattern
   Irregular schedule
   Extended time spent in bed

Illness
   Pain
   Respiratory disturbances
   Fatigue

Diet and drugs
   Hunger
   Sedatives and hypnotics
   Diuretics
   Alcohol
   Stimulants
      Caffeine—coffee, tea, chocolates, soft drinks
      Nicotine

Psychosocial factors
   Being institutionalized
   Anxiety, worry, tension
   Boredom, inactivity, monotony
   Isolation
   Changes in social patterns

Environmental factors
   Reduced exposure to daylight
   Lack of light or dark cues
   Excessive light and noise at night
   Room temperature too hot or too cold
   Uncomfortable bed or sleeping surface

1993; Prinz et al., 1990), and exposure to light has been found to help alleviate the problem (Campbell et al., 1993).

Adjustment to any change in the normal sleep-wake pattern takes longer in older people (Dement et al., 1982). Hospitalization or admission to a nursing home may impose a major disruption on an older person's normal sleep pattern and routine. In a study comparing the sleep patterns of hospitalized and non-hospitalized elderly people, Pacini and Fitzpatrick (1982) found that hospitalization quantitatively affected both nocturnal sleep time and sleep time during the day. Although care-related activities and the hospital environment caused some sleep problems, differences in the quality of sleep between hospitalized and nonhospitalized elderly people were most attributable to the patients' state of health, state of mind, and state of fatigue. Hospitalized patients were in a poorer state of health and had more worry, anxiety, tension, and fatigue than the nonhospitalized patients (Pacini and Fitzpatrick, 1982).

Clapin-French (1986) investigated sleep behavior in the elderly after their admission to a nursing home. The residents took more naps and had more sleep interruptions and slightly more difficulty in falling asleep. Ancoli-Israel and associates (1991) reported that nursing home residents had extremely fragmented sleep and were never asleep or awake for a full hour. This and other studies have reported that sleep difficulties can result from the following factors (Ancoli-Israel et al., 1991; Clapin-French, 1986; van Someren et al., 1993):

- Earlier bedtime
- Longer time in bed
- Proximity to others
- Nursing staff members giving medications and conducting other activities
- Timing of meals
- Limited time spent outdoors
- Lack of darkness at night

In both hospitals and nursing homes, sleep disturbances may result from the lack of usual social and environmental cues that distinguish day from night (Wooten, 1992). There is a higher level of noise, light, and activity during the normal hours of sleep. Older people experience a change in the usual and familiar daily routines, and they often have limited opportunity for social interaction and exercise, resulting in an increase in isolation, boredom, inactivity, and monotony. Medications, especially sedatives, hypnotics, and diuretics, interfere with the sleep-wake cycle. Inadequate attention to the relief of pain, cold, and hunger may also cause older people to experience poor sleep. Patients with dementia who are awakened during the night by nurses for various activities (e.g., a position change, toileting, or medications) suffer sleep fragmentation. This may result in increased agitation during the day and "sundowning" behavior in the late afternoon (Bliwise, 1994).

Prevention

Iatrogenic sleep disturbances can be minimized in elderly people who are hospitalized or in a nursing home. The sleep patterns of older people vary widely. Taking a detailed history and carefully assessing the 24-hour sleep-wake cycle will help direct and individualize nursing care. Iatrogenic sleep disturbances are best prevented through a consideration of age-related changes in sleep as well as the sleep problems secondary to illness and hospitalization (Vitello, 1997). Measures to improve and maintain sleep include the following:

- Providing a comfortable bed in a secure, quiet, darkened room
- Adjusting the room temperature for comfort
- Using additional blankets or putting socks on the feet to provide warmth
- Providing a gown or pajamas of the proper size and ensuring that the ties or other fasteners do not impede movement or cause discomfort
- Decreasing the amount of fluids taken after the evening meal
- Encouraging urination before going to bed
- Eliminating beverages containing alcohol or caffeine
- Providing a late evening snack
- Administering pain medication
- Carefully timing the administration of medications such as laxatives and diuretics

- Judiciously using sedatives and hypnotics

Careful explanations about tests, procedures, and the illness may also allay some worry and concern, improve the state of mind, and thereby improve the quality of sleep.

Older patients' circadian rhythms will be better maintained if attention is paid to providing social and environmental cues that indicate daytime or nighttime. Practices that may decrease the number of iatrogenic sleep disturbances experienced by nursing home residents include (1) providing clocks, regular mealtimes, and daytime activities with exposure to bright light; (2) discouraging patients from spending excessive time in bed or using the sleep environment for daytime activities; and (3) providing regular times for going to bed and getting up.

IATROGENIC DECLINE IN MOBILITY AND FUNCTION

As a result of their hospital experience, older people may be more debilitated, disabled, and dependent than is warranted by the primary illness. Functional disabilities increase with age and are experienced by a high proportion of the hospitalized and institutionalized older population (Guralnick & Simonsick, 1993). The delicate balance between independent functioning and dependence is further aggravated by hospital practices, such as keeping older patients on bedrest and inactive for an extended period and overlooking or delaying referral for physical rehabilitation. The deleterious effects of such practices include prolonged recovery with functional decline, reduced physiological reserve, and complications in many organ systems (Creditor, 1993; Hoenig & Rubenstein, 1991; Rousseau, 1993). Chapter 12 discusses the prevention and management of impaired mobility and deconditioning.

IATROGENIC PROBLEMS RELATED TO DRUGS

Drug-induced iatrogenesis is common among the elderly. Potential causes include age-related changes affecting pharmacokinetics and pharmacodynamics; inaccurate diagnosis; multiple health problems and polypharmacy, leading to medication errors, drug duplication, and drug reactions; changes in nutritional status resulting in drug-nutrient interactions; and poor communication between older adults and healthcare providers (Avorn & Gurwitz, 1997; Beers & Ouslander, 1989; Colley & Lucas, 1993; Cooper, 1994; Higbee, 1994). Chapter 26 presents a comprehensive discussion of drug-related problems in the elderly.

IATROGENIC EXCESS DISABILITY

Excess disability is defined as the failure of patients to perform cognitive and self-care tasks when they have the ability to do so (Kahn, 1965). Patients who exhibit this behavior often have self-care deficits that are incongruent with their medical diagnosis. The discrepancy between actual and potential function may be exhibited in many areas (Stone & Folks, 1992), including impairments in mobility, self-care, social relationships, family relationships, and performance of instrumental activities of daily living.

Factors Contributing to Excess Disability

Excess disability may be mitigated or exacerbated by depression, perceived locus of control, the constraints and expectations of the sick role, and learned helplessness. When combined with real helplessness from a physical impairment, these factors may create disability.

Depression. An important factor that may contribute to excess disability is depression (Reynolds, 1992). Elderly people who are depressed are more likely than others their age to perceive themselves as having a functional disability (Woo et al., 1994). There is also an indication that elderly people are more likely to be depressed than their younger counterparts. This might predispose them to developing *somatic depression*, in which their depression is manifest in physical symptoms and disability (Bleiker et al., 1993). The degree of disability is affected by the patient's support system, learned survival skills, and ability to adapt to new and demanding situations.

Locus of Control. This term encompasses the generalized expectations regarding who or what is responsible for any given outcome (Wallhagen et al., 1994). Those who perceive that they are able to regulate or direct situations are said to have an *internal locus of control.* In contrast, those who believe that external forces or authorities influence the course of their lives and the situations they find themselves in are said to have *external locus of control* (Lefcourt, 1976). People with an internal locus of control may feel that they play a role in maintaining and improving their health, whereas patients with an external locus of control may perceive others (i.e., medical personnel) as being responsible for their health. Recent studies, however, have raised questions about the relationship between locus of control and health. Researchers who interviewed elderly people about locus of control found that those who attributed negative outcomes to internal factors reported their health to be poorer than those who felt that external factors were more responsible for negative outcomes (Lachman, 1990).

The Sick Role. The role theory offers a plausible explanation for the presence of greater incapacity than is warranted by the severity of the disease. The *sick role* is defined as the extent to which a person perceives himself or herself to resemble a sick person with regard to worthiness, power, activity, and independence (Brown & Rawlinson, 1979). Elderly sick people are often socialized to the sick role by health professionals and family members who expect them to be dependent, inactive, and nonproductive for reasons of health or age (Slimmer et al., 1990).

There are times when the sick role is appropriate. Accepting the sick role enables the person to use the skills of others to achieve recovery. However, this role becomes disabling when the person is no longer clinically ill but remains dependent and relies on the aid and assistance of others. Patients who adopt the sick role may seek validation from their healthcare providers. Ohta and associates (1993) found that some elderly people experiencing

mental stress sought help from their physicians to alleviate physical symptoms rather than to relieve psychological symptoms. Patients with socioeconomic concerns are also more likely to perceive themselves as sicker and in need of help from their healthcare provider (Azzarto, 1993). When they accept the sick role, patients give up responsibility; as a result, the doctors and nurses gain more power, leaving patients feeling powerless.

Learned Helplessness. If patients repeatedly see themselves as powerless, they learn helplessness. The condition of helplessness develops in individuals who are exposed to uncontrollable events, who believe that they can do nothing to change the outcome of these events, and who develop the inappropriate expectation that the outcomes of these future events are beyond their control (Slimmer et al., 1990). Rather than engage in actions to change outcome, which they believe are futile, these patients simply give up. Elderly people most likely to develop learned helplessness are those who lack an influence over their own life, such as those with disability or who are dependent on others for care (Nystrom & Segesten, 1994). Often treated like children, these people have decisions made for them, which can reinforce feelings of powerlessness and helplessness.

Elderly patients who are passive and dependent are prone to depression, particularly in situations that are not likely to change (Baltes et al., 1994). Feelings of depression add to the patient's feelings of helplessness because depression is characterized by lack of motivation to try and change (de Figueiredo, 1993). Another component of learned helplessness is the patient's inability to make decisions, which forces family members or healthcare professionals to make decisions for them (Clements & Cummings, 1991).

Many nursing home residents suffer from learned helplessness. They live in environments in which personal choice is severely limited and routinized care is the norm. In a study on powerlessness in the nursing home, Nystrom and Segesten (1994) found that residents were expected to conform to the nursing home routine; those who did conform were rewarded with affection and privilege. Baltes and colleagues (1994) suggested another explanation for the inappropriate dependency of many nursing home residents: In their study, residents who acted dependent received more attention and social contact with staff members who cared for them than did the independent residents. Staff members in nursing homes often perform activities of daily living for the residents even when the resident can perform these tasks.

Prevention

Acute Care Settings. The level of dependency seen in hospitalized patients is a result of the acute illness or exacerbated chronic illness that led to their hospitalization as well as other preexisting conditions. Hospitalized patients need to be evaluated to determine what can be expected of them and to generate an individualized plan of care. Patients should be included in care planning as often as possible, especially to set goals that are important to them and to develop a timeline for accomplishing these goals. Nurses should keep in mind that their role is to do for the patients only what they cannot possibly do for themselves (Wilson, 1991).

Long-Term Care Settings. Residents in nursing homes are especially vulnerable to excess disability because of their physical and mental conditions and the nursing home environment. Residents have little choice over many aspects of their lives. They are frail and usually disabled, making it difficult for them to provide for their own needs. These conditions may lead to excessive disability as the residents perceive that nothing they do will change their situation. Staff members, however, can help to change these feelings of helplessness.

Certified nurse assistants, who provide most of the personal care for residents, sometimes provide this care in a manner that induces dependency. To prevent excess disability among nursing home residents, staff members should be encouraged to increase those behaviors that support independence and to decrease those behaviors that support dependence (Baltes et al., 1994). Emphasis should be given to treating residents politely and respectfully

and giving them a choice in how care is provided.

Staff members should speak to residents when delivering care so the residents will not feel that they are simply a source of work for their caregivers. Residents should be included in the care conference and be allowed to ventilate their own concerns about the care they receive. If these recommendations are followed, elderly people who live in long-term care facilities will remain as independent as possible.

SUMMARY

Iatrogenic complications cause distress for all people involved. They incur costs in both economic and human terms. For older people, iatrogenic complications may mean increased discomfort; the addition of another illness, injury, or disability; a prolonged recovery period; hospitalization or institutionalization; or even death. For healthcare professionals, questions arise about errors, misjudgment, or a lack of knowledge and skill.

The prevention of iatrogenesis is foremost in the provision of care for the elderly. Measures should be taken to reduce practices and events that are known to cause iatrogenic conditions. For older patients, such measures include setting accurate and realistic goals based on the initial and ongoing assessment of functional status as well as considering the risk-benefit ratio of a proposed approach to care. Caregivers can decrease the risk of iatrogenesis by increasing their knowledge and understanding of the circumstances that may impact negatively on the outcomes of care. It is critical that healthcare providers continuously review and analyze their practice to prevent the occurrence of iatrogenic complications.

REFERENCES

Altman, D. F. (1990). Changes in gastrointestinal, pancreatic, biliary, and hepatic function with aging. *Gastroenterology Clinics of North America, 19,* 227–234.

Ancoli-Israel, S., & Kripke, D. F. (1991). Prevalent sleep problems in the aged. *Biofeedback and Self-Regulation, 16,* 349–359.

Ancoli-Israel, S., Kripke, D. F., Jones, D. W., et al. (1991).

24-hour sleep and light rhythms in nursing home patients. *Sleep Research, 20A*, 410.

Arranz, E., O'Mahony, S., Baron, J. R., & Feguson, A. (1992). Immunosenescence and mucosal immunity: Significant effects of old age on secretory IgA concentrations and intraepithelial lymphocyte counts. *Gut, 33*, 882–886.

Avorn, J., & Gurwitz, J. (1997). Principles of pharmacology. In C. K. Cassel, H. J. Cohen, E. B. Larson et al. (Eds.), *Geriatric medicine* (3rd ed., pp. 55–70). New York: Springer-Verlag.

Azzarto, J. (1993). The socioemotional needs of elderly family practice patients: Can social workers help? *Health and Social Work, 18*, 40–48.

Baltes, M. M., Neumann, E. M., & Zank, S. (1994). Maintenance and rehabilitation of independence in old age: An intervention program for staff. *Psychology and Aging, 9*, 179–188.

Bartlett, J. G., & Froggatt, J. W. (1995). Antibiotic resistance. *Archives of Otolaryngology—Head and Neck Surgery, 121*, 392–396.

Bates, J. H., Campbell, G. D., & Barron, A. L. (1992). Microbial etiology of acute pneumonia in hospitalized patients. *Chest, 101*, 1005–1012.

Bates, J., Jorden, J. Z., & Griffiths, D. T. (1994). Farm animals as a putative reservoir for vancomycin-resistant enterococcal infection in man. *Journal of Antimicrobial Chemotherapy, 34*, 507–514.

Beck-Sague, C., Banerjee, S., & Jarvis, W. R. (1993). Infectious diseases and mortality among U.S. nursing home residents. *American Journal of Public Health, 83*, 1739–1742.

Beers, M. H., & Ouslander, J. G. (1989). Risk factors in geriatric drug prescribing: A practical guide to avoiding problems. *Drugs, 37*, 105–112.

Bell, G., Powell, K., Burridge, L., et al. (1993). Helibacter pylori eradication: Efficacy and side effect profile of a combination of omeprazole, amoxycillin and metronidazole compared with four alternative regimes. *Quarterly Journal of Medicine, 86*, 743–750.

Bleiker, E. M., van Der Ploeg, H. M., Mook, J., & Kleijn, W. C. (1993). Anxiety, anger and depression in elderly women. *Psychological Reports, 72*, 567–574.

Bliwise, D. L. (1994). What is sundowning? *Journal of the American Geriatrics Society, 42*, 1009–1011.

Bliwise, D. L. (1993). Sleep in normal aging and dementia. *Sleep, 16*, 40–81.

Bootzin, R. R., Lahmeyer, H., & Lillie, J. K. (1994). *Integrated approach to sleep management.* Belle Mead, MD: Calners Healthcare Communications.

Bradley, S. F. (1992). Methicillin-resistant *Staphlococcus aureus* infection. *Clinics in Geriatric Medicine, 8*, 853–868.

Brennan, T. A., Leape, L. L., Laird, N. M., et al. (1991). Incidence of adverse events and negligence in hospitalized patients. Results of the Harvard Medical Practice Study I. *New England Journal of Medicine, 324*(6), 370–376.

Brown, J. S., & Rawlinson, M. E. (1979). Sick role acceptance measure. In *Psychological instruments, vol. 1* (pp. 212–215). New York: American Psychological Association.

Buckler, D. A., Kelber, S. T., & Goodwin, J. S. (1994). The use of dietary restrictions in malnourished nursing home patients. *Journal of the American Geriatrics Society, 42*, 1100–1102.

Campbell, S. S., Dawson, D., & Anderson, M. W. (1993). Alleviation of sleep maintenance insomnia with timed exposure to bright light. *Journal of the American Geriatrics Society, 41*, 829–836.

Catchen, H. (1983). Repeaters: Inpatient accidents among hospitalized elderly. *Gerontologist, 23*, 273–276.

Cederholm, T., & Hellstrom, K. (1992). Nutritional status in recently hospitalized and free-living elderly subjects. *Gerontology, 38*, 105–110.

Cerimele, D., Celleno, L., & Serri, F. (1990). Physiological changes in ageing skin. *British Journal of Dermatology, 53*, 13–20.

Clapin-French, E. (1986). Sleep patterns of aged persons in long-term care facilities. *Journal of Advanced Nursing, 11*(1), 57–66.

Clements, S., & Cummings, S. (1991). Helplessness and powerlessness: Caring for clients in pain. *Holistic Nursing Practice, 6*, 76–85.

Colley, C. A., & Lucas, L. M. (1993). Polypharmacy: The treatment becomes the disease. *Journal of General Internal Medicine, 8*, 278–283.

Collinsworth, R. (1991). Determining nutritional status of the elderly surgical patient: Steps on the assessment process. *American Operating Room Nurses Journal, 54*, 622–631.

Constans, T., Baeq, Y., Brechot, J. F., et al. (1992). Protein-energy malnutrition in elderly medical patients. *Journal of the American Geriatrics Society, 40*, 263–268.

Cools, H. J. (1994). Twelve-year-old infection policy in a nursing home. *Nederlands Tijdschriftr voor Geneeskunde, 138*, 184–188.

Cooper, J. W. (1994). Drug-related problems in the elderly patient. *Generations, 18*(2), 19–27.

Creditor, M. C. (1993). Hazards of hospitalization of the elderly. *American College of Physicians, 118*, 119–223.

Crome, P., & Bruce-Jones, P. (1992). Infection in the elderly: Studies with lomefloxacin. *American Journal of Medicine, 92*(4A), 126S–129S.

de Figueiredo, J. M. (1993). Depression and demoralization: Phenomenologic differences and research perspectives. *Comprehensive Psychiatry, 34*, 308–311.

Dement, W. C., Miles, L. E., & Carskadon, M. A. (1982). "White paper" on sleep and aging. *Journal of the American Geriatrics Society, 30*, 25–50.

Ek, A., Larson, J., von Scheneck, H., et al. (1990). The correlation between anergy, malnutrition and clinical outcome in an elderly hospital population. *Clinical Nutrition, 9*, 185–189.

Emori, T., Banerjee, S. N., Culver, D. H., et al. (1991). Nosocomial infections in elderly patients in the United States, 1986–1990. National Nosocomial Infections Surveillance System. *American Journal of Medicine, 91*, 289S–293S.

Evans, B. D., & Rogers, A. E. (1994). 24-hour sleep/wake patterns in healthy elderly persons. *Applied Nursing Research, 7*(2), 75–83.

Fagiolo, U., Amadori, A., Cozzi, E., et al. (1993). Humoral and cellular immune reponse to influenza virus vaccination in aged humans. *Aging, 5*, 451–458.

Feinsilver, S. H., & Hertz, G. (1993). Sleep in the elderly patient. *Clinics in Chest Medicine, 14*, 405–411.

Flournoy, D. J. (1994). Antimicrobial susceptibilities of bacteria from nursing home residents in Oklahoma. *Gerontology, 40*, 53–56.

Frainow, H. S., Jungkind, D. L., Lander, D. W., et al. (1994). Urinary tract infection with an *Enterococcus faecalis* isolate that requires vancomycin for growth. *Annals of Internal Medicine, 121*, 22–26.

Gingrich, D. (1990). Infections in the hospitalized elderly. *Hospital Physician, 26*, 35–38.

Gleckman, R. A. (1992). Urinary tract infection. *Clinics in Geriatric Medicine, 8*, 793–803.

Gorbien, M. J., Bishop, J., Beers, M. H., et al. (1992). Iatrogenic illness in hospitalized elderly people. *Journal of the American Geriatrics Society, 40*, 1031–1042.

Govaert, T. M., Thijs, C. T., Masurel, N., et al. (1994). The efficacy of influenza vaccination in the elderly. A randomized double-blind placebo-controlled trial. *Journal of the American Medical Association, 272*, 1661–1700.

Gray, J., Marsh, P. J, Stewart, D., & Pedler, S. J. (1994). Enterococcal bacteremia: A prospective study of 125 episodes. *Journal of Hospital Infection, 27*, 179–186.

Griffith, M. C., & Schell, R. E. (1987). Nosocomial infections. *American Family Physician, 35*, 179–186.

Guralnik, J. M., & Simonsick, E. M. (1993). Physical disability in older Americans. *Journals of Gerontology, 48*(special issue), 3–10.

Gurwitz, J. H., Sanchez-Cross, M. T., Eckler, M. A., & Matulis, J. (1994). The epidemiology of adverse and unexpected events in the long-term care setting. *Journal of the American Geriatrics Society 42*(1), 33–38.

Henschke, P. J. (1993). Infections in the elderly. *Medical Journal of Australia, 58*, 830–834.

Higbee, M. D. (1994). Consumer guidelines for using medications wisely. *Generations, 17*(2), 43–47.

Hoenig, H. M., & Rubenstein, L. Z. (1991). Hospital-associated deconditioning and dysfunction. *Journal of the American Geriatrics Society, 39*, 220–222.

Hooten, T. (1990). The epidemiology of urinary tract infection. *Infection, 18*(suppl. 2), S40–S45.

Inamatsu, T., Ooshima, H., Masuda, Y., et al. (1992). Clinical spectrum of antibiotic-associated enterocolitis due to methicillin-resistant *Staphylococcus aureus. Japanese Journal of Clinical Medicine, 50*, 1087–1092.

Jones, S. R. (1990). Infections in frail and vulnerable elderly patients. *American Journal of Medicine, 88*(3C), 30S–33S.

Kahn, R. S. (1965). *Proceedings of the York House Institute on the mentally impaired aged.* Philadelphia: Philadelphia Geriatric Center.

Keller, H. H. (1993). Malnutrition in institutionalized elderly: How and why? *Journal of the American Geriatrics Society, 41*, 1212–1218.

Kotzmann, H., & Gisslinger, H. (1992). Treatment and prophylaxis of chemotherapy-induced gastrointestinal complaints. *Scandinavian Journal of Gastroenterology, 27*(suppl. 191), 12–15.

Krough, J., Jensen, J., Iversen, H. G., & Andersen, J. T. (1993). Age as a prognostic variable in patients undergoing transurethral prostatectomy. *Scandinavian Journal of Urology and Nephrology, 27*, 225–229.

Lachman, M. E. (1990). When bad things happen to older people: Age differences in attributional style. *Psychology and Aging, 5*, 617–619.

Larsson, J., Unosson, M., Ek, A. C., et al. (1990). Effect of dietary supplement on nutritional status and clinical outcome in 510 geriatric patients—A randomized study. *Clinical Nutrition, 9*, 179–184.

Leape, L. L., Brennan, T. A., Laird, N., et al. (1991). The nature of adverse events in hospitalized patients. *New England Journal of Medicine, 324*(6), 377–384.

Lefcourt, H. (1976). *Locus of control: Current trends in theory and research.* New York: John Wiley & Sons.

Lefevre, F., Feinglass, J., Potts, S., et al. (1992). Iatrogenic complications in high-risk elderly patients. *Archives of Internal Medicine, 152*, 2074–2080.

Lehmann, A. (1989). Review: Undernutrition in elderly people. *Age and Ageing, 18*, 339–353.

Lipschitz, D. A. (1997). Nutrition. In C. K. Cassel, H. J. Cohen, E. B. Larson et al. (Eds.), *Geriatric medicine* (3rd ed., pp. 801–813). New York: Springer-Verlag.

Lugger, K. E. (1994). Dysphagia in the elderly stroke patient. *Journal of Neuroscience Nursing, 26*, 78–84.

McWhirter, J., & Pennington, C. (1994). Incidence and recognition of malnutrition in hospital. *British Medical Journal, 308*, 945–948.

Mion, L., McDowell, J., & Heaney, L. (1994). Nutritional assessment of the elderly in the ambulatory care setting. *Nurse Practitioner Forum, 5*, 46–51.

Montecalvo, M. A., Horowitz, H., Gedris, C., et al. (1994). Outbreak of vancomycin-, ampicillin-, and aminoglycoside-resistant *Enterococcus faecium* bacteremia in an adult oncology unit. *Antimicrobial Agents and Chemotherapy, 38*, 1363–1367.

Moreno, F., Jorgensen, J., & Weiner, M. (1994). An old antibiotic for a new multiple-resistant *Enterococcus faecium? Diagnostic Microbiology and Infectious Disease, 20*, 41–43.

MRSA Interagency Advisory Committee in conjunction with the Connecticut Department of Public Health and Addiction Services (1993). Guidelines for management of patients with methicillin-resistant *Staphylococcus aureus* in acute care hospitals and long-term care facilities. *Connecticut Medicine, 57*, 611–617.

Niederman, M. S. (1993). Nosocomial pneumonia in the elderly patient. *Clinics in Chest Medicine, 3*, 479–490.

Nystrom, A. E., & Segesten, K. M. (1994). On sources of powerlessness in nursing home life. *Journal of Advanced Nursing, 19*, 124–133.

Ohta, Y., Tsukahara, M., Sugaski, H., et al. (1993). Mental and physical health of middle-aged and elderly women and psychosocial factors. *Japanese Journal of Psychiatry and Neurology, 47*, 735–742.

Pacini, C. M., & Fitzpatrick, J. J. (1982). Sleep patterns of hospitalized and nonhospitalized aged individuals. *Journal of Gerontological Nursing, 8*, 327–332.

Patterson, C. (1986). Iatrogenic disease in late life. *Clinics of Geriatric Medicine, 2*, 121–137.

Potts, S., Feinglass, J., Lefevere, F., et al. (1993). A quality-of-care analysis of cascade iatrogenesis in frail elderly. *Quality Review Bulletin, 19*(6), 199–205.

Powers, C. C. (1992). Immunological principles and emerging strategies for the elderly. *Journal of the American Geriatrics Society, 40*, 81–94.

Prasad, A. S., Fitzgerald, J., Hess, J., et al. (1993). Zinc deficiency in elderly patients. *Nutrition, 9*, 218–224.

Pressman, M., & Fry, J. (1988). What is normal sleep in the elderly? *Clinics in Geriatric Medicine, 4*(1), 71–81.

Prinz, P. N., Vitiello, M. V., Raskind, M. A., & Thorpy, M. J. (1990). Geriatrics: Sleep disorders and aging. *New England Journal of Medicine, 323*(8), 521–526.

Quick, R. E., Hoge, C. W., Hamilton, D. J., et al. (1993). Under-utilization of pneumococcal vaccine in nursing home in Washington state: Report of a serotype-specific outbreak and a survey. *American Journal of Medicine, 92,* 149–152.

Raju, L., & Khan, F. (1988). Pneumonia in the elderly: A review. *Geriatrics, 43*(10), 51–56, 59–62.

Reynolds, C. F. (1992). Treatment of depression in special populations. *Journal of Clinical Psychiatry, 53*(suppl.), 45–53.

Roe, D. A. (1994). Medications and nutrition in the elderly. *Primary Care: Clinics in Office Practice, 21,* 135–147.

Roebothan, B., & Chandra, R. (1994). Relationship between nutritional status and immune function of elderly people. *Age and Ageing, 23,* 49–53.

Rousseau, P. (1993). Immobility in the aged. *Archives of Family Medicine, 2*(2), 167–177.

Rubins, H. A., & Moskowitz, M. A. (1990). Complications of care in a medical intensive care unit. *Journal of General Internal Medicine, 5,* 104–109.

Satlin, A. (1994). Sleep disorders in dementia. *Psychiatric Annals, 24*(4), 186–191.

Schiff, G. (1993). Casade or facade: Focusing or obfuscating the pathogenesis of iatrogenesis? [editorial comment]. *Quality Review Bulletin, 19*(6), 196–198.

Schiffman, S. S. (1993). Perception of taste and smell in elderly persons. *Critical Reviews in Food Science and Nutrition, 33,* 17–26.

Shikora, S., & Blackburn, G. (1991). Nutritional consequences of major surgery. *Surgical Clinics of North America, 71,* 509–521.

Slimmer, L., Edwards-Beckett, J., LeSage, J., et al. (1990). Helping those who don't help themselves. *Geriatric Nursing, 11,* 20–22.

Smith, P. W. (1988). Infections in extended care facilities: Prevalence, problems and prevention. *Asepsis, 10,* 2–5.

Spera, R. V., & Farber, B. F. (1994). Multidrug-resistant *Enterococcus faecium.* An untreatable nosocomial pathogen. *Drugs, 48,* 678–688.

Stone, T., & Folks, D. G. (1992). Somatization in the elderly. *Psychiatric Medicine, 10,* 25–32.

Swartz, M. N. (1994). Hospital-acquired infections: Diseases with increasing limited therapies. *Proceedings of the National Academy of Sciences of the United States of America, 91,* 2420–2427.

Terpenning, M. S., & Bradley, S. F. (1991). Why aging leads to increased susceptibility to infections. *Geriatrics, 46,* 77–80.

Thomas, D., Verdery, R., Gardener, L. A., et al. (1991). A prospective study of outcome from protein-energy malnutrition in nursing home residents. *Journal of Parenteral and Enteral Nutrition, 15,* 400–404.

Tockman, M. S. (1995). The effects of age on the lung. In W. B. Abrams, M. H. Beers & R. Berkow (Eds.), *The Merck manual of geriatrics* (2nd ed., pp. 569–574). Whitehouse Station, NJ: Merck & Co., Inc.

van Someren, E. J., Mirmiran, M., & Swaab, D. F. (1993). Non-pharmacological treatment of sleep and wake disturbances in aging and Alzheimer's disease: Chronobiological perspectives. *Behavioral Brain Research, 57,* 235–253.

Varma, R. N. (1994). Risk for drug-induced malnutrition is unchecked in elderly patients in nursing homes. *Journal of the American Dietetic Association, 94,* 192–194.

Vitello, M. V. (1997). Sleep disorders and aging: Understanding the causes. *Journal of Gerontology: Medical Sciences, 52A,* M189–M191.

Volkert, D., Kruse, W., Oster, P., & Schlierf, G. (1992). Malnutrition in geriatric patients: Diagnostic and prognostic significance and nutritional parameters. *Annals of Nutrition and Metabolism, 36,* 97–112.

Wallhagen, M. I., Strawbridge, W. J., Kaplan, G. A., & Cohen, R. D. (1994). Impact of internal health locus of control on health outcomes for older men and women: A longitudinal perspective. *Gerontologist, 3,* 299–306.

Wauquier, A., van Sweden, B., Laggay, A. M., et al. (1992). Ambulatory monitoring of sleep-wakefulness patterns in healthy elderly males and females (>88 years): The "senieur" protocol. *Journal of the American Geriatrics Society, 40,* 109–114.

Wilson, J. S. (1991). Helplessness need not be a dirty word. *Home Healthcare Nurse, 9,* 47–48.

Woo, J., Ho, S. C., Lau, J., et al. (1994). The prevalence of depressive symptoms and predisposing factors in an elderly Chinese population. *Acta Psychiatrica Scandinavica, 89,* 8–14.

Wooten, V. (1992). Sleep disorders in geriatric patients. *Clinics in Geriatric Medicine, 8*(2), 427–439.

Wujick, D. (1992). Current research in side effects of high dose chemotherapy. *Seminars in Oncology Nursing, 8,* 102–112.

Yamaguchi, E., Valena, F., Smith, S. M., et al. (1994). Colonization pattern of vancomycin-resistant *Enterococcus faecium. American Journal of Infection Control, 22,* 202–206.

Zahler, L., Holdt, C., Gates, G., & Keiser, A. (1993). Nutritional care of ambulatory residents in special care units for Alzheimer's patients. *Journal of Nutrition for the Elderly, 12,* 5–19.

Nursing Management of Selected Illnesses

Depression

Kathleen C. Buckwalter
Mary Lynn Scotton Piven

Depression is one of the most common—and most treatable—of all mental disorders in older adults. It is a major health concern in this population and can be life threatening if unrecognized and untreated. Biological, psychological, and social changes place older adults at high risk for the development or recurrence of depression. Central nervous system (CNS) changes associated with normal aging, for example, may increase the risk for depression, and adjustments in lifestyle such as retirement, reduced income, or a decline in physical health can be stressful and have a negative impact on the older adult.

Although the National Institutes of Health (NIH) Consensus Development Panel on Depression in Late Life noted that "significant progress has been made in understanding the diagnosis, treatment, and design of systems for providing service for depression in late life," it also stated that many important questions remain unanswered (1992, p. 1018). Unfortunately, geropsychiatric disorders are still often misdiagnosed, mistreated, or simply overlooked, leading to high comorbidity, increased healthcare costs, unnecessary suffering, and diminished quality of life (Buckwalter, 1992). In addition, untreated depression may result in premature institutionalization or suicide; depression may not be recognized and appropriately treated because the signs and symptoms of depression in the elderly are different from those in the young (Gomez & Gomez, 1993).

Depression is among the mental disorders most commonly seen and treated by advanced-practice gerontological nurses. This chapter begins with an overview of the classification, prevalence, etiology, risk factors, and differential diagnosis of depression in later life. This is followed by a description of approaches to the assessment and management of depressive disorders, including research-based nursing interventions.

CLASSIFICATION AND PREVALENCE OF DEPRESSION

Definition

The term *depression* is used to describe many things, including a mood state, a disease, a syndrome, and a symptom (Buschmann & Rossen, 1993). For many years, controversy surrounded how to best classify depression. This controversy has continued in the psychiatric community through several editions of the American Psychiatric Association's (APA's) *Diagnostic and Statistical Manual of Mental Disorders* (DSM) since its first publication in the early 1950s (Kurlowicz, 1994).

As defined by the National Institutes of Health (NIH) Consensus Development Panel on Depression in Late Life, *depression* is used in a broad sense to describe "a syndrome that includes a constellation of physiological, affective, and cognitive manifestations" (1992, p. 1019). Current criteria provide a categorical approach to the diagnosis of mental disorders that is largely atheoretical (APA, 1994). The nomenclature includes several categories of depressive episodes and disorders under the category Mood Disorders, such as major depressive disorder, depressive disorder not otherwise specified, dysthymic disorder, bipolar I and II disorders, cyclothymic disorder, mood disorder due to a general medical condition, substance-induced mood disorder, and bipolar and mood disorders not otherwise specified (Table 17–1 lists the DSM-IV criteria). These

---

TABLE 17-1
DSM-IV Criteria for Major Depressive Episode

A. Five (or more) of the following symptoms have been present during the same 2-week period and represent a change from previous functioning; at least one of the symptoms is either (1) depressed mood or (2) loss of interest and pleasure.
Note: Do not include symptoms that are clearly due to a general medical condition, or mood-incongruent delusions or hallucinations.
  1. Depressed mood most of the day, nearly every day, as indicated by either subjective report or observation
  2. Markedly diminished interest or pleasure in all, or almost all, activities most of the day, nearly every day
  3. Significant weight loss when not dieting or weight gain (e.g., a change of more than 5% of body weight in a month) or increase or decrease in appetite nearly every day
  4. Insomnia or hypersomnia nearly every day
  5. Psychomotor agitation or retardation nearly every day
  6. Fatigue or loss of energy nearly every day
  7. Feelings of worthlessness or excessive or inappropriate guilt nearly every day (not merely self-reproach or guilt about being sick)
  8. Diminished ability to think or concentrate, or indecisiveness, nearly every day
  9. Recurrent thoughts of death, recurrent suicidal ideation without a specific plan, or a suicide attempt or a specific plan for committing suicide
B. The symptoms do not meet criteria for a Mixed Episode.
C. The symptoms cause clinically significant distress or impairment in social, occupational, or other important areas of functioning.
D. The symptoms are not due to the direct physiological effects of a substance (e.g., drug or alcohol abuse, medications) or a general medical condition.
E. The symptoms are not better accounted for by Bereavement.

Adapted from American Psychiatric Association (1994). *Diagnostic and statistical manual of mental disorders* (4th ed., p. 327). Washington, D.C.: American Psychiatric Association.

diagnostic categories differ in terms of onset, precipitating factors, symptoms, severity, and duration.

When empirical criteria such as those described in the DSM-IV are employed, depressive disorders are detected in the elderly population that have the same features and respond to the same interventions as depression in younger people. However, controversy exists over whether the symptomatic presentation of major depression in older adults is similar to that in other stages of life (Kurlowicz, 1994). Further, although impairment in social, occupational, or other vital areas of functioning is required to establish the diagnosis of depression, functional status remains largely ignored and is seldom measured in clinical practice.

Epidemiology

Findings from epidemiological studies vary considerably. Survey data from the Epidemiologic Catchment Area Project indicate that major depression is not more prevalent among the elderly than in other adults, with a 0.7% 1-month prevalence rate of major depressive disorder in people older than age 65 years (Myers et al., 1984). Other studies suggest that 15 to 25% of community-dwelling older adults suffer from depressive symptoms or emotional distress that adversely affect their quality of life (Blazer et al., 1987; NIH, 1992). The low rates of depression found in some studies likely reflect widespread but relatively mild (e.g., subsyndromal) symptoms of depression that fail to meet DSM-IV or research diagnostic criteria. Blazer (1991) has presented a strong case for minor depression as an important clinical entity that may resolve some of the epidemiological and diagnostic dilemmas currently surrounding late-life depression.

The prevalence of depression is thought to increase dramatically for those elderly people who are hospitalized for treatment of acute illness or who reside in institutions (Keilholz et al., 1989). Borson and colleagues (1986) reported a 24% prevalence rate of significant depressive symptoms in a primary care setting, with 10% of those identified as suffering from major depressive disorders. Similarly, major

depressive disorder in elderly patients hospitalized with a medical illness was estimated at 12 to 16%, with 20 to 30% suffering from depressive symptoms below the threshold of a syndromic diagnosis (Kitchell et al., 1982).

In a prospective study analyzing prevalence rates of major depressive disorders and depressive symptoms and their relationship to mortality, Rovner and colleagues (1991) confirmed that major depressive disorder in nursing home patients is a risk factor for mortality. Other significant predictors were poor scores on activity of daily living scales, male gender, and hospitalization within the previous year.

Symptoms

Depression can color every aspect of an elderly person's life. Most commonly, it is observed as changes in mood; disturbances in perceptions of oneself, the environment, and the future; and vegetative physical and behavioral signs. These three categories of symptoms are often referred to as the *depressive triad* (Table 17–2). As is the case throughout the lifespan, major depression in later life is characterized by remissions and exacerbations, with women affected more than men. The elderly differ from younger people with depression in that they are less likely to report feelings of worthlessness and guilt and are more prone to weight loss (Blazer, 1989). Approximately one third of those elders who recover from a depressive episode are expected to relapse within 1 year. The presence of a concurrent physical illness is a poor prognostic indicator, whereas a strong social support network suggests a more favorable outcome in late-life depression.

Types of Depression

Older adults suffer from varied types of depression, including primary depressions that occur for the first time in later life, recurring depressive episodes with onset earlier in life, dysthymia, bipolar affective disorders, and secondary depressions related to physical illnesses or the side effects of drugs (Table 17–3). The most common mood disorders listed in the

TABLE 17-2
The Depressive Triad

Symptoms	Behavioral Signs
Pervasive disturbance of mood	Sadness, discouragement Crying Anxiety, panic attacks Brooding Irritability Feeling sad, blue, depressed, low, down in the dumps; nothing is fun Paranoid
Disturbances in perception of self, environment, future	Withdrawal from usual activities Decreased sex drive Inability to express pleasure Feelings of worthlessness Unreasonable fears Self-reproach for minor failings Delusions of poverty Hallucinations (of short duration) Critical of self and others Passive
Vegetative	Increased or decreased body movements Pacing, wringing hands, pulling or rubbing hair, body, clothing Difficulty getting to sleep, staying awake, waking early Decreased or sometimes increased appetite Weight loss or sometimes gain Fatigue Preoccupation with physical health, especially fear of cancer Inability to concentrate, think, or make decisions Slowed speech, pauses before answering, decreased amount of speech, low or monotonous speech Thoughts of death Suicide or suicide attempts Constipation Tachycardia

From Smith, M., Buckwalter, K. C., & Mitchell, S. (1993). *Geriatric mental health training series.* New York: Springer. Copyright by K. C. Buckwalter.

DSM-IV (1994, pp. 317–319) of older adults are presented.

Major Depressive Disorder. This is characterized by one or more major depressive episodes (criteria listed in Table 17–1).

Dysthymic Disorder. This is characterized by at least 2 years of depressed mood for more days than not, accompanied by additional de-

pressive symptoms that do not meet the criteria for a major depressive episode. Older people with dysthymia usually have a long history of problems coping with life circumstances. In the hospitalized elderly, major depressive disorders are often superimposed on dysthymia (Koenig et al., 1988).

Bipolar Disorders. Bipolar I disorder is characterized by one or more manic or mixed episodes, usually accompanied by major depressive episodes. Bipolar II disorder is characterized by one or more major depressive episodes, accompanied by at least one hypomanic episode. The onset of bipolar disorders in old age is unusual, and these disorders are more likely to have occurred much earlier in life.

Mood Disorder Due to a General Medical Condition. This is characterized by a promi-

TABLE 17-3
Drugs and Physical Disorders Associated with Depression

Drugs Associated with Depression

Analgesics and anti-inflammatory agents
Antibiotics
Anticonvulsants
Antihistamines
Antihypertensives
Anti-Parkinsonian drugs
Cardiac drugs
Chemotherapeutic drugs
Hormones, especially steroids
Immunosuppressives
Sedatives and tranquilizers

Physical Disorders Associated with Depression

Cushing's syndrome
Hypothyroidism or hyperthyroidism
Hyperparathyroidism
Addison's disease
Cerebral tumors
Viral or other chronic infections
Stroke
Parkinson's disease
Pancreatic carcinoma
Vitamin B_{12} and folate deficiencies
Uremia

Adapted from American Geriatrics Society (1993). *Geriatric health care: A visual presentation and lecture guide* (p. 25). New York: American Geriatrics Society. Copyright by American Geriatrics Society.

nent and persistent disturbance in mood that is judged to be a direct physiological consequence of a general medical condition (see Table 17–3).

Substance-Induced Mood Disorder. This disorder is characterized by a prominent and persistent disturbance in mood that is judged to be a direct physiological consequence of a drug of abuse, a medication (see Table 17–3), another somatic treatment for depression, or toxin exposure.

Subsyndromal Depressive Symptoms. As noted previously, there is mounting research evidence to suggest that many older adults suffer from depressive symptoms that do not meet the criteria for major depression outlined (see Table 17–1) that nevertheless affect their quality of life and may lead to more severe mood disorder (Meyers, 1994). In a 1-year longitudinal study examining the incidence and persistence of depression among nursing home and congregate apartment residents, Parmelee and colleagues (1992) found that on initial evaluation, 15% of the 868 subjects displayed possible major depression and another 16.5% exhibited minor depressive symptoms. Follow-up of 448 residents 1 year later revealed that 40% of those with major depression had experienced no remission in symptoms and that a significant percentage (16.2%) of those categorized as *minor depressives* had developed major depression. This troubling finding suggests that minor, or subsyndromal, depression cannot necessarily be considered a transitory or easily managed disorder among the frail elderly.

Seasonal Affective Disorder (SAD). In the DSM-IV (1994, p. 389), SAD is classified under the category *specifiers describing course of recurrent episode* with a seasonal pattern, indicating that the onset and remission of major depression occurs at characteristic times of the year. This specifier can be applied to major depressive episodes, bipolar disorders, or recurrent major depressive disorder. SAD affects approximately 10 million Americans, and subsyndromal SAD (also referred to as the winter blues) another 25 million. The precise number of elderly people is not known. SAD is a cyclical illness characterized by depressed periods beginning in the fall and subsiding in the spring. About four times as many women are affected as men, with symptoms typically appearing in people's 30s. The most common symptoms in adults include decreased energy in the fall and winter months, tiredness and fatigue, usually increased appetite that leads to weight gain, craving of carbohydrates, difficulty concentrating and completing tasks, sadness, anxiety, and social withdrawal (National Institute of Mental Health [NIMH], 1993). SAD may be caused by variances in hormones and neurotransmitters as well as a response to changes in environmental light. The primary treatment is light therapy.

Suicide

During his life, the great Roman orator Seneca gave much thought to old age (Nuland, 1993, p. 151, copyright 1993 by Alfred A. Knopf):

I will not relinquish old age if it leaves my better part intact. But if it begins to shake my mind, if it destroys its faculties one by one, if it leaves me not life but breath, I will depart from the putrid or tottering edifice. I will not escape by death from disease so long as it may be healed, and leaves my mind unimpaired. I will not raise my hand against myself on account of pain, for so to die is to be conquered. But I know that if I must suffer without hope of relief, I will depart, not through fear of the pain itself, but because it prevents all for which I would live.

The risk associated with failure to detect or aggressively treat late-life depression is substantial. Suicide (especially in widowed white males living alone) is more common among the elderly, and the rate has been increasing. The old old, those 85 years and over, are particularly vulnerable (Manton et al., 1987), which may be explained by the increased proportion of people with severe disabilities or multiple chronic conditions that lead to the loss of autonomy and control. In fact, suicide ranks among the top 10 causes of death among the elderly. The national suicide rate for all ages is approximately 12.8 per 100,000, whereas among the elderly it is 21.6 per 100,000 (Koenig & Blazer, 1992). Barry Lebowitz (Chief, Mental Disorders, Aging Research Branch of the NIMH) has stated that if white males age 15 to 19 had a suicide rate as high as that for men ages 85 years and older, 356,000 men age 15 to 19 years would commit suicide every year, and we would declare a public health emergency (Lebowitz, 1994).

Regrettably, studies indicate that the majority of elderly people who commit suicide suffer from the most treatable kind of depression and yet do not receive needed mental health services. Lebowitz (1994) found that three fourths of elderly male suicide victims had seen their primary care physician within 1 month of taking their own life and had presented with diffuse, nonspecific complaints that were not properly diagnosed or treated as depression. This is particularly unfortunate in light of the fact that depression has been implicated in two thirds of all geriatric suicides (Allen & Blazer, 1991). The risk factors for suicide are listed in Table 17–4.

Organizations such as the Hemlock Society in the United States and the Voluntary Euthanasia Society in the United Kingdom support the idea that people who face "painful, disfiguring, or disabling terminal illness, should be given encouragement and assistance in thinking of suicide as a rational solution" (Brown et al., 1986). The current national debate concern-

ing euthanasia or assisted suicide must address the role of possible depressive illness. Although clinical depression can affect a patient's ability to make rational judgments, not all older people who long for death are suicidal. Since hopelessness and suicidal ideas can be symptoms of a treatable clinical depression, elderly patients who express ideas of death, suicide, or hopelessness should be evaluated by a psychiatrist for depression or another psychiatric disorder that may impair judgment (Conwell & Caine, 1991). In a study of patients ranging in age from 29 to 82 years old, 11 of 44 terminally ill patients were found to suffer from severe depression. Of the depressed patients, seven wished for death, but not by suicide; three had current or previous suicidal thoughts; and one had neither thoughts of death nor suicide. Patients who were not depressed experienced neither suicidal ideation nor wishes for premature death (Brown et al., 1986).

Advanced practice gerontological nurses who suspect that a depressed elderly person may be suicidal should conduct an assessment for suicidal risk, using a hierarchical questioning pattern such as the following:

1. Do you feel that life is not worth living?
2. Have you thought about harming yourself?
3. Are you thinking about suicide or taking your own life?
4. Do you have a plan in mind for killing yourself? What is it?
5. Have you ever attempted suicide?

THEORIES OF DEPRESSION

The present understanding of the etiology of depression hypothesizes that there are multiple independent or interacting biological and psychosocial factors. Although these factors underlie depressive disorders at all ages, age-specific differences likely exist in the etiology of depression. There is no single theory that best explains the onset of depression in later life. Rather, throughout the lifespan, depression probably represents a class of disorders with multiple causal pathways, which argues

---

TABLE 17-4
Risk Factors for Suicide in the Elderly

Depression
Suicide statements or threats
Having a definite plan
Having a readily available means of suicide
Previous suicide attempt(s)
Hopelessness or helplessness and feelings of emptiness, dejection, self-accusation
Sudden, marked change in behavior or personality
Neglect of responsibilities
Making final arrangements
Selection of reading material about death
Requests for sleeping pills
Divorced, separated, or widowed status
Socially isolated
Drug or alcohol use or abuse
Chronically or terminally ill

From Smith, M., Buckwalter, K. C., & Mitchell, S. (1993). *Geriatric mental health training series.* New York: Springer. Copyright by K. C. Buckwalter.

for an integrative etiological perspective (McNeal & Cimbolic, 1986). Understanding the causes of depression is important because they may influence the types of therapy that are most appropriate for a given group of depressed people.

Psychological Theories

Cognitive Theory. One of the best-known psychological theories proposed by Beck and colleagues (1979) postulated that cognitive styles and distortions contribute to the development of depression. The cognitive model holds that early experiences form the basis for the development of negative concepts. There are three main concepts in this theory of depression:

1. Cognitive triad, which includes an individual's negative view of the self, his or her world, and the future, which leads to negative automatic thinking
2. Rigid, unrealistically high basic assumptions or expectations and depressogenic schema or concepts; these are long-lasting attitudes about the world that represent the way an individual organizes the past and future and through which he or she "filters" and processes incoming information
3. Systematic logical errors of thinking that include arbitrary inference, overgeneralization, selective abstraction, magnification and minimization, and dichotomous (black and white, all or nothing) thinking

Learned Helplessness. This model of depression (Seligman, 1975), based on elements of attributional theory, argues that motivational and cognitive deficits and emotional changes follow when an individual learns that his or her behavior and outcomes are independent. Individuals learn that they cannot control future events, that depression may occur when they expect that something bad will happen, and that nothing can be done to prevent this event; they attribute the outcomes to internal, stable, and global factors.

Biological Theories

Neurobiological and Genetic Factors. Neurochemical changes, including the depletion of neurotransmitters in the CNS, may also predispose elderly people to depression. The increased sensitivity of CNS receptors may cause older adults to be more sensitive to CNS effects and the side effects of medications used to treat depression (American Geriatrics Society, 1993). Biological theories of depression have centered largely on the ability of selected medications to alter the release or uptake of monoamines and other neurotransmitters (e.g., norepinephrine, dopamine, indolamine, serotonin, and acetylcholine) into nerve terminals. As is discussed later, numerous psychosocial stressors may affect older adults and have been correlated with elevated blood cortisol levels. Twin and family studies offer compelling evidence of a genetic influence in depressive disorders, with the risk for developing an affective disorder almost four times greater among relatives of people with affective illness than in the general population (Blazer, 1993).

RISK FACTORS FOR DEPRESSION IN LATER LIFE

Another view of late-life depression has recently appeared in the popular literature. This view characterizes depression in old age as a natural response to the predictable losses of the elderly rather than as a clinical disorder (Jacobsen, 1995). Loss and change in later life represent threats to normal coping and may predispose older adults to depression (Table 17–5). In major depression, actual or perceived losses such as illness, impaired mobility, changes in sensory capacity, social isolation, death of a spouse or friends, economic hardship, and retirement are the most frequently associated stressors (Allen & Blazer, 1991). The impact of these stressors is compounded by the fact that many older adults lack the cognitive and psychic reserves to "bounce back" from multiple and cumulative losses quickly and effectively. The category *uncomplicated bereavement* is used when the focus of treatment is on the "normal" reaction to the death of a

---

TABLE 17-5
Threats to Normal Coping: Loss and Change

Health	Acute or chronic illnesses interfere with our ability to enjoy usual activities, function in familiar roles, or even perform simple activities of daily living. These illnesses can limit the ways we "achieve" and feel independent. Illness also interferes with our ability to maintain social relationships and the way we "feel close with" and joined to others (our dependency needs).
Mobility	Changes in our ability to move freely, to walk on our own, and to "do for ourselves" can reduce our ability to be independent and increase our dependency on others.
Sensory Changes	Changes in our hearing and sight may limit what we can "do for ourselves" and enjoy with other people. Not being able to hear the conversation or see what is going on can limit our ability to "be close with others."
Relocation	The loss of ability to live alone may cause us to move in with relatives or into a nursing facility. Typically, this relocation is accompanied by considerable stress and "misgivings," since the person wishes that he or she could continue to "get along on [his or her] own."
Finances	Loss of financial resources (that allow us to do what we want, when we want) can affect our ability to function independently.
Activity Level	Changes in our ability to participate in familiar activities may contribute to the loss of a sense of purpose, direction, and meaning in life. This can cause more problems if the person becomes depressed and, as a result, becomes even more dependent.
Loss of Loved One	Death, divorce, separation, relocation, or illness may remove people on whom we have depended for support, encouragement, and caring. The usual ways that we have achieved our dependency needs simply are no longer available.

Adapted from Smith, M., Buckwalter, K. C., & Mitchell, S. (1993). *Geriatric mental health training series*. New York: Springer. Copyright by K. C. Buckwalter.

---

loved one and shares many of the symptoms of a major depressive disorder (Kurlowicz, 1994). An important distinction from other types of depression is that bereaved individuals usually regard the depressed feelings as normal within the context of their loss and tend to maintain a positive self-image. Similarly, adjustment disorder with depressed mood, a maladaptive reaction to psychosocial stressors or illness that occurs within 3 months of the stressor, shares many symptoms with a major depressive disorder. Declines in social or occupational functioning or symptoms beyond those expected in response to the stressor help differentiate the diagnosis of adjustment disorder with depressed mood in the elderly, although the distinction is often difficult to make (APA, 1994; Kurlowicz, 1994).

Research suggests that those elderly people who live alone and have lower incomes are at the most risk for depression (O'Hara et al., 1985). Thus, social support, higher education, and married status are critical in lowering the risk for depression among the elderly. A complex cross-sectional study of important life events and depression among older adults (Ensel, 1991) found that undesirable major life events exacerbate the level of depression. Further, when controlling for both health-related (defined as major accident or injury, serious physical illness, frequent minor illness, and major dental work) and non–health-related (anything in the realm of home, love and marriage, family, personal change, work, finance, legal events, and school) undesirable events, Ensel found that psychological resources were more effective than social resources in predicting subsequent levels of depression for elderly people experiencing health-related events. However, for those elderly people who experienced non–health-related life events, social resources were found to be most important in predicting later symptomatology (Ensel, 1991).

As the elderly continue to confront developmental tasks in late adulthood, psychological factors may influence the risk for depression (Table 17–6). Approximately 800,000 people each year experience the death of a spouse, and research has confirmed that one third of these widows and widowers meet the criteria for major depression in the first month after the death. One year later, nearly half of these individuals remain clinically depressed (NIH, 1992). According to Erickson (1963), the final stage of life is characterized by a struggle to achieve ego integrity (i.e., acceptance of their life) versus despair. Other researchers (Butler, 1974) have identified *reminiscence,* the act or process of recalling the past, and *life review* as important psychological tasks of later life that

---

TABLE 17-6
Late Adulthood Developmental Tasks

Role changes related to retirement, widowhood, or disability of spouse

Normal biological changes and changes in physical appearance

Sense of finite time and one's own mortality

Losses related to health, death of family members and friends, or finances

Demands to modulate independence and dependence regarding medical systems and healthcare personnel

Intergenerational changes in relationships (i.e., being parented by adult children)

From Smith, M., Buckwalter, K. C., & Mitchell, S. (1993). *Geriatric mental health training series.* New York: Springer. Copyright by K. C. Buckwalter.

---

may assist older adults in reaffirming and rediscovering life (Soltys & Coats, 1994).

RELATIONSHIP AMONG DEPRESSION, ILLNESS, AND FUNCTION

Depression and Illness

Depression is associated with poor health in the elderly, and depressed elders use healthcare services more heavily than their nondepressed counterparts (Koenig et al., 1989). This relationship holds true for the elderly in both acute care and long-term care settings as well as cross-culturally. Poor ego strength and chronic medical problems were found to be common predictors of depression among black elderly men and women (Husaini et al., 1991).

In a previously cited study that examined the association between depression and mortality in nursing home and congregate living elders (Parmalee et al., 1992), the effects of depression on mortality were most attributable to the correlation of depression and ill health. In a large study of nursing home residents, Cohen-Mansfield and Marx (1993) corroborated the findings of Parmalee and colleagues and found that depressed residents were more likely to experience pain, whether or not they were cognitively impaired. Further, depressed affect was predicted by greater levels of pain, more medical diagnoses, and poor social networks.

Nurse investigators have also examined the relationship between physical health impairment and depression among older adults (Badger, 1993) and have found significant differences between those with mild impairments and those with moderate to severe impairments. Hierarchical multiple regression analyses revealed that mastery, social resources, and economic resources explained 58% of the variance on depression and were significant predictors of depression in older adults with physical health impairments.

In an excellent literature review on depression in the hospitalized medically ill elderly, Kurlowicz (1994) confirmed the high prevalence of depression in the elderly and presented consistent evidence that when depressive symptoms are combined with medical illness, they have an additive effect on patient function and well-being. This review highlights the difficulty in determining whether depressive symptoms are a symptom of the physical illness, a psychological reaction to the experience of the physical illness, or a part of a coexistent psychiatric disorder (Kurlowicz, 1994).

Depressive disorders often exist in association with medical conditions thought to be etiologically related to depression. Strokes, for example, which occur more commonly in the elderly, are believed to cause depression above and beyond their obvious disabling effects. They are thought to disrupt neurotransmitter pathways and result in biologically mediated depression (Robinson et al., 1984). Parkinson's disease, which also occurs more commonly in the elderly, similarly has a primary role in the pathogenesis of depression (Rodin & Voshart, 1986). Although 40% of patients with Parkinson's disease are thought to be depressed, perhaps due to a serotonin deficiency, their depressive symptoms are seldom treated, despite the fact that there is good support for the effectiveness of serotonin reuptake inhibitors and other antidepressant medications in the treatment of depression associated with Parkinson's disease. Thus, the cause of some depressive disorders in later life not only differs from that occurring at earlier ages but clearly results in differing patterns of comorbidity and impairment.

Among people seen in general medical settings, those with major depressive disorder have more pain and physical illness and decreased physical, social, and role functioning than those without depression. As many as 25% of individuals with diabetes, myocardial infarction, carcinomas, and stroke develop major depression during the course of their illness. Indeed, the management of the medical condition is more complex and the prognosis less favorable if depression is present (Dupont et al., 1988; Schleifer et al., 1989).

Chronic medical conditions are known to be a risk factor for more persistent episodes of depression (APA, 1994). For example, Mossey and colleagues (1990) followed the cases of 196 older women for 12 months after hip fracture and evaluated them using the Center for Epidemiology Studies-Depression Scale (CES-D). Controlling for age, prefracture physical condition, and cognitive status, people who reported persistently low levels of depressive symptoms were three times more likely than those with elevated depression scores to achieve independence in walking and nine times more likely to return to prefracture levels in physical functioning. The majority of people with persistently high depressive symptoms following hip fracture, however, also had a history of depressed mood *before* fracture, suggesting that depressive symptoms affected their recovery and were not simply a consequence of poor recovery. If depression does impede the recovery process, as this study indicates, then the general implications for healthcare are apparent, especially given the recent societal trends toward preventative healthcare and cutting healthcare costs.

Clearly, if depression is caused by a physical illness, as depicted in Table 17–3, every effort should be made to treat or control the illness. Similarly, if depressive symptoms are secondary to medications, the medication should be discontinued or reduced to the lowest clinically effective dose.

Depression and Function

Functional status is a multidimensional concept characterizing one's ability to provide for the necessities of life—defined as those socially influenced and individually determined activities that exist in the normal course of life to meet basic needs (Leidy, 1994). Medical and functional illness is clearly dynamic and varies with the acuity and severity of the diagnosis and individual and environmental characteristics. The functional impairment caused by chronic illness in the elderly, either physical or mental, can span a range from a declining ability to shop, cook, clean, and travel to difficulty dressing, grooming, bathing, and feeding oneself (see Chapter 9).

The DSM-IV (1994) criteria for major depressive disorder include impairment in work or social roles; however, the definition of impairment is vague and the empirical indicators are not well articulated. Functional limitations caused by depressive disorder are considered only secondary to the disorder, rather than as part of the definition (Wells et al., 1989). Moreover, older adults with higher levels of functional disability have been found to be at higher risk for depressive symptomatology (Turner & Noh, 1988), and both physical illness and depression are associated with restricted activity that results in disruptions in normal role functioning. Research has documented strong correlations between depression and decreased functional status in the general population (Blazer et al., 1991; Blumenthal & Dielman, 1975) and between depression and self-reported disability in community surveys (Berkman et al., 1986; Craig & Van Natta, 1993). Strong positive correlations have been found between mood and physical function in hospitalized patients (Harris et al., 1988) and between physical illness and depression in community samples (Aneshensel et al., 1984; Murrell et al., 1983) and rehabilitation settings (Harris et al., 1995).

The direction of causation between depression and functional status is unclear. Questions remain as to whether depressive symptoms contribute to functional impairment in medically ill older adults, whether functional status influences the patient's emotional response, or whether depression and functional status share a reciprocal and/or causal relationship (Kurlowicz, 1994). The biopsychosocial pathways and direction by which physical illness, depression, and functional impairment are related have yet to be elucidated. Further investigations and replications of some of the studies reported in this chapter are needed to determine whether declining health and increasing functional impairment also distinguish persistently depressed elderly from those who recover from depression.

Despite the known relationship between depression and functional status, the importance of functional status as an outcome measure in the treatment of depression has not been well developed in the research literature, the current psychiatric diagnostic system, or in nursing interventions. The future identification of any independent contributions that depressive symptoms make to late-life morbidity and mortality should spur the search for risk factors and the development and evaluation of more effective interventions. If depressive symptoms are related to slow recovery, prolonged hospitalization, increased risk of physical illness, and poor functional status, as appears to be the case, gerontological nurses and others must conduct prospective, controlled studies with valid and reliable measures to evaluate the relationship between depression, ill health, and functional status in the elderly.

DIFFERENTIAL DIAGNOSIS

The symptoms associated with depression are generally consistent throughout the lifespan. Depression in older adults, however, is often more difficult to diagnose: Although older adults may be preoccupied with a past event about which they feel guilty, they tend to verbalize less guilt than younger people suffering from depression. The elderly may also present with a *masked depression,* denying that they are depressed by covering up symptoms such as crying spells, apathy, and diminished appetite. In addition, depressed older adults are often more anxious and hypochondriacal and may present with vague, nonspecific complaints (often affecting the gastrointestinal, cardiac, and musculoskeletal systems) that cannot be confirmed on physical examination (American Geriatrics Society, 1993).

Another confounding factor is that older adults are more likely to experience cognitive dysfunction when depressed. This characteristic can confound efforts to differentiate between *pseudodementia*—the dementia associated with depression—and other irreversible dementias such as Alzheimer's disease (Table 17–7). Further, a major depression coexists in nearly one third of all cases of early to midstage dementia. The depression is often alleviated by antidepressants and brief psychotherapy and may improve both affective and functional status in the older patient; however, it does nothing to alter cognitive impairment. Finally, psychotic, or delusional, depressions are more common in later life, during which the older patient may experience paranoid ide-

| TABLE 17-7 |

Characteristics Distinguishing Pseudodementia from Dementia

Dementia	Pseudodementia
Insidious and indeterminate onset	Rapid onset
Symptoms usually of long duration	Symptoms usually of short duration
Mood and behavior fluctuate	Mood consistently depressed
"Near miss" answers typical	"Don't know" answers typical
Patient conceals disabilities	Patient highlights disabilities
Level of cognitive impairment relatively stable	Level of cognitive impairment fluctuates

Adapted from Allen, A., & Blazer, D. G. (1991). Mood disorders. In J. Sadavoy, L. Lazarus & L. Jarvik (Eds.), *Comprehensive review of geriatric psychiatry* (p. 345). Washington, D.C.: American Psychiatric Press.

ations and ideas of reference and a variety of delusional beliefs that make differential diagnosis with late-onset schizophrenia or other delusional disorders difficult. Elderly people experiencing psychotic depression seldom respond to antidepressant therapy alone and usually require the administration of either electroconvulsive therapy (ECT) or neuroleptics.

ASSESSMENT

There is no single diagnostic test recommended for the detection of depression in older adults. Rather, the assessment of depressed older adults is a challenging process of untangling the complex interplay among physical, mental, social, economic, spiritual, environmental, and treatment-related factors. It should begin with a thorough history, including a review of medications and alcohol use, a physical examination (including neurological function), and functional status and mental status evaluations.

Recommended laboratory tests are presented in Table 17–8. No laboratory findings have been identified that are diagnostic of a major depressive episode, although several values have been found to be abnormal in people with depression compared with controls. Further, laboratory test results are more likely to be abnormal in depressive episodes with melancholic or psychotic features as well as in individuals who are more severely depressed

TABLE 17-8

Laboratory Tests

Sequential Multiple Analyzer 20, Blood

Alanine aminotransferase
Albumin
Alkaline phosphatase
Aspartate aminotransferase
Total bilirubin
Calcium
Carbon dioxide
Chloride
Cholesterol
Creatine kinase
Creatinine
Gamma-glutamyl transpeptidase
Glucose
Lactate
Phosphorus
Potassium
Protein
Sodium
Triglycerides
Urea nitrogen
Uric acid

Complete Blood Count

Hematocrit
Hemoglobin
Red blood cells
    Mean cell volume
    Mean cell hemoglobin
    Mean cell hemoglobin concentration
White blood cells

Differential White Blood Cell Count

Granulocytes
    Segmented neutrophils
    Band neutrophils
    Eosinophils
    Basophils
Monocytes
Lymphocytes

Other Tests

Triiodothyronine radioimmunoassay
Thyroxine radioimmunoassay
Thyroid-stimulating hormone
Vitamin B_{12} (cyanocobalamin)
Folate (serum)
Rapid plasma reagin

(APA, 1994). In general, assessments that rely on biological markers (e.g., thyroid-stimulation hormone, platelet monoamine oxidase activity, platelet imipramine, and the dexamethasone suppression test) are not particularly helpful for discriminating among types of depression in older adults because of a high rate of false positives and negatives in elderly people—likely due to patients' chronic medical conditions, dietary habits, and current medications (American Geriatrics Society, 1993). Abnormal sleep electroencephalograms are evident in 40 to 60% of outpatients and 90% of inpatients with a major depressive episode (see Table 17–1), but polysomnographic findings may be confounded by normal age-related changes in rapid eye movement latency and stage 4 (slow wave) sleep in older adults.

Until recently, depression was often overlooked, especially among the elderly residing in long-term care facilities. Recent data, however, suggest that the implementation of federally mandated minimum data sets (MDS) with resident assessment protocol (RAP) summaries and problem area triggers has helped sensitize nursing home staff members to look for symptoms of depression and to intervene when appropriate (see Chapter 9 on functional assessment). The MDS is a standardized language for all long-term care settings that aids in resident assessment and screening in numerous areas of patient care. The RAP summary requires that for each RAP area triggered by the MDS assessment, care plan interventions be developed, and problems, complications, and risk factors documented in the patient's chart and care plan. In 1990, 35.7% of residents were triggered by the RAP for depression, and 62.1% had the problem addressed in their plan of care; in 1993, the figures were 29.1% and 72.6%, respectively (Brown University Long-Term Care Quality Newsletter, 1994).

Depression is also underrecognized in primary care settings (Callahan et al., 1994) and among the medically ill elderly (Black et al., 1987). The latter study found evidence to suggest that medically ill depressed patients were less likely to receive adequate treatment than were patients suffering from depression without a medical illness. In an effort to improve detection and treatment of depression overall, the Agency for Health Care Policy and Research has produced guidelines to assist primary care physicians and others to better recognize and treat depression (Kathol et al., 1994). This is an important step, because primary care and nonpsychiatric practitioners are most likely to be the first healthcare professionals to examine depressed patients. Volume 1 of the Clinical Practice Guidelines focuses on detection and diagnosis, and Volume 2, on the treatment of major depression (U.S. Department of Health and Human Services, 1993).

The advanced practice gerontological nurse must be knowledgeable of other illness and treatment parameters in the older patient and should obtain information about interpersonal relationships, role functioning, socialization, support systems, activities of daily living, and coping mechanisms and resources (Paulmeno, 1987). To accurately identify psychopathology, the gerontological nurse must obtain a comprehensive database that addresses the following factors (Paulmeno, 1987):

- Normal aging process
- Altered medication responses and tolerance
- Cognitive functioning alterations
- Altered, and often diverse, manifestations of physical and psychiatric illnesses
- Decreased rebound potential following losses and stressors (both physical and psychological)
- Increased risk potential
- Decreased stamina
- Sociocultural stressors
- Altered dietary needs and capabilities

Additional factors to consider in assessment are presented in Table 17–9.

INSTRUMENTS TO MEASURE DEPRESSION IN OLDER ADULTS

In recent years, the diagnostic procedures for mental disorders in late life have been developed with sufficient sensitivity and accuracy to enable clinicians to make diagnoses related to mental illness as well as other areas of healthcare (Lebowitz, 1994). Several depression scales (e.g., the Zung Self-Rating Depression

TABLE 17-9

Factors to Consider in Assessment

Lifelong Personality Traits:
Patterns of Relating with Others

What have they been like throughout their life?
What words do others use to describe them? (e.g., bossy, directive, hard to please, assertive, needy, insecure, overly sensitive)
What do we know about their "usual" way of relating with other people? Do they "make the first move," or do others?
Have they expected others to "look after" or anticipate their needs in the past?
Have they needed considerable support, direction, and encouragement from others?
Have they been very self-reliant—and comfortable taking care of themselves and others?
Are they able to accept help from others?
Do they seem to expect help, even when it is not really needed?

Self-Concept:
Values, Beliefs, Convictions About Oneself

What do they think about their abilities and characteristics?
Do they have a realistic view of their current abilities?
What do they seem to value—being cared for, or being able to care for themselves?
Do they seem to be thinking "I should be able to take care of myself" or "I deserve to be taken care of"?

Adapted from Smith, M., Buckwalter, K. C., & Mitchell, S. (1993). *Geriatric mental health training series.* New York: Springer. Copyright by K. C. Buckwalter.

Scale, the Beck Depression Inventory, the Hamilton Depression Rating Scale, and the Brief Psychiatric Rating Scale) have been used in both clinical and research contexts. It has been argued that depression symptom checklists in particular do not distinguish well between clinical syndromes of depression and other symptoms of diminished life satisfaction or response to chronic stress, and that they tend to elevate depression scores in older adults because of the prevalence of somatic (physical illness) symptoms in this population (Gatz & Hurwicz, 1990). Two of the most commonly used tools—the Center for Epidemiologic Studies Depression Scale (CES-D) and the Geriatric Depression Scale (GDS)—are discussed in this section.

Center for Epidemiologic Studies Depression Scale

The CES-D consists of 20 items that represent the symptoms of depressive disorder (Radloff, 1977). Response categories range from *rarely or none of the time*, which is scored as a 0, to *most of the time*, which is scored as a 3. The total score is the sum of all items and ranges from 0 to 60. Four subscales (depressed mood, psychomotor retardation, lack of well-being, and interpersonal difficulties) have also been identified (Gatz & Hurwicz, 1990). Depression is most commonly indicated by a score of 16 or greater. Respondents are asked to rate the frequency with which they experienced each symptom during the week before filling out the CES-D.

Geriatric Depression Scale

The GDS is an easily administered 30-item self-rating scale designed to serve as a screening tool for depression in the elderly (Yesavage & Brink, 1983). A major advantage of the GDS over other depression scales is that it excludes somatic items that may confound the detection of depression in older, physically ill people (Bolla-Wilson & Bleecker, 1989). The GDS has been validated using both normal elderly people and those undergoing treatment for depression in a variety of settings. A cut-off score of 11 yields a sensitivity of .84 and a specificity of .95, whereas a more stringent cut-off of 14 results in a sensitivity of .80 and 100% specificity. The GDS successfully discriminates depressed from nondepressed elderly people among the physically ill as well as those receiving treatment for cognitive impairments (Yesavage & Brink, 1983). A shorter 15-item version of the GDS has also been developed, but results are mixed regarding its ability to replace the original 30-item scale (Alden et al., 1989).

TREATMENT

The goals of treatment for an older depressed person include the improvement of quality of life and functional capacity and the reduction of morbidity and mortality (Lebowitz, 1994). Other treatment goals include improving medical health status and decreasing symptoms of depression, the risk of relapse and recurrence, and healthcare costs and mortality (NIH, 1992).

The elderly underuse mental health outpatient services and instead obtain care from their primary physicians (German et al., 1987). However, a meta-analysis of 58 controlled studies provided evidence of the cost-effectiveness of outpatient mental health treatment (Mumford et al., 1984), with the largest cost offset produced by decreased inpatient costs in the older population.

The lack of treatment of depression and other mental illnesses in older adults is probably caused by several factors, including the following:

1. Reluctance of many depressed elderly people to seek psychiatric care
2. Tendency of older adults to insist that physical ills rather than emotional problems are at the root of their distress
3. Ageism
4. Insufficient numbers of healthcare providers trained or interested in geropsychiatry
5. Nonreimbursement for care
6. Failure of many primary care practitioners to recognize that bodily (somatic) complaints may be masking an underlying depression and that depressive symptoms are not a "natural part of growing old"

Several types of therapies have been found to be beneficial in the treatment of older adults with depression. Although it is not known what specific aspects of therapy help the patient, beneficial effects may result from the caring, warm attitude of the therapist (Frank, 1973). The following section highlights some of the more common biological (somatic) and psychological treatments that have been shown to be effective in the treatment of late-life depression.

Biological Treatment (Somatic Therapies)

PHARMACOLOGICAL TREATMENT

Clinical trials have provided convincing evidence that antidepressants are effective in treating acute depression, although most of this research has been conducted with young or middle-aged subjects (NIH, 1992). About 60% of adult patients can expect to improve when treated with antidepressant therapy, but such a response requires adequate lengths of treatment, dosages, and blood levels. In the elderly, this response frequently occurs later than in younger patients, requiring 6 to 12 weeks of therapy (NIH, 1992).

Patients with certain symptom clusters respond positively to antidepressant medications. Seventy to 80% of patients exhibiting the following symptoms are likely to improve: vegetative symptoms, insomnia, diurnal rhythm (with mood worse in the morning hours), acute onset, positive family history of depression and response to either ECT or antidepressant medications, and prior positive response by the patient to antidepressant therapy (McNeal & Cimbolic, 1986). Conversely, patients who exhibit chronic symptoms, hypochondriacal features, or mood-incongruent psychotic symptoms or who have a family history of either schizophrenia or antidepressant drug failure are more apt to respond poorly to antidepressant therapy. Thus, medication should be selected by considering the specific symptoms experienced by the patient, his or her medical illnesses and other conditions, and the side effect profile.

Two types of antidepressant medications, monoamine oxidase inhibitors (MAOIs) and tricyclic antidepressants (TCAs), increase the activity of catecholamines in the brain. MAOIs prevent the breakdown of norepinephrine by monoamine oxidase, and TCAs block the uptake of amines released by the nerves and in so doing potentiate the effects of the neurotransmitters (McNeal & Cimbolic, 1986). However, the side effects of MAOIs and TCAs, especially hypotension, sedation, and anticholinergic effects, are particularly troublesome for many older adults.

Newer antidepressant compounds, such as bupropion hydrochloride (Wellbutrin), have fewer of these negative side effects and are safer in cases of overdose. Other new antidepressant medications known as selective serotonin reuptake inhibitors include fluoxetine (Prozac), sertraline (Zoloft), and paroxetine

(Paxil). These drugs act by preventing a neuron from taking serotonin back into the cell (Jacobs, 1994). Other promising new antidepressants have either been recently released or are undergoing clinical trials as part of the Federal Drug Administration (FDA) approval process. Venlafaxine HCl (Effexor) is a structurally novel antidepressant that has received recent FDA approval but does not yet have long-term clinical trial data. Venlafaxine inhibits the reuptake of serotonin and norepinephrine and requires that the patient's blood pressure be regularly monitored. Nefazodone HCl (Serzone), which has a pharmacological profile that is distinct from other antidepressants, is a relatively safe drug owing to its low cardiotoxicity. Flesinoxan (currently in phase II trials) has both antianxiety and antidepressant properties that may be of value in patients with difficult, treatment-resistant depressions. Mirtazapine (Remeron) is in the phase III approval process but appears to have weight gain and sleepiness as undesirable side effects (Walker, 1994).

PRINCIPLES OF MEDICATION MANAGEMENT

For many depressed elderly people, antidepressant medications "lift the veil of depression," allowing them to focus, attend, concentrate, express themselves, and process and resolve feelings of loss or grief that accompany later-life changes or bereavement (Smith & Buckwalter, 1992). The older adult may resist antidepressant medications, however, believing that they are "mind-altering," "mood elevators," or evidence that the elderly person is a "mental case." Thus, nurses must be extremely sensitive to labeling issues in providing patient education.

Any treatment with psychotropic medications must begin with consideration of age-related pharmacokinetic and pharmacodynamic changes (see Chapter 26). These physical changes serve to make the effects of drugs less predictable, especially many psychotropic drugs that are lipid soluble and thus become sequestered in fatty tissues (Smith & Buckwalter, 1992). Moreover, the consequences of polypharmacy are substantial and include the probability of interdrug reactions, drug-disease interactions, and adverse drug reactions

(Zanke & Hunter, 1986). For example, more than 40 interdrug reactions have been documented with commonly used antidepressant medications (Perry et al., 1991).

In general, the elderly require less medication to achieve therapeutic benefits than younger people suffering from depression. Therefore, the adage "Start low and go slow" is an appropriate principle to guide psychotropic medication management in this population; medications should be started at a low dose and increased by small increments over several weeks, watching closely for the development of any adverse side effects. Compliance can be a problem in elderly patients, with as many as three fourths of older patients failing to take some of their medications as prescribed.

An important role for advanced practice gerontological nurses is to provide information, guidance, and reassurance by encouraging depressed elderly people to take their prescribed medications, reminding them that these drugs do not work "overnight," and monitoring for symptoms of improvement as well as adverse side effects (Table 17–10) (Smith et al., 1993).

ELECTROCONVULSIVE THERAPY

Patients older than age 60 years now constitute the largest age group receiving ECT. Although there is strong evidence of its short-term efficacy in this population, the relapse rate is also quite high (NIH, 1992). ECT can be a rapid, safe, and in some cases lifesaving treatment for elderly people who are actively suicidal, psychotically depressed, or for whom antidepressant medications are contraindicated or ineffective. Older people who experience somatic delusions are likely to have a positive response to ECT (Blazer, 1989), as are those with psychomotor retardation, vegetative signs, and early insomnia (Gomez & Gomez, 1992). Unilateral administration (e.g., for seizures induced in the nondominant hemisphere) appears to decrease confusion and memory problems commonly associated with ECT, and a course of around 10 treatments is often sufficient to produce desired levels of improvement. Concurrent use of psychotrophic medication, a major medical illness, and preexisting cognitive impairment may increase the risk when undergoing ECT.

TABLE 17-10
Common Antidepressant Side Effects and Interventions

Blurred Vision	Fatigue, Weakness, Drowsiness
Reassure that it is a temporary side effect (it often resolves after being on the medication for several months and goes away when they stop taking the medication); provide support and assistance as necessary; check for environmental hazards if needed	Administer medication at hour of sleep to facilitate sleep and reduce daytime drowsiness; monitor level of sedation and fatigue over time (getting worse vs. getting better) to differentiate between medication side effects and symptoms of depression (fatigue caused by the depression should decrease with medication); assess activities of daily living and activity level for declines; monitor sleeping patterns for increased daytime sleeping; notify physician if symptoms seem to worsen as medication is increased
Constipation	
Increase water and fluid intake; suggest "natural" dietary laxative (prunes, fiber, etc.); request prescription softeners; monitor bowel habits to avoid impactions; use laxatives only as a last resort	**Tremors, Twitches, Jitteriness**
Dry Mouth	Monitor severity and interference with activities of daily living and other activities; assess subjective distress; provide information and encouragement that this is a medication side effect—not a permanent impairment—that will subside when the medication is discontinued; notify the physician if symptoms are prolonged or severe
Encourage fluids to reduce discomfort; check dentures for proper fit; monitor for sores or lesions that may cause discomfort and interfere with eating	
Urinary Retention	**Hallucinations, Delusions**
Monitor voiding patterns (scanty, difficulty starting, frequency) and assess for subjective distress (feeling of fullness or incomplete emptying, pain); monitor color and odor of urine (urinary stasis leads to infection); report findings to physician for possible catheterization and medication change	Establish onset to differentiate between "psychotic depression" and medication side effect; if associated with medication, hold additional doses and notify physician; monitor for safety and provide reassurance if hallucinations or delusions are frightening or upsetting; provide reality orientation: recognize that belief *seems* real to them but is actually an adverse side effect of the medication, that it will soon go away, and that you will keep them safe until then
Excessive Perspiration	
Offer comfort measures (dry clothes, handkerchiefs, tissues, etc.); inform residents that "sweating" is a side effect of medication	
Orthostatic Hypotension	
Take lying and standing blood pressures for 2–3 weeks when the medication is started; monitor for dizziness and light-headedness; inform resident that this is a side effect of the medication and that falls may occur if patient gets up too quickly; instruct patient to dangle feet over side of bed when getting up from a reclining position and to rise slowly and stand supported for a few minutes before walking	

Adapted from Smith, M., Buckwalter, K. C., & Mitchell, S. (1993). *Geriatric mental health training series.* New York: Springer. Copyright by K. C. Buckwalter.

PHOTOTHERAPY

The main treatment for SAD and subsyndromal SAD is phototherapy, which involves exposing SAD patients to levels of artificial light 5 to 20 times brighter than normal indoor lighting for 30 minutes to several hours in the morning. For about three fourths of adults who suffer from SAD, symptom relief is usually experienced from a few days to 2 weeks from the onset of treatment. The mechanism of action is believed to be that of light (entering the eye) modifying brain chemistry and physiology to correct abnormalities resulting from light deficiency. Side effects from light therapy include eyestrain, headaches, insomnia, and occasionally manic symptoms (NIMH, 1993). Other treatment recommendations for SAD include stress management and dietary changes, medications, and psychotherapy, although light therapy is the most effective approach.

Psychotherapy

Psychotherapies are designed to help patients develop more effective coping mechanisms. These treatment modes are best viewed on a continuum, with traditional psychodynamic psychotherapy and supportive psychotherapy the extremes. In psychodynamic therapy, anxiety is seen as a tool necessary for exposing the defenses of the patient, whereas in supportive therapy, anxiety is seen as an impediment to the goals of treatment. According to Lazarus and colleagues (1991), the choice of appropriate therapeutic goals depends on where the elderly individual is found on the functional continuum (Fig. 17–1). For example, in working with the developmental tasks of aging, one might consider psychodynamic psychotherapy because of an older adult's strong ego and ability to tolerate strong emotions. As the aging person experiences crisis or increasing frailty, however, an anxiety-reducing therapy such as supportive therapy may be more appropriate.

Although there have been few controlled studies on the efficacy of psychosocial interventions, cognitive, brief psychodynamic, and behavioral therapies have been found to be beneficial for the treatment of older adults with depression—for those with both melancholic as well as nonmelancholic features (Thompson & Gallagher, 1986; Thompson et al., 1987). Psychotherapies can be used as the sole mode of treatment or in conjunction with pharmacological interventions. Supportive psychotherapy in particular is helpful in reintegrating elderly people into their social networks and preventing the recurrence of depressive episodes. Individual, group, marital, and family therapy interventions can be used successfully with depressed elderly people.

Nurses can participate in a variety of psychosocial rehabilitative therapies for the elderly that can be implemented on a one-to-one or group basis (Table 17–11). The key component of these psychosocial interventions is the desire to bring about patient improvement that stimulates interest, good communication, and improved interpersonal relationships. Indeed, the precise method of intervention is often much less important than the process—that is, what happens between the nurse and the depressed older person (Smith et al., 1993). Gerontological nurses should be aware, however, that many of the reminiscence models currently in the nursing literature are not empirically derived or tested; rather, they are generated based on clinical experience and logic (Soltys & Coats, 1994).

BEHAVIORAL THERAPY

This is a brief, problem-oriented therapy that is focused on changing specific behaviors rather than thoughts or feelings. It is based on the belief that depression is a response to a self-limiting repertoire of behavioral choices and may be caused by a loss of positive reinforcement. A change in behavior can lead to a

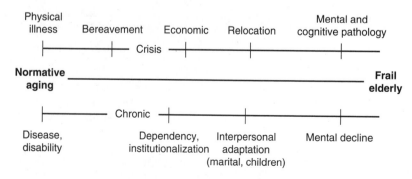

FIGURE 17–1. The continuum of functioning in old age. (Redrawn from Lazarus, L. W., Sadavoy, J., & Langley, P. R. [1991]. Individual psychotherapy. In J. Sadavoy, L. W. Lazarus & L. Jarvik [Eds.], *Comprehensive review of geriatric psychiatry* [p. 488]. Washington, D.C.: American Psychiatric Press.)

TABLE 17-11

Psychosocial Rehabilitative Therapies for the Elderly

Reminiscence and Life Review Methods

GOALS	PROCEDURES
Reexamine one's whole life and make sense of it Resolve old problems Make amends and restore harmony with friends and family Relive dreams of youth and come to terms with choices Understand and accept personal foibles Take responsibility for acts that caused real harm Differentiate between "real" and "neurotic" guilt Increase identification with past accomplishments Relive happy memories of the past to alleviate current depression Improve interaction and decrease withdrawal Reduce fear of death as they confront the myth of invulnerability	The critical component is *listening*! In general, the listener's tasks are the following: Enhance the natural and spontaneous process of "looking back" (e.g., make it conscious, deliberate, efficient) "Bear witness" to the older person's struggles Facilitate understanding of old conflicts or issues 　Promote a sense of peace about the past 　Reduce resentment, guilt, bitterness Increase identification with past competencies 　Accomplishments 　Personal characteristics Review and affirm past experiences that promote self-worth

INTERVENTIONS TO PROVOKE MEMORIES	GROUP INTERVENTIONS
Histories and interviewing Written or taped autobiographies Pilgrimages (in person or through correspondence) Reunions Scrapbooks, photo albums, letters, memorabilia Genealogy Summary of one's life work Renewal of ethnic identity Books and novels	Tangible reminders of the past stimulate reminiscing about specific events, eras, people: 　Pictures or letters 　Scrapbooks Focus on an historical event that acts as a stimulus for reminiscing: 　Childhood memories 　The Great Depression 　Military experiences 　Holiday celebrations 　Old-time songs, cars, etc. Encourage personalization of recalled events: 　Was this like the school you went to as a child? 　How did your family celebrate Thanksgiving? 　What were you doing when World War I began? Help identify positive elements in the recalled experiences Concentrate on identification and reinforcement of accomplishments: 　Did having so little as a child make you appreciate what you have more? 　That was quite an accomplishment to raise five children by yourself!

Music Therapy

GOALS	PROCEDURES
Stimulate interaction Encourage reminiscence Promote feelings of relatedness and cohesion Decrease agitation or aggression (demented)	Listening to music Music in the environment (soothing) Making music

Movement Therapy

GOALS	PROCEDURES
Promote trust Reinforce a sense of relatedness to others Provide sensory input through touch, vision, hearing Increase circulation (cardiovascular benefit)	Begin and end with a predictable activity Stand in a circle and hold hands Turn and rub the shoulders of the person next to you Stretching and reaching Mirror activity (e.g., "Simon Says" theme) leads to the following exchanges: 　Eye contact 　Facial expressions 　Postures 　Feelings 　Discussion following activity

Table continued on following page

TABLE 17-11

Psychosocial Rehabilitative Therapies for the Elderly *Continued*

Sensory Stimulation

GOALS	PROCEDURES
Increase contact with surroundings	Structured experiences involving five senses
Improve responsiveness to environment	Texture of fabrics and objects
Increase discrimination ability	Feel object in a sack where it is not seen
Catalyst to discussion and reminiscence	Play a tape of familiar sounds (e.g., train whistle, animal sounds)
	Smell of lemon, cinnamon, other spices
	Smell of candle or other scents
	Taste of hard candy, other foods

Pet Therapy

GOALS	PROCEDURES
Alleviate depression	Animal is used as a therapeutic catalyst
Enhance self-image and identity	Animal may live "in residence"
Help fulfill need to love and be loved	Animal "visitors" may be used
Help restore emotional equilibrium	

Remotivation Therapy

GOALS	PROCEDURES
Encourage renewed interest in surroundings	Welcoming—creating the climate of acceptance (5 min)
Stimulate thought and discussion of topics related to real world	Greet by name
Experience a sense of belonging	Appreciate attendance
Stimulate other-directed communication	Creating a bridge to reality—introduce subject of discussion (15 min)
Encourage to view self in relationship to others	Poetry (simple and rhythmic is best)
Increase feelings of self-worth	Pictures
	Newspaper articles
DESIRABLE BEHAVIORS	Questions to ponder
	Objects to examine (hobby items, animals, etc.)
Attentiveness to the leader and others	Sharing the world we live in (15 min)
Participation in discussion	Group pools their knowledge
Responsiveness to the material presented	Use 10–15 planned objective questions to stimulate
Appearance of enjoying the experience	Keep group on target
Realism in discussion	Use additional props to promote interest
Communication with others	The work of the world (15 min)
	Stimulate to think about work in relation to self
	Discuss jobs and tasks person used to perform
	Include current activity (e.g., occupational therapy) if possible
	Appreciation (5 min)
	Express appreciation for attendance and participation
	Plan for next meeting to increase continuity

Adapted from Smith, M., Buckwalter, K. C., & Mitchell, S. (1993). *Geriatric mental health training series.* New York: Springer. Copyright by K. C. Buckwalter.

change in thinking and feeling. The role of the therapist is that of an instructor of new skills: he or she teaches relaxation techniques, role playing, problem solving, assertive behavior techniques, and other skills and techniques that may help the elderly "take more control" of their actions (Wolpe, 1973).

COGNITIVE THERAPY

This is also a brief, focused, problem-oriented therapy, but it is based on the hypothesis that depression results from "negative automatic thoughts" that must be interrupted by helping the individual identify and correct these cognitive errors to integrate more realistic thinking patterns (Beck et al., 1979). The role of the therapist is that of teacher or coach—encouraging active patient participation in the completion of assignments in which patients record automatic thoughts and consider alternative perspectives, thereby becoming able to set more realistic personal goals. According to cognitive therapy, the recurrence of depression may be prevented by changing the way the person thinks.

BRIEF PSYCHODYNAMIC THERAPY

This is based on the theory that emotional distress is derived from unresolved, intrapsychic conflicts from early life. The origins of the patient's behavior in conflicts and traumas of earlier life are clarified, and treatment focuses on the resolution of intrapsychic conflicts and the restructuring of personality. Elderly patients suitable for psychodynamically oriented psychotherapy are motivated, capable of introspection and psychological insight, show evidence of good adaptation earlier in life, and are able to tolerate strong emotions (Davanloo, 1980).

INTERPERSONAL THERAPY

This is a time-limited, interpersonally oriented form of psychotherapy that has been shown to be effective in treating depression. Interpersonal therapy is focused on the patient's relationship to significant others as opposed to the intrapsychic focus of brief psychodynamic therapy. The approach is based on the notion that patients who experience social disruptions are at increased risk of developing depression. Interpersonal therapy thus targets patients' relationships as the locus of intervention and is designed to assist patients in modifying either their relationships or their expectations about those relationships. The therapist's goal is to provide a corrective or healthy relationship with the patient to supply a model of a satisfying, interpersonal relationship. In so doing, the therapist actively converses and empathizes with the patient and validates his or her thoughts and feelings (Peplau, 1952; Sullivan, 1954).

SUPPORTIVE THERAPY

Whereas the previous psychotherapies are tied to theories of psychopathology, supportive psychotherapy techniques are not theory driven. Rather, they are based on what works and what seems to make the patient feel and function better. Supportive psychotherapy involves evaluating the patient's psychological strengths and weaknesses and helping the individual make choices that increase his or her functional capacity. The therapist often strives to reduce the patient's anxiety, which may be interfering with the adequate use of typical coping devices. The therapist also supports the patient's healthy defenses and when the individual's own defenses are inadequate, helps him or her find ways of coping with stress. Appropriate elderly candidates for supportive psychotherapy include healthy, high-functioning patients undergoing extreme stress as well as frail elderly people with a limited capacity for insight and poor verbal skills (Winston et al., 1986).

NURSING CARE OF THE DEPRESSED OLDER ADULT

Gerontological nurses who care for depressed older adults can play an important role in their recovery, since every interaction has therapeutic potential. Even without extensive psychiatric training, gerontological nurses can assist depressed elderly patients by encouraging verbalizations, especially about the problems that may be contributing to the depressed state; encouraging participation in activities, including self-care; encouraging decision making to increase a sense of control; teaching elderly patients how to be more assertive and to speak up for themselves; enhancing their self-concept by introducing opportunities for achievement and mastery over current stressors; and creating opportunities for interaction with others. Leading or participating in various individual and group therapeutic modalities can also contribute to the treatment process (Smith et al., 1993).

Another important role for gerontological nurses who lack psychiatric training is that of making prompt and appropriate referrals to mental health professionals. Nurses should provide as much pertinent background information as possible regarding the length of time depressive symptoms have been present, patient and family history, potential precipitating factors such as recent death of a spouse, and relevant medical and medication history. Referral to a mental health specialist is particularly appropriate if the elderly patient expresses suicidal ideation, has poor judgment, demonstrates psychotic (delusional) or manic symptoms, or refuses compliance with prescribed treatment plan or medications.

First-Line Psychosocial Interventions

The following first-line psychosocial approaches foster therapeutic potential and can be used by nurses in any setting. They should be implemented on a consistent basis and should be an integral part of the elderly patient's plan of care, since these interventions offer support and encouragement, provide structure, and encourage interaction and involvement with others (Smith et al., 1993).

Nurses can communicate caring by telling depressed elderly patients that they care about and value them; by asking them how they feel and what they think; and by letting them talk about what is bothering them. Gerontological nurses should try to understand the situation from the patient's viewpoint and should recognize and accept that the patient may be experiencing great sadness. This calls for a nonjudgmental and nonpunitive attitude that conveys interest and permits the expression of strong, even negative, emotions.

Nurses can assist the elderly to see if they are unusually sad or blue by asking questions that may help them identify what they are feeling sad about or what they may have lost or are grieving over. Recalling past positive events may help them see that things have not always been this bad. Elderly people's sense of self-worth can be enhanced by telling them about the positive things that are observed or known about them.

Nurses can provide accurate information about depression by telling elderly patients that depression is a common, treatable illness and that the symptoms they are experiencing are part of the illness and are likely to disappear or diminish as the depression

lifts. It is helpful to remind them that they have lived a long life and have survived many difficulties and that they can draw on those past experiences to help them through this current crisis. An important nursing role is to explain that both the use of medications and talking about their feelings (psychotherapy) can assist the elderly in reducing or eliminating depression.

Nurses can modify the physical or social environment by increasing sensory input through enhanced lighting and an increased use of touch as well as ensuring that patients are wearing clean, functioning assistive devices such as hearing aids and glasses. Plants or gardening activities may increase the elderly patient's bond with others who "grow things," and affectionate, accepting pets can provide unconditional positive regard. Nurses can provide a sense of structure and security in the environment through anticipatory guidance and setting limits only when the latter is necessary for the depressed patient's well-being. In most instances, it is preferable to not "do things" for the patients when they can perform a task for themselves—even if it takes longer for the patient.

Research-Based Nursing Interventions for Depression

GROUP THERAPY

A modest amount of literature has been devoted to the topic of group therapy for late-life depression. Clark and Vorst (1994) described a framework for treating chronically depressed elderly patients in an inpatient setting with group therapy that was integrated in the patient's treatment plan. Interventions were focused on the physiological, cognitive, behavioral, and social aspects of chronic depression. Other nurse researchers have investigated group therapy approaches for treating late-life depression primarily in long-term care settings and have noted that modifications in group therapy may be necessary to address factors such as cognitive and physical limitations of the elderly.

The results from these and other group therapy studies have been at best equivocal and in many cases discouraging. Scanland and Emershaw (1993), for example, examined the effects of reality orientation and validation therapy on cognitive status, functional status, and the level of depression of elderly people in a nursing home. There were no significant differences in pretest and posttest scores of mental or functional status for either therapy group, although postdepression scores revealed a slightly higher degree of depression. Several limitations may have influenced these findings, including a short time frame for the lack of control for comorbidity, dementia subtypes, medications, and a small, nonrandomized sample with a high rate of subject attrition. Because of the contradictory findings in these studies, Scanland and Emershaw identified the need to develop and test a theoretical framework with older adults.

Abraham and colleagues (1992) tested the effects of cognitive-behavioral and focused visual imagery group therapy, along with an education-discussion control group, on cognitive functioning and depression among frail, depressed nursing home residents. In contrast to studies on younger adults and community-dwelling elderly people, neither the cognitive-behavioral nor the focused visual imagery group therapy affected depression and its psychoemotional correlates of hopelessness and life satisfaction. However, the cognitive performance of those elderly people receiving either type of experimental intervention significantly improved, with individuals in the visual imagery group demonstrating the greatest improvement. The researchers suggested that in old age, expressions of a lack of well-being may not represent hopelessness and depression but rather a coming to terms with constraints—that is, a realistic acceptance of limitations. More research on the differential impact of these therapies on depression and cognition is clearly needed.

On a more positive note, Zerhusen and colleagues (1991) studied nursing home residents to determine if the long-term care staff members (two registered nurses and one social worker) could function effectively as group leaders to improve depression levels among residents. Subjects in a cognitive treatment group were compared with those in a music therapy group and a third group receiving routine nursing care. In contrast to the findings reported by Abraham and colleagues (1992), these nurse researchers found that cognitive therapy was an effective intervention for depression in the institutionalized elderly. Follow-up of residents in the cognitive therapy group was recommended to determine if the treatment effects are lasting or are dependent on program stimulation and the effects of the group leader.

ALTERNATIVE TREATMENT APPROACHES

Recently, alternative interventions to treat or prevent depression in older adults have been tried, with mixed success. Leja (1989) used *guided imagery,* defined as using the imagination to project positive future images to produce favorable physical changes and psychological adjustments, as a discharge teaching approach to combat postsurgical depression. She found that older adults had significantly lower depression scores 1 week after guided imagery discharge teaching but that the depression scores of the treatment group were not significantly different from those of elderly control patients who received routine discharge teaching. Further controlled investigations are needed before a guided imagery teaching approach can be recommended.

Therapeutic touch and *massage* are other nursing interventions that have been in the literature for more than a decade (Rowlands, 1984), although the terms are sometimes erroneously used interchangeably. These approaches are especially popular in Australia and Great Britain. In an Australian study of depressed nursing home residents, therapeutic massage was found to be a valuable and acceptable form of contact between nurses and residents with a short-term effect of elevating mood (Rowlands, 1984).

SUMMARY

Depression in the elderly is an important problem because of its prevalence and complexity.

The differential diagnosis of depression in older adults is confounded by a variety of factors, including cognitive impairment, medical illness, medications, and normal age-related changes. According to the Agency for Health Care Policy and Research guidelines on the treatment of major depression (U.S. Department of Health and Human Services, 1993), most depressive disorders in later life are highly treatable, and the efficacy of various treatments (e.g., antidepressant medication, psychotherapy, ECT) is comparable to that found in younger adults. However, there is still a need for more methodologically rigorous studies of interventions with older depressed patients, especially those with comorbid medical disorders. The failure to recognize and treat depression in later life can lead to increased healthcare use and costs, longer hospital stays, a lack of compliance with treatment regimes, and heightened morbidity and mortality associated with both medical illnesses and suicide. Advanced practice gerontological nurses working in a variety of settings are in an ideal situation to improve the quality of life of older adults through a systematic assessment and research-based management of late-life depression.

REFERENCES

Abraham, I. L., Neundorfer, M. M., & Currie, L. J. (1992). Effects of group interventions on cognition and depression in nursing home residents. *Nursing Research, 41*(4), 196–202.

Alden, D., Austin, C., & Sturgeon, R. (1989). A correlation between Geriatric Depression Scale long and short forms. *Journal of Gerontology, 44*, 124–125.

Allen, A., & Blazer, D. G. (1991). Mood disorders. In J. Sadavoy, L. Lazarus & L. Jarvik (Eds.), *Comprehensive review of geriatric psychiatry* (pp. 337–351). Washington, D.C.: American Psychiatric Press.

American Geriatrics Society (1993). *Geriatric health care: A visual presentation and lecture guide.* New York: American Geriatrics Society.

American Psychiatric Association (1994). *Diagnostic and statistical manual of mental disorders* (4th ed.). Washington, D.C.: American Psychiatric Association.

Aneshensel, C. S., Frerichs, R. R., & Huba, G. J. (1984). Depression and physical illness: A multiwave, nonrecursive causal model. *Journal of Health and Social Behavior, 25*, 350–371.

Badger, T. (1993). Physical health impairment and depression among older adults. *Image: Journal of Nursing Scholarship, 25*(4), 325–330.

Beck, A. T., Rush, A. J., Shaw, B. F., & Emery, G. (1979). *Cognitive therapy of depression.* New York: Guilford.

Berkman, L. F., Berkman, C. S., Kasl, S., et al. (1986). Depressive symptoms in relation to physical health and functioning in the elderly. *American Journal of Epidemiology, 124*, 372–388.

Black, D. W., Winokur, G., & Nasrallah, A. (1987). Treatment and outcome in secondary depression: A naturalistic study of 1087 patients. *Journal of Clinical Psychiatry, 4*, 438–441.

Blazer, D. (1989). Depression in the elderly. *New England Journal of Medicine, 320*, 164–166.

Blazer, D. (1991). Clinical features in depression in old age: A case for minor depression. *Current Opinion in Psychiatry, 4*, 596–599.

Blazer, D. (1993). *Depression in late life* (2nd ed.). St. Louis: Mosby.

Blazer, D., Burchett, B., Service, C., & George, L. K. (1991). The association of age and depression among the elderly: An epidemiologic exploration. *Journal of Gerontology, 46*, M210–M215.

Blazer, D., Hughes, D., & George, L. (1987). The epidemiology of depression in any elderly community population. *Gerontologist, 27*(3), 281–287.

Blumenthal, M. D., & Dielman, T. E. (1975). Depressive symptomatology and role function in a general population. *Archives of General Psychiatry, 32*, 985–991.

Bolla-Wilson, K., & Bleecker, M. L. (1989). Absence of depression in elderly adults. *Journal of Gerontology, 44*, 53–55.

Borson, S., Barnes, R. A., Kukill, W. A., et al. (1986). Symptomatic depression in elderly outpatients. I: Prevalence demography, and health service utilization. *Journal of the American Geriatrics Society, 34*, 341–347.

Brown, J. H., Henteleff, P., Barakat, S., & Rowe, C. J. (1986). Is it normal for terminally ill patients to desire death? *American Journal of Psychiatry, 143*, 208–211.

Brown University Long-Term Care Quality Newsletter (1994, October 24), *6*, p. 20.

Buckwalter, K. C. (1992). *Geriatric mental health nursing: Current and future challenges.* Thorofare, NJ: Slack, Inc.

Buschmann, M., & Rossen, E. (1993). Depression in older women. *Journal of Women's Health, 2*(3), 317–322.

Butler, R. N. (1974). Successful aging and the role of life review. *Journal of the American Geriatrics Society, 22*, 529–535.

Callahan, C. M., Hendrie, H. C., Dittus, R. S., et al. (1994). Improving treatment of late-life depression in primary care: A randomized clinical trial. *Journal of the American Geriatrics Society, 42*, 839–846.

Clark, W. G., & Vorst, V. R. (1994). Group therapy with chronically depressed geriatric patients. *Journal of Psychosocial Nursing and Mental Health Services, 32*(5), 9–13.

Cohen-Mansfield, J., & Marx, M. (1993). Pain and depression in the nursing home: Corroborating results. *Journal of Gerontology, 48*(2), 96–97.

Conwell, Y., & Caine, E. D. (1991). Rational suicide and the right to die. *New England Journal of Medicine, 325*, 1100–1102.

Craig, T. J., & Van Nata, P. A. (1993). Disability and depressive symptoms in two communities. *American Journal of Psychiatry, 140*, 598–600.

Davanloo, H. (1980). A method of short-term psychotherapy. In H. Davanloo (Ed.), *Short-term dynamic psychotherapy* (pp. 43–71). New York: Aronson.

Dupont, R. M., Cullum, M., & Jeste, D. V. (1988). Poststroke depression and psychosis. *Psychiatric Clinics of North America, 11,* 133–149.

Ensel, W. M. (1991). "Important" life events and depression among older adults. *Journal of Aging and Health, 3*(4), 546–566.

Erikson, E. (1963). *Childhood and society.* New York: W. W. Norton.

Frank, J. (1973). *Persuasion and healing.* Baltimore: Johns Hopkins University Press.

Gatz, M., & Hurwicz, M. (1990). Are old people more depressed? Cross-sectional data on the Center for Epidemiological Studies depression scale factors. *Psychology and Aging, 5*(2), 284–290.

German, P., Shapiro, S., Skinner, E., et al. (1987). Detection and management of mental health problems of older patients by primary care providers. *Journal of the American Medical Association, 257,* 489–493.

Gomez, G. E., & Gomez, E. A. (1992). The use of antidepressants with elderly patients. *Journal of Psychosocial Nursing, 30*(11), 21–26.

Gomez, G. E., & Gomez, E. A. (1993). Depression in the elderly. *Journal of Psychosocial Nursing, 31*(5), 28–33.

Harris, R. E., Mion, L. C., Patterson, M. B., & Frengley, J. D. (1988). Severe illness in older patients: The association between depressive disorders and functional dependency during the recovery phase. *Journal of the American Geriatrics Society, 36,* 890–896.

Harris, R. E., O'Hara, P. A., & Harper, D. W. (1995). Functional status of geriatric rehabilitation patients: A one-year follow-up study. *Journal of the American Geriatrics Society, 43,* 51–55.

Husaini, B. A., Moore, S. T., Castor, R. S., et al. (1991). Social density, stressors, and depression: Gender differences among the black elderly. *Journal of Gerontology, 46*(5), 236–242.

Jacobs, B. (1994). Serotonin, motor activity and depression-related disorders. *American Scientist, 82,* 456–463.

Jacobsen, S. (1995). Overselling depression to the old folks. *Atlantic Monthly, 3*(1), 46–51.

Kathol, R., Katon, W., Smith, G. R., et al. (1994). Guidelines for the diagnosis and treatment of depression for primary care physicians. *Psychosomatics, 35,* 1–6.

Keilholz, L., Dettli, V. E., Eckert, V., & Waser, P. G. (1989). Dosage and side effects of psychotropic drugs in elderly patients. *International Review of Psychiatry, 1,* 167–168.

Kitchell, M. A., Barnes, R. F., Veith, R. C., et al. (1982). Screening for depression in hospitalized geriatric medical patients. *Journal of the American Geriatrics Society, 30,* 174–177.

Koenig, H., & Blazer, D. (1992). Mood disorders and suicide. In J. Birren, R. B. Sloane & G. Cohen (Eds.), *Handbook of mental health and aging* (pp. 379–407). San Diego: Academic Press.

Koenig, H. G., Meador, K. G., Cohen, H. J., & Blazer, D. G. (1988). Depression in elderly hospitalized patients with medical illness. *Archives of Internal Medicine, 148,* 1929–1936.

Koenig, H., Shelp, F., Goli, V., et al. (1989). Survival and health care utilization in elderly medical inpatients with major depression. *Journal of the American Geriatrics Society, 37,* 599–606.

Kurlowicz, L. H. (1994). Depression in hospitalized medically ill elders: Evolution of the concept. *Archives of Psychiatric Nursing, 8*(2), 124–136.

Lazarus, L. W., Sadavoy, J., & Langley, P. R. (1991). Individual psychotherapy. In J. Sadavoy, L. W. Lazarus & L. F. Jarvik (Eds.), *Comprehensive review of geriatric psychiatry* (pp. 487–511). Washington, D.C.: American Psychiatric Press.

Lebowitz, B. D. (1994). Depression is diabetes—demanding parity for mental health. *Aging Today Forum, 1,* 1–5.

Leja, A. M. (1989). Using guided imagery to combat post-surgical depression. *Journal of Gerontological Nursing, 15*(4), 7–11.

Leidy, N. K. (1994). Functional status and the forward progress of merry-go-rounds: Toward a coherent analytical framework. *Nursing Research, 43,* 196–202.

Manton, K. G., Blazer, D. G., & Woodbury, M. A. (1987). Suicide in middle age and later life: Sex and race specific life table and cohort analyses. *Journal of Gerontology, 42*(2), 219–227.

McNeal, E. T., & Cimbolic, P. (1986). Antidepressant and biochemical theories of depression. *Psychological Bulletin, 99*(3), 361–374.

Meyers, B. (1994). Epidemiology and clinical meaning of "significant" depressive symptoms in later life: The question of subsyndromal depression. *American Journal of Geriatric Psychiatry, 2,* 188–193.

Mossey, J. M., Knott, K., & Craik, R. (1990). The effects of persistent depressive symptoms on hip fracture recovery. *Journal of Gerontology, 45,* 163–168.

Mumford, E., Schlesinger, H. J., Glass, G. V., et al. (1984). A new look at evidence about reduced cost of medical utilization following mental health treatment. *American Journal of Psychiatry, 141,* 1145–1158.

Murrell, S. A., Himmelfarb, S., & Wright, K. (1983). Prevalence of depression and its correlates in older adults. *American Journal of Epidemiology, 117,* 173–185.

Myers, J., Weissman, M., Tischler, G., et al. (1984). Six-month prevalence of psychiatric disorders in three communities: 1980–1982. *Archives of General Psychiatry, 41,* 959–967.

National Institute of Mental Health (1993). *D/ART (depression/awareness, recognition and treatment) program fact sheet.* Rockville, MD: National Institute of Mental Health.

National Institutes of Health (1992). Consensus conference diagnosis and treatment of depression in late life. *Journal of the American Medical Association, 268*(8), 1018–1027.

Nuland, S. B. (1993). *How we die—reflections on life's final chapter.* New York: Alfred A. Knopf.

O'Hara, M., Kohut, F., & Wallace, R. B. (1985). Depression among the rural elderly: A study of prevalence and correlates. *Journal of Nervous and Mental Disease, 173*(10), 582–589.

Parmelee, P. A., Katz, I. R., & Lawton, M. P. (1992). Depression and mortality among institutionalized aged. *Journal of Gerontology, 47*(1), 3–10.

Paulmeno, S. R. (1987). Psychogeriatric care: A specialty within a specialty. *Nursing Management, 2,* 39–142.

Peplau, H. E. (1952). *Interpersonal relations in nursing.* New York: G. P. Putnam's Sons.

Perry, P. J., Alexander, B., & Liskow, B. I. (1991). *Psychotropic drug handbook*. Cincinnati, OH: Harvey Whitney Books.

Radloff, L. S. (1977). A self-report depression scale for research in the general population. *Applied Psychological Measurement, 1*, 385–401.

Robinson, R. G., Starr, L. B., & Price, T. R. (1984). A two-year longitudinal study of mood disorder following stroke: Prevalence and duration at six-month follow-up. *British Journal of Psychiatry, 144*, 256–261.

Rodin, G., & Voshart, B. (1986). Depression in the medically ill: An overview. *American Journal of Psychiatry, 143*, 696–705.

Rovner, B. W., Gerrman, P. S., Brant, L. J., et al. (1991). Depression and mortality in nursing homes. *Journal of the American Medical Association, 265*(8), 993–996.

Rowlands, D. (1984). Therapeutic touch: Its effects on the depressed elderly. *Australian Nurses Journal, 13*(11), 45–52.

Scanland, S. G., & Emershaw, L. E. (1993). Reality orientation and validation therapy. *Journal of Gerontological Nursing, 19*(6), 7–11.

Schleifer, S. J., Macari-Hinson, M. M., Coyle, D. A., et al. (1989). The nature and course of depression following myocardial infarction. *Archives of Internal Medicine, 149*, 1785–1789.

Seligman, M. (1975). *Helplessness: On depression, development and death*. San Francisco: W. H. Freeman.

Smith, M., & Buckwalter, K. C. (1992). Medication management, antidepressant drugs and the elderly: An overview. *Journal of Psychosocial Nursing, 30*(10), 30–36.

Smith, M., Buckwalter, K. C., & Mitchell, S. (1993). *Geriatric mental health training series*. New York: Springer.

Soltys, F. G., & Coats, L. (1994). The SolCos model: Facilitating reminiscence therapy. *Journal of Gerontological Nursing, 20*(11), 11–16.

Sullivan, H. S. (1954). *The psychiatric interview*. New York: W. W. Norton.

Thompson, L. W., & Gallagher, D. (1986). Psychotherapy for late-life depression. *Generations, 10*(3), 38–41.

Thompson, L. W., Gallagher, D., & Breckenridge, J. S. (1987). Comparative effectiveness of psychotherapies for depressed elders. *Journal of Consulting Clinical Psychology, 55*, 385–390.

Turner, R. J., & Noh, S. (1988). Physical disability and depression: A longitudinal analysis. *Journal of Health and Social Behavior, 29*, 23–37.

U.S. Department of Health and Human Services (1993). *Depression in Primary Care: Volume 1, Detection and Diagnosis; Volume 2, Treatment of Major Depression*. (Agency for Health Care Policy and Research Publ. No. 93-0550). Rockville, MD: U.S. Department of Health and Human Services.

Walker, T. (Ed.), *Alliance for the Mentally Ill of Johnson County Newsletter* (1994, November), pp. 1–3.

Wells, K. B., Stewart, A., Hays, R., et al. (1989). The functioning and well-being of depressed patients. *Journal of the American Medical Association, 262*, 914–919.

Winston, A., Pinsker, H., & McCullough, L. (1986). A review of supportive psychotherapy. *Hospital and Community Psychiatry, 37*, 1105–1114.

Wolpe, J. (1973). *The practice of behavior therapy* (2nd ed.). New York: Pergamon Press.

Yesavage, J., & Brink, T. L. (1983). Development and validation of a geriatric depression screening scale: A preliminary report. *Journal of Psychiatric Research, 17*, 37–49.

Zanke, D., & Hunter, T. S. (1986). Polypharmacy and altered pharmacokinetics in nursing homes (pp. 129–141). In M. S. Harper & B. D. Lebowitz (Eds.), *Mental illness in nursing homes: Agenda for research* (DHHS Publication No. ADM 86-1459). Rockville, MD: U.S. Department of Health and Human Resources, National Institute of Mental Health.

Zerhusen, J. D., Boyle, K., & Wilson, W. (1991). Out of the darkness: Group cognitive therapy for depressed elderly. *Journal of Psychosocial Nursing and Mental Health Services, 29*(9), 16–21.

Delirium and Dementia

Helen D. Davies

Disorders causing a decline in cognitive function affect approximately 15% of the population older than 65 years. Cognitive deficits are seen in 5% of the elderly older than 65 years and in 20% of the elderly older than 75 years who live in the community. One third to one half of hospitalized elderly people exhibit cognitive changes, and more than 50% of those residing in nursing homes are cognitively impaired (Kane et al., 1994). Depending on the degree of cognitive decline, the consequences for an older person can range from minor problems in performing day-to-day activities to devastation in terms of the person's self-identity, level of independence, relationships with others, and overall quality of life.

The most common conditions associated with cognitive decline in the elderly are dementia and delirium (Berkow et al., 1995). Other conditions affecting cognitive function include depression, paranoid states and other psychoses, amnestic syndromes, and age-associated memory impairment (benign senescent forgetfulness) (Kane et al., 1994; Mayeaux et al., 1993). This chapter addresses the causes, clinical presentation, assessment, and management of delirium and dementia.

DELIRIUM

Delirium, also referred to as *acute confusional states*, is a serious, often unrecognized neuro-psychiatric syndrome (Lipowski, 1994; Tune & Ross, 1994). It is especially prominent in older adults. Delirium is to the elderly what fever is to the young, in that the majority of individuals presenting with delirium suffer from a specific physical illness. Delirium may occur during the course of a dementing illness owing to the development of a new medical condition, which may evolve "silently" without a fever or other physical signs (Berkow et al., 1995). Table 18–1 lists the diagnostic criteria for delirium.

Epidemiology

Exact figures on the incidence of delirium are difficult to obtain for several reasons: the disorder is often undiagnosed, there is a failure to use consistent diagnostic criteria, terms are used inconsistently, and various methods of case finding are used by researchers (Francis, 1992; Lipowski, 1984; Miller & Lipowski, 1991).

TABLE 18-1
Diagnostic Criteria for Delirium

A. Disturbances of consciousness (i.e., reduced clarity of awareness of the environment) with reduced ability to focus, sustain, or shift attention.

B. A change in cognition (e.g., memory deficit, disorientation, language disturbance) or the development of a perceptual disturbance that is not accounted for by a preexisting, established, or evolving dementia.

C. The disturbance develops over a short period (usually hours or days) and tends to fluctuate during the course of the day.

D. There is evidence from the history, physical examination, or laboratory findings that the disturbance is caused by the direct physiological consequences of a general medical condition.

Adapted from American Psychiatric Association (1994). *Diagnostic and statistical manual of mental disorders* (4th ed., p. 129). Washington, D.C.: American Psychiatric Association. Copyright 1994, the American Psychiatric Association. Reprinted by permission.

In studies using the *Diagnostic and statistical manual of mental disorders* (DSM-III or DSM-IIR) criteria, prevalence rates of medical inpatients varied from 11 to 33%, and incidence rates varied from 4.2 to 10.4% (Levkoff et al., 1991; Tune & Ross, 1994). Acute confusional states have been reported in 10 to 15% of surgical patients, 30% of open heart surgical patients, and more than 50% of hip fracture patients (Francis, 1992).

Etiology

Causes of delirium can be classified as either predisposing or precipitating factors. Age itself is a predisposing factor. Thus, anything that affects brain function in the elderly can exacerbate the predisposition to delirium (Zisook & Braff, 1986). At high risk are people who have cardiac disorders or who abuse alcohol or drugs as well as elderly patients who have cognitive or memory disorders and have undergone trauma, surgery, or sudden environmental changes. Intoxication with medications, especially cholinergic drugs, is probably one of the most common causes of delirium in elderly people (Lipowski, 1994). Oncology patients are at risk owing to metabolic and nutritional imbalances, metastases, and infections. Patients with known neurological disturbances, such as strokes, head trauma, and brain tumors, and those with fever and dehydration are also at high risk. Table 18–2 presents some of the most frequent causes of delirium.

Clinical Presentation

People suffering from delirium have a decreased ability to attend to environmental stimuli and often show highly disruptive and variable behavior. The onset of delirium is acute, ranging from a few hours to a few weeks. Delirium is usually worse at night, and patients with delirium may have lucid intervals during which it is difficult to detect any disorder. Patients with delirium may present with a range of psychopathological symptoms, including delusions, hallucinations, confabulations, and a variety of emotions such as fear, anger, and apathy (Lipowski, 1994). Observers

TABLE 18-2
Systemic and Central Nervous System Causes of Delirium

Systemic Causes

Cardiovascular disease
  Congestive heart failure
  Arrhythmias
  Cardiac infarction
  Hypovolemia
  Aortic stenosis

Infections
  Pneumonia
  Urinary tract infection
  Bacteremia
  Septicemia

Medications
  Analgesics
  Anticholinergics
  Antidepressants
  Antihistamines
  Antiparkinsonian agents
  Cimetidine
  Digitalis glycosides
  Diuretics
  Neuroleptics
  Sedatives or hypnotics

Metabolic
  Electrolyte and fluid imbalance
  Hepatic, renal, or pulmonary failure
  Diabetes, hyperthyroidism or hypothyroidism, and other
    endocrinopathies
  Nutritional deficiencies
  Hypothermia and heat stroke

Neoplasm

Postoperative state

Substance abuse and
    poisons
  Alcohol
  Amphetamines
  Sedatives or hypnotics
  Heavy metals
  Solvents
  Pesticides
  Carbon monoxide

Trauma
  Head injury
  Burns
  Hip fracture

Central Nervous System Causes

Infection
  Meningitis
  Encephalitis
  Septic emboli
  Neurosyphilis
  Brain abscess

Neoplasm
  Primary intracranial
  Metastatic (bronchogenic or
    breast)

Trauma
  Subdural hematoma
  Extradural hematoma
  Contusion

Vascular disorder
  Transient ischemic episodes
  Stroke
  Chronic subdural hematoma
  Vasculitis
  Arteriosclerosis
  Hypertensive
    encephalopathy
  Subarachnoid hemorrhage

Seizure
  Ictal and postictal states

From Zisook, S., & Braff, D. L. (1986). Delirium: Recognition and management in the older patient. *Geriatrics, 41*(6), p. 73. Copyright 1986 by Edgell Communications, Inc.

have suggested that delirious patients differ in their levels of alertness. Some patients may be confused and unable to focus attention or respond to their environment appropriately but may nevertheless appear relatively alert. Other patients may be similarly confused but appear drowsy or stuporous (Tune & Ross, 1994). Several researchers have classified such patients as *active/somnolent* (Ross et al., 1991) or *hyperalert/hyperactive* and *hypoalert/hypoactive* (Lipowski, 1989). Characteristic features of delirium, such as clouding of consciousness, disorientation, memory impairment, incoherent speech, and perceptual disturbances, all give rise to behavior that appears confused. To ensure the early recognition and treatment of delirium, frequent assessments of mental status should be performed in high-risk patients at the first signs of inappropriate or labile behavior. Evidence of disturbances in attention and arousal as well as disorientation and abnormal behavior is essential in establishing the presence of delirium (Zisook & Braff, 1986). Sullivan and Fogel (1986) cautioned against overemphasizing disorientation as a presenting sign for the diagnosis of delirium. They described four early cases of delirium that masqueraded as a violent personality disorder, a factitious illness, uncooperative behavior, and psychotic suicidal ideas.

Differential Diagnosis

Dementia must be ruled out in the differential diagnosis of delirium. Dementia usually follows a relatively stable course of impairment, whereas delirium is often a variable waxing and waning syndrome (Lipowski, 1994). In a large study of admissions to a general medical service, Erkinjuntti and associates (1986) found that 41.4% of the patients with dementia had delirium on admission and that 24.9% of all delirium patients had a dementing illness (Tune & Ross, 1994). If in doubt, the syndrome should be treated provisionally as delirium. Dementia patients may become delirious, but when the delirium clears the dementia remains. Table 18–3 shows the characteristics used to distinguish delirium and dementia.

Management

Delirium can present a life-threatening situation and must be recognized and treated

TABLE 18-3

Differentiating Delirium from Dementia

	Delirium	Dementia
Onset	Sudden, acute	Insidious
Course	Marked contrasts in level of awareness	Not seen in such contrast Slow, progressive decline
Duration	Hours to weeks	In progress at least 1–2 yr
Level of awareness, alertness, and attention	Hypoalert or hyperalert and aware Level fluctuates	Not affected
Cognitive function, including orientation, thinking, and memory	Preserved during lucid intervals Focal cognitive deficits Orientation impaired for a time Immediate and recent memory impaired	Consistent loss and decline Global cognitive deficits Impaired orientation Recent and remote memory impairment
Affect	Intermittent fear, perplexity, or bewilderment	Flat or indifferent affect
Perceptual disturbances	Hallucinations often disturbing and very clearly defined	Hallucinations vague, fleeting, ill defined; in many cases, it is difficult to make a clear judgment that they exist
Thought disturbances Paranoid states	Prominent, while cognitive impairment is mild or variable	More consistent with degree of impairment; less-prominent paranoia
Persecutory delusions	Ordered and cohesive	Vague, random, contradictory
Cause	Usually medical illness or drugs	Alzheimer's disease and multiple infarcts are most common causes
Treatment	Requires immediate evaluation and treatment	Not required immediately Requires ongoing monitoring and evaluation with attention to preventable and treatable conditions that may occur

Data from Berkow et al. (1995); Cummings et al. (1997); and Kane et al. (1994).

promptly. It is essential to determine and treat the underlying medical causes and to provide supportive care. When treated promptly, delirium is usually completely reversible. If the underlying factor is not reversed, however, delirium can lead to chronic brain impairment and death. Studies estimate the in-hospital fatality rate for elderly patients with delirium to be 25 to 33% (Gottlieb et al., 1991; Inouye et al., 1990). Delirium itself is not the cause of death, but the underlying medical condition may be. Delirium should always be treated as a medical emergency.

Treatment efforts should focus on determining and treating the cause or causes of the delirium and maintaining physiological balance with hydration, nutrition, oxygen supply, and electrolyte balance. All unnecessary medications should be discontinued until the prob-

lem has been resolved. The use of a low-dose neuroleptic such as haloperidol (0.5–2.0 mg twice a day) may be necessary if the patient is agitated, but it should be discontinued as soon as the patient has recovered. *Neuroleptic malignant syndrome*, a rare, potentially lethal side effect of neuroleptics, can occur in elderly, delirious patients (Francis & Kapoor, 1990). Neuroleptic malignant syndrome is associated with a change in consciousness, fever, and rigidity. Careful monitoring of the patient's neurological state is essential to identify possible side effects. Owing to the fluctuating course of delirium, patients must be deemed stable for 48 hours before recovery can be considered certain (Zisook & Braff, 1986).

Nursing management of delirium may include prevention, detection, and intervention. Using knowledge of the predisposing factors as a guide, nurses can anticipate delirium and institute preventive measures. The following specific measures may benefit an elderly patient who is hospitalized with a preexisting dementia or whose cerebral function is compromised (Campbell et al., 1986; Tueth & Cheong, 1993):

1. If the patient is being hospitalized for scheduled elective surgery, family members should be encouraged to have a familiar person stay with the patient around the clock for the first few postoperative days. A familiar person can provide reality feedback, comfort, and a sense of continuity with the patient's life before hospitalization.
2. Attention should be paid to nonpharmaceutical comfort measures, as analgesic medications predispose patients to delirium, and medications with anticholinergic effects have cumulative effects and can cause delirium.
3. The patient's reliance on medication may be decreased through proper positioning, massage, maintaining comfortable temperature, and allowing maximum mobility.
4. The patient's orientation and alertness may be maximized by decreasing unnecessary noise, explaining all actions, providing orienting sensory input with brief but frequent contacts, and using staffing patterns that allow for continuity of care.
5. The incidence of dehydration or electrolyte imbalance will decrease with carefully monitored intake, output, skin turgor, and laboratory test results.

Patients in the community are equally susceptible to delirium. Particularly at risk are those patients who are frail, impaired, and living alone and those who have one or more chronic illnesses. Nurses may take an active role in caregiver education, teaching caregivers to be alert to subtle changes and to seek medical attention promptly for any sudden appearance of agitation, hallucinations, lethargy, somnolence, or sleep disturbance, even in patients with a preexisting dementia. The latter patients are particularly likely to have an undiagnosed delirium because the sudden change is interpreted simply as worsening of the existing dementia. Community health and homecare nurses should monitor frail, community-dwelling elderly people routinely for adequate nutrition and hydration, alcohol use, or misuse of medications. The same interventions are applicable to patients in long-term care settings.

Because nurses have continual contact with the elderly in many settings, they are often the first to detect delirium. The appearance of signs and symptoms that might indicate delirium should lead to immediate further investigation. These symptoms, all of which can fluctuate, can include difficulty with thinking and remembering, disoriented perception, disordered attention, and somnolence or night wakefulness. Vital signs should be taken and compared with baseline values. Assessment includes neurological, cardiovascular, and respiratory evaluations and a review of current medications. Findings from a mental status test should be compared with the patient's baseline function. The patient is screened for fluid volume deficit and hypoglycemia or hyperglycemia. Laboratory studies should include complete blood count with differential; blood urea nitrogen; and levels of creatinine, electrolytes, and glucose. If there are physical findings of respiratory insufficiency, a specimen for arterial blood gas should be drawn (Foreman, 1984). The presence of signs of delirium combined with positive findings in any of the above tests indicates that delirium is a likely diagnosis.

The first step in treating delirium is to find and treat or remove the causative factor. This process involves time. In the interval, providing nursing care for the patient with delirium presents a challenge. Primary nursing goals are to ensure patient safety and comfort and to intervene to mitigate psychiatric symptoms. Patients with delirium require hospitalization; if possible, they should be in a private room with continual supervision. The immediate environment should be quiet and as uncluttered and simple as possible. Patients with delirium are highly excitable and irritable and are prone to misinterpret stimuli. The presence of familiar objects, such as a large calendar and clock, is important. Ideally the room should have a view to provide cues to time and place. Lighting should be soft and diffuse to avoid sharp contrasts and shadows that can be misperceived. Patients who normally use hearing aids or glasses should be allowed to keep them (Levkoff et al., 1986; Tune & Ross 1994). The use of restraints should be avoided whenever possible (see Chapter 25).

Interactions with the patient should be kept to a minimum during periods of agitation. Medication may be used to treat symptoms of sleep-wake disturbance, hallucinations, and illusions present during agitated periods. Short–half-life benzodiazepines such as temazepam can be used to correct disturbed sleep-wake cycles. Because a patient with delirium is already impaired, care should be taken to use the lowest effective dose. As a rule of thumb, the starting dose should be one third the usual adult dose. The necessary nursing care, attending to hygiene, hydration, and nutrition should be given during periods of relative calm and lucidity. At these times the nurse can provide corrective sensory input while administering care.

The patient may need frequent reorientation to the surroundings and situation. Patients with delirium may not remember where or why they are hospitalized and may need to be retold the location and duration of the hospital stay and the events leading to it. Consider telling the patient that he or she is confused and disoriented. This can be done in a gently reassuring manner, emphasizing the positive aspects of the situation. Small improvements, such as a change from parenteral to oral nutrition, ambulating for greater distances, or taking a shower independently can be praised in a way that encourages the patient. A conversational tone and style by the nurse conveys respect and concern without being condescending. Successful nursing management of delirium includes monitoring and reporting the patient's condition and providing protection, support, and basic physical needs.

DEMENTIA

Clinicians have long recognized that dementia is a common clinical syndrome seen in the elderly; however, it is only in the past decade that the condition has been the subject of intensive systematic study (Katzman, 1992; Schoenberg, 1986). The knowledge gained has resulted in definitions and diagnostic criteria for this condition as well as a greater accuracy in its diagnosis.

Dementia is a symptom complex characterized by intellectual deterioration occurring in the presence of a clear state of consciousness. The intellectual deterioration is severe enough to interfere with social or occupational functioning and represents a decline from a previously higher level of functioning. Memory impairment, a prominent early symptom, is required to make the diagnosis of dementia. Dementia involves progressive deficits not only in memory but also in other cognitive areas, such as language, perception, praxis, learning, problem solving, abstract thinking, and judgment. Personality characteristics may be maintained or exaggerated in some patients and may be altered in others. Social withdrawal, fearfulness, and anxiety are common features. Paranoid symptoms and delusions can sometimes occur (American Psychiatric Association, 1994). Irritability, agitation, and verbal and physical aggression toward family members may develop as the dementia progresses and the individual experiences an increasing loss of control of his or her environment. Table 18–4 lists the diagnostic criteria for dementia.

Age-associated memory impairment (AAMI), also known as *benign senescent forgetfulness*, is distinctive from the changes caused by dementia. AAMI refers to the mild memory loss seen in elderly people. Memory loss in AAMI is not progressive, and other areas of cognitive function are not affected. Healthy older people with AAMI should be differentiated from those with early signs of a dementing illness. This important distinction can be made by observing over time for increased memory problems and cognitive decline as well as through psychometric testing (Kane et al., 1994; Mayeux et al., 1993). People with depression may appear demented; therefore, it is important to rule out depression in establishing the diagnosis of dementia (see Chapter 17). It is also critical to differentiate dementia from delirium, which is a more acute condition in which the level of

---

TABLE 18-4
Diagnostic Criteria for Dementia

A. Development of multiple cognitive deficits manifested by both
1. Memory impairment (impaired ability to learn new information or to recall previously learned information)
2. One (or more) of the following cognitive disturbances:
   a. Aphasia (language disturbance)
   b. Apraxia (impaired ability to carry out motor activities despite intact motor function)
   c. Agnosia (failure to recognize or identify objects despite intact sensory function)
   d. Disturbance in executive functioning (i.e., planning, organizing, sequencing, abstracting)
B. The cognitive deficits in criteria A1 and A2 each cause significant impairment in social or occupational functioning and represent a significant decline from a previous level of functioning.

Adapted from American Psychiatric Association (1994). *Diagnostic and statistical manual of mental disorders* (4th ed., pp. 142–143). Washington, D.C.: American Psychiatric Association. Copyright 1994, the American Psychiatric Association. Reprinted by permission.

---

alertness and awareness fluctuates (Berkow et al., 1995; Larson et al., 1992).

Recognizing the dementia is only the first step; to care for the patient, one must also understand the impact on the family and the environment. This chapter examines dementia not only as a diagnostic entity but also from a psychosocial perspective involving both patient and family.

Epidemiology

By the year 2040, an estimated 11.8 million people in the United States will be afflicted with some form of dementia (Evans, 1990). Similar trends are expected for many developed countries (Cooper, 1991; Schoenberg, 1986). The prevalence of dementia increases with age. Community surveys demonstrate that 4.6% of individuals older than 65 years have severe dementia and 10% have mild to moderate dementia. Prevalence rates vary significantly between the ages of 65 and 85 years. Severe dementia is thought to be present in fewer than 1% of those who are 65 years of

age but in more than 15% of those who are older than 85 years (Bachman et al., 1992). In the age range of 75 to 85 years, severe dementia is as frequent as myocardial infarction (Katzman, 1986).

Documenting the onset of dementia, as is required for studies of incidence or survival, is difficult because of the slow progressive nature of the condition. Mortality tabulations do not provide a reliable estimate, as deaths among demented individuals are often attributed to other underlying causes. Despite the prevalence of dementia in the elderly, the diagnosis is frequently missed (McCartney & Palmateer, 1985; U'Ren, 1987). Because many patients in the early stages of dementia may not be seen by a physician or are not diagnosed, the true magnitude of the problem may be underreported (Katzman, 1992).

Types of Dementias

Dementia can occur from a multitude of causes that may occur singly or in various combinations. These causes are broadly classified as *reversible* or *irreversible*. Table 18–5 lists the most common causes of dementia under these categories.

Some causes of dementia can be treated and ameliorated, whereas others are irreversible given the current state of knowledge. In a critical review of 32 studies investigating the prevalence of the causes of dementia, Clarfield (1988) found that 13.2% of all cases were potentially reversible. However, these studies did not always follow up the more important question of whether patients with potentially reversible causes actually achieved a reversal in their mental status. In 11 studies that did provide follow-up, 11% of dementias were resolved, either partially (8%) or fully (3%). The common reversible causes were drugs (28.2%), depression (26.2%), and metabolic disorders (15.5%). The true incidence of reversible dementias in the community is believed to be even lower (Clarfield, 1988, 1995).

Major Dementias in the Elderly

At present, it is estimated that more than 70 disorders cause dementia, with acquired im-

TABLE 18-5

Reversible and Irreversible Causes of Dementia

Potentially Reversible Causes

Cardiopulmonary disorders
   Hypertension
   Severe cardiac failure
   Cardiac arrest
Depression
Drug toxicity, including alcohol
Normal pressure hydrocephalus
Space-occupying lesions
   Subdural hematomas
   Primary brain tumor
Metabolic-endocrine derangements
   Hyperthyroidism or hypothyroidism
   Hyperparathyroidism
   Hypernatremia or hyponatremia
   Hypoglycemia
Nutritional deficiency states
   Thiamine deficiency
   Folate deficiency
   Cobalamin deficiency (vitamin B_{12})
Infections
   Bacterial meningitis or encephalitis
   Brain abscess
   Neurosyphilis

Probable Irreversible Causes

Alzheimer's disease
Dementia with Lewy bodies
Pick's disease
Huntington's disease
Multi-infarct dementia
Amyotrophic lateral sclerosis
Parkinson's disease
Cerebellar degenerations
Alcoholism—Korsakoff's syndrome
Infections
   Creutzfeldt-Jakob disease
   Acquired immunodeficiency syndrome

Data from Berkow et al. (1995); Feldman & Plum (1993); Kane et al. (1994); Katzman (1992); and Miller (1997).

mune deficiency syndrome being the latest cause identified (Katzman, 1992). The most common dementias seen in the elderly are Alzheimer's disease (AD), multi-infarct dementia (MID), and dementias secondary to metabolic endocrine derangements, with alcohol and medications being major contributors (Feldman & Plum, 1993; Katzman, 1992). AD accounts for 50 to 60% of all cases (Cummings, 1995), and vascular disease, specifically MID, accounts for 10 to 15%. Some patients may have both disorders. Other causes include alcoholic dementia (5–10%), normal pressure hydrocephalus (6%), intracranial masses (5%), and Huntington's chorea (3%). In 5% of the cases, the cause remains unknown (Chui et al., 1992; Kase, 1991; Katzman, 1992).

ALZHEIMER'S DISEASE

Alzheimer's disease, named after Alois Alzheimer, who first described its neuropathology in 1907, is a neurological disorder of the brain that occurs primarily in middle or late life, although it may occur earlier. Its primary characteristic is a progressive dementia. The pathology includes the degeneration and loss of nerve cells (neurons), particularly in those regions essential for memory and cognition, and the presence of neuritic plaques and neurofibrillary tangles. Aggregates of amyloid protein can be seen adjacent to and within the walls of many cerebral and leptomeningeal blood vessels (Brousseau et al., 1994; Selkoe, 1991). Alterations occur in the neurotransmitter and neuromodulator levels, especially in the cholinergic system and frequently in the somatostatinergic, glutamatergic, and noradrenergic systems (Ingram et al., 1994; Katzman, 1984).

Diagnostic criteria for AD were established by the National Institute of Neurological and Communicative Disorders and Stroke and the Alzheimer's Disease and Related Disorders Association (NINCDS-ADRDA) (Table 18–6). At present, a definitive diagnosis of AD can be made only through an examination of brain tissue obtained during either postmortem examination or a brain biopsy. In most cases, the risks of brain biopsy far outweigh the benefits. Therefore, the diagnosis is made by a systematic exclusion of all other possible causes of dementia. If the symptoms are progressive, follow a pattern over time, and are attributable to no other cause, a clinical diagnosis of probable AD should be made. In patients with an atypical presentation, a diagnosis of possible AD may be made and the patient followed at regular intervals to assist in clarifying the diagnosis (McKhann et al., 1984).

Epidemiology. The prevalence of AD in-

TABLE 18-6

NINCDS-ADRDA Criteria for Clinical Diagnosis of Alzheimer's Disease

I. The criteria for the clinical diagnosis of PROBABLE Alzheimer's disease:

Dementia established by clinical examination, documented by the Mini-Mental Test, Blessed Dementia Scale, or some similar examination, and confirmed by neuropsychological tests:

Deficits in two or more areas of cognition

Progressive worsening of memory and other cognitive functions

No disturbance of consciousness

Onset between the ages of 40 and 90 years, most often after age 65 years

Absence of systemic disorders or other brain diseases that in and of themselves could account for the progressive deficits in memory and cognition

II. The diagnosis of PROBABLE Alzheimer's disease is supported by the following:

Progressive deterioration of specific cognitive functions such as language (aphasia), motor skills (apraxia), and perception (agnosia)

Impaired activities of daily living and altered patterns of behavior

Family history of similar disorders, particularly if confirmed neuropathologically

Laboratory results of the following:

Normal lumbar puncture as evaluated by standard techniques

Normal pattern or nonspecific changes in electroencephalogram, such as increased slow-wave activity

Evidence of cerebral atrophy on computed tomography, with progression documented by serial observation

III. Other clinical features consistent with the diagnosis of PROBABLE Alzheimer's disease, after exclusion of causes of dementia other than Alzheimer's disease:

Plateaus in the course of progression of the illness

Associated symptoms of depression; insomnia; incontinence; delusions; illusions; hallucinations; catastrophic verbal, emotional, or physical outbursts; sexual disorders; and weight loss

Other neurological abnormalities in some patients, especially with more advanced disease, including motor signs such as increased muscle tone, myoclonus, or gait disorder

Seizures in advanced disease

Computed tomography normal for age

IV. Features that make the diagnosis of PROBABLE Alzheimer's disease uncertain or unlikely:

Sudden, apoplectic onset

Focal neurological findings such as hemiparesis, sensory loss, visual field deficits, and incoordination early in the course of the illness

Seizures or gait disturbances at the onset or very early in the course of the illness

V. Clinical diagnosis of POSSIBLE Alzheimer's disease:

May be made on the basis of the dementia syndrome, in the absence of other neurological, psychiatric, or systemic disorders sufficient to cause dementia, and in the presence of variations in the onset, in the presentation, or in the clinical course

May be made in the presence of a second systemic or brain disorder sufficient to produce dementia, which is not considered to be *the* cause of the dementia

Should be used in research studies when a single, gradually progressive severe cognitive deficit is identified in the absence of another identifiable cause

VI. Criteria for diagnosis of DEFINITE Alzheimer's disease:

Clinical criteria for probable Alzheimer's disease

Histopathologic evidence obtained from a biopsy or autopsy

VII. Classification of Alzheimer's disease for research purposes should specify features that may differentiate subtypes of the disorder, such as:

Familial occurrence

Onset before age of 65 years

Presence of trisomy-21

Coexistence of other relevant conditions such as Parkinson's disease

NINCDS-ADRDA, National Institute of Neurological and Communicative Disorders and Stroke and the Alzheimer's Disease and Related Disorders Association.
Adapted from McKhann, G., Drachman, D., Folstein, M., et al. (1984). Clinical diagnosis of Alzheimer's disease: Report of the NINCDS-ADRDA work group under the auspices of Department of Health and Human Services Task Force on Alzheimer's Disease. *Neurology, 34,* 940. Copyright 1984 by the American Neurological Association.

creases with age, and the rate more than doubles between the ages of 60 and 80 years (Mayeaux & Schofield, 1994). There is a higher prevalence of AD in women than in men. The underlying reason may be the longer life expectancy of women, although other factors may be involved (Berkow et al., 1995; Civil et al., 1993). A few studies have found that cultural or ethnic differences may exist in the prevalence and incidence of AD (Mayeaux & Schofield, 1994).

Theories of Causation. The cause of AD remains unknown. Several theories have been proposed and form the basis for current research:

1. Genetic theory (Levy-Lahad et al., 1995; Pericak-Vance et al., 1991; Reichman, 1994; St. George-Hislop et al., 1987; Schellenberg et al., 1992; Tanzi et al., 1992; Zoler, 1994)
2. Slow virus theory (Pruisner, 1984; Wurtman, 1985)
3. Aluminum theory (Bolla et al., 1992; Deary & Whalley, 1988)
4. Cholinergic theory (Bowen et al., 1976; Davies & Maloney, 1976; Ingram et al., 1994; Larson et al., 1992)
5. Amyloid theory (Beyreuther et al., 1991; Rosenberg, 1993; Rumble et al., 1989)
6. Autoimmune theory (Aisen & Davis, 1994; Wurtman, 1985)
7. Trauma theory (Clinton et al., 1991; Drachman & Lippa, 1992; Heyman et al., 1984; Mortimer et al., 1991; van Duijn et al., 1992)

Clinical Presentation. AD is a progressive neurological disorder that has an insidious onset and progresses over time, leaving the individual in a vegetative state. A wide variety of symptoms can progress. The most typical initial changes include lapses of recent memory, a decreased ability to learn new information, an altered attention span, agnosia, and a lack of spontaneity. Clinically, these patients show relatively good preservation of their ability to recall remote events, and they tend to more readily recall incidents that are associated with important life events, such as births, marriage, and wars (Fromholt & Larsen, 1991; Sagar & Sullivan, 1988). Sentence structure is not usu-

ally affected during the early stages, and there may be little or no evidence of a deficit in casual conversation.

Progression of the disease involves personality changes, mental status changes, social role dysfunction, difficulty with activities of daily living, language deterioration, visuoperceptual deficits, incontinence, and gait disorders. Drawing ability and the construction of three-dimensional figures become affected. Drawings are small and cramped, key features tend to be omitted, and patients may "close in" on figures (i.e., draw figures on top of the existing ones). Spatial disorientation, reading difficulties, and anomia are also noted when objects are presented visually (Huff et al., 1986). Figure 18–1 shows examples of constructional apraxias.

Rigidity of the extrapyramidal type occurs in about 30% of people with AD and may be associated with a greater severity of illness (Mayeux & Schofield, 1994; Sagar & Sullivan, 1988). Balance and gait disturbances are fairly frequent. The most frequent abnormalities seen are decreased arm swing, reduced stride length, and postural instability. Dyskinesia and myoclonus are common. Myoclonic jerks and generalized seizures may occur in the later stages of the disease (Katzman, 1992). Oculomotor function is typically impaired. There may be deficits in upward gaze, causing a perseveration of downward gaze, and severely impaired and demented patients show gaze perseveration (Sagar & Sullivan, 1988). During the advanced stages of the disease, the patient becomes mute, is unable to walk, is incontinent of bowel and bladder, and becomes dependent on others for all activities of daily living.

Patients with early dementia are often aware of and frightened by their deficits. Changes in affect and impulse control as well as motivational and general interest occur as the disease progresses. Behavioral symptoms frequently seen in patients with AD include wandering, aggressiveness, sleep disturbances, nocturnal confusion, tearfulness, and anxiety (Civil et al., 1993). Delusions have been reported in 13 to 53% of AD patients and tend to be primarily paranoid in nature, involving misbeliefs about infidelity or theft (Civil et al., 1993; Cummings & Benson, 1983). About 40% of AD pa-

| Original Figure | Closing In | Cramped Figures | Leaving Out Details |

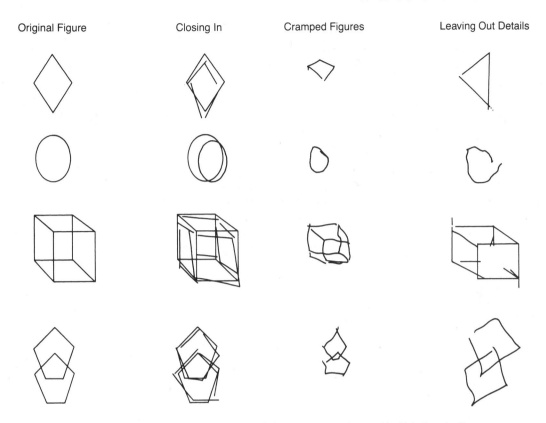

FIGURE 18–1. Examples of constructional deficits seen in patients with Alzheimer's disease.

tients have depressive features, usually early in the disease, which contribute to cognitive dysfunction (Rosser, 1993).

Approximately 10% of patients may have an atypical presentation, with a deficit predominately in one area of cognition. For example, the first presenting symptoms may be a difficulty with finding words, visuospatial deficits, isolated personality changes, or pure memory loss (Katzman, 1992). These focal symptoms may occur many years prior to the typical generalized progression seen in most AD patients. The rate of deterioration differs among patients and within patients over time. The Global Deterioration Scale developed by Reisberg and colleagues (1982) is one of several scales available to measure the changes and to identify the stage of the disease (Table 18–7).

When tested, patients in the early stages of

AD make continuous attempts to answer questions. In contrast, patients with depression complain of memory deficits and an inability to recall but, if encouraged, may do well on testing. Aware of their deficits, patients with AD frequently try hard to minimize or rationalize their errors in testing. Denial, confabulation, perseveration, and avoidance of questions are typical interview behaviors of patients in the later stages of AD.

Prognosis. Patients with AD have a reduced life expectancy (Terry & Katzman, 1992). The disease may have a course as short as 18 months or as long as 27 years, but the average duration of illness is 10 to 12 years (McLachlan et al., 1984; Miller et al., 1994). The leading causes of death in patients with AD have been found to be related to diseases of the heart (cardiopulmonary arrest, arrhythmia, myocar-

TABLE 18-7

Global Deterioration Scale for Age-Associated Cognitive Decline and Alzheimer's Disease

GDS Stage	Clinical Phase	Clinical Characteristics	Diagnosis
1 = No cognitive decline	Normal	No subjective complaints of memory deficit. No memory deficit evident on clinical interview.	Normal
2 = Very mild cognitive decline	Forgetfulness	Subjective complaints of memory deficits. No objective deficits in employment or social situations. Appropriate concern with respect to symptomatology.	Normal aged
3 = Mild cognitive decline	Early confusional	Earliest clear-cut deficits. Decreased performance in demanding employment and social settings. Objective evidence of memory deficit obtained only with an intensive interview. Mild to moderate anxiety accompanies symptoms.	Compatible with incipient Alzheimer's disease
4 = Moderate cognitive decline	Late confusional	Clear-cut deficit on careful interview. Inability to perform complex tasks. Denial is dominant defense mechanism. Flattening of affect and withdrawal from challenging situations occur.	Mild Alzheimer's disease
5 = Moderately severe cognitive decline	Early dementia	Patients can no longer survive without some assistance. Patients are unable during interview to recall a major relevant aspect of their current lives. People at this stage retain knowledge of many major facts regarding themselves and others. They invariably know their own names and generally know their spouse's and children's names. They require no assistance with toileting or eating but may have some difficulty choosing the proper clothing to wear.	Moderate Alzheimer's disease
6 = Severe cognitive decline	Middle dementia	May occasionally forget the name of the spouse on whom they are entirely dependent for survival. Patients are largely unaware of all recent events and experiences in their lives and require some assistance with activities of daily living. Personality and emotional changes occur.	Moderately severe Alzheimer's disease
7 = Very severe cognitive decline	Late dementia	All verbal abilities are lost. Frequently there is no speech at all—only grunting. Incontinent of urine; requires assistance toileting and feeding. Loses basic psychomotor skills (e.g., ability to walk).	Severe Alzheimer's disease

From Reisberg, B., Ferris, S. H., de Leon, M. J., et al. (1982). The global deterioration scale for assessment of primary dementia. *American Journal of Psychiatry, 139,* 1136–1139. Copyright 1982 by the American Psychiatric Association.

dial infarction) and to respiratory conditions or bronchopneumonia (Olichney et al., 1995). Chandra and associates (1986) reported that AD patients are at a greater risk for infections, trauma, nutritional deficiency, Parkinson's disease, and epilepsy. Although there is no cure for AD at present, there are many preventable and treatable conditions that, with appropriate management, may extend this population's life span and improve their quality of life (Kane et al., 1994; Katzman, 1992).

Research in Alzheimer's Disease. Clinical and research interest in dementia and its causes has greatly increased in recent years, and researchers have begun to study a broad spectrum of areas associated with the problem. It is still uncertain whether AD is an infectious process, a toxic disorder, a biochemical deficiency, or an exaggeration and acceleration of the normal aging process, with dementia appearing when the neural reserves are exhausted and compensatory mechanisms fail (Drachman & Lippa, 1992).

One of the most important research issues in AD is accurate diagnosis. The National Institute on Aging Task Force (1980) estimated incorrect diagnosis to be 10 to 30% in the general medical population. With the advent of newly developed diagnostic criteria, the reported diagnostic accuracy for dementia is now 95%, and the diagnostic accuracy of probable AD is approximately 90% (Katzman, 1990). Standardized criteria for the diagnosis of ischemic vascular dementia (VD) have been developed (Chui et al., 1992). An early and accurate diagnosis is essential for research on AD and other dementing disorders to progress.

The development of diagnostic criteria has in turn led to broader epidemiological studies. Longitudinal studies, which are necessary to advance research on the diagnosis of AD, are currently being conducted. Researchers in this area are collecting detailed information on people with the disease as well as on normal aging populations in an effort to identify premorbid events and conditions that may predispose some individuals to developing the disease and to gain a better understanding of the normal aging process. One of the major difficulties in diagnosing AD involves the variations in presentation and the need to understand the relationships among neuropsychological, neuropathological, and neuroradiological findings. Neuroimaging techniques and the development of more precise neuropsychological tests are high priorities.

The role of environmental factors is another central research theme. Memory loss was for many years considered a normal consequence of aging. However, the process of normal aging is not clearly understood, and until a better knowledge is gained in this area, diagnosing AD will continue to be a difficult and somewhat imprecise process. For some time, it has been clearly established that there is a serious defect in the cholinergic system of patients with AD. This finding has continued to generate a tremendous amount of interest. Research in this area has focused on understanding the

cause and effect of the defect and looking for pharmacological approaches to treat, prevent, or stop the disease process. Along with pharmacological studies, there is an interest in developing new ways of dispensing medications (e.g., by pumps and skin patches) that will be useful not only in AD but in many other disorders as well.

It is not yet known why brain cells die in AD. Many researchers are studying the chemistry of the neurofibrillary plaques and tangles found in the brains of AD patients. Data supporting a causal role of amyloid in AD have led to a wide range of studies aimed at delineating the biochemical pathways involved in the deposition of amyloid deposits in patients with AD or other dementias. Others are studying the membrane structures and how changes in the membrane influence transport and homeostasis of essential ions. Pedigree studies investigating the familial genetic aspects of AD are essential in understanding the disease and in helping predict which individuals are at risk for the disease. A high priority of current research is identifying genetic markers and biological correlates of AD. Recent animal studies have shown that nerve growth factor can promote the survival of central nervous neurons in adult life. Researchers are looking for therapeutic approaches that will use this information. Studies are currently investigating the use of estrogen, antioxidants, and nonsteroidal antiinflammatory or immunosuppressive drugs as a means of reducing the risk of and treating AD (Barrett-Connor & Kritz-Silverstein, 1993; Brietner, 1996; McGreer et al., 1992; Sano et al., 1997; Yaffe et al., 1998).

VASCULAR DEMENTIA

VD is a clinical syndrome of acquired intellectual and functional impairment resulting from the effects of cerebrovascular disease. After AD, cerebrovascular disease is the most common contributor to dementia. VD is characterized by a wide range of neurological and neuropsychological signs and symptoms that reflect the wide variety of responsible lesions. Depending on the cause of VD, the onset may be abrupt, insidious, static, remitting, or progressive (Reichman, 1994; Roman et al., 1993).

Ischemia, hemorrhage, and anoxia can all lead to dementia. Accumulations of ischemic cerebral infarctions can produce a condition in which dementia is the dominant symptom. Dementia resulting from the accumulation of ischemic cerebral infarctions is known as MID (multi-infarct dementia). Chronic ischemia, without frank infarction, may also contribute to cognitive deterioration, and ischemic changes may coexist with other pathology (Chui et al., 1992).

The extent and type of cognitive dysfunction found in patients with MID depend on the localization and size of the lesions. Small bilateral infarcts in the hippocampus or thalamus may produce considerable dysfunction in recent memory, whereas infarcts of the same size in the optic radiation may produce only minor visual field limitations. Some studies have found that multiple infarcts at times do not produce any cognitive dysfunction (Heyman, 1978; Kane et al., 1994; Kase, 1986). Patients with MID tend to have a more severe drop in motor functions than do patients with AD (Erkinjuntti et al., 1986, 1987).

There have been few reports of changes in specific cognitive function in patients with MID, probably because the nature of the deficit is so closely dependent on the location and size of the infarcts. To compound the difficulty in measuring dysfunction, AD and MID coexist in about 15% of patients with dementia (Berkow et al., 1995). The cognitive deficits of the two conditions may be additive, so that in patients who already have AD changes in the brain, higher cerebral dysfunction may be seen following a stroke (Sagar & Sullivan, 1988).

Epidemiology. As with most causes of dementia, the incidence of cerebrovascular disease increases with age. Neuropsychological studies have shown that approximately 12.5% of dementias in the elderly are caused by MID, and 13.6% by a combination of both MID and AD or a mixed dementia (Meyer et al., 1986). There is a higher incidence of MID in men than in women. Hypertension is a major risk factor (Marshall, 1993). In countries with a high incidence of hypertension, such as Japan and Finland, a higher proportion of dementia may be attributed to MID (Katzman, 1992).

Etiology. Several causes for vascular demen-

tia have been proposed. These are summarized in Table 18–8.

Clinical Presentation. The clinical features of VD depend on the underlying cause and/or the size and location of the responsible lesions. General features can include all or some of the following:

Abrupt onset
Fluctuating course
Focal neurological signs and symptoms
Depression
Emotional lability
Somatic complaints
Nocturnal confusion

TABLE 18-8

Multi-Infarct Dementia: Theories of Causation

Cause	Theory
Lacunae	Small focal infarcts result from occlusion of branch arteries that penetrate the brain. Accumulation of these lesions can cause progressive mental deterioration.
Binswanger's disease	Infarcts are limited to the subcortical white matter. Hypertension is thought to be major cause.
Multi-emboli	Any vessel can cause emboli, but extracranial arteries and the heart are most likely to produce the widely distributed lesions that produce multi-infarct dementia.
Vasculitis	May be idiopathic, infectious, granulomatous, or the result of toxins or immune complex. Lupus erythematosus is one of the most frequent causes.
Blood dyscrasias	Uncommon, but known to cause vascular lesions.
Hypoperfusion	Systemic hypotension, or occlusion of a major vessel, can cause damage to areas of the brain perfused by the most distal vessels.
Anoxic episodes	Caused by cardiac arrest, anesthesia, or other similar causes resulting in neuronal loss, leading to dementia without the presence of infarctions.

Data from Read & Jarvik (1984).

Patients with MID experience a stepwise decline with a fluctuating clinical course. The onset tends to be more acute with focal neurological signs and symptoms, and patchy cognitive losses are often seen (Marshall, 1993). Dysarthria, hemineglect of visual space, movement disorder, or a subtle paresis may be evident. Patients may exhibit an inability to distinguish left from right, to reproduce two-dimensional drawings, and to identify letters traced on the hand. Delusions may occur. Studies have found delusions in as many as 40% of patients with MID (Cummings et al., 1987). A history of transient ischemic attacks, hypertension, strokes, diabetes mellitus, vasculitis, and cardiac arrhythmias is frequently associated with MID. A family history of stroke or cardiovascular disease may be present (Read & Jarvik, 1984; Reichman, 1994).

A mental status examination is important in delineating patchy deficits. Focal slowing may be seen on electroencephalogram in patients with infarcts too small to be visible with computed tomography (Benson et al., 1982; Read & Jarvik, 1984). The Hachinski Ischemia Rating Scale is a useful tool in differentiating AD from MID (Table 18–9).

Disease Progression. The course of MID can be intermittent and fluctuating. Patients may have episodes of clouded sensorium or may plateau for long periods. Hypertension is the most important risk factor for stroke in patients with MID. Specific cardiovascular diagnosis and management are key to arresting progression and reducing mortality (Hachinski et al., 1974; Marshall, 1993). When deterioration proceeds rapidly following a single cerebrovascular accident, there has likely been slowly advancing subclinical change, now potentiated by infarction, which has served to push the neuronal damage beyond the threshold point.

Prognosis. The chances of social survival are thought to be better in patients with VD than in those with AD. Treatment of the underlying illness and the secondary psychiatric and medical conditions can substantially improve the prognosis. Selected patients with MID may benefit from anticoagulation therapy or surgery. Some cases of VD are remediable, and

---

TABLE 18-9

Hachinski Ischemic Rating Scale

Instructions: Record the presence or absence of the clinical features of dementia listed below and add the point values assigned each feature (value in parenthesis) whenever "Present" is checked. Summation of points produces an Ischemic Score. Scores of < +4 indicate patients with pure primary degenerative dementia (Alzheimer's type dementia). Scores of >4 indicate patients with multi-infarct dementia.

Feature	Absent	Present	Point Value
1. Abrupt feature	___	___	2
2. Stepwise deterioration	___	___	1
3. Fluctuating course	___	___	2
4. Nocturnal confusion	___	___	1
5. Relative preservation of personality	___	___	1
6. Depression	___	___	1
7. Somatic concern	___	___	1
8. Emotional incontinence	___	___	1
9. History of hypertension	___	___	1
10. History of strokes	___	___	2
11. History of associated atherosclerosis	___	___	1
12. Focal neurological symptoms	___	___	2
13. Focal neurological signs	___	___	2

From Hackinski, V. C., Iliff, L. D., Zilhka, E., et al. (1975). Cerebral blood flow in dementia. *Archives of Neurology, 32,* 634. Copyright 1975 by the American Medical Association.

occasionally some are reversible (Meyer et al., 1986; Read & Jarvik, 1984; Wade, 1991). Other individuals with VD may experience further cognitive decline.

ALCOHOLIC DEMENTIA

Alcohol abuse gives rise to a large and diverse group of mental disorders. Unfortunately, alcoholic dementia is not well studied, and confusion still exists concerning its diagnosis. Studies have shown that (1) mild forms of cerebral dysfunction are common in heavy drinkers, (2) a smaller but still significant proportion of heavy drinkers will have more severe dysfunction, and (3) a similar proportion of patients who present with dementia will have a history of heavy drinking or alcoholism (Willenbring, 1988). The effects of alcohol on the brain range from acute or reversible conditions (e.g., acute intoxication, alcoholic hallucinosis, and pathological intoxication) to withdrawal states (e.g., delirium tremens and withdrawal seizures) to chronic, largely irreversible conditions reflecting a long-term derangement of metabolism, as seen in Wernicke-Korsakoff's syndrome, alcoholic pellagra, and hepatic en-

cephalopathy (Feldman & Plum, 1993; Willenbring, 1988).

Wernicke-Korsakoff's syndrome is one of the major alcoholic dementias. Wernicke's encephalopathy and Korsakoff's syndrome are considered to be stages of one syndrome and not separate diseases (Victor, 1993). However, there may be cases of Korsakoff's syndrome with no apparent history of Wernicke's (Carlen & Neiman, 1990). Thiamine deficiency is the specific nutritional factor thought to be responsible for this condition. Neuropathological findings include lesions in the medial thalamic region, pons, medulla, and cerebellar cortex. The lesions responsible for memory loss are structural rather than biochemical. Korsakoff's syndrome is most often associated with alcohol but may be a symptom of various other disorders (Victor, 1993). Other alcoholic dementias are described in Table 18–10.

Epidemiology. Alcohol abuse is a major health problem. One out of eight adults is considered to be a heavy drinker. Alcohol contributes to nearly 7% of all dementias. Approximately 50% of excessive drinkers show neuropsychological impairment, and 3% of alcoholics have clinically defined dementia

TABLE 18-10
Alcoholic Dementias

Disease	Cause	Treatment	Progression	Prognosis
Wernicke-Korsakoff's	Thiamine deficiency	Thiamine, adequate diet	With treatment improvement begins in a few weeks to 3 months. Recovery is slow, 1 year or longer.	Varies. Complete or almost complete recovery in about 20% of patients. Small percentage show no recovery, and the majority fall in between.
Alcohol-induced pellagra	Poor nutrition over time; deficiency of niacin or tryptophan	Niacin, adequate diet	Degree of improvement depends on severity of brain lesions.	Aggressive treatment can produce considerable improvement. Fatal if untreated.
Hepatic encephalitis	Chronic alcoholism resulting in liver disease, leading to increased ammonemia	Treat liver disease	Symptoms evolve over days or weeks. Coma may occur. Symptoms may regress completely, become chronic, or worsen with repeated comas.	Symptoms are reversible if treatment is timely. Fatal if untreated.

(Feldman & Plum, 1993). The alcoholic dementias have a high mortality rate and can produce crippling effects.

Etiology. The role of alcohol is considered to be secondary in the pathogenesis of these dementias. The adverse effects on the nervous system are the result of nutritional and liver diseases engendered by the chronic abuse of alcohol. Alcoholic dementias are thought to differ in this respect from other pathological intoxication states that directly result from the effect of alcohol on the central nervous system or the withdrawal of alcohol following a period of chronic intoxication (Willenbring, 1988).

Clinical Presentation. In the chronic alcoholic patient, Korsakoff's syndrome (or Korsakoff's disease) usually begins with an acute attack of Wernicke's disease (presenting with global confusion, apathy, ataxia, and ocular abnormalities). With adequate diet and thiamine, patients become increasingly alert, responsive, and gradually less confused, and the major remaining impairment is a decreased retentive memory. If not treated, Wernicke's is thought to become chronic and persist as a Korsakoff's syndrome (Allen, 1994; Carlen & Neiman, 1990). Korsakoff's syndrome is unique and is characterized by two abnormalities that always occur together: *retrograde amnesia* (losing information acquired in the past) and *anterograde amnesia* (having a decreased ability to acquire new information). Confabulation is not consistently present and is not required for diagnosis. In an otherwise alert and responsive patient, retentive memory is impaired out of proportion to other cognitive functions. Other cognitive functions that are not memory dependent may be impaired but to a lesser degree. Limited insight, apathetic behavior, inertia, and indifference to people and events may also be present (Carlen & Neiman, 1990; Victor, 1993).

Prognosis. Improvement begins anywhere from a few weeks to 3 months after treatment, and the maximum degree of recovery may not be obtained for a year or longer. Recovery proceeds very slowly and is governed by both the inherent slowness of recovery of damaged brain tissue and the extent of damage present (Allen, 1994). Once Korsakoff's disease symptoms are established, complete or almost complete recovery occurs in approximately 20% of patients. A few patients show no recovery. The majority fall somewhere between slight and almost complete recovery (Carlen & Neiman, 1990; Victor, 1993). The syndrome is preventable.

The Dementia Workup

The workup for establishing a diagnosis of dementia and identifying its cause consists of a detailed medical and family history, a physical examination, a full mental status examination, and biochemical studies. Computed tomography or magnetic resonance imaging, neuropsychological evaluation, and additional diagnostic procedures may also be indicated in selected cases (Katzman, 1992; National Institutes of Health Consensus Conference, 1987). Even with this extensive workup, a definitive diagnosis may not be reached, and follow-up examinations for dementia may be required. A period of several months should be allowed between these evaluations to detect any progression or emergence of symptoms. Table 18–11 summarizes the dementia workup.

HISTORY

General Considerations. In the early stages of a dementing illness, many patients maintain their social skills and conversational abilities. Patients may be unaware of symptoms or deny that there is a problem. It is essential when taking a history to have someone present who knows the patient well to verify the patient's responses and supply additional information. If possible, clinicians should interview the patient with a family member present and also see the patient and the family member separately. This process gives the advantage of revealing the interactions between the patient and the family member and also provides each family member an opportunity to discuss information and concerns that he or she may be reluctant to divulge in the other's presence. The content of the history is listed in Table 18–11.

When working with the older population, it is of the utmost importance to be empathic, patient, and observant. Interviewers must wait for the patient's response to questions. Interviewers must *look as well as listen*, noting

TABLE 18-11
The Dementia Workup

History	Diagnostic Tests

Chronological account of current problem
  Onset
  Duration
  Specific cognitive, memory, and behavior changes
  Changes in functional status
	Standard
	  Complete blood count
	  Electrolyte panel
	  Screening metabolic panel
	  Thyroid gland function tests
	  Vitamin B_{12} and folate levels
	  Syphilis and additional tests based on history:
	    Human immunodeficiency virus titer
	    Lyme disease antibody titer
	  Urinalysis
	  Electrocardiogram
	  Chest roentgenogram

Medical history
  Relevant systemic diseases
  Trauma
  Surgery
  Psychiatric disorders
  Nutrition
  Alcohol and substance abuse
  Exposure to environmental toxins
  Medications—prescribed and nonprescribed	

Family history
  Dementia
  Down's syndrome
  Psychiatric disorders
	Other
	  Neuropsychological evaluation
	  Imaging
	    Computed tomography (without contrast)
	    Magnetic resonance imaging
	    Positron-emission tomography
	    Single photon emission computed
	      tomography

Physical Examination	Electroencephalogram Lumbar puncture
Neurological examination	
Mental status examination	

Data from Katzman (1992); Mayeaux & Schofield (1994); National Institutes of Health Consensus Conference (1987).

whether the patient is easily distracted and whether he or she can comprehend the question but is having difficulty with expressive speech. Does the person look depressed or restless and unable to sit still? Are there myoclonic movements, tremors, or gait disturbances?

Questions. Table 18–12 outlines some of the key questions asked in the dementia assessment. The dementia workup should include a detailed medical, social, and family history as well as a review of systems to identify infectious, metabolic, cardiovascular, and nutritional problems. Taking a detailed inventory of medications is also important, as they have long been known to cause fatigue, apathy, mental slowing, and confusion in the elderly (U'Ren, 1987).

Establishing the date of onset of symptoms may be difficult. Patients are often not aware of the changes, and family members may not note the early deficits or changes until the symptoms have become more pronounced.

Nevertheless, it is important to use specific questions to establish the date of onset as closely as possible, especially when there may be more than one condition present. A good way to assist families in establishing a date of onset is to ask of them, "Given what you now know about the individual's problems, think back and try to remember when you first may have seen changes but didn't think they were serious."

FUNCTIONAL STATUS

Three areas are crucial in assessing the patient: (1) cognitive state, (2) the ability to perform basic and instrumental activities of daily living, and (3) the frequency and quality of emotional symptoms and behaviors. Patients' strengths as well as weaknesses must be sought and used to assist them in compensating for their deficits. Patients need to maintain some power over their lives. Cognitive dysfunction does

TABLE 18-12
Questions for Assessing Dementia

Is there a history of hypertension, transient ischemic attacks, syncopal episodes, strokes, or cardiovascular disease?

Is there a family history of dementia, depression, psychiatric illness, or other neurological disorders?

Psychiatric signs and symptoms: Is there evidence of depressive symptoms, a sad mood or affect, lack of energy, loss of interest and enjoyment in former activities, changes in sleep patterns, loss of weight, loss of appetite?

Is there a past history of depression or psychiatric disorders?

Has the individual experienced any recent major losses, environmental changes, or traumas?

Have there been any changes in memory, intellect, or personality?

Did the memory loss come before the depression?

Did the personality changes occur before or after the stroke?

What medications is the patient taking?

What over-the-counter preparations and vitamins are used?

not mean a lack of feeling, and patients should be allowed to do as much as possible for as long as possible. Table 18–13 illustrates specific areas of functional ability that should be included in the assessment (see also Chapters 7 and 9).

FAMILY AND SOCIAL SUPPORT

Because the patient with a dementing illness increasingly relies on family support and assistance, assessment must of necessity include the family (see also Chapter 8). The five most critical areas to be covered when performing a family assessment are as follows:

1. Who is the family?
2. Who is the primary caregiver?
3. What is the family history?
4. What are the family coping styles?
5. What is the meaning of the illness and its symptoms?

PHYSICAL EXAMINATION

The physical examination should include a detailed neurological assessment to evaluate the presence or absence of focal neurological signs and symptoms and to assist in defining the cause of the dementia (Table 18–14). Patients in the early stages of AD are comparatively free of neurological changes, apart from the occasional presence of snout reflex, rigidity, and myoclonus. These symptoms may also be seen in nondemented elderly people (McKhann et al., 1984). As the disease progresses, myoclonic movements and rigidity increase, and patients in the later stages may develop seizures. MID patients show a higher frequency of focal neurological signs and symptoms and higher scores on the Hachinski Ischemic Rating Scale than patients with AD (Hachinski et al., 1974).

MENTAL STATUS EXAMINATION

The mental status examination plays a key role in the diagnosis of dementia. It is especially important during the early stages of impairment. Patients in the very early stages of cognitive decline may be able to carry on a normal conversation and answer questions about their personal history during an interview but may nevertheless show cognitive deficits on a mental status examination (Katzman, 1992; Sagar & Sullivan, 1988). The main components of the

TABLE 18-13
Functional Activities Assessment

Writing checks, paying bills, keeping records

Assembling tax records, making out business and insurance papers

Shopping alone for clothes, groceries, and household necessities

Playing a game of skill, such as bridge, other card games, or chess

Heating water for coffee or tea and turning off the stove

Preparing a balanced meal

Keeping track of current events

Paying attention to and understanding a television program, book, or magazine

Remembering appointments, family occasions, and medications

Traveling away from the neighborhood

TABLE 18-14
Neurological Examination

Cranial nerves II–XII
Motor (tone, bulk)
Sensory (pinprick, fine touch, position, vibration)
Cerebellar (finger to nose, heel to shin)
Frontal lobe (*Suck*—tap upper or lower lip. *Snout*—tap center of closed lips. *Grasp*—place fingers in patient's hand between thumb and forefinger. *Palmo-Mental*—scratch or stroke palm from base of thumb to wrist. *Glabellar*—tap root of nose.)
Gait (standard, tandem, Romberg)
Deep tendon reflexes and plantar response
Speech
Facial expression
Tremor at rest
Action or postural tremor of hands
Rigidity
Finger taps (tap thumb with index finger in rapid succession)
Hand movements (open and close hands in rapid succession)
Leg ability (tap heel on ground rapidly, picking up entire leg)
Arising from chair (rising from straight-backed chair with arms folded across chest)
Posture
Posture stability
Body bradykinesia and hypokinesia (slowness, hesitancy, decreased armswing, small amplitude, general poverty of movement)

mental status examination include orientation, memory, calculation, information and speech comprehension, concentration, and constructional ability. The goal is to not only identify the presence of cognitive deficits but also quantify the changes and establish a baseline to measure further changes over time. The basic strategy of the mental status examination is to start with very simple questions and advance to more complex questions that test the patient's basic cognitive abilities (Katzman, 1992).

Short-term memory and concentration are usually the first areas to be affected in individuals with dementia; other symptoms increase in severity and number as the condition progresses. In the very early stages of dementia, some highly trained individuals with premorbid intelligence quotients in the above-average range can continue to score well on a mental status examination. Impairment in one area by itself does not indicate the presence of demen-

tia. Decline from a premorbid level of function over time is more indicative of a progressive dementing illness than an isolated deficit. Many reliable and validated mental status examinations are available, ranging from the simple to the complex (see Chapter 7); of these, the Folstein Mini-Mental State Examination is the most frequently used by both clinicians and researchers (Folstein et al., 1975; Katzman, 1992). The clock test is also a useful screening instrument for identifying people with AD (Tuokko et al., 1992).

LABORATORY TESTS

The standard laboratory workup for dementia includes a complete blood cell count, electrolyte panel, metabolic screen, and syphilis serology (see Table 18–11). The use of additional laboratory tests depends on the history and clinical findings (Kane et al., 1994; Katzman, 1992). Blood chemistries should be obtained to identify abnormalities that could be contributing to or are the cause of the dementia. Elevated calcium levels and abnormal liver and kidney function can cause memory deficits. Abnormal thyroid function can contribute to memory loss and confusion. Correcting the abnormality may clear or improve the patient's difficulties. In the past, syphilitic dementia was a more common problem; however, the possibility of syphilitic infection should still be ruled out. Obtaining cerebral spinal fluid by means of a spinal tap should be considered where there is some question of infection, malignancy, or toxic substances contributing to the dementia (Berkow et al., 1995; McKhann et al., 1984).

OTHER DIAGNOSTIC TESTS

Neuropsychological Testing. Mental status examinations and neuropsychological testing are essential components of the dementia workup. Brief mental status tests such as the Folstein Mini-Mental State Examination are screening instruments used to detect cognitive impairment. Neuropsychological testing clarifies and refines the presence of cognitive impairment and provides additional information for the differential diagnosis of dementia. In addition, neuropsychological tests, because of their increasing complexity, are used to identify less severely impaired individuals. Patients may score normally on a Mini-Mental Status Examination, for example, but may show widespread cognitive impairment when tested by detailed neuropsychological examinations (Sagar & Sullivan, 1988). When used in longitudinal assessment, these tests can measure the progression of a disease through comparison with the individual's previous performance on the same test measures. Any correlations between clinical changes, test performance, and the findings of scanning or imaging procedures can be helpful in further identifying areas of deficit and in establishing a diagnosis in cases with atypical symptom presentation (Cronin-Golomb et al., 1993; McKhann et al., 1984).

Neuropsychological testing consists of a comprehensive battery of tests measuring various specific aspects of cognition, memory, language, sensory perception, motor function, visuospatial performance, and psychiatric evaluation (Cronin-Golomb et al., 1993; McKhann et al., 1984). More detailed information and standardized method summaries are provided in LaRue (1992), Lezak (1995), and Kolb and Whishaw (1985).

In progressive dementias such as AD, the range of deficits extends from a mild memory impairment to global brain failure virtually incompatible with life. This wide range creates an additional problem in testing patients over time and at different stages of the disease, as it is difficult to use a single clinical tool over the entire course of the illness. The Alzheimer's Disease Assessment Scale was developed specifically to evaluate the severity of cognitive and noncognitive behavioral dysfunctions characteristic of individuals with AD (Rosen et al., 1984). This standarized instrument is widely used in reporting AD research.

Imaging. Computed tomography and magnetic resonance imaging remain the most commonly used screening tools in establishing a diagnosis of dementia. Positron-emission tomography (PET) and single photon emission computed tomography (SPECT) add important data on the pathophysiology of dementia and assist in the differential diagnosis of more atypical presentations; their cost and availability, however, prevent their use in wide clinical ap-

plications at this time. Their ability to measure physiological changes in the brain over time may prove invaluable in the development of new treatment approaches. The electroencephalogram is useful in establishing a diagnosis of dementia in cases with atypical presentations and in clarifying the cause of a dementia.

Treatment Approaches

ALZHEIMER'S DISEASE

At present, there are no known cures for AD. Drug treatment for AD is divided into two types: *symptomatic treatment*, which concerns the management of emerging symptoms, and *specific drug therapies*, which focus on the presumed cause of the basic disorder (Hollister, 1985; Katzman, 1992**)**.

Symptomatic Treatment. Medications can be used to achieve either simple control or the symptomatic relief of behaviors such as aggression, agitation, restlessness, hyperboisterousness, hyperactivity, verbal hostility, and insomnia. Antipsychotic medications can be used to provide symptomatic relief of anxiety, depression, regressed behavior, hallucinations, and delusions (Table 18–15).

Patients with AD are acutely sensitive to central nervous system neurotransmitter alterations; small changes can produce significant effects. Many AD patients have idiosyncratic reactions to medications (Omar et al., 1995; Thornton et al., 1986), and thus medications must be initiated at very low doses and carefully titrated. Less emphasis should be placed on dosage than on the individual patient's clinical response (Maletta, 1990). Some behaviors can be managed or decreased by means of behavioral and environmental changes; these approaches should always be tried first and before medications. A concomitant medical illness or the use of contraindicated drugs must be determined before beginning medications. Clinicians should determine whether the patient had these behavioral problems in the past, whether any medications were effective, and if any side effects developed.

Neuroleptics remain the standard treatment for agitated behavior in patients with AD. Hal-

TABLE 18-15

Medications Used to Provide Symptom Relief

Drug (Generic)	Drug (Brand Name)	Daily Dosage
Antidepressants		
Sertraline	Zoloft	25–150 mg
Paroxetine	Paxil	10–50 mg
Desipramine	Norpramin	25–150 mg
Bupropion	Wellbutrin	75–300 mg
Fluoxetine	Prozac	5–20 mg
Nortriptyline	Aventyl or Pamelor	10–50 mg
Trazodone	Desyrel	25–200 mg
Sedative-Hypnotics		
Temazepam	Restoril	7.5–15 mg
Lorazepam	Ativan	0.5–1 mg
Zolpidem	Ambien	5–10 mg
Antipsychotics		
Haloperidol	Haldol	0.25–2 mg twice a day
Thiothixene	Navane	1–15 mg
Clozapine	Clozaril	75–100 mg
Risperidone	Risperdal	0.5–6 mg
Olanzapine	Zyprexa	2.5–20 mg
Quetiapine	Seroquel	100–250 mg
Antianxiety Agents		
Diazepam	Valium	2 mg every day or twice a day
Lorazepam	Ativan	0.5–1 mg twice a day
Alprazolam	Xanax	0.25 mg two or three times a day
Agents for Agitation or Aggressivity		
Buspirone	Buspar	5 mg twice a day
Trazodone	Desyrel	50 mg
Clonazepam	Klonopin	0.25–0.5 mg twice a day
Carbamazepine	Tegretol	50–100 mg twice a day
Valproate	Depakote	125–250 mg

Data from American Psychiatric Association (1997); Dubovsky (1994); Grossberg & Kumar (1998); Ham (1997); Jeste et al. (1998); Salzman (1998), and Small et al. (1997).

operidol (Haldol) is frequently used to control behavioral problems and has also been used with some success when augmented by buspirone (Buspar) (Caudiex, 1993). In very small doses, Haldol can be effective; however, some patients respond by becoming increasingly agi-tated, with increasing dosages only escalating the problem. Parkinsonian symptoms can become marked with the use of haloperidol, and the patient can rapidly become severely dysfunctional (Maletta, 1985; Mayeux & Schofield, 1994). Because of these side effects, the newer atypical antipsychotics should be the first drug of choice in this population. Risperidone (Risperdal) and olanzapine (Zyprexa) are the two most widely used. Clozapine (Clozaril) needs to be used with caution owing to the side effect of agranulocytosis, requiring weekly blood counts (Ham, 1997). A rule of thumb in drug therapy with these patients is to use the smallest possible doses and to temporarily discontinue the drug on a regular basis to evaluate response (Mayeux & Schofield, 1994).

Specific Drug Therapies. Specific drugs for AD are intended to treat the disease itself. Table 18–16 lists the specific strategies and medications used in treating AD. Most of these treatment approaches were conducted as clinical drug studies that strictly followed regulated research protocols. Although some studies found small changes in attention, mood, and concentration, there unfortunately have not been any major breakthroughs. Most drug trials are based on animal studies, and although some drugs appear promising in animal trials, the results have not been duplicated in humans. The recent development of transgenic mice with amyloid plaques similar to those seen in humans with AD is an important step in developing new treatment approaches.

OTHER DEMENTIAS

The management of dementia resulting from MID or alcohol abuse is focused primarily on treating the underlying condition and eliminating those factors that predispose or directly lead to the problem. The prognosis and quality of life for patients with MID can be improved by controlling hypertension, stabilizing the cardiovascular system, and treating secondary medical conditions or psychiatric disorders (Katzman, 1992; Read & Jarvik, 1984). Anticoagulation therapy and vascular surgery may benefit some patients with MID.

Shunts are sometimes the treatment of choice for patients with normal pressure hydroceph-

TABLE 18-16
Specific Drug Therapies for Alzheimer's Disease

Generic Name	Brand Name	Action
Tetrahydro-aminoacridine, tacrine	Cognex	Cholinesterase inhibitor
Donepezil	Aricept	Cholinesterase inhibitor
Velnacrine maleate	Mentane	Cholinesterase inhibitor
Physostigmine	Synapton	Cholinesterase inhibitor
E-2020		Cholinesterase inhibitor
Linopiridine	Aviva	Enhances release of acetylcholine, dopamine, and serotonin
Nimodipine	Nimotop	Calcium channel blocker
Sabeluzole		Calcium channel blocker; also effects serotonin
Acetyl-L-carnetine	Alcar	Enhances cell energy production—may help protect nerve cells from damage
Phosphatidylserine	Bovice Cortex-Phosphotydal-Serine	Helps maintain cell membrane integrity
L-deprenyl		Selective MAO B inhibitor
Lazabemide		Selective MAO B inhibitor
Desferrioxamine	Desferal	Reduces aluminum levels (chelation therapy)

MAO B, monoamine oxidase type B.
From The Alzheimer's Disease and Related Disorders Association (1992). *Theory to therapy: The development of drugs for Alzheimer's disease.* Chicago, IL: The Alzheimer's Disease and Related Disorders Association.

aly, although statistics show that the success rate for improvement is low and treatment complications are common (Beck et al., 1982; Graff-Radford et al., 1989). Studies indicate that in general, patients best suited for shunting are those who present with the classical triad—gait disturbance, incontinence, and dementia—who have a readily identifiable cause for NPH, and who have a relatively short duration of symptoms (Clarfield, 1989; Reichman, 1994). In alco-hol-related dementias, the standard treatments of choice include eliminating alcohol use, improving nutrition, stabilizing the patient's medical status, and using high doses of thiamin, niacin, and vitamin B_{12} (Willenbring, 1988). The pharmacological management of secondary symptoms and behaviors was discussed in the preceding section covering the treatment of AD, and nonpharmacological approaches are discussed later (see *Management of Dementia*).

ALTERNATIVE TREATMENT APPROACHES

Chelation therapy and megavitamin therapy have been promoted as alternative approaches in the treatment of dementias. Statistics have not shown any basis for their therapeutic claims, however, and in fact, the use of megavitamins may cause more difficulties and adverse reactions than improvement (Funkenstein et al., 1981; Thal, 1988). Some preliminary studies (Gold & Stone, 1988; Hall et al., 1989) have shown that circulating glucose may control acetylcholine synthesis and enhance memory in older individuals. Many AD patients develop cravings for sweets, and PET and SPECT data show deficits in glucose metabolism in the brains of these patients. Age-related memory deficits in some elderly individuals might be alleviated by better control of blood glucose levels achieved through dietary control or medications; however, the mechanisms for doing this have yet to be developed. The high intake of glucose on a regular basis has not been effective, and there is no evidence that this would be beneficial in patients with AD. It is important to maintain a balanced nutritional status for the patient, and families should be taught to do so.

Management of Dementia

Dementia is a multifaceted problem. Integrated management focuses not only on the individual but also on the family, the environment, and the community. Assessment and planning must begin early, and planning, implementation, and evaluation should be concurrent and longitudinal. Because of the complexity of the problem, a multidisciplinary approach should be used to provide diagnosis, pharmacological management, nursing management, and resource management. In working with this population, a commitment to long-term relationships among the patient, family, staff members, and health professionals is essential. Learning to live with a dementing illness is also learning to live with uncertainty. The course of the disease varies among individual patients and may be unpredictable. Families frequently ask the following questions: How long will the patient live? How soon will changes take place? Will the patient become assaultive? Will he or she wander? Will he or she hallucinate? Will our children get the disease? Unfortunately there are no firm answers. Although the outcome of dementia is known, many factors and variations can influence its progression. Some patients have a more gradual decline with periods of plateauing, whereas others have a more rapid rate of decline with more severe behavioral changes.

The responsibilities of the advanced practice nurse are threefold: assessment, planning, and the coordination of care. Plans must be realistic, tailored to the individual, consistent with the psychosocial environment, and financially feasible. Because of the progressive nature of the disease, planning should anticipate and accommodate the patient's decline, with the support system increasingly activated to the escalating need for assistance (American Medical

---

TABLE 18-18
Environmental Safety Checks

Keep environment simple; remove knickknacks or clutter that may distract or confuse
Remove items that can prove dangerous (e.g., car keys, knives, iron, power tools, matches, cleaning solvents)
Keep all medications out of reach and under lock and key
Install gates on stairs; check handrails
Install grab-bars
Reduce temperature on water heater
Remove rugs that slip
Remove glass tables and unsteady or delicate furniture
If possible, arrange an outside area that is safe and accessible where the patient can walk or sit
Put bright reflector tape on steps

Data from Mace & Rabins (1991).

Association Council on Scientific Affairs, 1993; Eisdorfer & Cohen, 1981; Teri & Logsdon, 1990).

BEHAVIORAL MANAGEMENT

There are no magic tricks for dealing with problem behaviors. Dementia patients are extremely sensitive to nonverbal cues and tend to mirror the affective behavior of those around them. Nurses can serve as role models to other caregivers in helping to soothe the patient; patience, gentleness, and calmness can be very effective. Models such as the Progressively Lowered Stress Threshold (Hall et al., 1995) can be used in planning and evaluating the management of behavioral symptoms in these patients. Table 18–17 lists effective communication techniques, and Chapter 27 provides additional information on managing problem behaviors.

Although all dementia patients exhibit some form of behavioral disturbance, the exact type and extent of behavioral problems are quite variable. A specific and thorough behavioral assessment is essential for identifying and treating behavioral problems in AD patients (Teri & Logsdon, 1990). Supportive psychotherapy may be helpful in disrupting a cycle of frustration, anger, anxiety, and rage in patients with mild to moderate dementia (Haggerty, 1990; Verwoerdt, 1981).

TABLE 18-17
Communication Techniques

Avoid arguments—dementia patients reason by a different set of rules and arguments, usually resulting in aggravation for both parties.

Use distractors—the patient's memory deficits can frequently be used to advantage to distract and redirect attention.

Communicate nonverbally—by touching or holding hands.

Praise desired behavior—and make it emotionally meaningful.

Ignore undesired behaviors—only if it is safe to do so.

Data from Thornton et al. (1986).

SAFETY

Individuals with a dementing illness experience changes not only in memory and learning but also in visuoperceptual areas, smell, taste, and balance and gait. Dysphagia is frequently a problem. Table 18–18 notes areas of environmental safety that must be assessed and taken into consideration when caring for these patients.

CAREGIVER EDUCATION AND SUPPORT

Families must be taught to respond to their loved ones' catastrophic and massive emotional overresponses to minor stress; they should remain calm and remove the patient from the threatening situation. Caregivers must learn to work on specific solvable problems within a general framework. By developing strategies for dealing with problems in advance, caregivers can gain a measure of control and thus not approach each problem behavior as a crisis. This also helps stabilize the environment for the patient. Teaching families to remain calm and improve nonverbal communication often helps reduce behavioral disturbances in the patient (Thornton et al., 1986). Responding to feelings rather than to the content of the patient's words is an important practice for caregivers and families and an effective way of dealing with the frequent repetition of questions.

Fear and uncertainty cause caregivers to dread the future. Families can accept uncertainty and be better prepared for emergencies by learning about the disease; learning how to handle specific contingencies as they arise; breaking down dilemmas into smaller, solvable problems; and, most important, taking care of themselves by allowing others to provide support for the patient. Learning that a family member has AD or a related dementing illness is shocking, but once families have made the appropriate legal and financial adjustments (see Chapter 3), they should be encouraged to focus not on the disease and its disabilities but on positive experiences. With early diagnosis and supportive therapies, patients are capable of enjoying many family activities and intima-

cies for a considerable period. It is tragic when fear and anxiety in both the patient and the family are allowed to deprive them of these years.

Counselors and support groups should be made available to all patients with dementia and their families. For these individuals, there is nothing worse than to be told that "there is nothing to be done" and to be left without any additional support. Families are often tremendously relieved and helped by meeting others who are sharing the same experiences and problems. Several nationally and regionally organized groups provide information, assistance, and regularly held support meetings throughout the country. These groups are often tailored to the type of caregiver or the setting of the care recipient. One of the most helpful things clinicians can do for patients and families is to put them in contact with these groups. More than one group is frequently required as patients and their families move along the various stages of the disease process. The Alzheimer's Disease Association, a national organization with chapters in most major areas of the country, is an excellent resource for information regarding support groups and services (see Appendix 18–1).

Impact of a Dementia Diagnosis

People who have a dementing illness must cope simultaneously with associated psychopathological states, such as depression, anxiety, and paranoia, as well as a number of losses. The loss of memory, loss of a job, loss of a role as head of a household or breadwinner, and loss of a future are only a few of the losses experienced by individuals with a dementing illness. In addition, these people must cope with the reactions of others toward them, perhaps overprotective spouses, or distant children and friends. They may feel embarrassment and shame. The nuclear family may experience fear, anger, helplessness, and hopelessness. Feelings of abandonment and isolation are frequent. Criticism by relatives is a common occurrence, wherein they have difficulty accepting the diagnosis and try to rationalize the patient's symptoms in the earlier stages of the disease by attributing blame to family members. The patient may deal with fears and anxiety by becoming verbally and physically abusive toward family members.

Spouses are in social limbo; they cannot mourn decently because the patient is still alive and frequently shows few outward signs of change. They cannot divorce with dignity, even if they wish to do so, and are left with no acceptable outlets for their sexual frustrations and emotional needs.

Young children living in the home are frequently ignored by the patient and neglected by the caregiver, who is mentally and physically drained in attempting to cope with the meaning of the diagnosis and the changes in the patient. The patient may bully the children or vie for attention with them. This is seen more often in fathers whose teenage sons try to assume the parent's role and are viewed as a threat by the patient. Younger children frequently incorporate and misinterpret the family's frustrations, fears, and self-recriminations (Lezak, 1978).

Older children living away from home must cope with feelings of guilt, fear, and loss. Torn between conflicting needs, they may become actively involved or distance themselves from the parent and the disease. Some may become oversolicitous to obtain previously unreceived love from a parent. As the disease progresses in the parent, the adolescent and young adult children engage in a sociopsychological process with distinct stages and phases. The stages of this process of sequential resolving are as follows (Davies et al., 1988):

1. Awareness, in which the child comes to realize that something is truly wrong
2. Exploration, in which the child seeks a reason for the parent's behavior and deals with the physical and psychosocial consequences of the diagnosis
3. Definition, in which the child separates the *patient that is* from the *parent that was*

Factors that influence the adjustment process are family dynamics and each child's age, developmental stage, and personal coping style. Compounding these difficulties, the disease can affect insight, judgment, and decision-making abilities. Attempts by caregivers and pro-

fessionals to deal with evolving deficits may be viewed by the patient as obstructive, interfering, and manipulative (Lezak, 1978).

FAMILY STAGES AFTER DIAGNOSIS

A diagnosis of dementia in a family member results in many changes in the family system. Roles, family expectations, and alliances are altered. In order to cope, families must learn to deal with many new demands. This author's clinical practice has identified several stages that families must move through following a diagnosis; Table 18–19 delineates these stages.

The assessment of a family's ability to care is essential. This assessment should include (1) the organization or disorganization of the family system; (2) individual family members' levels of sophistication about medical and psychological problems; (3) the degree of cooperation; (4) the existence in family members of major chronic or recurring physical illness; (5) the presence of psychiatric problems in any family members; and (6) the dynamics of patient interaction with individual family members (Cohen, 1994).

INSTITUTIONALIZATION AS A FAMILY CRISIS

The decision to seek nursing home placement frequently presents a crisis in the family. Family members often disagree as to the need for and timing of placement. Feelings of anger, guilt, self-recrimination, and failure are common. Most people, particularly older people, have a fear of and deep aversion to nursing homes; in addition, patients often extract promises from their spouses and families that

---

TABLE 18-19

Family Stages After Diagnosis of Dementia

Coping with diagnosis
Beginning to look at management
  Deciding what to do
  Coping maximally
Making the transition to institutionalization
  Making the decision
  Acting on the decision

they will never be placed in a nursing home. Clinicians, therefore, are often faced with a situation in which a spouse insists on caring for the patient at home even though the patient's needs for care far exceed the resources of the caregiver or family—and even if in reality this situation is against both the patient's and family's best interests (Meier & Cassel, 1986). This situation is highly complex for the family and may be compounded by financial issues, a scarcity of resources, and the clinician's own biases and feelings. The sense of guilt and personal responsibility felt when contemplating nursing home placement can be devastating, especially if there is disagreement within the family as to what should be done.

Clinicians should be aware of all these factors when assisting families in making the decision to institutionalize. Important questions to be considered are the patient's needs and preferences (if known), the caregivers' needs, and the needs of the overburdened family. Have all other alternatives been thoroughly explored? Emotional support, reassurance, and assistance in evaluating existing resources are essential at this time. The use of respite and hospice care is gaining acceptance and may provide an alternative to institutionalization. It is helpful to let the patient and family know that they will not be cut adrift from their previous support systems. Ideally, the issue of possible future placement should be discussed with the patient and family early in the disease process when the patient may be able to discuss concerns and preferences and designate a surrogate decision maker.

SUMMARY

Delirium and dementia are major concerns in geriatric care. They represent two of the most common mental disorders encountered in older adults. Basic and clinical research have resulted in improved diagnostic methods and the clinical management of delirium and dementia.

Delirium is a neuropsychiatric syndrome characterized by reversible changes in attention (clouding of consciousness) and cognition. Onset is relatively rapid and the course typically fluctuates. Some patients may have increased levels of arousal accompanied by hallucinations and delusions, whereas others may appear confused, drowsy, or stuporous. The most consistent high-risk factors for developing delirium are age, concurrent cognitive impairment (dementia), and drug toxicity. Clinical examination and consistent observation are the most important factors in detecting and diagnosing delirium. Delirium can present as a life-threatening situation and should always be treated as a medical emergency.

Dementia is a devastating problem for everyone concerned. A conservative estimate of the cost of AD to society is about $90 to 113 billion per year in medical bills, nursing home costs, homecare costs, and lost productivity (Cramer, 1993; Cummings & Mega, 1996). Prolonging patients' stay in the community and providing social support systems for the family add to the quality of life for both the individual and family. But prolonging the inevitable is not enough. With the rapid changes occurring in the healthcare system, widely recognized standards of care for dementia patients and their families are essential and are currently being developed (California Workgroup for Alzheimer's Disease Management Guidelines, in progress). Additional research is needed for effective treatments, including the prevention of underlying causes of the disorder.

REFERENCES

Allen, A. (1994). Alcohol and other toxic dementias. In J.R.M. Copeland, M. T. Abou-Saleh & D. G. Blazer (Eds.), *Principles and practice of geriatric psychiatry* (pp. 385–388). New York: John Wiley & Sons.

Aisen, P. S., & Davis, K. L. (1994). Inflammatory mechanisms in Alzheimer's disease: Implications for therapy. *American Journal of Psychiatry, 151*, 1105–1113.

American Medical Association Council on Scientific Affairs (1993). Physicians and family caregivers: A model for partnership. *Journal of the American Medical Association, 269*, 1282–1284.

American Psychiatric Association (1994). *Diagnostic and statistical manual of mental disorders* (4th ed.). Washington, D.C.: American Psychiatric Association.

American Psychiatric Association (1997). APA practice guidelines for the treatment of patients with Alzheimer's Disease and other dementias of late life. *American Journal of Psychiatry, 154*(suppl.), 1–39.

Bachman, D. L., Wolf, P. A., Linn, R., et al. (1992). Prevalence of dementia and probable senile dementia of the

Alzheimer's type in the Framingham study. *Neurology, 42*, 115–119.

Barrett-Connor, E., & Kritz-Silverstein, D. (1993). Estrogen replacement therapy and cognitive function in older women. *Journal of the American Medical Association, 269*(20), 2637–2641.

Beck, J. C., Benson, D. F., Scheibel, A. B., et al. (1982). Dementia in the elderly: The silent epidemic. *Annals of Internal Medicine, 97*, 231–241.

Benson, D. F., Cummings, J. F., & Tsai, S. Y. (1982). Angular gyrus syndrome simulating Alzheimer's disease. *Archives of Neurology, 39*, 616–620.

Berkow, R., Butler, R. N., & Sunderlund, T. (1995). Cognitive failure: Delirium and dementia. In W. B. Abrams, M. H. Beers & R. Berkow (Eds.), *The Merck manual of geriatrics* (2nd ed., pp. 1139–1161). Whitehouse Station, NJ: Merck & Co., Inc.

Beyreuther, K., Bush, A. I., Dyrks., T., et al. (1991). Mechanisms of amyloid deposition in Alzheimer's disease. *Annals of New York Academy of Science, 640*, 129–139.

Bolla, K. I., Briefel, G., Spector, D., et al. (1992). Neurocognitive effects of aluminum. *Archives of Neurology, 49*, 1021–1026.

Bowen, D. M., Smith, C. B., White, P., & Davison, A. N. (1976). Neurotransmitter-related enzymes and indices of hypoxia in senile dementia and other abiatrophies. *Brain, 99*, 459–496.

Breitner, J.C.S. (1996). Inflammatory processes and anti-inflammatory drugs in Alzheimer's disease: A current appraisal. *Neurobiology of Aging, 17*(5), 789–794.

Brousseau, T., Legrain, S., Berr, C., et al. (1994). Confirmation of the e4 allele of the apolipoprotein E gene as a risk factor for late-onset Alzheimer's disease. *Neurology, 44*, 342–344.

California Workgroup for Alzheimer's Disease Management Guidelines. Sacramento, CA: Department of Health Services, Alzheimer Programs (in progress).

Campbell, E. B., Williams, M. A., & Mlynarczyk, S. M. (1986). After the fall confusion. *American Journal of Nursing, 86*(2), 151–154.

Carlen, P. L., & Neiman, J. (1990). Wernicke's encephalopathy and alcohol-related nutritional disease. In R. Johnson (Ed.), *Current therapy in neurologic disease* (3rd ed., pp. 361–364). Philadelphia: B. C. Decker.

Caudiex, R. J. (1993). Geriatric psychopharmacology. A primary care challenge. *Postgraduate Medicine, 93*(4), 281–301.

Chandra, V., Bharucha, N. E., & Schoenberg, B. S. (1986). Conditions associated with Alzheimer's disease at death: Case control study. *Neurology, 36*, 209–211.

Chui, H. C., Victoroff, J. I., Margolin, D., et al. (1992). Criteria for the diagnosis of ischemic vascular dementia proposed by the state of California Alzheimer's disease diagnostic and treatment centers. *Neurology, 42*, 473–480.

Civil, R. H., Whitehouse, P. J., Lanska, D. J., & Mayeux, R. (1993). Degenerative dementias. In P. J. Whitehouse (Ed.), *Dementia* (pp. 167–214). Philadelphia: F. A. Davis.

Clarfield, A. M. (1988). The reversible dementias: Do they reverse? *Annals of Internal Medicine, 109*(6), 476–486.

Clarfield, A. M. (1989). Normal-pressure hydrocephalus: Saga or swamp? *Journal of the American Medical Association, 262*, 2592–2593.

Clarfield, A. M. (1995). The reversible dementias. *Neurology, 45*(3), 601.

Clinton, J., Ambler, M. W., & Roberts, G. W. (1991). Post-traumatic Alzheimer's disease: Preponderance of a single plaque type. *Neuropathology and Applied Neurobiology, 17*(1), 69–74.

Cohen, D. (1994). A primary checklist for effective family management. *Medical Clinics of North America, 78*(4), 795–809.

Cooper, B. (1991). The epidemiology of primary degenerative dementia and related neurological disorders. *European Archives of Psychiatry and Clinical Neurosciences, 240*, 223–233.

Cramer, D. (Ed.). (1993). *Perspectives in health promotion and aging. 8* (4), 1–12. Washington, D.C.: National Eldercare Institute on Health Promotion, American Association of Retired Persons.

Cronin-Golomb, A., Corkin, S., & Rosen, T. J. (1993). Neuropsychological assessment of dementia. In P. J. Whitehouse (Ed.), *Dementia* (pp. 130–164). Philadelphia: F. A. Davis.

Cummings, J. L. (1995). Dementia: The failing brain. *Lancet, 345*, 1481–1484.

Cummings, J. L., & Benson, D. F. (1983). *Dementia: A clinical approach*. Woburn, MA: Butterworth.

Cummings, J. L., & Mega, M. (1996). Alzheimer's Disease: Etiologies and pathogenesis. *Consultant Pharmacist* (suppl. E), 8–15.

Cummings, J. L., Arsland, D., & Jarvik, L. (1997). Dementia. In C. K. Cassel, H. J. Cohen, E. B. Larson, et al. (Eds.), *Textbook of geriatric medicine* (3rd ed., pp. 897–916). New York: Springer.

Cummings, J. L., Miller, B., Hill, M. A., & Neshkles, R. (1987). Neuropsychiatric aspects of multi-infarct dementia and dementia of the Alzheimer's type. *Archives of Neurology, 41*, 874–879.

Davies, H. D., Ingram, L., Priddy, J. M., & Tinklenberg, J. R. (1988). *Responding to the loss of a parent over time: Experiences of young-adult children of Alzheimer's patients.* Paper presented at the annual meeting of the Gerontological Society of America, San Francisco, CA.

Davies, P., & Maloney, A. J. F. (1976). Selective loss of central cholinergic neurons in Alzheimer's disease. *Lancet, 2*, 1403.

Deary, I. J., & Whalley, L. J. (1988). Recent research on the causes of Alzheimer's disease. *British Medical Journal, 297*, 807–810.

Drachman, D. A., & Lippa, C. F. (1992). The etiology of Alzheimer's disease: The pathogenesis of dementia. *Annals of the New York Academy of Sciences, 648*, 176–186.

Dubovsky, S. L. (1994). Geriatric neuropsychopharmacology. In C. E. Coffey & J. L. Cummings (Eds.), *Textbook of geriatric neuropsychiatry* (pp. 596–631). Washington, D.C.: American Psychiatric Press.

Eisdorfer, C., & Cohen, D. (1981). Management of the patient and family coping with dementing illness. *Journal of Family Practice, 12*, 831–837.

Erkinjuntti, T., Ketonen, L., Sulkava, R., et al. (1987). Do white matter changes on MRI and CT differentiate vascular dementia from Alzheimer's disease? *Journal of Neurology, Neurosurgery, and Psychiatry, 50*, 37–42.

Erkinjuntti, T., Laaksonen, R., Sulkava, R., et al. (1986).

Neuropsychological differentiation between normal aging, Alzheimer's disease and vascular dementia. *Acta Neurologica Scandinavica, 74,* 393–403.

Evans, D. (1990). Estimated prevalence of Alzheimer's disease in the United States. *Milbank Memorial Fund Quarterly, 68,* 267–289.

Feldman, E., & Plum, F. (1993). Metabolic dementia. In P. Whitehouse (Ed.), *Dementia* (pp. 307–336). Philadelphia: F. A. Davis.

Folstein, M. F., Folstein, S. E., & McHugh, P. R. (1975). Mini-Mental State: A practical method for grading the cognitive state of patients for the clinician. *Journal of Psychiatric Research, 12,* 189–198.

Foreman, M. (1984). Acute confusional states in the elderly: An algorithm. *Dimensions of Critical Care Nursing, 3*(4), 207–215.

Francis, J. (1992). Delirium in older patients. *Journal of American Geriatrics Society, 40,* 829–838.

Francis, J., & Kapoor, W. N. (1990). Delirium in hospitalized elderly. *Journal of General Internal Medicine, 5,* 65–79.

Fromholt, P., & Larsen, S. F. (1991). Autobiographical memory in normal aging and dementia. *Journal of Gerontology, 46*(3), 85–91.

Funkenstein, H. H., Hicks, R., Dysken, M. W., & Davis, J. M. (1981). Drug treatment of cognitive impairment in Alzheimer's disease and the late life dementias. In N. E. Miller & G. D. Cohen (Eds.), *Clinical aspects of Alzheimer's disease and senile dementia, vol. 15* (pp. 139–160). New York: Raven Press.

Gold, P. E., & Stone, W. S. (1988). Neuroendocrine effects on memory in aged rodents and humans. *Neurobiology of Aging, 9,* 709–717.

Gottlieb, G. L., Johnson, J., Wanich, C., & Sullivan, E. (1991). Delirium in the medically ill elderly: Operationalizing the DSM-III criteria. *International Psychogeriatrics, 3,* 181–196.

Graff-Radford, N. R., Godersky, J. C, & Jones, M. P. (1989). Variables predicting surgical outcome in symptomatic hydrocephalus in the elderly. *Neurology, 39,* 1601–1604.

Grossberg, G. T., & Kumar, V. (Eds.). (1998). Psychotherapeutic agents in older adults [entire issue]. *Clinics in Geriatric Medicine, 14*(1).

Hachinski, V. C., Lassen, N. A., & Marshall, J. (1974). Multi-infarct dementia: A cause of mental deterioration in the elderly. *Lancet, 2,* 207–209.

Haggerty, A. D. (1990). Psychotherapy for patients with Alzheimer's disease. *Advances, 7*(1), 55–60.

Hall, J. L., Gonder-Frederick, L. A., Chewning, W. W., et al. (1989). Glucose enhancement of memory in young and aged humans. *Neuropsychologia, 27,* 1129–1138.

Hall, G. R., Gerdner, L., Zwygart-Stauffacher, M., & Buckwalter, K. (1995). Principles of nonpharmacological management: Caring for people with Alzheimer's disease using a conceptual model. *Psychiatric Annals, 25*(7), 432–440.

Ham, R. (1997). After the diagnosis: Supporting Alzheimer's patients and their families. *Postgraduate Medicine, 101*(6), 57–70.

Heyman, A. (1978). Differentiation of Alzheimer's disease from multi-infarct dementia. In R. Katzman, R. D. Terry & K. L. Brick (Eds.), *Alzheimer's disease: Senile dementia and related disorders, vol. 7* (pp. 109–110). New York: Raven Press.

Heyman, A., Wilkinson, W. E., Stafford, J. A., et al. (1984). Alzheimer's disease. A study of the epidemiological aspects. *Annals of Neurology, 15,* 335–341.

Hollister, L. E. (1985). Alzheimer's disease. Is it worth treating? *Drugs, 29*(6), 335–341.

Huff, F. J., Corkin, S., & Growdown, J. H. (1986). Semantic impairment and anomia in Alzheimer's disease. *Brain Language, 28,* 235–249.

Ingram, D. K., Spangler, E. L., IIjima, S., et al. (1994). Rodent models of memory dysfunction in Alzheimer's disease and normal aging: Moving beyond the cholinergic hypothesis. *Life Sciences, 55*(25/26), 2037–2049.

Inouye, S. K., van Dyck, C. H., Alessi, C., et al. (1990). Clarifying confusion: The confusion assessment method. *Annals of Internal Medicine, 113,* 941–948.

Jeste, D. V., Eastham, J. H., Lohr, J. B., & Salzman, C. (1998). Treatment of disordered behavior and psychosis. In C. Salzman (Ed.), *Clinical geriatric psychopharmacology* (3rd ed., pp. 106–149). Baltimore: Williams & Wilkins.

Kane, R. L., Ouslander, J. G., & Abrass I. B. (1994). *Essentials of clinical geriatrics* (3rd ed., pp. 83–114). New York: McGraw-Hill.

Kase, C. S. (1986). Multi-infarct dementia. A real entity? *Journal of American Geriatrics Society, 34,* 482–484.

Kase, C. S. (1991). Epidemiology of multi-infarct dementia. *Alzheimer Disease and Associated Disorders, 5*(2), 71–76.

Katzman, R. (1984). Dementia. In S. H. Apple (Ed.), *Current Neurology, vol. 5* (pp. 91–110). New York: John Wiley & Sons.

Katzman, R. (1986). Alzheimer's disease. *New England Journal of Medicine, 4,* 964–972.

Katzman, R. (1990). Should a major imaging procedure (CT or MRI) be required in the workup of dementia? *Journal of Family Practice, 31*(4), 401–410.

Katzman, R. (1992). Diagnosis and management of dementia. In R. Katzman & J. W. Rowe (Eds.), *Principles of geriatric neurology* (pp. 167–206). Philadelphia: F. A. Davis.

Kolb, B., & Whishaw, I. Q. (1985). *Fundamentals of human neuropsychology* (2nd ed.). New York: W. W. Freeman.

Larson, E. B., Kukull, W. A., & Katzman, R. L. (1992). Cognitive impairment: Dementia and Alzheimer's disease. *Annual Review of Public Health, 13,* 431–439.

LaRue, A. (1992). *Aging and neuropsychological assessment.* New York: Plenum.

Levkoff, S. E., Besdine, R. W., & Wetle, T. (1986). Acute confusional states in hospitalized elderly. In C. Eisdorfer (Ed.), *Annual review of gerontology and geriatrics, vol. 6* (pp. 1–26). New York: Springer.

Levkoff, S. E., Cleary, P., Liptzin, B., & Evans, D. A. (1991). Epidemiology of delirium: An overview of research issues and findings. *International Psychogeriatrics, 3,* 149–167.

Levy-Lahad, E., Wijsman, E. M., Nemens, E., et al. (1995). A familial Alzheimer's disease locus on chromosome 1. *Science, 269*(5226), 970–973.

Lezak, M. D. (1995). *Neuropsychological assessment* (3rd ed.). New York: Oxford University Press.

Lezak, M. D. (1978). Living with the characterologically altered brain injured patient. *Journal of Clinical Psychiatry, 39,* 592–598.

Lipowski, Z. J. (1984). Acute confusion states in the elderly.

In M. N. Albert (Ed.), *Clinical neurology of aging* (pp. 279–297). New York: Oxford University Press.

Lipowski, Z. J., (1989). Delirium in the elderly patient. *New England Journal of Medicine, 320,* 578–582.

Lipowski, Z. J. (1994). Delirium (acute confusional states). In W. R. Hazzard, E. L. Bierman, J. P. Blass, et al. (Eds.), *Principles of geriatric medicine and gerontology* (3rd ed., pp. 1021–1026). New York: McGraw-Hill.

Mace, N. L., & Rabins, P. V. (1991). *The 36-hour day* (2nd ed.). Baltimore: Johns Hopkins University Press.

Maletta, G. J. (1985). Medications to modify at home behavior of Alzheimer's disease patients. *Geriatrics, 40*(12), 31–42.

Maletta, G. J. (1990). Pharmacological treatment and management of the aggressive demented patient. *Psychiatric Annals, 20,* 446–455.

Marshall, J. (1993). Vascular dementias. In P. J. Whitehouse (Ed.), *Dementia* (pp. 215–236). Philadelphia: F. A. Davis.

Mayeux, R., Foster, N. L., Rossor, M., & Whitehouse, P. J. (1993). The clinical evaluation of patients with dementia. In P. J. Whitehouse (Ed.), *Dementia* (pp. 92–129). Philadelphia: F. A. Davis.

Mayeux, R., & Schofeld, P. W. (1994). Alzheimer's disease. In W. R. Hazzard, E. L. Bierman, J. P. Blass, et al. (Eds.), *Principles of geriatric medicine and gerontology* (3rd ed., pp. 1035–1050). New York: McGraw-Hill.

McCartney, J. R., & Palmateer, L. M. (1985). Assessment of cognitive deficit in geriatric patients: A study of physician behavior. *Journal of the American Geriatrics Society, 33,* 467–471.

McGreer, P. L., McGreer, E. G., Rogers, J., & Sibley, J. (1992). Does anti-inflammatory treatment protect against Alzheimer's disease? In Z. S. Khachaturian & J. P. Blass (Eds.), *Alzheimer's disease: New treatment strategies.* New York: Marcel Dekker.

McKhann, G., Drachman, D., Folstein, M., et al. (1984). Clinical diagnosis of Alzheimer's disease: Report of the NINCDS-ADRDA work group under the auspices of Department of Health and Human Services Task Force on Alzheimer's Disease. *Neurology, 34,* 939–944.

McLachlan, D. R., Dalton, A. J., Galin, H., et al. (1984). Alzheimer's disease: Clinical course and cognitive disturbances. *Acta Neurologica Scandinavica, 99,* 83–89.

Meier, D. E., & Cassel, C. K. (1986). Nursing home placement and the demented patient. *Annals of Internal Medicine, 104,* 98–105.

Meyer, J. S., Judd, B. W., Tawakina T., et al. (1986). Improved cognition after control of risk factors for multi-infarct dementia. *Journal of the American Medical Association, 256,* 2203–2209.

Miller, B. L. (1997). Clinical advances in degenerative dementias. *British Journal of Psychiatry, 171,* 1–3.

Miller, B. L., Chang, L., Oropilla, G., & Mena, I. (1994). Alzheimer's disease and frontal lobe dementias. In C. E. Coffey & J. L. Cummings (Eds.), *Textbook of geriatric neuropsychiatry* (pp. 390–404). Washington, D.C.: American Psychiatric Press.

Miller, N. E., & Lipowski, Z. J. (1991). Advancing age and the syndrome of delirium: Ancient conundrums and modern research advances. *International Psychogeriatrics, 3*(2), 103–113.

Mortimer, J. A., van Dijn, C. M., Chandra, V., et al. (1991). Head trauma as a risk factor for Alzheimer's disease: A collaborative reanalysis of case control studies. EURO-DEM risk factors research group. *International Journal of Epidemiology, 20*(suppl. 2), S28–S35.

National Institute on Aging Task Force (1980). Senility reconsidered: Treatment possibilities for mental impairment in the elderly. *Journal of the American Medical Association, 244,* 259–263.

National Institutes of Health Consensus Conference (1987). Differentiating diagnosis of dementing diseases. *Journal of the American Medical Association, 258,* 3411–3416.

Olichney, J. M., Hofstetter, C. R., Galasko, D., et al. (1995). Death certificate reporting of dementia and mortality in an Alzheimer's Disease Research Center. *Journal of the American Geriatrics Society, 48,* 890–893.

Omar, S. J., Robinson, D., Davies, H. D., et al. (1995). Fluoxetine and visual hallucinations in dementia. *Biological Psychiatry, 38,* 556–558.

Pericak-Vance, M. A., Bedout, J. L., Gaskell, P. C., et al. (1991). Linkage studies in familial Alzheimer's disease—evidence for chromosome 19 linkage. *American Journal of Human Genetics, 48,* 1034–1050.

Pruisner, S. B. (1984). Some speculations about prions, amyloid and Alzheimer's disease. *New England Journal of Medicine, 310,* 661–663.

Read, S. L., & Jarvik, L. F. (1984). Cerebrovascular disease in the differential diagnosis of dementia. *Psychiatric Annals, 14*(2), 100–108.

Reichman, W. E. (1994). Nondegenerative dementing disorders. In C. E. Coffey & J. L. Cummings (Eds.), *Textbook of geriatric neuropsychiatry* (pp. 370–388). Washington, D.C.: American Psychiatric Press.

Reisberg, B., Ferris, S. H., de Leon, M. J., & Crook, T. (1982). The global deterioration scale for assessment of primary degenerative dementia. *American Journal of Psychiatry, 139,* 1136–1139.

Roman, G. C., Tatemichi, T. K., Erkinjuntti, T., et al. (1993). Vascular dementia: Diagnostic criteria for research studies. Report of the NINCDS-AIREN International Workshop. *Neurology, 43,* 250–260.

Rosen, W. G., Mohs, R. C., & Davis, K. L. (1984). A new rating scale for Alzheimer's disease. *American Journal of Psychiatry, 141*(11), 1356–1364.

Rosenberg, R. N. (1993). A causal role for amyloid in Alzheimer's disease: The end of the beginning. 1993 American Academy of Neurology presidential address. *Neurology, 43,* 851–856.

Ross, C. A., Peyser, C. E., Shapiro, I., & Folstein, M. F. (1991). Delirium: Phenomenologic and etiologic subtypes. *International Psychogeriatrics, 3*(2), 135–147.

Rosser, M. (1993). Alzheimer's disease. *British Medical Journal, 307,* 779–782.

Rumble, B., Retallack, R., Hilbich, C., et al. (1989). Amyloid A4 protein and its precursor in Down's syndrome and Alzheimer's disease. *New England Journal of Medicine, 320,* 1446–1452.

Sagar, H. J., & Sullivan, E. V. (1988). Patterns of cognitive impairment in dementia. In C. Kennard (Ed.), *Recent advances in clinical neurology, 5,* 47–86.

St. George-Hyslop, P. H., Tanzi, R. E., Polinsky, R. J., et al. (1987). The genetic defect causing Alzheimer's disease maps on chromosome 21. *Science, 235,* 885–890.

Salzman, C. (1998). Appendix A: Prescribing information. In C. Salzman (Ed.), *Clinical geriatric psychopharmacology* (3rd ed., pp. 543–546). Baltimore: Williams & Wilkins.

Sano, M., Ernesto, C., Thomas, R. G., et al. (1997). A controlled trial of selegiline, alpha-tocopherol, or both as treatment for Alzheimer's disease. *New England Journal of Medicine, 336,* 1216–1222.

Schellenberg, G. D., Bird, T. D., Wijsman, E. M., et al. (1992). Genetic linkage evidence for a familial Alzheimer's disease locus on chromosome 14. *Science, 258,* 668–671.

Schoenberg, B. S. (1986). Epidemiology of Alzheimer's disease and other dementing illnesses. *Journal of Chronic Diseases, 39*(12), 1095–1104.

Selkoe, D. J. (1991). The molecular pathology of Alzheimer's disease. *Neuron, 6,* 487–498.

Small, G., Rabins, P., Barry, P., et al. (1997). Diagnosis and treatment of Alzheimer Disease and related disorders: Consensus Statement of the American Association for Geriatric Psychiatry, the Alzheimer's Association, and the American Geriatrics Society. *Journal of the American Medical Association, 278,* 1363–1371.

Sullivan, N., & Fogel, B. (1986). Could this be delirium? *American Journal of Nursing, 12,* 1359–1363.

Tanzi, R. E., Vaula, G., Romano, D. M., et al. (1992). Assessment of amyloid beta protein precursor gene mutations in large set of familial and sporadic Alzheimer disease cases. *American Journal of Human Genetics, 51,* 273–282.

Teri, L., & Logsdon, R. (1990). Assessment and management of behavioral disturbances in Alzheimer's disease. *Comprehensive Therapy, 16*(5), 36–42.

Terry, R., & Katzman, R. (1992). Alzheimer's disease and cognitive loss. In R. Katzman & J. W. Rowe (Eds.), *Principles of geriatric neurology* (pp. 207–265). Philadelphia: F. A. Davis.

Thal, L. J. (1988). Treatment strategies: Present and future. In M. K. Aronson (Ed.), *Understanding Alzheimer's disease* (pp. 55–60). New York: Charles Scribner's Sons.

Thornton, J. E., Davies, H. D., & Tinklenberg, J. R. (1986).

Alzheimer's disease syndrome. *Journal of Psychosocial Nursing and Mental Health Services, 24*(5), 16–22.

Tueth, M. J., & Cheong, J. A. (1993). Delirium: Diagnosis and treatment in the older patient. *Geriatrics, 48,* 75–80.

Tune, L., & Ross, C. (1994). Delirium. In E. C. Coffey & J. L. Cummings (Eds.), *Textbook of geriatric neuropsychiatry* (pp. 352–365). Washington, D.C.: American Psychiatric Press.

Tuokko, H., Hadjistravopoulos, T., Miller, J. A., & Beattie, B. L. (1992). The Clock Test: A sensitive measure to differentiate normal elderly from those with Alzheimer's disease. *Journal of the American Geriatrics Society, 40,* 579–584.

U'Ren, R. C. (1987). Testing older patient's mental status: Practical office-based approach. *Geriatrics, 42*(3), 49–56.

van Duijn, C. M., Tanja, T. A., Haaxma, R., et al. (1992). Head trauma and the risk of Alzheimer's disease. *American Journal of Epidemiology, 135*(7), 775–782.

Verwoerdt, A. (1981). Individual psychotherapy in senile dementia. In N. E. Miller & G. E. Cohen (Eds.), *Clinical aspects of Alzheimer's disease and senile dementia* (pp. 187–208). New York: Raven Press.

Victor, M. (1993). Persistent altered mentation due to ethanol. *Neurologic Clinics, 11,* 639–661.

Wade, J. P. H. (1991). Multi-infarct dementia: Prevention and treatment. *Alzheimer Disease and Associated Disorders, 5*(2), 144–148.

Willenbring, M. L. (1988). Organic mental disorders associated with heavy drinking and alcohol dependence. *Clinics in Geriatric Medicine, 4*(4), 869–887.

Wurtman, R. J. (1985). Alzheimer's disease. *Scientific American, 252*(1), 62–74.

Yaffe, K., Sawaya, G., Leiberburg, I., & Grady, D. (1998). Estrogen therapy in postmenopausal women: Effects on cognitive function and dementia. *Journal of the American Medical Association, 279*(9), 688–695.

Zisook, S., & Braff, D. L. (1986). Delirium: Recognition and management in the older patient. *Geriatrics, 41*(6), 67–78.

Zoler, M. L. (1994, September 15). Genetic puzzle taking shape, but many pieces still missing. *Internal Medicine News & Cardiology News,* p. 15.

APPENDIX 18 – 1

Resources

ORGANIZATIONS

Alzheimer's Disease and Related Disorders
Association (ADRDA)
919 N. Michigan Avenue, Suite 1000
Chicago, IL 60611-1676
Phone: (800) 272-3900

The ADRDA is an excellent source of help
for patients and their families. The national
office maintains an 800 number and provides
informational material on specific questions of
concern to a caregiver or family and refers
them to the local chapter of the association.
Local chapters provide direct information from
experienced caregivers or staff members and
maintain a variety of support groups and services.

Alzheimer's Disease Education and
Referral Center
P.O. Box 8250
Silver Springs, MD 20907
Phone: (800) 438-4380
http://www.alzheimers.org/adear

Excellent source for current information on all
aspects of Alzheimer's disease.

AREA AGENCIES ON AGING

In addition to voluntary organizations, state
governmental agencies such as the local area
agencies on aging are often involved in providing information and assistance to dementia patients and their families. To identify resources
in your community, contact the National Association of Area Agencies on Aging, phone:
(202) 296–8130

DIAGNOSTIC AND TREATMENT CENTERS

In a number of states diagnostic and treatment
centers have been established. Most are affili-
ated with University Medical Centers. In addition to diagnostic evaluations these centers
provide social services and other related resources.

ALZHEIMER'S DISEASE RESEARCH CENTERS

A number of centers are supported by grants
from the National Institute on Aging and the
National Institute of Mental Health. These centers have a responsibility to provide education
to professionals and caregivers. Most centers
also provide a variety of formal courses open
to family members as well as professionals.

BOOKS

Mace, N. L., & Rabins, P. V. (1991). *The 36
hour day* (2nd ed.). Baltimore: Johns Hopkins
University Press.
Written for caregivers. Covers all aspects of
Alzheimer's disease and is an excellent resource for managing the day-to-day care of
dementia patients.

Aronson, M. K. (Ed.). (1988). *Understanding Alzheimer's disease*. New York: Charles Scribner's.
Covers all aspects of the disease, the diagnostic
process, and management of the dementia patient. Appropriate for both lay members and
professionals. Recommended as a first line of
information for newly diagnosed patients and
their families.

Cohen, D., & Eisdorfer, C. (1987). *The loss of
self*. New York: New American Library.
Lends additional insights into the psychological issues of Alzheimer's patients and their
families.

Davies, H. D., & Jensen, M. P. (1998). *Alzheimer's: The answers you need.* Forest Knolls, CA: Elder Books.
Written for individuals in the early stages of Alzheimer's disease and their caregivers. The book provides helpful answers, in an easy-to-read format, to the questions frequently raised by newly diagnosed individuals.

Gwyther, L. P. (1985). *Care of Alzheimer's patients: A manual for nursing home staff.* Chicago: American Health Care Association and ADRDA.
Care guide for nursing home staff; a useful resource for caregivers and professionals.

A wide variety of other educational materials is also available, including video and audio for professionals and caregivers. The ADRDA maintains a current list.

Parkinson's Disease

Glenna A. Dowling

DEFINITION

Parkinson's disease (PD) is a progressive neurological disorder that results from cell death in a region of the brain called the *substantia nigra* (SN). The progressive loss of nigrostriatal dopaminergic function leads to a constellation of symptoms that usually includes resting tremor, bradykinesia (from the Greek *brady*, meaning slow, and *kinesis*, meaning movement), muscle rigidity, and postural instability. PD is one of the most common neurological diseases, and an estimated one in three individuals reaching 80 years of age will be affected (Aminoff, 1994). Currently, more than 1 million people in the United States have PD, and as the population ages, this figure will increase significantly. The course of the disease is unpredictable, and there is great variation in individual disabilities and needs. Responses to medication are also variable and somewhat unpredictable. In some patients, with appropriate drug therapy the disease can be well controlled for long periods and may never progress to severe disability. In other cases, however, patients can become extremely rigid and bradykinetic, rendering them nearly immobile (Mastrian, 1984).

As with many degenerative, neurological diseases that involve gradual deterioration in motor and behavioral activities, PD is often difficult to identify at its onset or to diagnose in its early stages. There is currently no laboratory test to definitively diagnose PD, and the diagnosis remains one based on clinical assessment (Standaert & Stern, 1993). Positron-emission tomography can demonstrate the disruption of regional cerebral metabolism and neurotransmitter systems that underlie the symptoms of PD (Brooks, 1993); however, widespread use of this technology is probably not warranted, as such data would not significantly alter the course of clinical treatment.

PATHOPHYSIOLOGY

Dopaminergic cells function as inhibitory nerve fibers in the central nervous system. In PD, massive death of the SN dopaminergic cells decreases activity that normally modulates impulses leaving the striatum (Finch et al., 1981). This decrease in input to the striatum and the resulting imbalance in dopaminergic and cholinergic activity contribute to the symptoms manifested in PD. The neurons of the SN have many different projection pathways and show topographic organization. The lateral neurons project principally to the putamen and are involved in motor performance. The medial neurons project primarily to the caudate nucleus and frontal and limbic areas and are involved with psychomotor functions (Rinne, 1993). In classical PD, there is preferential loss of SN neurons in the ventrolateral region, with the more medial region being relatively well preserved (Rinne, 1993). Striatal signals, unmodified by inhibitory input from the SN, are transmitted through the ventral thalamus to the motor cortex and spinal motor neurons, resulting in oscillating electrical signals that produce the involuntary rhythmic muscular movements (tremor), muscle rigidity, and bradykinesia that are the three classic symptoms of PD.

A deficiency of brain dopamine can result from a variety of causes, and various neurological problems therefore manifest symptoms similar to those of PD. The term *parkinsonism* refers to any condition marked predominantly by the symptoms of rigidity, tremor, and bradykinesia that result from a brain dopamine deficiency. This deficiency can result from injury to the SN by, for example, a stroke, a tumor, certain neurotoxic drugs, or a virus. A functionally similar state can result from any condition that blocks the action of dopamine in the striatum or renders these neurons incapable of receiving messages.

The most prevalent type of parkinsonism is PD, first described by James Parkinson in 1817 in his *Essay on the shaking palsy*. This type of parkinsonism, also known as *paralysis agitans*, is termed idiopathic because its cause is unknown. Several types of parkinsonism are known, including degenerative, symptomatic, and vascular parkinsonism. *Degenerative parkinsonism* results from neuronal death in multiple regions of the brain, including the striatum, and is usually seen in elderly individuals. The major tranquilizer drugs (e.g., phenothiazines) used to treat psychiatric conditions can induce parkinsonism. These drugs block the action of dopamine in the brain and thereby induce the constellation of symptoms seen in PD. Metoclopramide (Reglan), a drug prescribed for a variety of stomach disorders, acts in the same way as the phenothiazines and can also induce parkinsonism. In the early 20th century, a viral encephalitis epidemic resulted in many affected individuals developing parkinsonism. This particular type of viral encephalitis became known as *encephalitis lethargica* because its first symptom was extreme and prolonged sleepiness. Patients subsequently developed a variety of other symptoms, including parkinsonian symptoms, which often remained throughout their lives.

Symptomatic parkinsonism results from traumatic injury to the basal ganglia, from the repeated head injuries sustained by boxers, for example. *Vascular parkinsonism* can result from small infarcts in the cerebral arteries that leave patients with residual deficits such as stiffness, slowness, the tendency to walk with short shuffling steps, and difficulty speaking clearly. Finally, in many chronic progressive neurological disorders, parkinsonian symptoms can occur in conjunction with other symptoms. These conditions are termed *parkinsonism plus,* as the additional symptoms do not occur in classical PD. Examples of these disorders include olivopontocerebellar atrophy, striatonigral degeneration, and Shy-Drager syndrome.

The remainder of this chapter deals primarily with classical PD, but many of the management strategies may be useful in other types of parkinsonism as well.

INCIDENCE AND PREVALENCE

As mentioned previously, PD is one of the most common neurological diseases affecting people older than 50 years (Boller, 1984; Schoenberg, 1987). Community-based studies to assess the incidence and prevalence of PD were not undertaken until the late 1950s. These studies have yielded prevalence (i.e., the total number of affected individuals in a given population at a given time) estimates ranging from 31 per 100,000 to 328 per 100,000. Incidence (i.e., the number of new cases diagnosed during a specific period) estimates range from 4.5 per 100,000 to 20.5 per 100,000 (Mayeux et al., 1995; Tanner, 1992; Tanner & Goldman, 1996). Methodological, geographical, and diagnostic variability across these studies accounts for the large differences in findings.

RISK FACTORS

Although the definitive cause of PD is not known, it is likely that a combination of factors contributes to this disorder; these factors can include aging, exposure to toxins, genetic predisposition, and oxidative mechanisms (Jankovic, 1993b).

Aging. An important risk factor that is unequivocally associated with PD is increasing age. PD is rare in individuals younger than 30 years, and the incidence and prevalence increase exponentially through middle and late life (Jenner et al., 1992; Tanner, 1992). As individuals age, significant changes occur in the basal ganglia that may be responsible for the movement disorders characteristic of even healthy elderly people, such as slower movement, greater difficulty in coordination, and a decreased ability to perform finely controlled movements. Changes in the basal ganglia with age are implicated in the development of PD (Finch et al., 1981). In normally aging individuals, the SN loses 30 to 50% of its neurons. The concentration of dopamine, the neurotransmitter released from SN cells, shows parallel decreases. The normal loss of cells during aging, although leading to some slowing in motor activities, is not sufficient to result in PD. Age, however, in conjunction with exposure to environmental toxins or cumulative oxidative stress caused by dopamine metabolism throughout life, can contribute to the development of PD (Jenner et al., 1992).

Toxic Exposure. Positive correlations have been reported between the incidence of PD and the use of pesticides in communities (Lewin, 1985). The fact that PD was first described in 1817 (Critchley, 1955), as the Industrial Revolution was beginning, suggests that PD may be caused by chronic exposure to environmental toxins (Spencer et al., 1987). In addition, a number of young narcotic users exposed to the toxin MPTP (1-methyl-4-phenyl-1,2,3,6-tetrahydropyridine) developed parkinsonism, suggesting that exposure to an exogenous agent may cause PD in some instances (Langston, 1986).

Genetics. Several studies (e.g., Golbe et al., 1990) have reported that PD has a hereditary component. However, genetic studies of monozygotic twins have shown that there is no strongly dominant genetic factor in determining susceptibility to or the onset of PD (Jenner et al., 1992; Ward et al., 1983). Some investigators have identified specific subtypes of PD— a tremor-associated form and a juvenile form—in which a weak familial association has been demonstrated. Genetic variation exists in human responses to environmental chemicals, a possible cause of idiopathic PD. Patients with drug-induced parkinsonism characteristically have lower amounts of the liver enzymes that detoxify foreign compounds than do normal subjects (Barbeau et al., 1985). Recent studies confirm that the first-degree relatives of PD patients have a higher incidence of PD than do the first-degree relatives of control subjects (Lazzarini et al., 1994; Payami et al., 1994, 1995). A genetically based susceptibility to toxins might contribute to the development of PD, or a genetic defect might impair the body's ability to deal with exogenous toxic substances or generate endogenous neurotoxins (Jenner et al., 1992).

Recently, the genetic linkage of a large pedigree of a family with a rare autosomal dominant form of PD was identifed (Polymeropoulos et al., 1997). The role of this genetic mutation in sporadic PD has yet to be determined.

Other. In most studies, the prevalence of PD is the same in men and women; however, at least one study has found an increased prevalence in men (Tanner, 1992). Trauma is often listed as a risk factor for PD, as associations have been reported in retrospective case-control studies. However, prospectively collected data do not show this association. The reported associations between PD and head trauma likely reflect biased recall and not a cause-and-effect relationship (Tanner, 1992).

CARDINAL FEATURES

Tremor

Resting tremor is the most characteristic symptom of PD and the initial symptom in 70% of patients (Standaert & Stern, 1993). The tremor is usually a rhythmic, involuntary movement of the thumb and fingers in a rocking motion called *pill rolling,* but it may also occur in the feet, head, jaw, lips, or tongue. It is usually unilateral at onset and spreads as the disease progresses. Patients often feel the tremor before it is visible to an observer and may describe it as a quivering or vibrating sensation. This is

often the case for patients who experience tremors in the abdominal muscles or diaphragm. The tremor usually disappears during sleep or when the patient is resting quietly. It may be present only intermittently and is exacerbated by any kind of stress. The variable and unpredictable nature of the tremor is disconcerting to patients and may result in embarrassment and social isolation. Tremors occur in a variety of neurological conditions, and the tremor of PD is often confused with benign essential tremor, also called familial tremor. The characteristics of benign essential tremor are quite distinct, however, as essential tremor is one of intention and is not present at rest.

Rigidity

Rigidity is characterized by a passive resistance to stretching or movement. This condition is present in nearly all patients with PD and can be detected by moving the patient's joints so as to stretch the skeletal muscles. Resistance of a plastic quality is felt during the movement, often together with jerky, intermittent resistance called *cogwheel rigidity.* The patient often experiences this symptom as a kind of stiffness, and the continuous muscle tension can lead to sensations of aching, soreness, cramping, or pain. The essential motor deficit in rigidity is an inability to activate or relax muscles selectively. Rigidity of the back and neck muscles is often experienced as a headache, of the spinal muscles as a backache, of the leg as a "charley horse," and of the chest and shoulders as chest pain. Common over-the-counter analgesics (e.g., aspirin) are not very effective in relieving the discomfort associated with rigidity, but massage and heat may be helpful for short periods. The best relief is gained from the antiparkinsonian medications discussed later in this chapter.

Bradykinesia and Akinesia

Bradykinesia (slowness of movement) and akinesia (absence of movement) are among the most incapacitating and least understood of all the disabilities encountered in PD (Stem & Lees, 1982). Akinesia occurs because of an inability to convert the will to move into actual motion; it is often experienced by patients as "freezing" or being stuck in place. Akinesia is independent of muscle rigidity and tremor (Birkmayer & Riederer, 1983), but when these symptoms are combined, they produce major changes in overall appearance and behavior. The most common manifestation of bradykinesia is the loss of automatic movements usually taken for granted, for example, swinging the arms while walking, blinking the eyes, swallowing saliva, postural corrections while sitting or walking, and expressive movements of the hands and face. As with tremor and rigidity, akinesia may be symmetric or asymmetric. Patients with asymmetric symptoms tend to turn toward the unaffected side, which disrupts their balance.

The effects of bradykinesia can be quite debilitating and can contribute to patients' decreased ability to perform simple acts, such as getting up out of a chair or car and performing repetitive movements with sustained speed and amplitude (e.g., walking, writing). The severity of the bradykinesia is unpredictable and, like tremor, it is influenced by mood and greatly increased by emotional stress and can almost disappear for brief periods. The ability of a patient to perform a task at one minute but not the next can be very frustrating for both the patient and caregivers. It is crucial to educate the patient, family, caregivers, and others as to validity of the disability.

Postural Instability

Postural instability is another of the extremely disabling features of PD. Poor control of voluntary movement and altered postural reflexes contribute to the problem. Normal postural responses can be classified as *passive* or *active* (Bloem, 1992). The passive elastic properties of muscles, tendons, and ligaments constitute the first response to disturbances of equilibrium and help compensate for small perturbations in balance. Active muscular responses are, however, required to counteract large perturbations. These active responses consist of automatic and voluntary postural responses that are activated sequentially to counteract a displacement of the center of gravity. People with

PD exhibit abnormal postural strategies, reflex amplitudes, latencies, and anticipatory reflexes. Antiparkinsonian medications are usually ineffective in treating this problem, and medication side effects (e.g., dyskinesias) can actually exacerbate the problem. Other symptoms of PD, including altered visuospatial perception, orthostatic hypotension, gait abnormalities, decreased muscle strength, and other non–PD factors related to aging in general can also contribute to postural instability (Bloem, 1992).

ASSOCIATED PROBLEMS

Depression

Reported rates of depression in the PD literature range from 4 to 70%, with a mean frequency of 40% (Celesia & Wanamaker, 1972; Cummings, 1992; Goodwin, 1971; Hoehn & Yahr, 1967; Lieberman et al., 1979; Mayeux et al., 1984). The diagnosis of depression in PD may be difficult because some of the symptoms of depression are similar to the behavioral manifestations of the disease (Guze & Barrio, 1991; Ring, 1993). Some studies have found that patients with PD are significantly more depressed than other chronically ill patients such as those with cancer, multiple sclerosis, and stroke. These findings are especially significant because the patients in the comparison groups were more physically disabled than the patients with PD (Dakof & Mendelsohn, 1986). It is now generally agreed that the depression and often associated anxiety in people with PD are not primarily a psychological reaction or a side effect of treatment but rather manifestations of the underlying neurochemical changes in PD (Menza et al., 1993).

Depression in PD is somewhat different than that reported in idiopathic depression: PD patients tend to have a dysphoric mood and high levels of anxiety but less guilt and self-punitive ideation than do non–PD patients (Brown et al., 1988; Levin et al., 1988). Although the cause of the depression is not fully understood, changes in dopamine and serotonin probably play a major role. Approximately half of the PD patients with depression meet the criteria for a major depressive episode, and half meet the criteria for dysthymia or minor depression

(Cummings, 1992). Depression has a significant clinical impact, as PD patients who are depressed tend to become more disabled than those who are not depressed. Treatment with antidepressant medication or electroconvulsive therapy can provide great relief for the patient (Cummings, 1992; Guze & Barrio, 1991; Rasmussen & Abrams, 1991).

Dementia

Cognitive impairment and dementia are relatively common in patients with PD, but the actual prevalence estimates vary considerably, ranging from 10 to 80%. Recent studies indicate that the incidence of dementia in PD is probably much less common than previously thought. A more realistic estimate is probably a 10 to 20% lifetime risk of moderate to severe dementia as defined by the *Diagnostic and statistical manual of mental disorders* (3rd ed., DSM-III) (Ring, 1993). The pathophysiological basis of the cognitive changes in PD are not well understood, but the clinical picture is often quite different from that seen in other dementias such as Alzheimer's disease (Cummings, 1988).

Specific cognitive deficits associated with PD are an inability to encode, comprehend, and analyze new material; to remember recent events; to follow instructions; and to shift behavior to meet new task requirements (Cools et al., 1984). *Bradyphrenia*, a slowing of thinking processes, is the most commonly reported cognitive impairment. Characteristics that remain intact include long-term memory, social judgment, social manners, verbal fluency, object recognition, auditory attention, and rhythmic pattern discrimination (Loranger et al., 1972; Matthews & Haaland, 1979; Pirozzolo et al., 1982; Talland, 1962).

Degeneration of the brain's dopaminergic system is probably not the major factor responsible for cognitive impairment (Mayeux & Stern, 1983; Rinne, 1993). Studies of PD patients with dementia have shown the additional presence of cortical atrophy, cell loss in the nucleus basalis, plaques and Alzheimer-type tangles, and decreased concentrations of the acetylcholine-synthesizing enzyme choline acetyltransferase. These findings suggest that

there may be a clinical and pathological continuum ranging from predominant dementia with motor dysfunction in Alzheimer's disease to predominant motor dysfunction with dementia in PD (Boller, 1984; Levin et al., 1992). In addition, cognitive impairment and depression frequently coexist in PD, and the severity of the depression is related to the severity of cognitive impairment. This relationship has important therapeutic implications if the treatment of depression can reverse cognitive decline (Gannon, 1992). More research is needed to clarify these issues.

Autonomic Disturbances

Changes in the function of the autonomic nervous system lead to a variety of additional symptoms. Gastrointestinal dysfunction includes delayed gastric emptying, small intestine motor dysfunction, increased colon transit time, and disordered salivary clearance due to altered swallowing. Although the pathophysiology of these symptoms is poorly understood, contributing factors likely include autonomic dysfunction, reduced physical activity, alterations in diet, and medication side effects (Edwards et al., 1992). In addition, autonomic disturbances probably play a role in such symptoms as (1) a decreased ability to regulate blood pressure, particularly when going from a lying to a standing position (resulting in orthostatic hypotension); (2) bladder dysfunction, sometimes termed *neurogenic bladder*; (3) changes in sexual functioning; (4) altered temperature regulation; (5) excessive secretion by the sebaceous glands, resulting in a seborrheic dermatitis; (6) loss of appetite; and (7) profuse perspiration.

Other Symptoms

As previously mentioned, complaints of aches and pains are often associated with rigidity and bradykinesia, and persistent tremor can result in symptoms of muscular fatigue. Changes in posture occur, with the patient tending to bend the trunk forward with the knees flexed, especially while walking. One or both of the upper extremities may also be carried in a slightly abducted position and flexed at the elbow and/or wrist (Duvoisin, 1992). Speech tends to become soft and poorly modulated, making it progressively more difficult for the patient with PD to communicate. Swallowing abnormalities and resultant silent aspiration are common. Ankle edema occurs and is particularly problematic in severely bradykinetic patients owing to decreased movement. Conjunctivitis caused by a decreased frequency of eye blinking may cause the patient to complain of burning or itching eyes. The characteristic tendency of patients with PD to write progressively smaller-sized letters (*micrographia*) can be useful in diagnosing the disease and as a tool to track the effect of treatment.

Impaired visuospatial perception is common among patients with PD (Boller, 1984). Patients typically experience difficulty in accurately identifying the relative position of objects in space, in orienting objects or body parts in specific directions, and in performing other mental tasks involving spatial relationships. Patients with PD have been found to have difficulty in shifting from one type of perceptual organization to another, which results in an inability to perform sequential or predictive voluntary movements. Studies suggest that perceptual motor impairment in PD may result from an inability to use incoming sensory information to generate the spatial perception necessary for expected movements (Mayeux & Stern, 1983). Oculomotor problems may contribute to visuoperceptual spatial and constructional problems, making it difficult for the patient to perceive objects in the peripheral field of vision.

Finally, research indicates that people with PD tend to have more disturbed sleep than do age-matched controls. The most commonly reported sleep-related problems are an inability to sleep through the night and difficulty returning to sleep after awakening. People with PD also report daytime sleepiness, very different kinds of dreams than they experienced before they had PD, nightmares or night terrors, nighttime vocalizations, leg movements or jerking, painful leg cramps, difficulty with or an inability to turn over in bed, and waking up to go to the bathroom. Very little research has been conducted on sleep in people with PD, and the reasons for the observed changes are unknown. Potential explanations include reactions to or side effects of medications (especially levodopa) and awakening due to symptoms such as pain, stiffness, urinary frequency, or disease effects on the internal clock (Askenasy, 1993; Dowling, 1995; Nausieda et al., 1984).

PHARMACOLOGICAL TREATMENTS AND THEIR NURSING IMPLICATIONS

The management of PD is primarily pharmacological in conjunction with supportive medical and nursing care and a variety of therapies (e.g., physical, speech, swallowing). Symptomatic pharmacological treatment is aimed at re-establishing normal brain neurotransmitter levels and relationships. Additional preventive drugs may also be prescribed. The patient usually receives a combination of medications, which may include one or several of those discussed in this section (Fig. 19–1). (See Olanow & Koller [1998] for a thorough review.)

Levodopa

The administration of levodopa is based on scientific evidence that the characteristic pathology of PD is a degeneration of the SN cells and the resultant loss of dopamine. In the majority of patients with classical PD, replacement of dopamine by therapeutic administration of its precursor levodopa results in symptomatic benefit (Aminoff, 1994). Approximately 15% of patients fail to improve with levodopa therapy, and it is hypothesized that these nonresponders probably do not have classical PD but instead have one of the other forms of parkinsonism (Jankovic, 1993a). As experience with levodopa therapy has accumulated, various controversies have emerged. The optimal time to institute therapy has come into question because levodopa may lose its effectiveness over time or even exert deleterious consequences on the course of the disease itself. Treatment with levodopa should be initiated in response to the patient's clinical picture of functional impairment, and the dose should be kept to a minimum to reduce the risk of developing long-term complications (Aminoff,

No functional impairment

↓

Education and support
No symptomatic pharmacotherapy
? Preventive pharmacotherapy (selegiline)

Mild functional impairment

↓

As above but commence symptomatic treatment
Dopamine agonists, anticholinergic drugs (for tremor),
or amantadine

Mild to moderate functional impairment

↓

Commence dopaminergic treatment
Low-dose Sinemet (levodopa and carbidopa)
+/-
dopamine agonist

↓

Declining ← Good → Response
response   response   fluctuations

Declining response	Good response	Response fluctuations
Ensure Sinemet is taken 1 hour before or 2 hours after meals Add selegiline and/or Increase Sinemet and/or Add dopamine agonist and/or Add COMT inhibitor and/or Consider pallidotomy	Continue above regimen	Restrict protein intake Main protein meal at night Increase dosing of Sinemet and/or Switch to controlled-release Sinemet and/or Add dopamine agonist and/or Add selegiline and/or Consider pallidotomy

FIGURE 19–1. The selection of treatment for Parkinson's disease. (Redrawn from Aminoff, M. J. [1994]. Treatment of Parkinson's disease. *Western Journal of Medicine, 161*[3], 305. Additional data from Olanow & Koller [1998].)

1994). Levodopa is usually administered in combination with a dopa-decarboxylase inhibitor to both decrease the amount of levodopa converted to dopamine in the intestinal mucosa and increase the amount of levodopa reaching the brain. The combination medication produces fewer side effects of nausea and vomiting. This preparation is marketed in the United States as Sinemet.

After 5 to 10 years of levodopa therapy, most patients (50–90%) who initially experienced great benefit typically begin to have adverse reactions (Jankovic, 1993a; Olanow & Koller, 1998). These reactions include a *wearing-off effect* that necessitates more frequent dosing to maintain a given level of function as well as response fluctuations (*on-off phenomena*) that often bear no relationship to the timing of the medication. These problems can be quite disabling and are often difficult to treat. Fluctuations of the delivery of levodopa to the site where it exerts its effect can be caused by erratic gastric emptying and intestinal absorption in addition to competition between amino acids and levodopa for active transport across the blood-brain barrier. Thus, a more constant drug blood level and decreased dosing frequency may be achieved by advising patients to take their levodopa on an empty stomach (i.e., 1 hour before or 2 hours after meals) and to restrict protein intake to the minimal daily requirement, eaten primarily in the last meal of the day. Controlled-release preparations of levodopa (Sinemet CR) are now available and deliver a more constant amount of dopamine to the receptors and more closely approximate physiological conditions (Koller & Pahwa, 1994; Stern, 1993). In cases of response fluctuation or dyskinesia, this form of levodopa is worth a trial (Stern, 1993). Continuous infusion of levodopa either intravenously or directly into the duodenum is also a possibility (Chase et al., 1994; Fowler & Bergen, 1993).

Dyskinesias, defined as abnormal involuntary movements, often occur as a side effect of levodopa therapy. Management of these dyskinesias can be difficult and depends on an accurate assessment of their temporal patterning (Aminoff, 1994). Dyskinesias can occur constantly, at peak plasma levodopa concentrations, or at a specific levodopa concentration but not above or below this concentration (Jankovic, 1993a). If dyskinesias appear at peak dose levels, an overall reduction of dose should relieve the symptom. If the dyskinesias occur at a submaximal plasma concentration, keeping the level above this level can alleviate the problem. Dyskinesias are thought to result from a supersensitivity of the postsynaptic dopamine receptor, and dopamine agonist drugs may lessen these symptoms by directly stimulating central dopamine receptors (see the subsequent discussion of dopamine agonists).

Dopamine Agonists

Unlike levodopa, dopamine agonists directly stimulate postsynaptic dopamine receptors and do not require enzymatic conversion, neuronal presynaptic storage, or active transport across the blood-brain barrier. Considerable evidence suggests that these drugs may be useful for treatment early in the course of PD, and their use may delay the need to introduce levodopa. As adjunctive therapy, they provide functional improvement at lower doses of levodopa and have the potential to delay the occurrence of the side effects associated with long-term levodopa therapy. When given at advanced stages of the disease, dopamine agonists can alleviate or lessen some of the motor complications observed with levodopa treatment, especially the wearing-off phenomena (Montastruc et al., 1993). Bromocriptine and pergolide have been available for many years in the United States, and lisuride and apomorphine are used widely elsewhere.

Data from large-scale studies on two new dopamine agonists (pramipexole and ropinirole) were recently reviewed and approved by the Food and Drug Administration (FDA). These newer dopamine agonists are more selective in their site of action, and it is hoped that this specificity will produce greater antiparkinsonian benefit with fewer side effects than the agonists previously available (see Gottwald et al., 1997, for a thorough review). Methods of continuous subcutaneous administration of dopamine agonists via a portable minipump or a transdermal patch also hold promise as delivery mechanisms that can maintain constant drug plasma levels and thereby prevent or delay some of the long-term complications that are common today.

COMT Inhibitors

Several clinical studies have recently been completed, and others are currently under way to investigate the effectiveness of catechol-*O*-methyltransferase (COMT) inhibitors as therapeutic agents. These agents should enhance the benefit of levodopa therapy by reducing its conversion to 3-*O*-methyldopa, which competes with levodopa for transport (Aminoff, 1994). COMT inhibitors act to increase the availability and transfer of levodopa into the brain. Both tolcapone (recently approved by the FDA) and entacapone (currently under review by the FDA) increase the plasma levodopa half-life, thereby providing more stable plasma levels and enhanced and smoother levodopa availability to the brain (Olanow & Koller, 1998).

Monoamine Oxidase Inhibitors

Another means by which to increase the level of dopamine is to inhibit its oxidation by monoamine oxidase type B (MAO B) in the synaptic cleft. Selegiline (e.g., deprenyl, Eldepryl), an MAO B inhibitor, has been used in Europe for this purpose. It can be used in the early phase of PD as monotherapy or later as adjuvant therapy in patients whose response to levodopa has waned or who are experiencing response fluctuations (Nutt, 1993; Rinne, 1993). Although the research results to date have been ambivalent, there is concern that levodopa therapy may accelerate the rate of dopaminergic neuron degeneration as a result of toxic metabolites that are generated during its oxidative metabolism (Olanow, 1993a, 1993b). Selegiline is hypothesized to decrease the enzymatic breakdown of dopamine, thereby decreasing free radical formation and possibly reducing related neuronal damage (Parkinson Study Group, 1989). In the United States, selegiline is often prescribed as a preventive therapy for this reason (Rinne, 1993).

The metabolites of selegiline (l-amphetamine and l-methamphetamine) can occasionally induce insomnia in patients, and it is recommended that the standard dosage of 5 mg twice daily be given at breakfast and lunch. Unlike the nonselective MAO inhibitors, selegiline in the recommended dose does not have the potential to precipitate a hypertensive crisis. However, if taken in higher doses (e.g., 30 mg or more), the selectivity is lost and hypertension becomes a risk. Like other MAO inhibitors, selegiline can have potentially life-threatening interactions with meperidine hydrochloride (Demerol), and these medications should never be used simultaneously (Ahlskog, 1994). Somerset Pharmaceuticals, Inc. also warns against the use of selegiline with serotonin reuptake inhibitors (e.g., fluoxetine) and tricyclic antidepressants (e.g., amitriptyline), owing to the potential for serious toxicity.

Anticholinergics

For many years the only symptomatic treatment available for PD was with anticholinergic drugs. The anticholinergics act by correcting the balance between dopamine and acetylcholine, which is shifted toward cholinergic dominance in the striatum of patients with PD (Calne, 1993). These drugs are still used and can in some cases be important additions to the drug regimen. They are particularly useful when tremor is a predominant and troublesome symptom and is not adequately controlled by levodopa. These drugs are, however, often poorly tolerated in the elderly, and side effects include blurry vision, dry mouth, constipation, urinary retention (especially in men with prostate hypertrophy), decreased sweating, memory impairment, confusion, and hallucinations.

Amantadine

Amantadine, an antiviral agent, was found in the 1960s to have antiparkinsonian effects. Although the mechanism of action is not clearly understood, amantadine increases dopamine release, decreases dopamine reuptake, stimulates dopamine receptors, and acts peripherally as an anticholinergic. Amantadine, unlike most antiparkinsonian medications, is usually taken in a standard dose (100 mg twice daily); it is effective in probably only half of patients, and the effects may be short lived. An unusual and sometimes alarming but harmless side effect of this drug is the appearance of a purplish mottling of the skin, called *livedo reticularis*, which is sometimes accompanied by lower extremity edema. These symptoms disappear when the medication is discontinued. Other side effects include confusion, hallucinations, insomnia, and nightmares (Olanow & Koller, 1998) (Table 19–1).

Treatments on the Horizon

Preclinical studies indicate that gene therapy may be valuable in the treatment of PD (Bresden, 1993). Other neurotransmitters and peptides are also affected in PD. For example, overactivity by glutaminergic neurons may be important in producing some parkinsonian deficits. Glutamate antagonist therapeutic strategies may prove beneficial in the future (Aminoff, 1994).

TABLE 19-1

Pharmacological Treatments

Drug	Action	Effect	Administration Issues	Common Side Effects
Levodopa (Sinemet)	Replacement of dopamine by therapeutic administration of its precursor levodopa	Symptomatic (physical and cognitive) benefit in the majority of patients with classical Parkinson's disease (PD)	Begin treatment when patient needs symptomatic relief; usually administered in combination with a dopa-decarboxylase inhibitor (carbidopa) to decrease the amount of levodopa converted to dopamine in the intestinal mucosa and to increase the amount of levodopa reaching the brain; should be taken on an empty stomach	Nausea and vomiting especially with initial treatment, "wearing-off," "on-off," dyskinesias, orthostatic hypotension, confusion, hallucinations, nightmares, reversal of sleep-wake patterns
Dopamine agonists (bromocriptine, pergolide)	Do not require enzymatic conversion to an active metabolite; consequently, absorption and delivery to the brain are more constant	May be useful for treatment early in the course of PD and may delay the need to introduce levodopa or provide functional improvement at lower doses of levodopa; therefore, may delay the occurrence of the side effects associated with long-term levodopa therapy	For symptomatic treatment, may be used alone or in combination with levodopa	Nausea and vomiting, dyskinesias, orthostatic hypotension, hallucinations, confusion
COMT inhibitors (tolcapone, entacapone)	Increase availability and transfer of levodopa into the brain; increase plasma levodopa half-life and thereby provide more stable plasma levels and enhanced and smoother levodopa availability to the brain	Enhance the antiparkinsonian effect of levodopa in both nonfluctuating and fluctuating patients; improve "on" time and decrease "off" time	Used as adjunctive therapy with levodopa in doses of either 100 or 200 mg three times a day, administered at the same time as levodopa	Increased incidence of dopaminergic side effects, especially dyskinesia and neuropsychiatric effects; side effects are usually easily managed by a 20–30% reduction in total daily levodopa dose; severe diarrhea and increase in liver transaminase are less common but serious side effects
Monoamine oxidase inhibitors (selegiline)	Increases dopamine levels by inhibiting its oxidation by monoamine oxidase type B in the synaptic cleft	Often no benefit noticed, but may improve symptoms or enhance effect of levodopa	Used in the early phase of PD as monotherapy or later as adjuvant therapy in patients whose response to levodopa has waned or who are experiencing response fluctuations	Insomnia, nausea, may exacerbate dyskinesia
Anticholinergics (trihexyphenidyl, benztropine mesylate)	Correcting the balance between dopamine and acetylcholine, which is shifted toward cholinergic dominance in the striatum of patients with PD	Particularly useful when tremor is a predominant and troublesome symptom and is not adequately controlled by levodopa	Often poorly tolerated in the elderly	Blurry vision, dry mouth, constipation, urinary retention (especially in men with prostate hypertrophy), decreasing sweating, memory impairment, confusion, hallucinations
Amantadine	Antiviral agent	Mechanism of action is not clearly understood; some of its side effects (e.g., blurry vision, constipation, dry mouth) suggest that it may act as an anticholinergic drug	Unlike most antiparkinsonian medications, is usually taken in a standard dose (100 mg twice daily); it is effective in probably only half of patients; the effects may be short lived, but if stopped for a short time, it may regain its effectiveness	Confusion, hallucinations, insomnia, nightmares; livedo reticularis, sometimes accompanied by lower extremity edema

Nursing Management Issues

To achieve the ideal therapeutic range, medications must be continuously monitored. Nursing care related to pharmacological treatment should focus on educating the patient about potential side effects, drug interactions, and dietary modifications. The patient needs specific written information as to the dosage, frequency, possible side effects, and expected outcome of medications.

Side effects are common with all antiparkinsonian medications. Long-term management of the treatment regimen is challenging and requires excellent communication among patients, their significant others, and healthcare providers. Drug toxicity to levodopa and anticholinergics may occur, with confusion, loss of drug effectiveness, hallucinations, nightmares, dyskinesias, dystonia, and a reversal of sleep-wake patterns. A reduction in dosage or change in the timing of administration may lead to an improvement of symptoms. Treatment with atypical antipsychotic agents such as clozapine or olanzapine may be useful in lessening some of the psychiatric side effects associated with antiparkinsonian drug therapy (e.g., hallucinations, delusions, paranoia) (Factor & Brown, 1992; Friedman, 1991; Olanow & Koller, 1998). These agents provide antipsychotic benefit without the extrapyramidal side effects associated with other drugs in this class. In addition, they may be useful in suppressing levodopa-induced dyskinesias (Bennett et al., 1993). For a more thorough discussion of the behavioral, neuropsychological, and psychiatric complications of drug treatment in PD, see Cummings (1991) or Saint-Cyr and colleagues (1993).

NONPHARMACOLOGICAL TREATMENTS

Diet

The pharmacokinetic properties of levodopa cause its levels in the blood to fluctuate. Dietary intake affects both the absorption of levodopa from the gastrointestinal tract and its transport within the body. Early in the disease course, fluctuating levodopa levels result in fewer response fluctuations than occur later on, when the disease has progressed. Therefore, in patients with advanced disease and motor response fluctuations, food intake can be modified to minimize its negative effect on levodopa pharmacokinetics (Kempster & Wahlquist, 1994). A high-protein diet can block the effects of levodopa. This blocking can occur whether levodopa is given alone or in combination with an inhibitor such as carbidopa. Patients receiving the inhibitor, however, are less susceptible to blocking. In addition, alkaline products such as antacids and milk slow the absorption of drugs, and patients may therefore experience a delay between taking their medication and noticing an improvement in symptoms (Garrett, 1982). Patient recommendations should include taking levodopa on an empty stomach, keeping protein to the recommended daily allowance, and redistributing protein intake to the last meal of the day. For a thorough review of these issues, see Kempster and Wahlquist (1994).

Exercise and Physical Therapy

Few studies have examined the efficacy of physical therapy (PT) in PD. Although research needs to be done on the outcomes of PT, it is generally accepted that in PD patients PT helps prevent the complications of immobility, reduce tone abnormalities, and maintain or improve overall muscle ability (e.g., strength, speed, and initiation). Training techniques should be used that take into account the specific aspects and motor deficits in PD. Helpful techniques include cueing to facilitate rhythmic movement patterns and emphasizing large-amplitude movements (Homberg, 1993).

Surgery and Transplants

Surgical procedures to treat parkinsonism have been used since the 1950s but fell into disfavor after the discovery of levodopa therapy. Recently, however, there has been renewed interest in these procedures in patients who respond poorly to pharmacological management

(Aminoff, 1994). Posteroventral pallidotomy has been found effective in relieving bradykinesia, rigidity, and tremor (Laitinen et al., 1992), and thalamotomy can reduce or abolish tremor (Olanow et al., 1994; Tasker et al., 1983).

Other Treatments

Assistance from other therapeutic specialists such as speech and language therapists can positively affect swallowing abnormalities and decrease the incidence of silent aspiration and pneumonia. These therapies can also improve patients' communication skills so that they are able to maintain work or social activities for longer periods. Individual and family psychotherapy, music therapy, and involvement in support groups can all benefit patients and their significant others.

NURSING MANAGEMENT

Nurses may encounter PD patients in the home, daycare centers, outpatient clinics, acute care hospitals, and, in the later stages of the illness, in long-term care facilities. Working collaboratively with physicians and other healthcare providers, nurses can plan and coordinate the care of patients in these multiple settings. The major components of nursing care for PD patients fall into five categories: (1) assessment of patient and family needs and education; (2) functional assessment of the patient; (3) psychological and cognitive assessment of the patient; (4) promotion and maintenance of autonomy and independence; and (5) prevention of complications. These categories are each discussed separately but are also interrelated. As a result, addressing a problem in one area may achieve a positive outcome in another; for example, providing patients with assistive devices so that they can remain mobile contributes to autonomy and independence but also improves morale, thus promoting psychological well-being. Exercises such as walking improve muscle tone, thus preventing or at least delaying the immobility that may occur in advanced PD.

Assessment of Patient and Family Needs and Education

Patients newly diagnosed with PD and their families are faced with a new, unknown, and somewhat frightening situation. Nurses can be instrumental in helping patients accept the reality of PD and realize that with adaptation, planning, treatment, and supportive services, they can live meaningful lives (Calne, 1984). Initially, nurses should assess the level of knowledge about the disease process and the treatment regimen and should provide patients and their families with accurate information regarding treatment and the nature of the disease. It is also important, early in the course of the disease, to assess the patient's and caregiver's abilities to cope with PD and to anticipate how they will be able to manage the progressive disability that occurs. A home visit is valuable in assessing the family members' knowledge of the disease process, their support of the patient, and their awareness of supportive community services. During the home visit, nurses can evaluate the patient's understanding of the medical regimen, inquire about any over-the-counter drugs in the home, discuss the danger of self-medication, and evaluate the home to determine if any changes are necessary to provide a safe environment.

Drug therapy can bring about a dramatic improvement in the patient's condition. However, drug therapy is complex and must be monitored carefully to achieve maximal benefit. If possible, patients should take their medications independently; however, because forgetfulness, depression, or dementia can contribute to medication errors, significant others should be included when instructing patients about treatment regimens. Antiparkinsonian medication regimens must be individually tailored to each patient, as almost none of these drugs is given in a standard dose, and the regimen evolves over time depending on clinical response. Therefore, it is necessary for nurses to develop a specific teaching plan for each patient, even though some general principles apply to all patients. Patients should be advised, for example, that medication doses must not be omitted or altered without first checking with their healthcare provider. Over-the-counter drugs should not be taken unless recommended by the physician, and it is essential that the physician or nurse conduct a periodic evaluation of the treatment regimen. A teaching plan that includes a complete written and verbal explanation of the treatment regimen, possible side effects, and recommendations for accurate administration of medications is essential. Nurses may suggest, for example, that medications for each day be placed in medication cups or envelopes in the morning so that a dose is not duplicated or forgotten. Practices that are extremely helpful to patients and their families, giving them some control in managing the disease, include explaining the therapeutic effects and possible side effects of each drug and making recommendations to counter the adverse effects of the drug.

Patient and family education depends on effective communication skills by all individuals involved in the patient's care. Important principles to use when teaching patients and their families include appraising the ability of patients and significant others to understand, assessing their readiness for learning, and allowing time to repeat the information at a later time.

Functional Assessment of the Patient

The Unified Parkinson's Disease Rating Scale (UPDRS) (Fahn et al., 1987) is an instrument used to assess the overall functional status of patients with PD. The scale can be completed by an experienced clinician in 10 to 20 minutes, depending on the extent of the patient's bradykinesia. The first three parts are quantitative five-point scales that measure the following:

I. Mentation, behavior, and mood
II. Activities of daily living (ADL) in both the "on" and "off" phases
III. Motor functioning

Part IV assesses the complications of therapy, including dyskinesias and clinical fluctuations; part V is a stage of disease assessment using the Modified Hoehn and Yahr scale; and part VI yields a percentage score based on the Modified Schwab and England ADL Scale. Each

subsection can be summed independently, and all sections can be combined into a total numerical score. In addition to a comprehensive geriatric assessment, a specific PD assessment is essential for planning nursing management strategies. A general ADL assessment scale does not provide essential information about the time required to perform ADL, and a patient may therefore appear more functional than he or she really is. For example, a patient with PD may be able to carry out a particular ADL but only during an extremely protracted period. The use of standardized scales such as the UPDRS also enables clinicians and researchers at many different sites to assess patients in the same way and to communicate meaningfully with each other.

Psychological and Cognitive Assessment of the Patient

Psychological and cognitive assessment should be undertaken as described earlier in this text (see Chapters 7 and 17). An accurate assessment of the psychological and cognitive status of the patient is essential, and an important goal should be developing a plan of care that maintains and strengthens the patient's remaining abilities. The physical and psychological symptoms of PD are interdependent, and symptoms such as tremor, drooling, masked facies, and impaired visuoperceptual and motor coordination can lead to psychological problems. In turn, psychological problems such as depression can contribute to malnutrition and weight loss, and malnutrition can precipitate respiratory infections. Nurses should keep in mind the interrelationship of the problems surrounding patient care.

Patients with PD are in great need of emotional support; as the disease progresses, the body image changes, and patients therefore need an understanding, supportive network to help deal with these alterations. Many of the symptoms of PD, such as tremor, drooling, a loss of facial expression, and a shuffling gait, may cause embarrassment and discourage patients from engaging in social activities. Tremor, for example, is rarely a physically disabling symptom; however, it can have serious psychological consequences. If people stare at this involuntary movement, it may be embarrassing and stressful to the patient and may deter him or her from attending social gatherings. Further, when discomfort in a social gathering occurs and is stressful to the person with PD, the tremor is aggravated by the stress. Because it is important for patients to be active socially, nurses must work with patients and their families to reduce stress and to encourage them to attend social functions, despite a fear of embarrassment.

It is important for people with PD to be active socially for as long as possible. If a person with PD tends to withdraw from social engagements, the spouse, if the patient has one, also tends to socialize less at a time when social support is necessary. Social activities may need to be planned around the energy level of the patient or during "on" periods. Many people with PD tend to be very tired at the end of the day. To maintain an active social life, activities such as brunch, luncheons, or movies can be planned early in the day, before fatigue begins.

Eating is a social activity, and family members should be encouraged to have their meals with the patient. They can reduce embarrassment by providing tissues to wipe saliva and providing enough time for the patient to eat comfortably. In an institutional setting, the patient should also be encouraged to eat in the company of others, and again the nurse should provide assistive devices that facilitate independent eating.

Nurses can be instrumental in relieving some of the symptoms of depression and in helping patients cope. As mentioned earlier, some of the physical symptoms of PD are similar to the neuropsychological symptoms of this disease. Unfortunately, nursing staff and patients' friends and family members may tend to withdraw from patients who are cognitively impaired or depressed. It is important for nurses to spend quality time with PD patients. Sitting at the bedside and engaging the patient in conversation demonstrate acceptance, which is a primary need (Fischbach, 1978). Most patients enjoy talking about earlier life experiences, and because long-term memory is not usually impaired, this can be a meaningful experience for them. If patients are no longer able

to walk, nurses should take them out of their room at least once a day to a pleasant environment where they can observe other people and outdoor scenery or engage in enjoyable social activities.

Nurses can strengthen their patients' remaining abilities and help prevent depression by promoting autonomy, treating patients with dignity and respect, and helping them maintain a strong sense of individuality and identity. While conducting research in a nursing home, Kayser-Jones (1984) observed that a man with PD who had been a pianist in a fashionable urban hotel was lying in his bed for hours without access to music. Providing him with a radio and headphones allowed him to pleasantly fill long hours when his wife could not be with him. Being able to listen to music at will gave him a sense of autonomy and helped diminish the feelings of helplessness that were contributing to depression. People's sense of identity derives from their belief that they possess unique characteristics that set them apart from others; this sense of identity is an important aspect of psychological health. Music was an integral part of this man's identity, and providing him with music helped him maintain his identity and individuality.

As the disease progresses, patients will need considerable help with physical activities. Most of the burden for providing this support and care falls on the primary caregiver, who is often a spouse or a daughter. Meeting the dependency needs of a person whose physical and cognitive status continues to decline is physically and psychologically demanding, and caregivers should realize that the demands for care will increase as the disease progresses. As the burden for providing care increases, social isolation can become a problem for the caregiver as well as for the patient. Important roles for the nurse include showing sensitivity to the needs of caregivers, counseling them in regard to their needs, assessing their emotional status to determine if outside supportive services are necessary, and directing them to agencies in the community that provide these services. For a discussion of social support, see Chapter 8.

Promotion and Maintenance of Autonomy and Independence

Although we are all to some degree dependent on others during our lives, our society places a high value on autonomy and independence. Clark and Anderson (1967) found that the elderly feared dependency and would endure great hardships to remain independent. When a chronic illness such as PD begins to erode independence, it can have a devastating effect on the patient's morale. Owing to the clinical symptoms of tremor, rigidity, bradykinesia, and akinesia, independence and autonomy begin to decline as patients experience difficulty in walking, talking, eating, dressing, bathing, and performing other ADL. Nurses can provide a tremendous service to patients by helping them identify their remaining strengths and resources and by adapting the environment to prolong independence. For example, rigidity of the trunk muscles contributes to an inability to roll over in bed or to rise to a sitting position. Some patients find that satin sheets facilitate movement in bed and that maneuvering using a rope tied to the foot of the bed assists them in turning and getting out of bed independently (Calne, 1984). Further, gentle range-of-motion exercises for 10 minutes four times a day will help maintain full range of motion, delay rigidity, and prevent contractures.

Tremor can make it difficult for patients to eat independently. Eating can be made easier with the use of assistive devices such as utensils with large handles (the handles of cutlery can be enlarged with foam rubber secured with tape), and patients can more easily drink without assistance using straws and cups designed to prevent spillage. Food should be prepared and served so that patients can eat as independently as possible; for example, meat should be cut before it is served, and fruit should be sliced into small pieces. Rigidity of the facial and pharyngeal muscles contributes to difficulty with mastication and swallowing; the rate of swallowing is decreased and eating may become slower and assume a deliberate quality. As the disease progresses, eating may become increasingly difficult. Both liquids and solids are difficult to swallow, whereas soft foods are swallowed more easily. Patients should be instructed to take small bites, chew thoroughly, and swallow slowly; they should be allowed as much time as necessary to eat

(Mastrian, 1984). Patients with swallowing difficulty should be supervised during meals.

Communication may become a problem for patients with PD. The patient's voice may become low and speech sometimes slurred, making it difficult to understand what is being said. There may be a delayed response time when the patient attempts to speak. Nurse-patient communication will be facilitated through exercising patience, listening carefully, and assigning the same nurse to a patient for a given period.

Physical exercise prevents muscle atrophy, helps prevent contractures, and also improves patients' morale. In general, it is wise for patients to be as active as possible without becoming unduly fatigued. Walking is perhaps the most beneficial activity. Frequent and regular short walks in a quiet park or neighborhood are preferable to long, irregular walks on a crowded, noisy street. The physical symptoms of PD may discourage independent physical activities. If, however, patients anticipate situations that are likely to cause an episode of akinesia (freezing), they can plan accordingly and have some sense of control over the situation. The mechanisms that underlie the execution of normal movement can be prodded by visual and auditory cues. Attention to lines on a carpet or cracks in the pavement, for example, can facilitate the initiation and maintenance of rhythmic stride and prevent freezing episodes. Some patients have found that counting while walking helps, and others have reported that listening to marching music on a small headset stereo is helpful. When freezing occurs, another technique is to take a small step either backwards or sideways to initiate rhythmical movement. If the patient is walking with a companion, it may be helpful to have the companion place one foot in front of the patient's and ask the patient to step over the obstacle. Families should be advised against attempting to pull the person forward, as this only increases the problem and may result in a fall (Stern & Lees, 1982).

Tremor, rigidity, and bradykinesia interfere with the normal performance of ADL; given enough time, however, patients can often successfully dress, bathe, and feed themselves. Simple modifications help the person with PD remain independent. Velcro closures, elastic shoelaces, and loose-fitting clothing help make dressing a manageable activity; handrails in the bathroom, raised toilet seats, and shower chairs are also helpful (Mastrian, 1984).

Dependency may be fostered by staff members or family caregivers who, perhaps unconsciously, do things for the patient that he or she could do independently rather than allow the patient to care for himself or herself. Nurses and families have a tendency to help as they watch a person struggle to accomplish ADL and other difficult tasks. It is important to withhold unnecessary help, as being able to complete tasks independently will contribute immeasurably to patients' self-esteem. Medical treatment is most effective when patients remain active physically and strive for independence in their daily routine (Lannon et al., 1986).

Prevention of Complications

Preventing complications is an important aspect in the management of PD. Infections, gastrointestinal problems, and falls are the most commonly occurring complications.

INFECTIONS

Upper respiratory infections are among the most dangerous complications of PD; bronchopneumonia is the second leading cause of death in advanced PD. Dysphagia or choking due to poor muscle tone and rigidity of the pharyngeal muscles contributes to the aspiration of food and fluids, which can result in aspiration pneumonia. In advanced PD, a nasogastric tube may be inserted for feeding; aspiration pneumonia is a complication that commonly occurs when nasogastric tubes are in place. The use of tube feeding is controversial; however, if tube feedings are indicated, a gastrostomy tube causes fewer complications, is more comfortable, and is psychologically more acceptable to the patient and family than a nasogastric tube. If dysphagia occurs, the physician should be consulted regarding the need for diagnostic studies, such as laryngoscopy, to rule out the possibility of an obstruction.

Providing the patient with soft and semisoft foods diminishes the risk of aspiration.

Respiratory function must be carefully assessed on an ongoing basis, and patients must be observed and monitored for signs of respiratory infections. Nursing measures such as encouraging regular deep-breathing exercises, getting the patient out of bed regularly, and changing the position of the bedfast patient all decrease the risk of respiratory infections. Breathing exercises, which consist of deep inspirations with maximal chest expansion, stretch the chest wall and carry oxygen to poorly aerated parts of the lung. Personnel with respiratory infections should not care for the patient, and family and friends with respiratory infections should be discouraged from visiting. Nurses should advise the patient's family that a low-grade fever may not necessarily be an indication of infection; however, if the patient develops a fever, the family should be instructed to notify the nurse or physician so that the source of fever can be determined.

Urinary tract infections (UTIs) are common. Anticholinergic drugs may cause urinary retention, and urinary retention and urinary stasis contribute to UTIs. A lack of mobility as well as insufficient fluid intake may also precipitate UTIs (Robinson, 1974). Fluids should be readily available and offered frequently. Tremor may make drinking difficult, but patients can usually manage to drink with the use of a flexible drinking straw. Foods high in water content such as fresh fruits (e.g., melons and apples) are also a good source of water and may be easier for the patient to swallow than liquids.

Seborrhea is commonly found in patients with PD and may contribute to the incidence of external eye infections. Frequent showers and hair washing with antidandruff shampoos are necessary, and the patient should be taught good eye hygiene. Eye problems may be prevented by gently washing the eyelids, eyelid margins, and eye lashes with a small amount of a "no tears" shampoo on a moist cotton ball and then rinsing the eyes with warm water. Vigorous cleaning must be avoided so as not to cause a mechanical conjunctivitis.

GASTROINTESTINAL COMPLICATIONS

Gastrointestinal motility is slowed as a result of PD and antiparkinsonian agents (Hahn, 1982).

Decreased motility of the gastrointestinal tract, a lack of saliva in the gastrointestinal tract (lost through drooling), and dehydration contribute to constipation. A diet high in fiber, adequate fluid intake, daily exercise, and the use of bulking agents and stool softeners all help prevent constipation.

Anorexia, nausea, and vomiting are common side effects of drugs such as levodopa, and this problem combined with dysphagia may result in severe weight loss. Patients should be weighed periodically; high-calorie supplemental feeding may be necessary to prevent weight loss.

FALLS

Postural instability with falling affects about 25% of patients with PD, and serious injury along with fractures occurs in about 15% of patients (Hahn, 1982). Falling is most likely to occur when the patient is turning, backing up, reaching for an object, getting out of a chair, or attempting to move unassisted from one location to another.

Many falls can be prevented by encouraging the patient to use a cane, tripod, or walker; by teaching the patient how to ambulate safely; and by providing assistive devices such as handrails in the bathroom. The environment at home and in institutional settings should be carefully assessed to prevent falls. Rubber mats in the tub and shower are mandatory, small throw rugs should be removed, and electrical cords and telephone cords should be eliminated in any area where the patient may be walking.

SUMMARY

Long-term management of PD requires the cooperative efforts of a multidisciplinary team. Working collaboratively with the physician, the nurse can plan and coordinate the services of all healthcare providers. A physical therapist, for example, can design a specific program of exercise and mobility training to help reduce the symptoms of PD and to encourage functional independence. An occupational therapist can assess skills such as bathing, dressing,

feeding, and swallowing and can work closely with the family to suggest adaptive equipment and devices. A speech therapist can evaluate the swallowing and communication status of the patient, and a social worker can assess the psychosocial situation of the patient and family and make appropriate suggestions. A social worker may suggest individual counseling sessions or support group meetings with patients and their families (Lannon et al., 1986).

In summary, the optimal management of patients with PD is a difficult and challenging task. The nurse is, however, in a position to coordinate the efforts of professional interdisciplinary team members, the patient, and the patient's support network to ensure maximal functioning and quality of life for people with PD. Appendix 19–1 lists several national organizations whose focus is on PD–related activities, as well as relevant publications.

REFERENCES

Ahlskog, J. E. (1994). Treatment of Parkinson's disease: From theory to practice. *Postgraduate Medicine, 95*(5), 52–69.

Aminoff, M. J. (1994). Treatment of Parkinson's disease. *Western Journal of Medicine, 161*(3), 303–308.

Askenasy, J. J. (1993). Sleep in Parkinson's disease. *Acta Neurologica Scandinavica, 87*, 167–170.

Barbeau, A., Cloutier, T., Roy, M., et al. (1985). Ecogenetics of Parkinson's disease: 6-hydroxylation of debrisoquine. *Lancet, 2*(8466), 1213–1215.

Bennett, J. P., Landow, E. R., & Schuh, L. A. (1993). Supression of dyskinesias in advanced Parkinson's disease. *Neurology, 43*, 1551–1555.

Birkmayer, W., & Riederer, P. (1983). *Parkinson's disease.* New York: Springer-Verlag.

Bloem, B. R. (1992). Postural instability in Parkinson's disease. *Clinical Neurology and Neurosurgery, 94*(suppl.), S41–S45.

Boller, F. (1984). Parkinson's disease and Alzheimer's disease: Are they associated? In J. T. Hutton & A. D. Kenny (Eds.), *Senile dementia of the Alzheimer type: Neurology and neurobiology, vol. 18* (pp. 119–129). New York: Alan R. Liss.

Bredsen, D. E. (1993). Potential role of gene therapy in the treatment of Parkinson's disease. *Clinical Neuroscience, 1*(1), 45–52.

Brooks, D. J.(1993). PET studies on the early and differential diagnosis of Parkinson's disease. *Neurology, 43*(suppl. 6), S6–S16.

Brown, R. G., MacCarthy, B., Gotham, A. M., et al., (1988). Depression and disability in Parkinson's disease: A follow-up study of 132 cases. *Psychological Medicine, 18*, 49–55.

Calne, D. B. (1993). Treatment of Parkinson's disease. *New England Journal of Medicine, 329*(14), 1021–1027.

Calne, S. (1984). Parkinson's disease—helping the patient with a movement disorder. *Canadian Nurse, 80*(11), 35–37.

Celesia, G. G., & Wanamaker, W. M. (1972). Psychiatric disturbances in Parkinson's disease. *Diseases of the Nervous System, 33*(9), 577–583.

Chase, T. N., Engber, T. M., & Mouradian, M. (1994). Palliative and prophylactic benefits of continuously administered dopaminomimetics in Parkinson's disease. *Neurology, 44*(suppl. 6), S15–S18.

Clark, M., & Anderson, B. (1967). *Culture and aging: An anthropological study of older Americans.* Springfield, IL: Charles C. Thomas.

Cools, A. R., Van Den Bercken, J. H. L., Horstink, M. W. I., et al. (1984). Cognitive and motor shifting aptitude disorder in Parkinson's disease. *Journal of Neurology, Neurosurgery and Psychiatry, 47*, 443–453.

Critchley, M. (Ed.). (1955). *James Parkinson (1755–1824).* London: MacMillan.

Cummings, J. L. (1988). The dementias of Parkinson's disease: Prevalence, characteristics, neurobiology and comparison with dementia of the Alzheimer type. *European Neurology, 28*(suppl. 1), 15–23.

Cummings, J. L. (1991). Behavioral complications of drug treatment of Parkinson's disease. *Journal of the American Geriatrics Society, 39*, 708–716.

Cummings, J. L. (1992). Depression and Parkinson's disease: A review. *American Journal of Psychiatry, 149*(4), 443–454.

Dakof, G. A., & Mendelsohn, G. A. (1986). Parkinson's disease: The psychological aspects of a chronic illness. *Psychological Bulletin, 99*(3), 375–387.

Dowling, G. A. (1995). Sleep changes with aging and Parkinson's disease. *Parkinson Report, 16*(1), 8–9.

Duvoisin, R. C. (1992). Overview of Parkinson's disease. *Annals of the New York Academy of Sciences, 648*, 187–193.

Edwards L. L., Quigley, E. M., & Pfeiffer, R. F. (1992). Gastrointestinal dysfunction in Parkinson's disease: Frequency and pathophysiology. *Neurology, 42*, 726–732.

Factor, S. A., & Brown, D. (1992). Clozapine prevents recurrence of psychosis in Parkinson's disease. *Movement Disorders, 7*(2), 125–131.

Fahn, S., Elton, R.L., & Members of the UPDRS Committee (1987). Unified Parkinson's disease rating scale. In S. Fahn, C. D. Marsden, M. Goldstein & D. B. Calne (Eds.), *Recent developments in Parkinson's disease* (pp. 153–163). Florham, NJ: Macmillan Healthcare Information.

Finch, C. E., Randall, P. K., & Marshall, J. F. (1981). Aging and basal ganglia functions. *Annual Review of Gerontology and Geriatrics, 2*, 49–87.

Fischbach, F. R. (1978). Easing adjustment to Parkinson's disease. *American Journal of Nursing, 78*(1), 66–69.

Fowler, S. B., & Bergen, M. (1993). Continuous duodenal infusions of levodopa. *Journal of Neuroscience Nursing, 25*(5), 317–320.

Friedman, J. H. (1991). The management of levodopa psychosis. *Clinical Neuropharmacology, 12*(4), 283–295.

Gannon, M. (1992). Psychiatric disorders in Parkinson's disease. *British Journal of Hospital Medicine, 47*(9), 663–666.

Garrett, E. (1982). Parkinsonism: Forgotten considerations in medical treatment and nursing care. *Journal of Neurosurgery Nursing, 14*(1), 13–17.

Golbe, L. I., Farrell, T. M., & Davie, P. H. (1990). Follow-up study of early life protective and risk factors in Parkinson's disease. *Movement Disorders, 5*, 66–70.

Goodwin, F. K. (1971). Psychiatric side effects of levodopa in man. *Journal of the American Medical Association, 218*(13), 1915–1920.

Gottwald, M. D., Bainbridge, J. L., Dowling, G. A., et al. (1997). New drug development in Parkinson's disease. *Annals of Pharmacotherapy, 31*, 1205–1217.

Guze, B. H., & Barrio, J. C. (1991). The etiology of depression in Parkinson's disease patients. *Psychosomatics, 32*(4), 390–395.

Hahn, K. (1982). Management of Parkinson's disease. *Nurse Practitioner, 7*(1), 13–25, 50.

Hoehn, M. M., & Yahr, M. D. (1967). Parkinsonism: Onset, progression, and mortality. *Neurology, 17*, 427–442.

Homberg, V. (1993). Motor training in the therapy of Parkinson's disease. *Neurology, 43*(suppl. 6), S45–S46.

Jankovic, J. (1993a). Natural course and limitations of levodopa therapy. *Neurology, 43*(2), S1-14–S1-17.

Jankovic, J. (1993b). Theories on the etiology and pathogenesis of Parkinson's disease. *Neurology, 43*(suppl. 1), S1-21–S1-23.

Jenner, P., Schapira, A. H., & Marsden, C. D. (1992). New insights into the cause of Parkinson's disease. *Neurology, 42*, 2241–2250.

Kayser-Jones, J. (1984). Psychosocial care of nursing home patients. In B. A. Hall (Ed.), *Mental health and the elderly* (pp. 205–219). New York: Grune & Stratton.

Kempster, P. D., & Wahlquist, M. L. (1994). Dietary factors in the management of Parkinson's disease. *Nutrition Review, 52*(2), 15–58.

Koller, W. C. & Pahwa, R. (1994). Treating motor-fluctuations with controlled-release levodopa preparations. *Neurology, 44*(suppl. 6), S2–S28.

Laitinen, L. V., Bergenheim, A. T., & Hariz, M. I. (1992). Leskell's posteroventral pallidotomy in the treatment of Parkinson's disease. *Journal of Neurosurgery, 76*, 53–61.

Langston, J. W. (1986). MPTP–induced parkinsonism: How good a model is it? In S. Fahn, C. D. Marsden & P. Jenner (Eds.), *Recent developments in Parkinson's disease* (pp. 119–126). New York: Raven Press.

Lannon, M. C., Thomas, C. A., Bratton, M., et al. (1986). Comprehensive care of the patient with Parkinson's disease. *Journal of Neuroscience Nursing, 18*(3), 121–131.

Lazzarini, A. M., Myers, R. H., & Zimmerman, T. R. (1994). A clinical genetic study of Parkinson's disease: Evidence for dominant transmission. *Neurology, 44*, 499–506.

Levin, B. E., Llabre, M. M., & Weiner, W. J. (1988). Parkinson's disease and depression: Psychometric properties of the Beck Depression Inventory. *Journal of Neurology Neurosurgery and Psychiatry, 51*, 1401–1404.

Levin, B. E., Tomer, R., & Rey, G. J. (1992). Cognitive impairments in Parkinson's disease. *Neurologic Clinics, 100*(2), 471–485.

Lewin, R. (1985). Parkinson's disease: An environmental cause? *Science, 229*, 257–258.

Lieberman, A., Dziatolowski, N., Kupersmith, M., et al. (1979). Dementia in Parkinson's disease. *Annals of Neurology, 6*(4), 355–359.

Loranger, A., Goodell, H., McDowell, F. H., et al. (1972). Intellectual impairment in Parkinson's syndrome. *Brain, 95,* 402–412.

Mastrian, K. G. (1984). The patient with a degenerative disease of the nervous system. In E. B. Rudy (Ed.), *Advanced neurological and neurosurgical nursing* (pp. 265–287). St. Louis: C. V. Mosby.

Matthews, C. G., & Haaland, K. Y. (1979). The effects of a symptom duration on cognitive and motor performance in parkinsonism. *Neurology, 29,* 951–956.

Mayeux, R., Marder, K., Cote, L., et al. (1995). The frequency of idiopathic Parkinson's disease by age, ethnic group, and sex in northern Manhattan, 1988–1993. *American Journal of Epidemiology, 142*(8), 820–827.

Mayeux, R., & Stern, Y. (1983). Intellectual dysfunction and dementia in Parkinson's disease. In R. Mayeux & W. G. Rosen (Eds.), *Advances in Neurology, vol. 38* (pp. 211–227). New York: Raven Press.

Mayeux, R., Stern, Y., Cote, L., & Williams, J. B. (1984). Altered serotonin metabolism in depressed patients with Parkinson's disease. *Neurology, 34,* 642–646.

Menza, M. A., Robertson-Hoffman, D. E., & Bonapace, A. S. (1993). Parkinson's disease and anxiety: Comorbidity with depression. *Biological Psychiatry, 34,* 465–470.

Montastruc, J. L., Rascol, O., & Senard, J. M. (1993). Current status of dopamine agonists in Parkinson's disease management. *Drugs, 46*(3), 384–393.

Nausieda, P., Glantz, R., Weber, S., et al. (1984). Psychiatric complications of levodopa therapy of Parkinson's disease. *Advances in Neurology, 40,* 271–277.

Nutt, J. G. (1993). Pharmacotherapy of Parkinson's disease. *Clinical Neuroscience, 1*(1), 64–68.

Olanow, C. W. (1993a). A rationale for monoamine oxidase inhibitions as neuroprotective therapy for Parkinson's disease. *Movement Disorders, 8*(suppl. 1), S1–S7.

Olanow, C. W. (1993b). The early treatment of Parkinson's disease. *Neurology, 43*(suppl. 1), S1-30–S1-31.

Olanow, C., & Koller, W. (1998). An algorithm (decision tree) for the management of Parkinson's disease: Treatment guidelines. *Neurology, 50*(suppl. 3), S1–S57.

Olanow, C. W., Marsden, C. D., Lang, A. E., & Goetz, C. G. (1994). The role of surgery in Parkinson's disease mangement. *Neurology, 44*(suppl. 1), S17–S20.

Parkinson Study Group (1989). Effect of deprenyl on the progression of disability in early Parkinson's disease. *New England Journal of Medicine, 321,* 1364–1371.

Payami, H., Bernard, S., Larsen, K., et al. (1995). Genetic anticipation in Parkinson's disease. *Neurology, 45*(1), 135–138.

Payami, H., Larsen, K., Bernard, S., & Nutt, J. (1994). Increased risk of Parkinson's disease in parents and siblings of patients. *Annals of Neurology, 36*(4), 659–661.

Pirozzolo, F. J., Hansch, E. C., Mortimer, J. A., et al. (1982). Dementia in Parkinson's disease: A neuropsychological analysis. *Brain and Cognition, 1,* 71–83.

Polymeropoulos, M., Lavedan, C., Leroy, E., et al. (1997). Mutation in the alpha-synuclein gene identified in families with Parkinson's disease. *Science, 276*(5321), 2045–2047.

Rasmussen, K., & Abrams, R. (1991). Treatment of Parkinson's disease with electroconvulsive therapy. *Psychiatric Clinics of North America, 14*(4), 925–933.

Ring, H. (1993). Psychological and social problems of Parkinson's disease. *British Journal of Hospital Medicine, 49*(2), 111–116.

Rinne, J. O. (1993). Nigral degeneration in Parkinson's disease. *Movement Disorders, 8*(suppl. 1), S31–S35.

Robinson, M. B. (1974). Levodopa and parkinsonism. *American Journal of Nursing, 74*(4), 656–651.

Saint-Cyr, J. A., Taylor, A. E., & Lang, A. E. (1993). Neuropsychological and psychiatric side effects in the treatment of Parkinson's disease. *Neurology, 43*(suppl. 6), S47–S452.

Schoenberg, B. S. (1987). Descriptive epidemiology of Parkinson's disease: Disease distribution and hypothesis formulation. *Advances in Neurology, 45,* 277–283.

Spencer, P. S., Nunn, P. B., Hugon, J., et al. (1987). Guam amyotrophic lateral sclerosis-Parkinsonism-dementia linked to a plant excitant neurotoxin. *Science, 237,* 517–522.

Standaert, D. G., & Stern, M. B. (1993). Update on the management of Parkinson's disease. *Medical Clinics of North America, 77*(1), 169–183.

Stem, G., & Lees, A. (1982). *Parkinson's disease: The facts.* New York: Oxford University Press.

Stern, G. (1993). Sinemet CR: Rationale and clinical experience. *Neurology, 43*(suppl. 1), S1-34–S1-35.

Talland, G. A. (1962). Cognitive functioning in Parkinson's disease. *Journal of Nervous and Mental Disorders, 135*(3), 196–205.

Tanner, C. M. (1992). Epidemiology of Parkinson's disease. *Neurologic Clinics, 10*(2), 317–329.

Tanner, C., & Goldman, S. (1996). Epidemiology of Parkinson's disease. *Neurologic Clinics, 14*(2), 317–335.

Tasker, R. R., Siqueira, J., Hawrylyshyn, P., & Organ, L. W. (1983). What happened to VIM thalamotomy for Parkinson's disease? *Applied Neurophysiology, 46,* 68–83.

Ward, C. D., Duvoisin, R. C., Ince, S. E., et al. (1983). Parkinson's disease in 65 pairs of twins and in a set of quadruplets. *Neurology, 33,* 815–824.

APPENDIX 19 - 1

Patient and Family Resources

ORGANIZATIONS

American Parkinson Disease Association, Inc.
(APDA)
116 John Street
New York, NY 10034
1–800–684–2732

APDA National Young Parkinson's
Information and Referral Center
1–800–223–9776

National Parkinson Foundation, Inc.
1501 N.W. 9th Avenue
Miami, FL 33136
1–800–327–4545

Parkinson's Disease Foundation
650 West 168th Street
New York, NY 10032
1–800–457–6676

United Parkinson Foundation
360 West Superior Street
Chicago, IL 60610

GENERAL INFORMATION BOOKS

Duvoisin, R. C., & Sage, J. (1996). *Parkinson's disease: A guide for patient and family* (4th ed.). New York: Raven Press.

Liberman, A., & Williams, F. (1993). *Parkinson's disease: Complete guide for patient and caregiver.* New York: Simon and Schuster.

McGoon, D. (1990). *The Parkinson's handbook.* New York: W. W. Norton & Company.

Arthritis

Rebecca Lee Burrage
Cynthia A. Sutter

The prevalence of arthritis and its resulting limitations in physical activities increase with age. In the Longitudinal Study on Aging, 55% of community-dwelling people aged 70 years and older reported having arthritis (Yelin, 1992). Of these people, 78% described a secondary limitation in physical activity. More than one third had a limitation in at least one activity of daily living. Those elderly people with at least one physical limitation were 50% more likely to die and four times more likely to be in a nursing home at the end of 1 year. The arthritic involvement of feet, knees, and ankles may cause an unstable gait and an increased risk of falling. If osteoporosis is present, especially if steroids have been used to treat rheumatoid arthritis (RA), the risk of fractures increases (Miller-Blair & Robbins, 1993). Emotional and social problems also arise in coping with chronicity, pain, and the social and physical limitations associated with arthritis (Wallston et al., 1989). This chapter presents information on the assessment and management of the most prevalent forms of arthritis.

PREVALENCE AND DIAGNOSIS OF COMMON TYPES OF ARTHRITIS

Rheumatoid Arthritis. RA often begins between the ages of 30 and 50 years; however, 10 to 30% of patients develop the disease after the age of 60 years. People can have a genetic predisposition for the disease. Although women are two to three times more prone to develop the problem, the difference between sexes is less marked after the age of 60 years (Nesher & Moore, 1993). RA is a chronic inflammatory system disease that affects *diarthrodial* (synovial-lined) joints and is characterized by persistent inflammatory synovitis. Extraarticular manifestations may involve the pulmonary, cardiac, nervous, integumentary, and reticuloendothelial systems. As many as 80% of patients with RA have *rheumatoid factor* (an autoantibody directed at portions of human immunoglobulin) in their serum (Murphy, 1992). Although useful in diagnosis, laboratory tests are not specific for the disease, and diagnosis is therefore made chiefly through clinical examination findings (Harris, 1993). The America Rheumatism Association has published criteria for use in epidemiological studies of RA, which can be useful to clinicians (Table 20–1). Common signs and symptoms of the disease and a list of disorders resembling RA are described in Table 20–2. Figures 20–1 through 20–3 illustrate abnormalities associated with RA.

Osteoarthritis. Osteoarthritis (OA) is the most common form of arthritis, affecting 40 million Americans and 30 to 60% of people older than 65 years (Fife, 1994). The disease is no longer considered to be only a normal consequence of aging. The number of cartilage cells diminishes, cartilage becomes ulcerated and thinned, subchondral bone is exposed, bony surfaces rub together, and joint destruction results. Risk factors for OA include obesity (Felson et al., 1992), repetitive mechanical overuse of a joint, and heredity (Fife, 1994). The signs and symptoms of OA are described in Table 20–3. Figures 20–4 and 20–5 show abnormalities commonly found in patients with OA.

Crystal-Induced Arthropathies. Gout occurs at a rate of 1.5 to 2.2 per 1000 people, and calcium pyrophosphate deposition disease

---

TABLE 20-1
1988 Revised ARA Criteria for Classification of Rheumatoid Arthritis*

Criteria	Definition
Morning stiffness	Morning stiffness in and around the joints lasting at least 1 hour before maximal improvement
Arthritis of three or more joint areas	At least three joint areas have simultaneously had soft tissue swelling or fluid (not bony overgrowth alone) observed by a physician; the 14 possible joint areas are (right or left) PIP, MCP, wrist, elbow, knee, ankle, and MTP joints
Arthritis of hand joints	At least one joint area swollen as above in wrist, MCP, or PIP joint
Symmetric arthritis	Simultaneous involvement of the same joint areas (as in 2) on both sides of the body (bilateral involvement of PIP, MCP, or MTP joints is acceptable without absolute symmetry)
Rheumatoid nodules	Subcutaneous nodules, overbony prominences, or extensor surfaces, or in juxtaarticular regions, observed by a physician
Serum rheumatoid factor	Demonstration of abnormal amounts of serum rheumatoid factor by any method that has been positive in less than 5% of normal control subjects
Radiographic changes	Radiographic changes typical of RA on posteroanterior hand and wrist radiographs, which must include erosions or unequivocal bony decalcification localized to or most marked adjacent to the involved joints (osteoarthritis changes alone do not qualify)

ARA, American Rheumatism Association; MCP, metacarpophalangeal; MTP, metatarsophalangeal; PIP, proximal interphalangeal; RA, rheumatoid arthritis.

*For classification purposes, a patient is said to have RA if he or she has satisfied at least four of the above seven criteria. Criteria 1 through 4 must be present for at least 6 weeks. Patients with two clinical diagnoses are not excluded. Designation as classic, definite, or probable rheumatoid arthritis is *not* to be made.

From Harris, E. D. (1993). Clinical features of rheumatoid arthritis. In W. N. Kelley, E. D. Harris, S. Ruddy & C. B. Sledge (Eds.), *Textbook of rheumatology, vol. 1* (4th ed., p. 874). Philadelphia: W. B. Saunders.

TABLE 20-2
Rheumatoid Arthritis

History

Onset: Usually slow; initial symptoms systemic or articular
Course: Possibly more benign after age 60 years
Pain/Stiffness: In and around joints for at least 1 hour in A.M.
Systemic Symptoms: Often present (malaise, fatigue, anorexia, weight loss, myalgia, vasomotor instability, depression)
Joint Distribution: Multiple joints, often symmetrical; small joints commonly involved first (PIP, MCP, wrist, rarely DIP); shoulder, cervical spine common in older people; hip; cricothyroid joints (hoarseness); ossicles of middle ear (deafness); temporomandibular joint
Disorders Resembling RA: Ankylosing spondylitis; calcium pyrophosphate dihydrate deposition disease, chronic fatigue syndrome, diffuse connective tissue diseases (e.g., systemic lupus erythematosus, scleroderma), infectious arthritis, intermittent hydrarthrosis, malignancy, osteoarthritis, fibromyalgia, glucocorticoid withdrawal syndrome, gout, Parkinson's disease, polymyalgia rheumatica, giant cell arteritis

Examination

Possible low-grade fever and soft, small lymph nodes
Movement guarded, of limited range
Early localized muscle atrophy; strength/function impaired
Joints warm (not usually red); soft tissue and synovial fluid swelling (diffuse boggy swelling common over age 60 years)
Subcutaneous nodules over bony prominences and extensor surfaces or in juxtaarticular positions (less common in older people)
Palmar erythema and prominent veins on dorsum of hands common
Flexion contractures or deformities (e.g., swan neck—DIP flexion and PIP extension; Boutonniere—DIP extension and PIP flexion; ulnar deviation at MCP).

Laboratory Tests

Erythrocyte sedimentation rate: ≥30 mm/hour
Rheumatoid factor positive (lower frequency of positive tests after age 60 years; titers above 1:256 more diagnostic)
Lupus erythematosus factor: occasionally positive (more often with increased age)
Complete blood count: mild anemia common (normochromic and either normocytic or microcytic); slight leukocytosis or higher with very active disease and with corticosteroid therapy; thrombocytosis
Serum uric acid: normal (before salicylates)
Antinuclear antibodies: negative
Serum complement level: normal or elevated
Synovial fluid: decreased viscosity; white blood count 3000–25,000 (rarely 50,000)

Radiography

Juxtaarticular osteoporosis
Marginal erosions
Uniform narrowing of joint spaces
Subluxation

DIP, distal interphalangeal; MCP, metacarpophalangeal; PIP, proximal interphalangeal; RA, rheumatoid arthritis.
Data from Calkins et al. (1994); and Harris (1993).

(CPDD) occurs at a rate of 0.9 per 1000 people. CPDD is also referred to as *chondrocalcinosis* and *pseudogout*. Gout is most commonly found in men aged 50 years and older and in women after menopause (Moskowitz, 1993). Both types of arthritis begin with the deposition of aggregated crystals in and around the joints. Gout results from monosodium urate monohydrate crystals, and pyrophosphate gout is caused by crystals of calcium pyrophosphate dihydrate. Although crystals may be present without symptoms, a painful inflammatory response occurs if neutrophils are attracted into the joint space and begin crystal phagocytosis. The incidence of gout increases with rising serum urate levels, and the cumulative incidence of gout is 22% if serum urate levels are greater than 7 mg per dL for 5 years (Kelley & Schumacher, 1993).

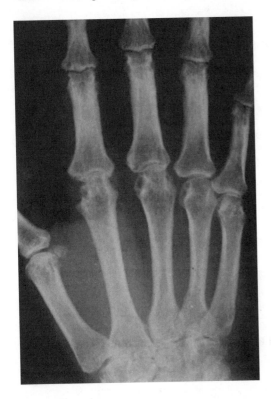

FIGURE 20–1. Posteroanterior roentgenograph of the hand showing the typical changes of rheumatoid arthritis. Mild juxtaarticular osteoporosis, cartilage loss, most evident at the metacarpophalangeal (MCP) joints; marginal erosion, particularly proximal to the second MCP joint; and several cysts in the carpals and adjacent to proximal interphalangeal joints are present. (From Hardin, J. G. [1986]. Rheumatoid arthritis. In G. V. Ball & W. N. Koopman [Eds.], *Clinical rheumatology* [p. 66]. Philadelphia: W. B. Saunders.)

Gouty arthritis also occurs with normal levels of serum uric acid, so the presence of normal levels should not be used to exclude a diagnosis of gout (McCarty, 1994). Common signs and symptoms of these types of arthritis are described in Tables 20–4 and 20–5. Figure 20–6 shows chronic gouty arthropathy of the great toe.

Septic Arthritis. Although infrequent in occurrence, septic arthritis can result in irreversible cartilage and bone destruction and can be life threatening. Occult infections of deep joints such as the hip may present with minimal signs and symptoms in patients who have systemic risk factors (such as immunosuppression or diabetes) or difficulty communicating

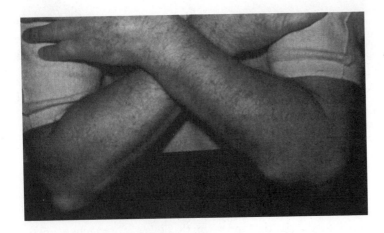

FIGURE 20–2. Subcutaneous rheumatoid nodules over both olecranon processes and distal to the left elbow on the extensor surface of the forearm. (From Hardin, J. G. [1986]. Rheumatoid arthritis. In G. V. Ball & W. N. Koopman [Eds.], *Clinical rheumatology* [p. 67]. Philadelphia: W. B. Saunders.)

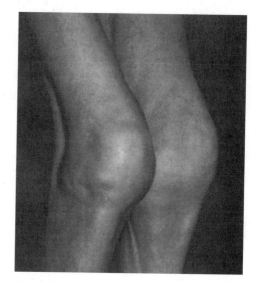

FIGURE 20–3. Soft tissue complications about the rheumatoid knee. Soft tissue swelling, flexion contractures, and marked muscle wasting are apparent; valgus deformities are present but not demonstrated by this photograph. (From Hardin, J. G. [1986]. Rheumatoid arthritis. In G. V. Ball & W. N. Koopman [Eds.], *Clinical rheumatology* [p. 74]. Philadelphia: W. B. Saunders.)

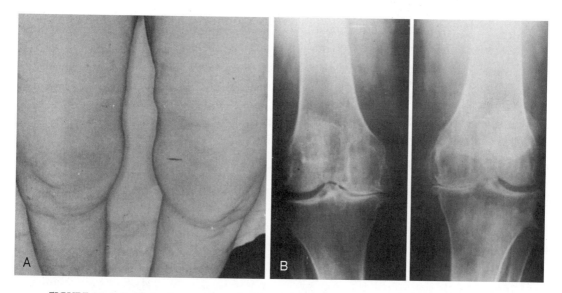

FIGURE 20–4. A, Bilateral genu varum (bowleg deformity) caused by osteoarthritis. B, Roentgenogram of right and left knees. The genu varum seen clinically is related to marked cartilage loss with narrowed joint spaces at the medial femorotibial compartments of both knees. Osteophyte formation, which is most marked at the distal aspect of the medial femoral condyle, is also seen. (From Moskowitz, R. W. [1992]. Osteoarthritis: Signs and symptoms. In R. W. Moskowitz, D. S. Howell, V. M. Goldberg & H. J. Mankin [Eds.], *Osteoarthritis: Diagnosis and medical/surgical treatment* [2nd ed., p. 258]. Philadelphia: W. B. Saunders.)

TABLE 20-3
Osteoarthritis

History

Onset: Usually gradual
Pain/Stiffness: Mild to moderate; dull, aching; brief (10–45 min) A.M. stiffness (may become fixed); limbering with mild exercise; worsens with activity; relieved partially with rest
Systemic Complaints: Possible fatigue
Joints: Few usually; commonly hips, knees, first MTP (great toe), hands (DIP, PIP, MCP of thumb), wrist, shoulder, spine
Common Complaints:
Enlarged joints, crepitation, restricted range of motion, mobility or gait problems
Grasp problems
Elbow extension restricted; possible paresthesia and hand weakness (with osteophyte ulnar nerve compression)
Knee pain with stairs
Hip pain while standing up, climbing, often unilateral and worse at night, may refer to knee, groin, buttocks
Cervical spine pain into back of head, shoulders, and arms and enhanced by movement
Possible paresthesias, sensory loss, weakness, atrophy of arms and hands (with cervical nerve root compression)
Lumbar spine pain worse on prolonged standing, relieved by reclining
Possible acute pain or paresthesia to buttock, leg, calf, ankle (with lumbar disc prolapse or osteophyte involvement of nerve root foramina)

Examination

General: Pain with pressure or movement; crepitus; restricted movement; possible joint enlargement (effusion, osteophytes, bony hypertrophy) or joint redness, warmth, diffuse tenderness (swollen synovium and soft tissue)
Joint Deformity: Abnormal position, subluxation; gait disturbances
Hands: Heberden nodes (DIP), Bouchard's nodes (PIP), thenar wasting, adduction deformity (rectangular appearance); subluxation of DIP, PIP joints
Wrists, Elbows, Shoulders: Little deformity; elbow extension restricted
Knees: Quadriceps wasting; loss of extremes of flexion, extension (stiff knee gait); joint instability; possible synovial thickening, effusion; varus, valgus deformity
Hips: Restricted flexion, internal rotation, abduction, leg shortening, asymmetry of gait, altered cadence
Feet/Ankles: Rare except first MTP joint; hallux valgus deformity
Spine: Loss of lumbar curve, possible nerve root compression signs (muscle wasting, weakness, diminished tendon reflexes, sensory changes, straight leg-raise test), slow shuffling gait with spinal stenosis

Laboratory Tests

Usually normal; synovial fluid: clear, normal viscosity and white cell count (<3000; may be bloody), calcium pyrophosphate crystals may be seen

Radiography

Asymmetric narrowing of joint space; dense sclerosis of subchondral bone; cysts; osteophytes

---

DIP, distal interphalangeal; MCP, metacarpophalangeal; MTP, metatarsophalangeal; PIP, proximal interphalangeal.
Data from Calkins et al. (1994); and Mankin (1993).

(McCune, 1993). Synovial joints may become infected with a wide variety of viruses, bacteria, and fungi. People with other forms of arthritis, particularly RA, have a greater risk of developing pyogenic arthritis. Monarticular pain with onset over seconds or minutes suggests problems such as a fracture, loose body, trauma, or internal derangement. If the onset of pain occurs over hours to a week, the differential should include inflammatory arthritis, especially from a bacterial infection, or a crys-

tal-induced synovitis (McCune, 1993). Tuberculosis and fungal arthritis have a more insidious onset (Grahame, 1994). Signs and symptoms of septic arthritis are described in Table 20–6.

Other. Other forms of arthritis that may occur in older people are mentioned here briefly. Hypertrophic osteoarthropathy is an example of an articular manifestation of a malignant disease that is associated with intrathoracic tumors. This condition causes clubbing of the fingers and toes, periosteal thickening, enlarge-

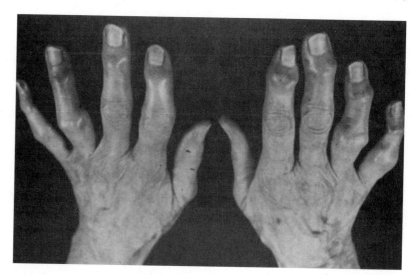

FIGURE 20–5. Osteoarthritis involving the distal and proximal interphalangeal joints in characteristic distribution. (From Moskowitz, R. W., & Bluestone, R. [1992]. General aspects of differential diagnosis. In R. W. Moskowitz, D. S. Howell, V. M. Goldberg & H. J. Mankin [Eds.], *Osteoarthritis: Diagnosis and medical/surgical treatment* [2nd ed., p. 418]. Philadelphia: W. B. Saunders.)

TABLE 20-4
Gout: Clinical Features and Stages

Asymptomatic Hyperuricemia

Laboratory: Serum urate level about 70 mg/dL
Arthritic Symptoms: none
Duration: Until first attack of gouty arthritis or urolithiasis (usually at least 20–30 years)

Acute Gouty Arthritis

Precipitating Factors: Increased serum urate levels (due to drugs such as diuretics, heparin, cyclosporin), traumatic events, dietary or alcoholic excess, previously damaged joints, family history
Associated Disorders: Renal disease, vascular disease, hemolytic anemia, myeloproliferative diseases, psoriasis, endocrine abnormalities
Onset: Acute, often at night
Course: If untreated, hours to weeks; symptoms resolve between attacks; later attacks more severe and frequent
Symptoms: Severe pain, fever
Joints: Commonly single joint initially, then asymmetrical distribution, mostly in lower extremities; first MTP joint (great toe) in 50–60% of initial attacks; also commonly instep, ankle, heel, knee, wrist, fingers, elbow; may cause bursitis
Examination: Varying degrees of erythema, heat, extreme tenderness (may resemble cellulitis); desquamation possible as attack subsides; possible fever; seldom lymphadenopathy
Laboratory: Complete blood count: possible leukocytosis and elevated erythrocyte sedimentation rate; usually hyperuricemia; synovial fluid: intracellular needle or rod-shaped, bifringent crystals; negative elongation with compensated polarized light
Radiography: Soft tissue swelling

Intercritical Gout (intervals between gouty attacks)

Length of Interval: Usually 6 months to 2 years
Laboratory: Synovial fluid with monosodium urate crystals in 12.5–58% of asymptomatic knees and 52% of MTP joints and often with leukocytosis; 24-hour urinary excretion of uric acid and creatinine: normal uric acid of 600 mg

Chronic Tophaceous Gout (chronic symptoms or visible tophi)

Onset: Average of 11.6 years after initial attack
Precipitating Factors: Elevated serum urate, long duration; may occur without prior gouty arthritis
Course: Acute attacks become less frequent, milder
Systemic Symptoms: None
Joints: Any joint; common in helix of ear, fingers, hands, knees, feet, ulnar surface forearm, olecranon bursae, achilles tendon, subcutaneous tibial surface
Examination: Tense, shiny, thin skin over tophus may ulcerate and extrude chalky/pasty material; rare bony ankylosis; marked limitation of joint movement with deformities, crippling
Radiography: Erosions similar to rheumatoid arthritis; calcification possible

MTP, metatarsophalangeal.
Data from Kelley & Schumacher (1993); and McCarty (1994).

TABLE 20-5

Calcium Pyrophosphate Deposition Disease: Clinical Presentations

Pseudogout

Precipitating Factors: Trauma, severe illness, diuretic therapy
Symptoms: Acute attacks 1 day to several weeks; similar to gout; possible fever, confusion (likely with aged)
Joints: Monoarticular or polyarticular; knee, wrist, shoulder, occasionally metatarsophalangeal

Pseudo Rheumatoid Arthritis

Symptoms: Morning stiffness; fatigue; fever (102–104°F), confusion (likely with aged)
Joints: Multiple (less than with rheumatoid arthritis); varying degrees of inflammation; often large joints (knee, wrist, elbow); synovial thickening, subacute or chronic synovitis, local pitting edema, limited range of motion
Laboratory Tests: Leukocytosis (marked in aged); possible elevated erythrocyte sedimentation rate

Pseudo Osteoarthritis

Symptoms: Low-grade chronic symptoms, with or without acute attacks
Joints: Multiple joints, symmetrical bilaterally; most often knee (also wrist, metacarpophalangeal, hip, spine, shoulders, elbow, ankle)

Lanathanic (Asymptomatic) Pyrophosphate Gout

Symptoms: Most joints with deposits are asymptomatic

Pseudo Neuropathic Pyrophosphate Gout

Joints: Severe degeneration of the neuropathic type in absence of neurological abnormalities
Clinical: Presentation as above
Radiography: Evidence of chondrocalcinosis
Laboratory Tests: Synovial fluid: presence of weakly positive birefringent rhomboid or rodlike crystals by compensated polarized light microscopy; fewer than 50,000 leukocytes/mm³; glucose low. Screening studies recommended to rule out metabolic disorders: serum calcium, phosphorus, alkaline phosphatase, iron

Other names for calcium pyrophosphate deposition disease include pyrophosphate gout and chondrocalcinosis.
Data from Seegmiller (1994).

ment of extremities, and possible swelling, heat, and pain. Myeloproliferative disorders and malignant lymphoma may result in joint conditions from hyperuricemia and the deposition of amyloid or malignant tissue in the area. Neuropathic arthropathy is a severe destructive lesion of the joint that results from abnormal stresses placed on a joint in people who are unable to perceive pain normally. Causes of this problem include tabes dorsalis (Charcot's joints), syringomyelia, diabetic neuropathy, and long-standing indifference to pain (Grahame, 1994).

DIFFERENTIAL DIAGNOSIS

By accurately diagnosing the type of arthritis present, proper treatment can be initiated more promptly, thereby preventing unnecessary suffering, disability, and cost. For example, irre-

versible osteoarticular lesions are found only after RA has been present for 4 months (Caruso et al., 1990). Diagnosis by history and examination alone is difficult, as one type of arthritis may mimic or occur in conjunction with another type.

Plain radiographs of the affected and the contralateral joints are generally recommended. Films provide baseline information for later comparison and useful information about the possible type of arthritis; they may also detect unsuspected bony lesions (McCune, 1993). Radiographic findings of OA do not always correlate well with clinical signs and symptoms (Chan et al., 1991; Fife, 1994; Marino & McDonald, 1991; McCune, 1993).

Laboratory findings in older people are often confusing. For instance, elevated erythrocyte sedimentation rates (ESR) and the presence of rheumatoid factor are common findings in older people who do not have RA. Table 20–7

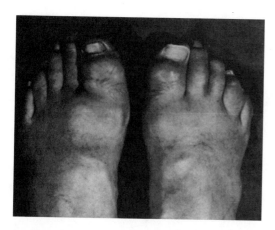

FIGURE 20–6. Chronic gouty arthropathy of both great toes. Roentgenograms revealed tophaceous joint destruction. (From Moskowitz, R. W., & Bluestone, R. [1992]. General aspects of differential diagnosis. In R. W. Moskowitz, D. S. Howell, V. M. Goldberg & H. J. Mankin [Eds.], *Osteoarthritis: Diagnosis and medical/surgical treatment* [2nd ed., p. 421]. Philadelphia: W. B. Saunders.)

compares major differential diagnosis findings in older people with common types of arthritis.

The synovial fluid of all newly inflammatory joints should be examined with a Gram's stain and culture, cell count, and examination for crystals. Synovial fluid examination is particularly useful in differentiating septic and crystal-induced forms of arthritis. This is an important diagnosis to make because untreated joint infections can lead to osteomyelitis, joint destruction, and permanent disability (Kane et al., 1994). Conversely, incorrectly using antibiotics to treat a patient who has gout exposes the person to possible adverse drug reactions. In a study of 67 hospitalized patients with a diagnosis of acute gout or CPDD, a quarter of them experienced errors in diagnosis, treatment, or both before a rheumatologist was consulted (Ho & Denuccio, 1993). Septic arthritis and pyrophosphate gout closely resemble each other and may coexist.

Nonarticular conditions masquerading as arthritis, such as tendinitis and bursitis, can often be treated differently than arthritis, such as with local corticosteroid injections (Kane et al., 1994). Bursitis may occur in conjunction with RA, OA, gout, or CPDD. Acute olecranon bursitis with CPDD deposition may appear very similar to acute septic or gouty arthritis. Tro-

chanteric bursitis should be considered if night pain becomes a major complaint in an older person with OA of the hip. Tendinitis of the rotator cuff of the shoulder may be caused by OA or RA. Carpal tunnel syndrome, caused by a median nerve impingement, may be mistaken for OA when a patient complains of numbness, tingling, or burning pain in the median nerve distribution (thumb, index finger, middle finger, and radial half of the ring finger). Tarsal tunnel syndrome, an entrapment neuropathy of the posterior tibial nerve, may be found in patients with RA. It results in complaints of burning or aching pain and paresthesia in the sole of the foot and toes (Semble, 1994).

Polymyalgia rheumatica (PMR) imitates RA. It is an inflammatory disorder of the muscles, affecting people older than 55 years and occurring more often in women than in men. The clinical signs and symptoms of PMR—onset abrupt or after a mild infection; systemic signs; morning stiffness; increased ESR; and possible

---

TABLE 20–6
Septic Arthritis

History

Onset: Rapid
Pain: Generally severe
Systemic Symptoms: Severity of fever, chills varies with host and organism
Joint Distribution: More often monarticular; commonly large joints, in absence of trauma or peripheral vascular disease

Examination

Fever: Superficial joints tender, warm, may be red; cellulitis common; limited range of motion; deep joints with less obvious signs. General examination: possible source of infection (e.g., lungs, skin, urinary or gastrointestinal tract)

Laboratory Tests

Leukocytosis common
Synovial fluid: white blood count often more than 50,000 organisms on smear or culture; low glucose

Radiography

Radionuclide scans help identify deep joint infection

Data from McCune (1993); Schumacher (1993); and Stevens (1988).

TABLE 20-7
Brief Guide to Diagnosing Rheumatic Disease in the Elderly

	OA	RA	Carpal Tunnel Syndrome	PMR	Gout	Pseudo-gout	Drug-Induced Lupus
Gradual onset	+ + +	+ + +	+ + +	+ + +	0	+	+ + +
Joint swelling or effusion	+ + +	+ + + +	+	+	+ + + +	+ + + +	+ +
Joint pain	+ + + +	+ + + +	+	+	+ + + +	+ + + +	+ + +
Symmetric involvement	+	+ + +	+ +	+ + + +	+	+	+ + +
Muscle pain	+	+	+	+ + +	+	+	+
Abnormal x-ray	+ + + +	+ + +	0	0	+	+ + +	0
Synovial fluid crystals	+	+	0	0	+ + +	+ + +	0
Elevated ESR	+	+ + +	+	+ + + +	+	+	+ + +
Anemia	0	+ +	0	+ + +	0	0	+ +
Positive FANA	0	+	+	+	0	0	+ + + +
High serum uric acid	0	0	0	0	+ + +	0	0
Positive RF test	0	+ + +	0	+	0	0	+

0 = Does not occur
+ = Occurs occasionally
+ + = Occurs frequently
+ + + = Occurs almost always
+ + + + = Difficult to make diagnosis without it

ESR, erythrocyte sedimentation rate; FANA, fluorescent antinuclear antibody; OA, osteoarthritis; PMR, polymyalgia rheumatica; RA, rheumatoid arthritis; RF, rheumatoid factor.
Adapted from Reich, M. L. (1982). Arthritis: Avoiding diagnostic pitfalls. *Geriatrics, 37*(6), 47.

mild thickening of the synovium of the wrists, knees, and finger joints—are often similar to those of RA. With PMR, however, symmetrical muscle aches and stiffness occur particularly in the shoulders but also in the back and thighs. The ESR is usually more elevated than in RA (usually >40 mm/hr). Patients with PMR generally respond within hours or a day to a short trial of prednisone. A disease frequently associated with PMR is temporal arteritis, which can result in blindness. Symptoms such as a headache or recent vision changes in combination with an ESR of greater than 75 mm per hour should prompt a temporal artery biopsy (Calkins et al., 1994).

TREATMENT

Osteoarthritis and Rheumatoid Arthritis

The goals of therapy for both OA and RA are focused on pain control, the preservation of function and mobility, and patient education. Additional goals for RA include the prevention of tissue destruction in involved joints, the re-

duction of joint inflammation, and the restoration of joint function, all of which support increased quality of life in the elderly RA patient (Nesher & Moore, 1993; Williams, 1993). The importance of individualizing treatment strategies cannot be overemphasized, especially in the elderly for whom concurrent chronic illness frequently complicates treatment.

PHARMACOLOGICAL THERAPY

For OA patients, the regular use of acetaminophen may provide adequate analgesia with minimal side effects (Moskowitz & Goldberg, 1993; Schnitzer, 1993). The use of nonsteroidal antiinflammatory drugs (NSAIDs) is controversial because they may contribute to joint damage (Doherty, 1989) and because of their lack of effect beyond analgesic properties (Bradley et al., 1991; Dieppe et al., 1993). Capsaicin, a recently approved topical medication, has been shown to be effective in treating of OA pain while avoiding the systemic effects of NSAIDs (Altman et al., 1994).

RA patients with mild generalized disease may respond well to an analgesic or to analgesic antiinflammatory drugs alone. In patients with more severe disease, however, these drugs should be used as an adjunct to other treatments. Acetaminophen, alone or in combination with codeine, may control symptoms in some patients, but care must be taken to monitor for constipation and confusion when narcotics are used in the elderly (Goode, 1993). Although NSAIDs are indicated to control the inflammatory processes of RA, they pose a special risk for those elderly who experience altered absorption, distribution, and elimination of drugs. These alterations are a direct result of decreases in gastrointestinal, hepatic, and renal blood flow; increased gastric pH; and reduced serum albumin (Ouslander, 1981). Shorter-acting NSAIDs such as naproxen (Naprosyn) and ibuprofen (Advil, Medipren, Motrin, Nuprin, and Rufen) are safer for use in the elderly, as are the pro-drugs nabumetone (Relafen) and sulindac (Clinoril) (Goode, 1993). Monitoring of salicylate levels, with a target range of 20 to 30 mL per dL is recommended to avoid toxicity (Anderson et al., 1976; Dromgoole et al., 1981). The selection of particular NSAIDs may be based on several factors, including cost, availability, dosing frequency, and prescriber familiarity with particular drugs (Williams, 1993). See Table 20–8 for a list of selected NSAIDs.

The advent of cytoprotective agents has helped mitigate the gastrointestinal damage of NSAID therapy. However, the addition of any drug must be weighed against compliance problems owing to cost and the increased complexity of therapy. Prophylactic therapy may be indicated for patients who have an increased risk of gastropathy; these patients include the elderly (especially women older than 75 years) as well as individuals with a history of ulcers, gastrointestinal bleeding, prior NSAID gastrointestinal side effects, concurrent prednisone use, and high-dose NSAID use (Fries et al., 1991; Griffin et al., 1991; Piper et al., 1991; Roth, 1988). Misoprostol (Cytotec) may reduce the risk of gastric ulceration in high-risk patients but may also require a reduction in dosage to 0.1 mg four times daily to reduce the side effects of dyspepsia and diarrhea (Graham et al., 1988; Lanza et al., 1981). The prescribing information also recommends titrating the drug when initiating therapy.

When NSAID therapy is inadequate for RA management, slow-acting antirheumatic drugs (SAARDs) should be added. These drugs are also referred to as *disease-modifying antirheumatic drugs*. Although the mechanism of action of SAARDs is not known, they do have demonstrated efficacy over placebos in controlled trials (Furst, 1990). Patients requiring these therapies should be managed in conjunction with a rheumatologist (McCarty, 1993b). The use of and precautions for selected SAARDs are outlined in Table 20–9. Owing to the loss of effectiveness, the median time to discontinuation of most SAARDs is about 2 years (McCarty, 1993b). Methotrexate may be the exception to this, with studies showing sustained efficacy over a mean period of 90 months (Kremer & Phelps, 1992). The simultaneous use of multiple SAARDs is controversial (Healey & Wilske, 1991; McCarty, 1993b; Paulus, 1990; Wilske & Healey, 1989).

RA patients may require corticosteroid therapy to decrease inflammation and to allow them to maintain activity or improve functioning pending the onset of other therapies. However, it may be difficult or impossible to completely discontinue steroid therapy once it has been started in RA patients (McCarty, 1993b; Williams, 1993). Systemic steroids are not indicated in the treatment of OA (Moskowitz & Goldberg, 1993). Intraarticular injection of steroids may be beneficial for controlling isolated joint inflammation in patients with RA and, to a lesser extent, with OA (McCarty, 1993a; Schnitzer, 1993; Williams, 1993). When joint injection is used, care should be taken to ensure that the joint is not infected and that injections are not used to mask pain, which can lead to overuse and increased joint damage (McCarty, 1993a; Schnitzer, 1993).

Recent studies with minocycline have demonstrated its effectiveness and safety for patients with mildly to moderately active RA. In doses of 100 mg/day, treated patients showed significant improvement in joint swelling and laboratory measures when compared with control groups. The onset of improvement occurred after 12 weeks, with effectiveness maintained for the 48 weeks of the study. Although infrequent and similar to those effects seen in the control group, adverse effects of particular concern in the elderly included dizziness, increased liver function test results, and in-

TABLE 20-8
Nonsteroidal Antiinflammatory Drugs

Generic Name	Trade Name	Total Daily Dose for RA (mg)	Recommended Number of Divided Daily Doses	Plasma Half-Life (hr)
Aspirin compounds	Anacin, Ascriptin, Bayer, Bufferin, Ecotrin, Excedrin	4000	3	12
Diclofenac	Voltaren	200–300	4	1–2
Diflunisal	Dolobid	1000	2	10
Fenoprofen	Nalfon	2400	4	2
Flurbiprofen	Ansaid	200	3	3
Ibuprofen	Advil, Medipren, Motrin, Nuprin, Rufen	2400	4	2
Indomethacin	Indocin	150–200	3	5
Ketoprofen	Orudis	200	3	1.5
Meclofenamate	Meclomen	400	4	2
Nabumetone	Relafen	1000	1	22–30
Naproxen	Naprosyn	750	2	13
Piroxicam	Feldene	20	1	45
Sulindac	Clinoril	400	2	16
Tolmetin	Tolectin	1600	4	1

Adapted from Payne, D. G. (1992). Nonsteroidal anti-inflammatory drugs; nonopioid analgesics; drugs used in gout. In B. G. Katzung (Ed.), *Basic and clinical pharmacology* (5th ed., pp. 491–501). Stamford, CT: Appleton & Lange.

creased bilirubin and creatinine levels (Tilley et al., 1995). Cyclosporin has been used experimentally in RA, but its usefulness may be limited owing to nephrotoxicity (Wilder, 1988). Gamma interferon has shown a significant initial effect on RA, but the effect was not sustained after 2 years (Cannon et al., 1990). Biological therapies including interleukin-2 and anti-CD4 monoclonal antibodies are also under investigation (Horneff et al., 1991; Murphy, 1992).

Owing to the naturally varying course of RA, the effectiveness of therapy may be difficult to monitor. Some indicators that are useful in monitoring the disease over time include functional self-assessment, counts of involved joints, grip strength, walking time, ADL questionnaires, and laboratory tests such as ESR, rheumatoid titer, and radiographic evaluation of joints (Murphy, 1992). Periodic monitoring of functional status is equally appropriate in the OA patient.

NONPHARMACOLOGICAL THERAPY

Education. As it is for any chronic condition, patient education is the cornerstone for manag-

ing arthritis, both OA and RA. The goals of arthritis education in the elderly include the improvement or maintenance of function, psychosocial status, pain, and symptoms as well as satisfaction with management (Bombardier et al., 1982; Dacher, 1989). Important outcomes of educational intervention include behavioral changes, increased knowledge, ability to communicate with caregivers, and sense of control (Daltroy & Liang, 1993). Some of the behaviors believed to affect arthritis patients' health and psychological status include exercise, relaxation, joint protection, and adherence to medication regimens (Daltroy & Liang, 1993). When working with the geriatric patient, it may be helpful to have the patient identify how he or she best mastered skills or learning in the past and to try to build on those successes (Dacher, 1989).

Patient education should include an appropriate review of pathophysiology, including the chronic nature of the disease and the patient's role in monitoring and managing the disease. Self-management techniques may include stress management, coping strategies, and problem-solving techniques as well as re-

TABLE 20-9

Slow-Acting, Antirheumatic Drugs

Drug	Dose	Onset	Side Effects	Monitoring	Special Considerations
Auranofin (oral gold)	6 mg/d; maximum 9 mg/d	2–6 mo	Abdominal discomfort, diarrhea	CBC weekly initially, then monthly	May switch to injectable gold if oral ineffective or side effects a problem
Sodium aurothiomalate (IM gold)	Test dose 10 mg followed by 25 mg the next week then 50 mg/wk for 3–6 months May decrease frequency to 2–4 wk with response Total dose 1 g cumulative or symptoms of toxicity	3–4 mo	Thrombocytopenia Proteinuria Skin rash Oral ulcers	UA, CBC, platelets prior to each injection Check for ulcers and rash	Generally not self-administered Compliance easily monitored
D-penicillamine	125 or 250 mg/d increase 125–250 every month Most respond to 500–750 mg	6 wk or more after reaching effective dose	Thrombocytopenia Proteinuria Skin rash Alteration of taste	UA, CBC, platelets weekly for 4 wk, then monthly LFTs, muscle enzyme every 6 mo	Must give on an empty stomach to avoid inactivation or drug interaction Consider pyridoxine supplement
Hydroxychloroquine	400 mg/d in single or divided dose Decrease to 200 mg/d once response achieved	Up to 6 mo	Retinal change GI disturbance Skin rash	Baseline eye and slit lamp exam with follow-up every 3–6 mo	Avoid concurrent use of thioridazine descending to similar pattern of maculopathy
Methotrexate	Oral or injection 5–7.5 mg/wk single or divided; may increase to 15 mg/wk	4–8 wk	Oral ulcers GI symptoms Hepatotoxicity Pneumonitis	CBC, LFTs weekly, monthly, then 2–3 mo Renal function and chest x-ray or PFTs baseline then every 6–12 mo	Contraindicated with concurrent use of sulfa containing antibiotics or in presence of HIV infection Alcohol use, obesity, and diabetes may aggravate hepatotoxicity
*Sulfasalazine	0.5 g/d increase weekly to 2 g/d divided	Approximately 1 mo after full dose	Malaise Nausea Hepatotoxicity	CBC, UA, LFTs biweekly then every 1–3 mo	Contraindicated in patients with known sulfa allergy

*Not approved by the Food and Drug Administration for use with rheumatoid arthritis.
CBC, complete blood count; GI, gastrointestinal; HIV, human immunodeficiency virus; IM, intramuscular; LFT, liver function test; PFT, pulmonary function test; UA, urinalysis.
Data from Goode (1993); Nesher & Moore (1993); and Williams (1993).

laxation, distraction, or visualization for pain control. The inclusion of family members or care providers in the patient's education can enhance these individuals' understanding of the impact of arthritis on the patient and can also facilitate communication and overall patient management. Focusing initial educational efforts on the patient's self-identified priorities will also facilitate patient participation in the overall plan of care. Lorig and Fries's *The arthritis helpbook: A tested self-management program for coping with your arthritis* (1990) serves as an excellent reference for patients and is readily available at bookstores nationwide.

Rest and Exercise. Although rest and exercise are recognized therapies in arthritis, they pose special risks in the elderly. Rest may relieve fatigue, help decrease inflammation in affected joints, and facilitate pain control; however, after even a few days of bed rest, elderly patients may lose muscle strength and have difficulty resuming ambulation (Nesher & Moore, 1993). All joints, even those with active disease and inflammation, should be put through their full range of motion daily to preserve function (McCarty, 1993b). Recent studies have shown that elderly RA patients on steroid therapy can tolerate physical training in individualized programs without increasing disease activity (Lyngberg et al., 1994). High-intensity strength training exercise has also been shown to preserve bone mass and increase muscle mass, strength, and balance in postmenopausal women (Nelson et al., 1994).

Elderly patients should maintain a balanced program of exercise, including flexibility, strengthening, and cardiovascular conditioning. Although the program needs to be tailored to meet the individual patient's needs and limitations, all patients should be advised that pain lasting more than 2 hours after a specific activity is excessive and indicates the need to decrease the activity level. The Arthritis Foundation offers the Aquatic Program and the Young Men's Christian Association Aquatic Program throughout the United States to assist with patients who are more comfortable with or prefer water exercise. Discussion of the patient's usual routine may help establish a balanced program that allows for necessary activities, regular exercise, and structured rest or relax-

ation periods. Identification of usual activities also offers the opportunity to instruct the patient in joint protection and energy conservation techniques.

Physical therapists can provide patients with exercise programs specific to their needs as well as instruction in the use of therapies to augment pain control, such as heat, cold, traction, or electrical stimulation (Swezey, 1993). Physical therapists are also excellent resources for the evaluation of or instruction in transfer techniques and ambulation (Hyde, 1980). Occupational therapists can evaluate the patient's functional capacity, identify the need for adaptive or safety equipment, and counsel patients on energy conservation and joint protection in their daily activities. Occupational therapists can also provide splinting to ensure rest for specific joints while preserving function (Swezey, 1993). An in-home evaluation of the patient by the physical or occupational therapist is frequently of great assistance in developing adaptive strategies for a specific patient.

Diet. Questions about the role of diet in arthritis are frequently asked, but answers are far from clear. This is especially true in the elderly, for whom concurrent disease processes can complicate dietary recommendations. Although some studies suggest that food allergies may play a role for some RA patients, the current recommendations are to follow a balanced, healthy diet and to avoid fad dietary practices (Panush, 1993). Achieving and maintaining one's ideal body weight helps relieve joint stress and enhances overall health (Goode, 1993). Specific dietary precautions may apply to patients on medications such as NSAIDs, steroids, or methotrexate. Patients with specific dietary needs due to arthritis or other conditions may benefit from consultation with a registered dietitian to develop a comprehensive nutritional plan.

MANAGEMENT OF COMPLICATIONS

When other therapies have proved unsatisfactory, patients may benefit from joint surgery to relieve symptoms and improve function. The presence of concurrent disease is a more significant factor than age in predicting poor surgical outcomes (Nesher & Moore, 1993). Available surgical interventions include joint replacement, tendon repair, carpal tunnel release, and synovectomy (Bently & Dowd, 1986). Joint replacement may be preferable to alternative therapies that require prolonged immobilization in RA patients (Herndon & Hubbard, 1983).

The occurrence of vasculitis, Felty's syndrome, and rheumatoid lung disease require consultation because modification of drug therapy and the use of high-dose steroids are usually indicated. Atlantoaxial subluxation may require surgical interventions if a soft cervical collar fails to provide symptomatic relief. Synovial cysts, most frequently seen in the popliteal space, may require synovectomy if steroid injection fails. Rheumatoid nodules should be surgically removed only if they become infected or interfere with function (Williams, 1993).

GENERAL CONSIDERATIONS

Compliance in the elderly may be enhanced by simplifying the treatment regimen as much as possible, giving specific written instruction on medications, encouraging the use of medication boxes that can be prefilled, and eliciting the support of family members or involved significant others. One study also showed that telephone contacts by trained lay personnel were a cost-effective intervention that supported increased physical health and decreased pain in OA patients (Weinburger et al., 1993).

Gout and Pseudogout

ACUTE MANAGEMENT

The acute management of both gout and pseudogout consists of analgesia and splinting for pain control as well as definitive treatment to promptly restore joint function. Colchicine, although effective in both conditions when started promptly after the onset of symptoms, has significant adverse effects. This is especially true in the elderly, who may develop diarrhea from oral colchicine therapy, resulting in severe electrolyte imbalances. Acute oral treatment is 0.5 mg/hr until relief or side ef-

fects occur. The maximum dose is 10 to 12 tablets for younger people and less in the elderly (Spilberg et al., 1980). When oral medications or NSAIDs are contraindicated, such as in the immediate postoperative period or with severe congestive heart failure, intravenous colchicine may be appropriate. The drug is prepared by mixing 1 mg in 20 mL of normal saline and administering slowly over a minimum of 10 minutes. Extreme care must be used to avoid extravasation. The intravenous colchicine dose should be reduced by 50% in the elderly. Therefore, no more than 1 mg should be administered in a single dose, not more than 2 mg should be administered in a total dose, and repeated administrations should not be given beyond 24 hours for a single attack. Additional colchicine should not be given for at least 7 days (Wallace & Singer, 1988a, 1988b). Intravenous colchicine should also be avoided in patients with prior use of oral colchicine for therapeutic or prophylactic reasons (Terkeltaub, 1993). Joint aspiration followed by the injection of microcrystalline adrenocorticosteroid esters is also effective in managing single joint inflammation in both gout and pseudogout and provides almost immediate relief (Spilberg et al., 1980; Terkeltaub, 1993).

CHRONIC MANAGEMENT

Gout should not be treated prophylactically until the patient establishes a pattern of frequency of attacks. Many patients can effectively manage their disease by being educated about recognizing joint pain, tenderness, or swelling as the earliest signs of disease flair so that treatment can be initiated and the attack aborted (Pratt & Ball, 1993). Allopurinol may be required, but the starting dose should be 100 mg/day or less, rather than the usual 300 mg/day (Wallace & Singer, 1988a). Owing to decreased glomerular filtration rates, most patients older than 60 to 65 years do not respond to the uricosuric drugs traditionally used for gout. There is no means of removing the CPPD crystals of pseudogout from the joints, and treating the underlying conditions does not alter the crystal deposits (McCarty, 1993a).

Septic Arthritis

Septic arthritis is managed through hospitalization and aggressive antibiotic treatment. Initial antibiotic therapy should be based on Gram's stain results of the synovial fluid or of other known infective organisms in the individual. Subsequent therapy can be modified by initial and repeat culture and sensitivity studies as well as through evidence of clinical responses to therapy (Mahowald, 1993; Schmid, 1993). The patient's renal function must be taken into account in determining the appropriate antibiotic dosing and should be monitored carefully throughout therapy. Calculated creatinine clearance is generally a more reliable indicator of renal function than is serum creatinine alone. A 10-year study on septic arthritis in the elderly identified *Staphylococcus aureus* as the most frequent infecting organism. The same study identified the usefulness of the ESR as both a diagnostic tool and a means to monitor the effectiveness of therapy in a population that frequently fails to manifest classic signs of infection (Vincent & Amirault, 1990).

Accumulations of synovial fluid in the infected joint must be removed through needle aspiration or surgical drainage. Repeated aspiration with an analysis of fluid serves as an adjunct in monitoring the effectiveness of treatment and also helps preserve joint function (Schmid, 1993). Once the initial effusion has been treated, passive and active range of motion should be initiated to preserve long-term joint function (Goldenberg & Reed, 1985; Salter, 1981). Weight bearing should be avoided while signs of acute inflammation are present. When pain control is necessary, antiinflammatory drugs should be avoided until the effectiveness of antibiotic therapy is well established. Once started, antiinflammatory drugs should be continued for the duration of antibiotic therapy (Schmid, 1993). The length of parenteral and oral antibiotic therapy should be adjusted based on the clinical response of the individual patient (Smith, 1990).

Outcomes in septic arthritis are directly related to the timeliness of the diagnosis and initiation of therapy. Delayed or inadequate therapy leads to permanent destruction of joint structures with a resultant loss of function. Pre-existing joint damage, such as a rheumatoid joint, and multiple joint involvement are also poor prognostic indicators (Gardner & Weisman, 1990; Mahowald, 1993; Schmid, 1993; Vincent & Amirault, 1990).

RESOURCES FOR CLIENTS AND FAMILIES

Aging services and the American Association of Retired Persons can provide a variety of services relating to housing, transportation, and government services for elderly clients with arthritis or other disabling illness (see Appendix 20–1). The Arthritis Foundation provides a variety of services at the local and national level. Arthritis educational materials covering general and specific topics are available and can be ordered in bulk for distribution. Topics covered include specific disease types, general medication management, specific drug information, exercise options, coping strategies, and pain and stress management. Local Arthritis Foundation chapters can provide information on health professionals specializing in arthritis, the location for obtaining specialized equipment, and the availability of community facilities such as warm-water pools. Many chapters also have a speaker's bureau for interested groups. Courses such as the Arthritis Self-Help Course (ASHC) and People with Arthritis Can Exercise (PACE) are also available. Research has shown that patients who complete the ASHC show a decrease in pain and physician visits, even with increased physical disability. These improvements, sustained over a 4-year period, are attributed to these patients' feelings of enhanced self-efficacy (Lorig et al., 1993).

Professional education and research funding are also available through the Arthritis Foundation.

SUMMARY

This chapter described common types of arthritis in older adults. Information was provided on the differential diagnosis and treatment of arthritis, including nonpharmacological therapies and community resources.

REFERENCES

Altman, R. D., Aven, A., Holmburg, C. E., et al. (1994). Capsaicin cream 0.025% as monotherapy for osteoarthritis: A double-blind study. *Seminars in Arthritis and Rheumatism, 23*(6, suppl. 3), 25–33.

Anderson, R. J., Potts, D. E., Gabow, P. A., et al. (1976). Unrecognized adult salicylate intoxication. *Annals of Internal Medicine, 85,* 745–748.

Bently, G., & Dowd, G. S. E. (1986). Surgical treatment of arthritis in the elderly. *Clinics in Rheumatic Diseases, 12,* 291–327.

Bombardier, C., Tugwell, P., Sinclair, A., et al. (1982). Preference for endpoint measures in clinical trials: Results of structured workshops. *Journal of Rheumatology, 9,* 798–801.

Bradley, J. D., Brandt, K. D., Katz, B. P., et al. (1991). Comparison of an anti-inflammatory dose of ibuprofen, an analgesic dose of ibuprofen, and acetaminophen in the treatment of patients with osteoarthritis of the knee. *New England Journal of Medicine, 325,* 87–91.

Calkins, E., Reinhard, J. D., & Vladutiu, A. O. (1994). Rheumatoid arthritis and the autoimmune rheumatic diseases in the older patient. In W. R. Hazzard, E. L Bierman, J. P. Blass, et al. (Eds.), *Principles of geriatric medicine and gerontology* (3rd ed., pp. 965–979). New York: McGraw-Hill.

Cannon, G. W., Emkey, R. D., Denes, A., et al. (1990). Prospective two-year follow-up of recombinant interferon-Y in rheumatoid arthritis. *Journal of Rheumatology, 17,* 304–310.

Caruso, I., Santandrea, S., Puttni, P. S., et al. (1990). Clinical, laboratory and radiographic features in early rheumatoid arthritis. *Journal of Rheumatology, 17,* 1263–1266.

Chan, W. P., Lang, P., Stevens, M. P., et al. (1991). Osteoarthritis of the knee: Comparison of radiography, CT, and MR imaging to assess extent and severity. *American Journal of Roentgenology, 157,* 799–806.

Dacher, J. E. (1989). Rehabilitation and the geriatric patient. *Nursing Clinics of North America, 24*(1), 225–237.

Daltroy, L. H., & Liang, M. H. (1993). Arthritis education: Opportunities and state of the art. *Health Education Quarterly, 20*(1), 3–16.

Dieppe, P. A., Frankel, S. J., & Toth, B. (1993). Is research into the treatment of osteoarthritis with non-steroidal anti-inflammatory drugs misdirected? *Lancet, 341,* 353–354.

Doherty, M. (1989). 'Chondroprotection' by non-steroidal anti-inflammatory drugs. *Annals of Rheumatologic Disease, 48,* 619–621.

Dromgoole, S. H., Furst, D. E., & Paulus, H. E. (1981). Rational approaches to the use of salicylates in the treatment of rheumatoid arthritis. *Seminars in Arthritis Rheumatism, 11,* 257–283.

Felson, D. T., Zhang, Y., Anthony, J. M., et al. (1992). Weight loss reduces the risk for symptomatic knee osteoarthritis in women: The Framingham study. *Annals of Internal Medicine, 116*(7), 535–539.

Fife, R. (1994). Osteoarthritis. In W. R. Hazzard, E. L. Bierman, J. P. Blass, et al. (Eds.), *Principals of geriatric medicine and gerontology* (3rd ed., pp. 981–994). New York: McGraw-Hill.

Fries, J. F., Williams, C. A., Block, D. A., & Michel, B. A. (1991). Nonsteroids anti-inflammatory drug-associated gastropathy: Incidence and risk factor models. *American Journal of Medicine, 91,* 213–222.

Furst, D. E. (1990). Rationale use of disease modifying antirheumatic drugs. *Drugs, 39,* 19–37.

Gardner, G. C., & Weisman, M. H. (1990). Pyarthrosis in rheumatoid arthritis: 13 cases and a review of the literature from the last 40 years. *American Journal of Medicine, 88,* 503–522.

Goldenberg, D. L., & Reed, J. I. (1985). Bacterial arthritis. *New England Journal of Medicine, 312,* 764–771.

Goode, J. D. (1993). Anti-rheumatic treatment in the elderly. *Zeitschrift für gerontologie, 26*(1), 39–43.

Graham, D. Y., Agrawal, N. M., & Roth, S. H. (1988). Prevention of NSAID-induced gastric ulcer with misoprostol: A multicenter, double-blind, placebo-controlled trial. *Lancet, 2,* 1277–1280.

Grahame, R. (1994). Joint disease in old age. In J. C. Brocklehurst, R. C. Tallis & H. M. Fillit (Eds), *Textbook of geriatric medicine & gerontology* (4th ed., pp. 813–833). Edinburgh: Churchill Livingstone.

Griffin, M. R., Piper, J. M., Daugherty, J. R., et al. (1991). Nonsteroidal anti-inflammatory drug use and increased risk for peptic ulcer disease in elderly persons. *Annals of Internal Medicine, 114,* 257–263.

Harris, E. D. (1993). Clinical features of rheumatoid arthritis. In W. N. Kelly, E. D. Harris, S. Ruddy & C. B. Sledge (Eds.), *Textbook of rheumatology, vol. 1* (4th ed., pp. 874–911). Philadelphia: W. B. Saunders.

Healey, L. A., & Wilske, K. R. (1991). Evaluating combination drug therapy in rheumatoid arthritis. *Journal of Rheumatology, 18,* 641–642.

Herndon, J. H., & Hubbard, L. F. (1993). Total joint replacement in the upper extremity. *Surgical Clinics of North America, 63*(3), 715–735.

Ho, G., & DeNuccio, M. (1993). Gout and pseudogout in hospitalized patients. *Archives of Internal Medicine, 153*(24), 2787–2790.

Horneff, G., Burmester, G. R., Emmrich, F., & Kalden, J. R. (1991). Treatment of rheumatoid arthritis with anti-CD4 monoclonal antibody. *Arthritis and Rheumatism, 34,* 129–140.

Hyde, S. A. (1980). *Physiotherapy in rheumatology.* Oxford: Blackwell Scientific Publications.

Kane, R. L., Ouslander, J. G., & Abrass, I. B. (1994). *Essentials of clinical geriatrics* (3rd ed., pp. 228–230). New York: McGraw-Hill.

Kelley, W. N., & Schumacher, H. R. (1993). Gout. In W. N. Kelley, E. D. Harris, S. Ruddy & C. B. Sledge (Eds.), *Textbook of rheumatology, vol. 2* (4th ed., pp. 1291–1336). Philadelphia: W. B. Saunders.

Kremer, J. M., & Phelps, C. T. (1992). Long-term prospective study of the use of methotrexate in the treatment of rheumatoid arthritis—update after a mean of 90 months. *Arthritis and Rheumatism, 35*(2), 138–145.

Lanza, F. L., Royer, G. L., Nelson, R. S., et al. (1981). A comparative endoscopic evaluation of the damaging effects of non-steroidal anti-inflammatory agents on the gastric and duodenal mucosa. *American Journal of Gastroenterology, 75,* 17–21.

Lorig, K., & Fries, J. F. (1990). *The arthritis helpbook: A tested self-management program for coping with your arthritis* (3rd ed.). New York: Addison-Wesley Publishing.

Lorig, K. R., Mazonson, P. D., & Holman, H. R. (1993). Evidence suggesting that health education for self-management in patients with chronic arthritis has sustained health benefits while reducing health care costs. *Arthritis and Rheumatism, 36*(4), 439–446.

Lyngberg, K. K., Harreby, M., Bentzen, H., et al. (1994). Elderly rheumatoid arthritis patients on steroid treatment tolerate physical training without an increase in disease activity. *Archives of Physical Medicine and Rehabilitation, 75,* 1189–1195.

Mahowald, M. L. (1993). Infectious arthritis. In H. R. Schumacher (Ed.), *Primer on rheumatic diseases* (10th ed., pp. 192–197). Atlanta: Arthritis Foundation.

Mankin, H. J. (1993). Clinical features of osteoarthritis. In W. N. Kelley, E. D. Harris, S. Ruddy & C. B. Sledge (Eds.), *Textbook of rheumatology, vol. 2* (4th ed., pp. 1374–1384). Philadelphia: W. B. Saunders.

Marino, C., & McDonald, E. (1991). Osteoarthritis and rheumatoid arthritis in elderly patients. *Postgraduate Medicine, 90*(5), 237–243.

McCarty, D. J. (1993a). Calcium pyrophosphate dihydrate crystal deposition disease. In H. R. Schumacher (Ed.), *Primer on rheumatic diseases* (10th ed., pp. 219–222). Atlanta: Arthritis Foundation.

McCarty, D. J. (1993b). Treatment of rheumatoid arthritis. In D. J. McCarty & W. J. Koopman (Eds.), *Arthritis and allied conditions—A textbook of rheumatology* (12th ed., pp. 877–886). Philadelphia: Lea & Febiger.

McCarty, D. J. (1994). Gout without hyperuricemia. *Journal of the American Medical Association, 271*(4), 302–303.

McCune, W. J. (1993). Monarticular arthritis. In W. N. Kelley, E. D. Harris, S. Ruddy & C. B. Sledge (Eds.), *Textbook of rheumatology, vol. 1* (4th ed., pp. 368–380). Philadelphia: W. B. Saunders.

Miller-Blair, D. J., & Robbins, D. L. (1993). Rheumatoid arthritis: New science, new treatment. *Geriatrics, 48*(6), 28–38.

Moskowitz, R. W. (1993). Diseases associated with the deposition of calcium pyrophosphate or hydroxyapatite. In W. N. Kelley, E. D. Harris, S. Ruddy & C. B. Sledge (Eds.), *Textbook of rheumatology, vol. 2* (4th ed., pp. 1337–1354). Philadelphia: W. B. Saunders.

Moskowitz, R. W., & Goldberg, V. M. (1993). Osteoarthritis—clinical features and treatment. In H. R. Schumaker (Ed.), *Primer on rheumatic diseases* (10th ed., pp. 188–190). Atlanta: Arthritis Foundation.

Murphy, N. G. (1992). Current concepts in the management of rheumatoid arthritis. *Delaware Medical Journal, 64*(4), 257–265.

Nelson, M. E., Fiatarone, M. A., Morganti, C. M., et al. (1994). Effects of high-intensity strength training on multiple risk factors for osteoporotic fractures—a randomized controlled trial. *Journal of the American Medical Association, 272*(24), 1909–1914.

Nesher, G., & Moore, T. L. (1993). Rheumatoid arthritis in the aged—incidence and optimal management. *Drugs & Aging, 3*(6), 487–501.

Ouslander, J. G. (1981). Drug therapy in the elderly. *Annals of Internal Medicine, 95,* 711–722.

Panush, R. S. (1993). Arthritis, food allergy, diets, and nutrition. In D. J. McCarty & W. J. Koopman (Eds.), *Arthritis and allied conditions—A textbook of rheumatology* (12th ed., pp. 139–146). Philadelphia: Lea & Febiger.

Paulus, H. E. (1990). The use of combinations of disease modifying antirheumatic agents in rheumatoid arthritis. *Arthritis and Rheumatism, 33,* 113–120.

Piper, J. M., Ray, W. A., Daugherty, J. R, & Griffin, M. R. (1991). Corticosteroid use and peptic ulcer disease: Role of non-steroidal anti-inflammatory drugs. *Annals of Internal Medicine, 114,* 735–740.

Pratt, P. W., & Ball, G. V. (1993). Gout-treatment. In H. R. Schumaker (Ed.), *Primer on rheumatic diseases* (10th ed., pp. 216–219). Atlanta: Arthritis Foundation.

Reich, M. L. (1982). Arthritis: Avoiding diagnostic pitfalls. *Geriatrics, 37*(6), 46–54.

Roth, S. H. (1988). NSAID and gastropathy: A rheumatologist's review. *Journal of Rheumatology, 15,* 912–919.

Salter, R. B. (1981). The protective effect of continuous passive motion on living articular cartilage in acute septic arthritis: An experimental investigation in the rabbit. *Clinical Orthopaedics and Related Research, 159,* 223–247.

Schmid, F. R. (1993). Principles of diagnosis and treatment of bone and joint infection. In D. J. McCarty & W. J. Koopman (Eds.), *Arthritis and allied conditions—A textbook of rheumatology* (12th ed., pp. 1975–2001). Philadelphia: Lea & Febiger.

Schnitzer, T. J. (1993). Management of osteoarthritis. In D. J. McCarty & W. J. Koopman (Eds.), *Arthritis and allied conditions—A textbook of rheumatology* (12th ed., pp 1761–1769). Philadelphia: Lea & Febiger.

Schumacher, H. R. (1993). Synovial fluid analysis and synovial biopsy. In W. N. Kelley, E. D. Harris, S. Ruddy & C. B. Sledge (Eds.), *Textbook of rheumatology, vol. 1* (4th ed., pp. 562–578). Philadelphia: W. B. Saunders.

Seegmiller, J. E. (1994). Gout and pyrophosphate gout (chondrocalcinosis). In W. R. Hazzard, E. L. Bierman, J. P. Blass, et al. (Eds.), *Principles of geriatric medicine and gerontology* (3rd ed., pp. 987–994). New York: McGraw-Hill.

Semble, E. L. (1994). Bursitis, tendinitis, and related disorders. In W. R. Hazzard, E. L . Bierman, J. P. Blass, et al. (Eds.), *Principles of geriatric medicine and gerontology* (3rd ed., pp. 995–1003). New York: McGraw-Hill.

Smith, J. (1990). Infectious arthritis. *Infectious Disease Clinics of North America, 4,* 523–538.

Spilberg, I., McLain, D., Simchowitz, & Berrey, S. (1980). Colchicine and pseudogout. *Arthritis and Rheumatism, 23,* 1062–1063.

Stevens, M. B. (1988). The differential diagnosis of arthritis. In A. M. Harvey, R. J. Johns, V. A. McKusick, et al. (Eds.), *The principles and practice of medicine* (22nd ed., pp. 535–542). New York: Appleton-Century-Crofts.

Swezey, R. L. (1993). Rehabilitation medicine and arthritis. In D. J. McCarty & W. J. Koopman (Eds.), *Arthritis and allied conditions—A textbook of rheumatology* (12th ed., pp. 887–917). Philadelphia: Lea & Febiger.

Terkeltaub, R. A. (1993). Pathogenesis and treatment of crystal induced inflammation. In D. J. McCarty & W. J. Koopman (Eds.), *Arthritis and allied conditions—A textbook of rheumatology* (12th ed., pp. 1819–1833). Philadelphia: Lea & Febiger.

Tilley, B. C., Alarcon, G. S., Heyse, S. P., et al. (1995). Minocycline in rheumatoid arthritis—A 48-week, double-blind, placebo-controlled trial. *Annals of Internal Medicine, 122*(2), 81–89.

Vincent, G. M., & Amirault, J. D. (1990). Septic arthritis in the elderly. *Clinical Orthopedics and Related Research, 251,* 241–245.

Wallace, S. L., & Singer, J. Z. (1988a). Review: Systemic toxicity associated with intravenous administration of colchicine—Guidelines for use. *Journal of Rheumatology, 15,* 495–499.

Wallace, S. L., & Singer, J. Z. (1988b). Therapy in gout. *Rheumatic Disease Clinics of North America, 14,* 441–458.

Wallston, K. A., Brown, G. K., Stein, M. J., & Dobbins, C. J. (1989). Comparing the short and long versions of the arthritis impact measurement scales. *Journal of Rheumatology, 16*(8), 1105–1109.

Weinberger, M., Tierney, W. M., Cowper, P. A., et al. (1993). Cost-effectiveness of increased telephone contacts for patients with osteoarthritis—A randomized, controlled trial. *Arthritis and Rheumatism, 36*(2), 243–246.

Wilder, R. L. (1988). Treatment of the patient with rheumatoid arthritis refractory to standard therapy. *Journal of the American Medical Association, 259,* 2446–2449.

Williams, H. J. (1993). Rheumatoid arthritis and treatment. In H. R. Schumacher (Ed.), *Primer on the rheumatic diseases* (10th ed., pp. 96–99). Atlanta: Arthritis Foundation.

Wilske, K. R., & Healey, L. A. (1989). Remodeling the pyramid—a concept whose time has come. *Journal of Rheumatology, 16,* 565–567.

Yelin, E. (1992). Arthritis: The cumulative impact of a common chronic condition. *Arthritis and Rheumatism, 35*(5), 489–497.

Resources

Local Arthritis Foundation Chapter (listed in the phone book)
or
Arthritis Foundation
P.O. Box 1900
Atlanta, GA 30326
1-800-283-7800

American Association of Retired Persons (AARP)
601 E Street N.W.
Washington, D.C. 20049
1-202-434-2277

Local County Aging Services (e.g. Salt Lake County Aging Services)
2001 S. State
Salt Lake City, UT 84115
1-801-468-2480

Includes: Legal services, Meals on Wheels, nutrition, outreach, healthy aging, and other programs for seniors

CHAPTER 21

Cardiovascular Conditions

Mary Ann Johnson

Cardiovascular disease continues to be the most common cause of death and acute problems requiring hospitalization for older adults (Wolfel, 1990). The actual prevalence of cardiovascular disease in older adults is unknown, and several factors may be responsible for the lack of prevalence data. First, age selection for surveys such as the National Health and Nutrition Examination Survey-I from 1971 to 1975 failed to include the *old old*, those people older than 80 years. Second, most of the studies conducted relied on self-report, which tends to underestimate the actual prevalence of the disease (Mittelmark, 1993). Older adults who live in a long-term care facility or who are disabled or seriously ill usually are not included in these self-reported surveys. Another factor in the underestimation of cardiovascular disease is the difficulty differentiating between normal, or expected, and pathological changes of aging (Lakatta, 1995). When self-reports are the primary source of data, older adults may mistakenly believe that the cardiovascular symptoms they are experiencing are to be expected with aging; as a result, these symptoms simply are not recognized as pathology.

This chapter focuses on the advanced practice nurse's assessment and management of cardiovascular conditions in older adults. Age-related changes in the cardiovascular system are delineated, and the impact of these changes on the diagnosis and management of cardiovascular conditions is presented. Three major chronic conditions—hypertension, congestive heart failure (CHF), and ischemic cardiovascular illnesses—are discussed in depth.

AGE-RELATED CHANGES

Impact on Diagnosis and Treatment

In older adults, it can be difficult to differentiate age-related changes caused by pathology of the cardiovascular system from changes in function caused by disuse or a sedentary lifestyle. Table 21–1 presents a summary of changes in the cardiovascular system usually associated with aging.

Determining a diagnosis may be complicated by the fact that some common diagnostic measures do not indicate the presence of cardiac pathology. For example, a resting electrocardiogram (ECG) may not show the presence of coronary disease. Modern technology has produced increasingly sophisticated equipment and tests to help with diagnosis, such as an echocardiogram with or without Doppler, exercise or pharmacological stress testing, and radioisotope studies. However, many of these high technology–based diagnostic tests and procedures are not available in every practice site.

General Risk Factors

Several factors place the older person at risk for cardiovascular problems. First, age itself is a risk factor for the development of cardiovascular disorders. With increasing age, conditions such as atherosclerosis that have probably been present for many years express themselves in overt illness. A critical factor in the continued

TABLE 21–1

Age-Related Physiological and Anatomical Changes

At-rest heart adequate in healthy older adults to meet needs related to pressure changes and flow; cardiac output at rest unchanged

Increased thickness of heart wall

Increased force of atrial contraction compensates for decreased ventricular filling during early diastole to maintain stroke volume

Systolic pressure increases gradually, beginning in early adult life

Diastolic pressure increases until seventh decade, then decreases

End diastolic and systolic volumes at rest essentially unchanged

Increased aortic pulse wave velocity results in later peak of aortic root pressure, changing the contour of the pressure pulse

Blunting of baroreflex response

Oxygen consumption (measured by work capacity) unchanged in healthy individuals

Decreased response to beta-adrenergic stimulation to increased cardiac work under stress

Little to no change in response to alpha-adrenergic stimulation

Decreased maximal obtainable heart rate with exercise

Increased cardiac volumes, both end diastolic and end systolic, with exercise

Data from Kane et al. (1994); and Lakatta (1995).

development of atherosclerotic changes over the years is the lifestyle pattern of the individual (Hopkins & Williams, 1986). Lifestyle risk factors for younger people apply to the older age group; these include tobacco use or exposure to tobacco smoke, inappropriate nutritional patterns, and a lack of exercise. Individuals at risk for cardiovascular disease include males, postmenopausal females, and those who have a positive family history for cardiac problems. One study found that women older than 62 years demonstrated a greater increase in systolic, mean, and pulse pressures than did younger women or men of any age (Gardner & Poehlman, 1995). The development of cardiovascular problems is further exacerbated by chronic conditions such as diabetes mellitus, obesity, and hyperlipidemia (Benfante et al., 1991, 1992; Sorkin et al., 1992; Wong et al., 1991). Low-level high-density lipoprotein (HDL) in association with high-level low-density lipoprotein (LDL) especially increases the potential for developing cardiac disorders

(Wolfel, 1990). The presence of one cardiovascular condition—hypertension, for example—can lead to the development of other cardiovascular problems such as CHF and other organ failure.

Relationship Between Cardiovascular System and Other Systems

The effect of cardiac or vascular pathological changes on other organs, such as the brain, kidney, and eyes, has been readily demonstrated. Results of the Systolic Hypertension in the Elderly Program (SHEP) trial (1991) demonstrated that active treatment of isolated systolic hypertension (ISH) decreased the risk of stroke by 36%. The Framingham Study (Kannel et al., 1976; Vokonas et al., 1988) demonstrated that systolic hypertension was a strong predictor of atherosclerotic brain infarction in men between the ages of 65 and 74 years. Atherosclerotic changes occurring in blood vessels as well as hypertensive effects on blood vessels supplying the retina have long been implicated in a loss of vision. Laboratory data have been useful in evaluating renal function and detecting possible parenchymal disease in the presence of congestive heart disease or hypertension.

Awareness of the effects of hypertension on morbidity has apparently created changes in treatment as well as prevention. The Fifth Report of the Joint National Committee on Detection, Evaluation, and Treatment of High Blood Pressure (National Institutes of Health, 1993) reported a decrease of about 48% in deaths caused by coronary heart disease and a 57% decrease for deaths caused by stroke over the past 18 years. These decreases were attributed partially to the detection and control of hypertension.

Pharmacokinetic and Pharmacodynamic Changes

Specific issues related to use of medications with the elderly are discussed elsewhere (see Chapter 26). The Pharmaceutical Assistance Contract for the Elderly in Pennsylvania found

that cardiovascular drugs were the most commonly prescribed of all drugs (Schechter et al., 1990). This finding indicates that close attention should be given to the potential occurrence of drug interactions and adverse events with the use of drugs to treat hypertension, chronic ischemic heart disease, heart failure, dysrhythmias, and hypertensive heart disease.

Age-related changes in the gastrointestinal, renal, and cardiovascular systems affect the pharmacokinetics of drugs. In the presence of decreased vascular volume, altered vasomotor controls, and decreased cardiac output, a lack of vigilance to drug dosing can lead to adverse events. The decreased ability of the kidney to respond to metabolic changes with aging underscores the need to evaluate kidney function when treating an elderly person with cardiovascular problems. Determining a person's estimated creatinine clearance and reviewing all medications the patient is taking will guide appropriate drug therapy.

Management of Chronic Conditions

Aging is associated with an increase in chronic conditions, some of which could be avoided with screening for risk factors at an earlier age. Chronic disease conditions require a different approach for management than do acute problems. The term *chronic* implies a situation that has persisted for more than 6 months and includes "one or more of the following characteristics: permanency, residual disability, non-reversible pathological alteration, special training of patient for rehabilitation, and a long period of supervision, observation or care" (Mayo, 1956, p. 5). According to this definition, many of the cardiovascular conditions seen in older adults can be considered chronic. The approach to diagnosing and managing chronic cardiovascular conditions is delineated in Table 21–2 and is discussed further in the following section.

SELECTED CHRONIC CARDIOVASCULAR CONDITIONS: ASSESSMENT, DIAGNOSIS, AND MANAGEMENT

Hypertension

Following arthritis and hearing impairment, hypertension is the third most frequent chronic

TABLE 21-2

Diagnosis and Management of Chronic Cardiovascular Conditions

Chronic Condition	Diagnosis	Management

Hypertension	Accurate baseline pressure
	  Average of two or more readings on
	    separate occasions after 5 min of
	    rest
	  Supine and standing
	  Proper cuff size
	  Arm at heart level
	  No tobacco or caffeine for 30 min
	    preceding
	Assess end-organ damage
	Assess coexisting conditions
	  Renal
	  Neurological
	  Hematological
	  Drug effects
	  Lifestyle
	Identify isolated systolic hypertension
		Nonpharmacological
		  Exercise
		  Weight reduction
		  Decrease salt and alcohol
		Drug regimens
		  Diuretics
		  Beta-blockers
		  Alpha-blocker
		  Alpha$_2$-agonist
		  Angiotensin-converting
		    enzyme inhibitor
		  Calcium channel blocker
		  Involve patient in decision for
		    treatment and care

Congestive heart failure	Identify related conditions
	  Ischemia
	  Hypertension
	  Valvular disease
	Assess individual factors leading to or
	  exacerbating failure
	  Medication interactions or failure to
	    use medications as directed
	  Anemia, hypoxia, thyroid disease,
	    arrhythmias, infections, sodium
	    intake
		Enable the person for self-care;
		  provide information
		  Management of illness
		  Diet, activity, medications
		  Prevention of complications
		  Available resources
		Reevaluate program and effect
		  of drugs
		  Digitalis
		  Angiotensin-converting
		    enzyme inhibitors
		  Calcium channel blockers

Ischemia: peripheral	Assess status of vessels: pulse and
	  return venous flow
	Assess for complications and functional
	  status
		Arterial: prevention of
		  complications
		Venous: support blood return;
		  anticoagulate

Data from Jones & Fagan (1993); Lindenfeld (1990); and Wolfel (1990).

health problem for people older than 65 years. Systolic hypertension is commonly seen in older adults. The incidence of essential hypertension also increases with age, from 5% at age 20 years to 45% at age 70 years (Barkis, 1993). The prevalence rate of ISH is approximately 60% in people older than 65 years and approximately 10% in those younger than 55 years (Tjoa & Kaplan, 1990). African American men have the highest rate of hypertension, although socioeconomic level, geographical locale, and education also influence these rates.

CLASSIFICATION

There is no concise definition for hypertension (Rocella et al., 1987). Different classifications have been used, based on the association of either systolic or diastolic blood pressure levels with the risk of cardiovascular complications. The most recent classifications published by the Joint National Committee on Prevention, Detection, Evaluation, and Treatment of High Blood Pressure (1997) use normal, high normal, and hypertension stages 1 through 3 in association with risk factors as a basis for treatment decisions as well as follow-up evaluations (Table 21–3).

In addition to diastolic and systolic hypertension, another form of hypertension is pseudohypertension. This condition is associated with rigid arteries caused by calcification or thickening of the arterial wall, which results in

TABLE 21-3

Blood Pressure Classifications for Adults Aged 18 Years and Older*

Category	Systolic (mm Hg)		Diastolic (mm Hg)
Normal	<130	and	<85
High normal	130–139	or	85–89
Hypertension			
Stage 1	140–159	or	90–99
Stage 2	160–179	or	100–109
Stage 3	≥180	or	≥110

*Older adults should be categorized in same fashion, with more than 140/90 as hypertension; however, treatment may not be instituted if pressure remains in this range.

From Joint National Committee on Prevention, Detection, Evaluation, and Treatment of High Blood Pressure (1997). The sixth report of the Joint National Committee on Prevention, Detection, Evaluation, and Treatment of High Blood Pressure. *Archives of Internal Medicine, 157*(21), 2417.

falsely elevated blood pressure readings (Applegate, 1994). The percentage of older adults who have this condition is not known; however, the differential diagnosis of pseudo-hypertension should be kept in mind for people who do not respond to therapy despite having undergone multiple adjustments, especially in drug therapy.

SCREENING AND DIAGNOSIS

A family history of high blood pressure and the presence of high blood pressure in childhood are important components in screening for the presence or risk of developing hypertension; longitudinal studies have demonstrated these factors to be predictors of hypertension in later life. In addition to family history, clues that a person may be at risk for developing hypertension include his or her lifestyle history (e.g., the use of tobacco and alcohol), extent and type of exercise, and dietary and weight patterns. Important factors to assess for primary prevention are the use of prescription and over-the-counter medications; a medical history of renal, endocrine (glucose intolerance, thyroid), cerebrovascular, or cardiovascular problems previously identified

and treated; and the presence of stressors and the methods used to control them.

A thorough physical examination should be conducted, with special attention given to the signs and symptoms of cardiovascular risk factors, problems, and associated complications. Of special concern are the presence of vascular abnormalities (e.g., bruits or retinopathy) as well as evidence of peripheral edema in the lower extremities, lungs, abdomen, and sacral and periorbital areas. Basic laboratory testing should include a complete blood count; blood chemistries; cholesterol and lipid profile; and liver, kidney (preferably fasting), and thyroid function tests. The evaluation of blood pressure for a new patient should ideally include a determination of pressure in all extremities to rule out obstruction. A reading of supine, sitting, and standing pressures in both arms is needed to rule out orthostasis. The initial examination should be followed by repeated blood pressure readings taken either in the office or at home. An average of at least two or three pressure readings (obtained on separate occasions) and two readings obtained during one visit are needed to accurately diagnose hypertension. When a discrepancy occurs between office and home blood pressure readings, blood pressure monitoring devices similar to the Holter Monitor should be used. The use of a Holter Monitor helps identify falsely elevated readings caused by anxiety associated with the office environment as well as variations associated with the time of day (e.g., nocturnal variations). This type of monitoring is also beneficial following the institution of treatment.

Disease prevention is an important role for the advanced practice nurse. Based on the knowledge of the prevalence of hypertension in older adults, the advanced practice nurse teaches the older person about this condition and ways to prevent its occurrence. (Teaching is considered a *primary prevention* technique; see the section on prevention and health promotion.) When the patient's history reveals a risk of developing hypertension, additional preventive measures are indicated. The focus of interventions (*secondary prevention* techniques) is based on those factors identified from the person's history that may contribute to the development of hypertension, such as inadequate or inappropriate exercise, a lack of knowledge about the dynamics of blood pressure, and poor diet. Use of the guidelines in *Healthy People 2000* (U.S. Department of Health and Human Services [USDHHS], 1988) can help older adults understand the impact of lifestyle on maintaining normal blood pressure. Return visits to the clinic should be focused on assisting the patient in assuming responsibility for self-care and instituting appropriate behavior changes. However, complete reliance on the individual may not be appropriate, especially when economic factors, lifestyle stressors, or educational background indicate inadequate support to change behavior. The use of community resources such as a local heart association or home health referral may be helpful. In communities where these resources do not exist, the advanced practice nurse may need to work with community leaders to develop needed programs, such as support groups or educational programs through the local school or public health system.

When a diagnosis of hypertension is established, active treatment (*tertiary prevention*) is indicated to prevent mortality and morbidity. The goal of treatment is the prevention of damage to several target organ systems, including the retina and the cardiovascular, cerebrovascular, renal, and peripheral vascular systems.

The results of the SHEP study (SHEP Cooperative Research Group, 1991) demonstrated that ISH is a risk factor for stroke and coronary heart disease in older adults. ISH is defined as a systolic pressure greater than 160 mm Hg that persists in the presence of a normal diastolic pressure. The underlying pathology of this condition is the loss of elasticity of the aorta and large arteries. The elevated systolic pressure is considered to result from the loss of compliance and greater rigidity of the vessel. The incidence of ISH increases with age, with as many as 20% of people older than 80 years experiencing this condition.

The SHEP trial was a multicentered, double-blind, randomized, placebo-controlled study that enrolled over 4700 men and women for treatment. Treatments included either placebo or a stepped-care intervention using a thiazide diuretic such as chlorthalidone (Hygroton) as well as atenolol (Tenormin) or reserpine (Serpasil) if needed. When blood pressure was not controlled for subjects receiving either placebo or treatment, other antihypertensive drugs were used. The subjects underwent follow-up over a 5-year period. The goal of treatment was to reduce systolic blood pressure below 160 mm Hg in those people with a baseline pressure of 180 mm Hg or above, or to reduce systolic blood pressure by at least 20 mm Hg in those people with a baseline systolic pressure of 160 to 179 mm Hg. In the treatment group, there was a 36% decrease in nonfatal and fatal stroke and a 27% decrease in fatal and nonfatal myocardial infarctions (MIs) (NIH, 1993; SHEP Cooperative Research Group, 1991). Approximately 95% of the subjects in the SHEP trial were fully capable of performing all activities of daily living. Therefore, the results of this study may not be extrapolated to those older adults who have added disabilities or comorbid conditions.

TREATMENT

To decrease even moderate risks of cardiovascular complications, older adults with a systolic blood pressure between 140 and 159 mm Hg should be treated for hypertension. The efficacy of treating diastolic pressures 90 to 99 mm Hg is not as clear, however (Applegate & Rutan, 1992). The differences in opinion found in the literature regarding the treatment of systolic and diastolic hypertension emphasize the need for advanced practice nurses to individualize treatment to each patient's assessment and needs. Factors that compound decisions for intervention, for example, include comorbid diagnoses, the complexity of the drug or nonpharmacological regimen used to treat hypertension and concomitant conditions, side effects of the medications, and the patient's financial or personal ability to follow a prescribed plan of care.

Health maintenance or nonpharmacological therapy is still considered to be an appropriate first-line intervention for both mild ISH that is uncomplicated by other vascular pathology as well as diastolic hypertension. Teaching and attention to health maintenance techniques are two approaches that may be benefit patients, regardless of their age. Attention especially to diet and exercise may help control, if not alleviate, ISH. Some people particularly benefit from controlling their intake of sodium and total calories from fat; those who are apparently most sensitive to the control of sodium are the older population, African Americans, and people with hypertension (Flack et al., 1991; Grobbee, 1991). A lack of financial resources or socialization may result in an inadequate nutritional pattern, especially if the person relies on convenient sources of nutrition such as canned or processed foods.

An exercise prescription may benefit older adults, regardless of their living arrangements. Postmenopausal women with centrally distributed body fat in particular appear to benefit from controlling elevated blood pressure through diet modification and aerobic exercise (Gardner & Poehlman, 1995). Errors that many people make when exercising are attempting to progress too rapidly and allowing insufficient time to warm up and cool down (Gillett et al., 1993). Older people tend to need a 10- to 15-minute warm-up period to safely achieve an aerobic level at 75% of their maximum heart rate. When the person has been inactive, exercise should start at 5 to 10 minutes 2 to 3 days per week and gradually increase to 20 to 30 minutes 3 to 4 days per week. Walking is the best aerobic activity for older adults because they can control the intensity, location (indoors or outdoors), and time of day for the activity with less chance of injury.

The use of hormone replacement therapy (HRT) for postmenopausal women is thought to provide continued protection from severe cardiac pathology. Some women may experience an increase in blood pressure after instituting HRT. Therefore, a good health maintenance practice is to monitor blood pressure for women using HRT more frequently (i.e., at least every 4 to 6 months) (Grady et al., 1992; Greendale & Judd, 1993).

Pharmacological Therapy

Pharmacological therapy is indicated when preventive techniques have been ineffective. Multiple medications are available for the treatment of hypertension. The use of diuretics as a first-level drug intervention continues to be recommended by the Joint National Committee on Prevention, Detection, Evaluation, and Treatment of High Blood Pressure (1997). However, the specific drug treatment used does need to be individualized based on the guidelines previously noted, such as comorbid conditions. A summary of antihypertensive medications and their advantages and disadvantages is presented in Table 21–4, in which examples of each class of drugs are provided. The reader is referred to other references for more complete details of these drugs.

To determine the effectiveness of treatment and need for alterations in therapy, patients should be continuously monitored. Three essential factors to include in follow-up visits are (1) a repeat chemistry profile 6 weeks after the initiation of medications; (2) a physical examination and review of the patient's history to detect any side effects of drug therapy, including signs and symptoms of orthostasis; and (3) a determination of the patient's ability to follow nonpharmacological and drug management. A change in medication or addition of a second medication may be needed if there is no response, or an inadequate response, to initial therapy. Referral to a medical internist or cardiologist may be needed for more severe situations.

Congestive Heart Failure

CHF is a complex of symptoms, rather than a disease, that results from multiple cardiac and noncardiac sources. Differences have been found in the prevalence of CHF in the older population, possibly owing to the populations sampled (Mittelmark, 1993; Phillips et al., 1990). The causes of CHF include cardiomyopathies (restrictive, idiopathic, or hypertrophic) and ischemic and hypertensive heart diseases, all of which account for approximately 90% of CHF. Other causes include valvular heart disease; endocarditis; cor pulmonale; and concomitant noncardiac pathologies such as thyrotoxicosis or hypothyroidism, anemia, infections, and an acute sodium chloride overload. A failure to maintain the medication routine for treating hypertension can precipitate CHF, as can the use of medications that affect cardiac

TABLE 21-4

Pharmacological Therapy for Hypertension

Drug	Advantages	Disadvantages
Thiazide Diuretics		
Hydrochlorothiazide (Hydrodiuril) 12.5–25 mg q.d.	Inexpensive Well tolerated Q.d. to b.i.d. dosing Decreases extracellular fluid volume Excreted unchanged in renal tubule	Slow onset Increases fasting uric acid, glucose Decreases potassium Alters HDL/total cholesterol ratio Ineffective with serum creatinine >2 mg/dL
Beta-Blockers		
Metoprolol (Lopressor): 25–300 mg/d Pindolol (Visken): 5–60 mg/d Atenolol (Tenormin): 25–100 mg/d	Multiple actions Antiarrhythmic Antianginal Improves LVH Good for secondary prevention of MI Can be given q.d.	Bronchospasm, masks hypoglycemia Rate of blood pressure control less than with thiazides May cause impotence, claudication, dreams, fatigue, heart failure, confusion, depression
Calcium Channel Blockers		
Nifedipine (Procardia): 10–40 mg t.i.d. Amlodipine besylate (Norvasc): 2.5–10 mg q.d.	Coronary vasodilation Does not affect lipid profiles Q.d. dosing for amlodipine	Expensive May worsen CHF owing to negative inotropism Bradycardia with beta-blockers, or alpha-agonists Constipation Edema
ACE Inhibitors		
Enalapril (Vasotec): 2.5–40 mg/d Captopril (Capoten): 6.25–12.5 mg every 8–12 hr initially	Long acting, q.d. dosing Reduces peripheral vascular resistance No change in cardiac output	Cough Expensive Hyperkalemia

ACE, angiotensin-converting enzyme; b.i.d., twice a day; CHF, congestive heart failure; HDL, high-density lipoprotein; LVH, left ventricular hypertrophy; MI, myocardial infarction; q.d., every day; t.i.d., three times a day.

All medications should be started at lowest dose possible and increased gradually. Effects should be monitored with home and office blood pressure readings and an assessment of side effects and changes in blood chemistries. One side effect to monitor for all antihypertensive medications is orthostatic blood pressure changes, which can potentiate falls.

Data from Jones & Fagan (1993); and Joint National Committee on Prevention, Detection, Evaluation, and Treatment of High Blood Pressure (1997).

output by depressing myocardial function or by increasing sodium and thus fluid retention. CHF is often considered to represent simply the inability of the heart to supply oxygen to the body. For older people, the inability to maintain function in the presence of pulmonary or systemic congestion may be the precipitating factor for a vicious cycle of decreased activity that in turn leads to a reduction in the ability for self-care.

CHF may originate from either systolic or diastolic dysfunction. Systolic dysfunction is characterized by pathology associated with a loss of functional myocardial units caused by ischemic heart disease or cardiomyopathy; cardiac decompensation results from an increased workload on the heart that can accompany hypertensive heart disease or valvular lesions. In contrast, diastolic CHF is characterized by a noncompliant muscle. The diastolic form of CHF may be a consequence of obstructive cardiomyopathies or constrictive processes such as pericarditis that interfere with ventricular filling.

Inadequate performance of the heart may be related to four factors: preload, afterload, contractility, and heart rate. All have an effect on cardiac output. Preload and afterload are based on Laplace's law and are determined by myocardial wall thickness and internal radius. *Preload* refers to the myocardial wall stress that balances transmural pressure prior to contraction. Although preload does not change markedly with aging, the rate of diastolic filling has been found to slow with aging, apparently owing to prolonged relaxation (Lakatta, 1995). *Afterload* refers to the muscle tension that is required for ejection during systole. This factor is somewhat increased in older adults; however, no substantive studies have resolved whether the increased size of myocytes resulting in cardiac hypertrophy represents pathological changes or is simply an adaptation to changes in the arterial system. Studies regarding changes in the contractility of the myocardium in older people do not clearly differentiate if deficits related to action potential and calcium exchange are adaptive processes or precursors to pathology. The heart rate for older people fluctuates more during activity than during rest and is dependent on both sympathetic and parasympathetic tone.

DIAGNOSIS

The diagnosis of CHF begins with a history and physical examination. Four categories are usually used to differentiate the clinical severity of disease (Lindenfeld, 1990):

Class I patients have no physical limitation
Class II patients experience symptoms with ordinary physical activity
Class III patients sustain symptoms with less than normal activity
Class IV patients suffer symptoms with any activity and at times during rest

As noted in the recent Agency for Health Care Policy and Research (AHCPR) Guidelines for heart failure (Konstam et al., 1994), all presenting symptoms that may pertain to CHF are not specific for that diagnosis. Differential diagnoses related to pulmonary, cardiovascular, renal, or metabolic sources must be considered when an older person complains of various forms of dyspnea (orthopnea, dyspnea on exertion, or paroxysmal nocturnal dyspnea), weight gain, cough, increasing fatigue, or lower extremity edema. Hausdorff and associates (1994) found that the presence of jugular venous distention and a third heart sound were more suggestive of heart failure than either inspiratory crackles or pitting pedal edema. Consideration should be given to a person's activity level, as the presence of a sedentary lifestyle and inadequate nutrition are predisposing factors for these latter symptoms. Bittner and colleagues (1993) suggested that the distance a person with CHF can walk is both a useful diagnostic tool and a predictor of morbidity and mortality. Changes in gait (including velocity), the distance walked, and the length of time a person is able to walk are important indicators of CHF. The maximum distance that people older than 65 years could walk was found to be significantly shorter in those with severe CHF than in those with mild or no CHF (Hausdorff et al., 1994).

The AHCPR guidelines (Konstam et al., 1994) recommend the following tests when a chest x-ray as well as signs and symptoms are suggestive of CHF:

1. ECG to detect previous MI or acute ST wave changes; tachyarrhythmias or bradyarrhythmias; left ventricular hypertrophy; or low voltage, indicating pericardial effusion
2. Complete blood count to rule out anemia
3. Urinalysis and serum creatinine to detect renal damage
4. Serum albumin to differentiate edema caused by hypoalbuminemia
5. Thyroid tests (T_4 and thyroid-stimulating hormone) to rule out hypothyroidism or

hyperthyroidism as the underlying cause, especially if atrial fibrillation is also present

In addition to the basic tests named here, an echocardiograph or radionuclide ventriculograph is needed to determine left ventricular ejection fraction. Those people with left ventricular systolic CHF have an ejection fraction below 40%. These tests aid in determining whether the source of malfunction is cardiomyopathy, valvular heart disease, diastolic pathology, or noncardiac sources.

TREATMENT

The treatment of CHF consists of three components intended to minimize exacerbations of the condition: patient and family counseling and teaching, the use of medications to control symptoms, and clinical monitoring of patient therapy. Patient and family counseling can become part of both secondary and tertiary prevention as family members are informed about the causes and symptoms of CHF and the patient is instructed on ways to control symptoms and prevent complications. Medications are used to promote function and decrease morbidity and mortality. By monitoring the management strategies used, the healthcare provider can periodically assess the effectiveness of treatment and evaluate the patient's willingness and ability to follow a treatment regimen.

The primary goal of patient and family counseling is to enable the patient to live with and maintain control over a chronic condition. Education begins with a discussion about CHF, including those symptoms that may indicate exacerbation of the condition as well as when to call the healthcare provider should these symptoms occur. The patient's prescribed diet, activity level, and medication regimen should be reviewed. Based on how well the patient is adhering to these changes, he or she should be given suggestions regarding ways to maintain the treatment plan.

Teaching and counseling tend to be least effective when provided in one long session. The use of repeated or spaced sessions, based on priority of information needed, can prevent either the patient or family members from feeling overwhelmed. Redundancy in teaching is appropriate for an older person who may feel uncertain about his or her ability to manage the necessary changes in lifestyle. Written information and plans for telephone follow-up are essential to obtain tangible evidence of the treatment plan and to offer ongoing support so that the patient does not feel alone in managing CHF. The Emory University Hospital Center for Heart Failure has developed a plan of teaching that meets the above requirements (see Appendices 21–1 to 21–3 for examples). Although these instructions pertain to hospital discharge, the principles represented apply to any situation involving CHF.

To reduce the cardiac workload, patients should balance their time between activity and rest or sleep and should also limit their use of salt. An evaluation of sleep patterns, including daytime naps and activities within energy capacity, can guide planning for a balanced day. Teaching about sleep hygiene may be beneficial to ensure adequate nighttime sleep. Substitutions for sodium chloride include herbs and spices such as lemon pepper, garlic powder, basil, thyme, rosemary, oregano, cumin, and cinnamon. Removal of the salt shaker from the table is also advised. Written information and a chart on the sodium content of foods is helpful to identify items often not suspected as being high in sodium; these can include processed foods, over-the-counter medications such as antacids and laxatives, and condiments such as mustard. In addition to restricting salt intake, the patient may also need to limit fluid intake to less than 1 L per day and to monitor weight daily or weekly. Providing instructions that use common household items such as a quart pitcher to measure water intake per day can assist the patient and family in more accurately following the plan of care. Important pharmacological information includes untoward side effects of the medications prescribed as well as a list of over-the-counter preparations to be avoided. Referrals to occupational and physical therapy are appropriate for evaluation and teaching methods that promote low energy expenditure in daily activity. Home health services may be needed when the person has little caregiver support, has a complex treatment regimen, or requires monitoring of the treatment plan at home to ensure compliance with that plan and to avoid frequent exacerbations of CHF.

Medications for CHF are specific to the type of heart failure (i.e., diastolic or systolic). Table 21–5 presents examples of the classes of medications used and their expected results.

The use of digitalis to treat systolic failure in older adults is often inappropriate, as the toxic effects persist and the desired inotropic effects are not as effective as those of other drugs. Digoxin (Lanoxin) may be indicated in con-

junction with an angiotensin-converting enzyme inhibitor (ACEI) such as enalapril (Vasotec) and a diuretic such as furosemide (Lasix) for those patients in acute or severe failure or with atrial fibrillation. Symptoms in most patients can be controlled with the use of an ACEI that interferes with the conversion of angiotensin I to angiotensin II and a loop diuretic. Vasodilators (other than ACEI) such as nitroglycerin transdermal patches, isosorbide (Isordil), or hydralazine (Apresoline) may also

TABLE 21-5

Medications for Congestive Heart Failure*

Drug	Desired Action	Adverse Effects
Drugs Indicated for Diastolic Dysfunction		
Calcium Channel Blockers		
Verapamil hydrochloride (Calan): 40–120 mg every 12 hr	Vasodilation	Negative inotropic, heart block
Diltiazem hydrochloride (Cardizem): 30–120 mg every 8 hr	Vasodilation	
Drugs Indicated for Systolic Dysfunction		
Diuretics		
Furosemide (Lasix): 10–80 mg q.d.	Control fluid overload Preload reduction	Hypokalemia, dehydration, incontinence, postural hypotension
Hydrochlorothiazide (Hydrodiuril): 12.5–50 mg q.d.		
Angiotensin-Converting Enzyme Inhibitors†		
Captopril (Capoten): 6.25–12.5 mg t.i.d.	Useful for prevention Preload and afterload reduction	Hypotension, azotemia hyperkalemia, cough, skin rash, neutropenia
Enalapril (Vasotec): 2.5 mg b.i.d. to start		
Vasodilators		
Isosorbide dinitrate (Isordil): 10 mg t.i.d.	Preload reduction Dosage can be increased to maximum of 80 mg t.i.d.	Headache, hypotension
Cardiac Glycosides		
Digoxin (Lanoxin): 0.125 mg q.d.	Used for severe heart failure, unresponsiveness to ACE inhibitor May increase dose to 0.25 mg q.d.	Toxicity: confusion, nausea, anorexia

*Anticoagulants generally indicated when atrial fibrillation or pulmonary embolism present.
†Avoid the use of potassium-sparing diuretics with ACE inhibitors.
ACE, angiotensin-converting enzyme; b.i.d., twice a day; q.d., every day; t.i.d., three times a day.
Data from Gambert (1987); Konstam et al. (1994); and Selma et al. (1997).

be indicated to reduce afterload. The AHCPR guidelines (Konstam et al., 1994) recommend that patients with asymptomatic CHF who have a left-ventricular ejection fraction below 35 to 40% be treated with an ACEI as a prevention measure. Pharmacological intervention for diastolic heart failure usually involves calcium channel blockers such as diltiazem (Cardizem). Acute management of diastolic CHF requiring hospitalization may include other medications such as nonglycoside inotropes (e.g., dopamine) or phosphodiesterase inhibitors such as amrinone (Inocor).

The advanced practice nurse should monitor CHF treatment using patient-kept records of daily to weekly weight, activity level and type, fatigue, and daily functioning (e.g., sleep patterns, sexual activity, management of stressors, appetite or anorexia, and socialization). Involving the patient and family in these monitoring parameters promotes personal investment in treatment, which can enhance the control of symptoms. Return visits to the clinic should include an assessment for dyspnea (including orthopnea and paroxysmal nocturnal dyspnea as well as dyspnea on exertion) and a physical examination for the presence of peripheral edema (including increased jugular venous pressure, pulmonary adventitious sounds, and abdominal and lower extremity edema). Cardiac rate, rhythm, the presence of an S3, and blood pressure should also be documented. Laboratory tests should be used to periodically monitor responses to the diuretic and ACEI. The effectiveness of treatment is also indicated by the following: serum electrolytes (to determine sodium and potassium levels); magnesium levels (especially if thiazide diuretics are used); blood urea nitrogen and creatinine levels (to monitor renal status); and digoxin levels.

Several factors influence the monitoring plan and frequency of laboratory tests for older adults. These include (1) an expected age-related decrease of the glomerular filtration rate, (2) the presence of comorbid conditions that require medications that may interact with the medications prescribed to treat CHF, (3) self-medication with over-the-counter drugs such as nonsteroidal antiinflammatory drugs, and (4) the severity and duration of CHF. A person who has been newly diagnosed should be monitored once a week to every other week and will be frequently hospitalized for this. In contrast, a person with stable CHF may need monitoring every 3 to 6 months depending on his or her treatment regimen, ability for self-monitoring, and access to care providers. When concomitant conditions such as hypertension, thyroid disease, or anemia are present, the treatment plan must address these variables, and the effect of treatment on these conditions should be continuously monitored. A referral to home health nurses is appropriate when the complexity of treatment might create problems for patient management. Planned clinic visits, with patient access to the advanced practice nurse as needed, may be satisfactory for patients whose condition is stable.

When a treatment regimen involves marked changes in activity and meal planning, the patient's ability to follow the regimen may be limited. Alteration of the treatment plan and more frequent follow-up evaluations may be indicated if the patient has difficulty managing the plan of care. When acute symptoms are not present, the incentive to follow a plan may not be high. Advanced practice nurses should reinforce the need for patients to pay daily attention to the details of controlling CHF; they can do this by providing support and encouragement to keep records and achieve goals such as improved sleep or weight loss.

Ischemic Cardiovascular Conditions

Ischemia, defined as an interference of blood flow to the myocardium and the peripheral vascular system, is associated with increased morbidity and mortality in older adults. As the problems worsen, the ability to manage personal care tends to decline. There has been a slight decrease in mortality due to atherosclerosis, primarily in white men. However, the death rate in the United States due to coronary heart disease for Blacks and for Asian and Pacific Islander groups has not decreased to the same extent. In fact, heart disease is the leading cause of death for the latter group (Secretary's Task Force on Black and Minority Health, 1985; Sempos et al., 1988). Coronary artery disease (CAD) and peripheral vascular disease (PVD) are the two ischemic cardiovascular system conditions discussed in this section.

CORONARY ARTERY DISEASE

CAD may present as ischemia, angina, or MI. Although ischemia is present in older people, they may not have the typical presentation of chest pain, owing to their limited engagement in activity that would ordinarily stimulate chest pain. Ambepitiya and associates (1994) reported a time lag in anginal perceptual threshold with treadmill testing for those aged 70 to 82 years. This delay from the time of 1 mm ST depression to the individual's perception of anginal pain reinforces the fact that anginal pain cannot be used as the sole indicator of myocardial ischemia for older people. Neuropathies or changes in pain recognition may also limit the use of this symptom as an indication of ischemia. Instead, dyspnea or confusion may be the initial presenting symptom. When a person complains of chest pain or pain with exertion (angina), a search for other causes (e.g., musculoskeletal or gastrointestinal) is indicated.

Attempts to diagnose coronary disease on the basis of symptoms alone appear to be misguided. A fatal myocardial infarct in the older individual may be directly related to age-associated structural and functional changes in the cardiovascular system that do not present as chest pain (Rich et al., 1992). Unrecognized myocardial infarcts lead to damage and precipitate the complications of heart failure and pulmonary edema.

The Framingham Study (Kannel et al., 1976) found that the risk factors associated with CAD in older adults are similar to those identified for younger people. These factors include current cigarette use, which may be correlated with higher leukocyte levels (Phillips et al., 1992); elevated LDL levels; low HDL levels; a high LDL/HDL ratio; systolic blood pressure above 195 mm Hg; and left ventricular hypertrophy on ECG. However, the contradictory results of different studies cast uncertainty on the absolute effects of lipid levels, cigarette use (Benfante et al., 1992; Sorkin et al., 1992), and gender differences (Wolfel, 1990). Differences

between the sexes apparently modulate as people reach their mid-70s, at which age the incidence and prevalence of CAD appear to be the same for men and women. Gilligan and coworkers (1994) suggested, however, that estrogen replacement may also protect postmenopausal women from developing CAD by promoting vasodilation of the coronary microvascular.

Diagnosis

The epidemiological data for people older than 74 years reinforce the need to consider the presence of CAD in all older adults, especially those with known risk factors. CAD should be suspected if the person has also been diagnosed with peripheral or cerebrovascular ischemia. When symptoms typical of angina are present, the predictive probability of CAD for people older than 60 years is 94% for men and 91% for women (Diamond & Forrester, 1979). Symptoms of angina include burning, pressure, and a squeezing pain in the midsternal region (with or without radiation) that is brought on by exertion, lasts 1 to 15 minutes, and is relieved by rest or nitroglycerin.

In the presence of symptoms, a resting ECG may be indicated. However, many older adults show nonspecific ST wave abnormalities on a resting ECG. Unless there is prior pathology, such as a transmural infarct, the ECG alone may not be a good indicator of CAD. The resting ECG is not appropriate as a screening device for asymptomatic individuals and does not localize the ischemic region or identify the lesion; referral for other diagnostic tests may be indicated. More advanced diagnostic tests include exercise ECG testing, stress echocardiography, thallium perfusion (with or without exercise), and radionuclide angiography. A major limitation of tests requiring exercise is that many older adults are not able to exercise to their maximum ability owing to both musculoskeletal and pulmonary conditions. Therefore, these results may be inaccurate. Another limiting factor may be the added cost of an advanced diagnostic test.

Treatment

The basis of treating CAD in both older and younger adults is the use of nitrates, beta-blockers, calcium channel blockers, and aspirin (Table 21–6). Invasive treatment, such as cardiac catheterization, angioplasty, or coronary artery bypass surgery, is usually reserved for those older adults who have intractable angina. Noninvasive and nonpharmacological interventions mean a change in lifestyle, including an exercise program suitable to the individual (Fleury, 1992).

Myocardial Infarction

Another presentation of CAD is MI. All efforts should be made to prevent this condition; for example, nitrates should be used as an early intervention in the treatment of angina, and unstable angina should be treated with aspirin. Historically, efforts to diagnose a silent MI were warranted; the Framingham Study (Kannel & Abbott, 1984), for example, found that 36% of men and 46% of women with a new MI showed no ECG changes. Approximately 45% of new MI cases were in people older than 65 years. Age is a dramatic variable for survival beyond the initial episode. Udvarhelyi and associates (1992) found that 30-day mortality increased from 19% for those age 65 to 74

years to 38% for those age 85 years and older. They attributed this increase in part to a lack of aggressive treatment of older adults with acute MI, especially women and Blacks.

As with angina, the presenting symptom of an MI may be dyspnea rather than chest pain, especially in people older than 80 years. Neurological disturbances (e.g., confusion and syncope) and gastrointestinal complaints are also common presenting symptoms of an MI. Diagnosis may be hampered for older adults as a result of subtle ECG changes and different cardiac enzyme laboratory values. Morbidity and mortality tend to be higher for older people than for younger people. A prolonged hospital stay may be required for older adults, with the potential for problems related to disuse. Cardiac sequelae of an MI include CHF, arrhythmias and conduction disturbances, pneumonia, and phlebitis. These occur more frequently in older than in younger patients.

Treatment. The management of an acute MI in older adults is proposed to be similar to that for younger individuals. Treatment includes admission to a coronary care unit, anticoagulation, the use of beta-blockers, and postrecovery cardiac rehabilitation. Rosenthal and Fortinsky

TABLE 21-6

Medical Treatment of Angina

Drug	Action	Adverse Events
Nitrates, nitroglycerin	Decrease preload by decreasing venous return Intermittent dosing (e.g., remove transdermal patch at night)	Orthostatic hypotension; falls Decreased effect with steady dosing
Beta-blockers	Decrease heart rate, blood pressure, contractility of heart, oxygen demand; increase oxygen supply with decrease of heart rate	Heart block, bradycardia, fatigue, depression, heart failure, bronchospasm More common with preexisting pathology May be less effective with older adults owing to decreased reliance on catecholamines with aging
Calcium channel blockers	Decrease coronary and peripheral vascular resistance	Hypotension, negative inotropic effect, bradycardia Some cause heart block, edema, constipation

Aspirin, 325 mg daily, has also been shown to decrease mortality and reinfarction with myocardial infarction for people with unstable angina.
Data from Gambert (1987); and Gerstenblith (1995).

(1994) noted that older adults are frequently excluded from clinical trials, however. This exclusion can result in uncertainty about the effectiveness of angioplasty, angiograms, or thrombolytic therapy. In their retrospective study, these authors found that the elderly received these interventions less frequently than did people younger than 65 years; they were 7 times less likely to have angioplasty or angiograms and 12 times less likely to receive thrombolytic therapy. Coronary artery bypass surgery for people older than 65 years has gained popularity with the recognition that their functional capacity can be improved; age is not an automatic exclusion from this surgery. Increased morbidity is usually related to a greater incidence of comorbid conditions, the presence of hypertension or peripheral vascular conditions, and increased primary risk factors (Naunheim et al., 1987).

The advanced practice nurse may not be involved in the care and treatment of the patient while the patient is hospitalized. Prevention and follow-up care, however, which involve monitoring for the appearance of complications such as CHF and assessing the effects of cardiac rehabilitation, do fall within the advanced practice nurse's purview.

PERIPHERAL VASCULAR DISEASE

PVD may be arterial or venous. The cardinal symptom of peripheral arterial ischemic angina is intermittent claudication. Claudication has also been implicated as a primary risk factor for the development of or death from cardiovascular and cerebrovascular conditions (Simonsick et al., 1995). Four related factors are similar between peripheral arterial ischemia and angina pectoris:

1. Relationship of pain with activity, but pain occurring in the lower extremity or buttock due to hypoxia to skeletal muscle (intermittent claudication)
2. Effect of rest in relieving the pain
3. Association of the pathology with atherosclerosis
4. Risk factors for developing peripheral ischemia: diabetes mellitus, tobacco use, hypertension, and family history

Usually the patient has adequate perfusion and pulsation in the femoral arteries but diminished dorsalis pedis and posterior tibial pulses. The symptoms of peripheral disease do not typically occur in isolation, however; the person may have concomitant cardiac or cerebrovascular atherosclerotic lesions. When the individual is more sedentary, the association of pain with activity may be absent. Instead, discomfort and aching in the supine position and associated ischemic signs such as skin atrophy, lack of hair on the feet, and nail and skin discoloration are more common.

In contrast to arterial disease, venous involvement is associated with inactivity, heart failure, and dehydration, among other precipitating causes. The usual presenting sign is edema of the involved dependent extremity. The most important risk factor is immobility—from any cause. The veins of the lower extremities are dependent on skeletal muscle contraction to maintain blood flow. The older adult is at special risk when he or she is affected by any condition that results in decreased activity, such as orthopedic surgery. In addition to inactivity, increased blood viscosity resulting from the use of diuretics or inadequate fluid intake can predispose individuals to peripheral intravascular clotting.

Diagnosis

The diagnosis of PVD differs for arterial and venous involvement (Table 21–7).

Treatment

The treatment of both arterial and venous peripheral vascular problems begins with trying to prevent complications. Older adults should strive to maintain their previous activity level; this may require referral to physical therapy to evaluate the need for gait training and muscle strengthening exercises.

The general guidelines of caring for patients with diabetes mellitus may be used for people with arterial insufficiency. These guidelines include the avoidance of temperature extremes and irritating local self-treatments (often over-the-counter preparations), daily washing and inspection of the feet and lower legs, the prevention of dryness and breakdown of skin, and

TABLE 21-7

Diagnosing Arterial and Venous Peripheral Vascular Disease

Arterial	Venous
1. History: heart conditions including atherosclerosis, atrial fibrillation, distance walked without stopping*	1. History: immobility, congestive heart failure; family history of varicosities (chronic phase)
2. Symptoms: acute onset of pain, loss of sensation including position sense, loss of function	2. Symptoms: vein engorgement, unilateral or bilateral-dependent edema, heavy feeling in legs
3. Examination: palpation of popliteal, posterior tibial, and dorsalis pedal pulses; cardiac irregularity; pallor, or cyanosis of extremity; texture of skin	3. Examination: skin color of legs, presence of vein engorgement, palpable cords, edema
4. Other examinations: Doppler ultrasound arterial studies needed to localize the site	4. Refer for venous impedance plethysmography
5. Treatment: anticoagulation, possible surgery (e.g., embolectomy); control risk factors such as hyperlipedemia, tobacco use	5. Treatment: elastic compression stockings, elevate legs, avoid diuretics; treat ulcers (e.g., with Unna boot or zinc oxide ointment)

*Chronic arterial occlusive disease may be asymptomatic with older people.
Data from Pham & Robinson (1993).

periodic assistance from a podiatrist or other qualified person to trim toenails and treat corns or calluses. Some patients may profit from vasodilator drugs, but the main benefit is found in the self-care measures just defined. People with severe ischemia may need referral for bypass surgery or angioplasty.

The goal for treating venous conditions is the prevention of pulmonary embolism and chronic venous insufficiency through the use of anticoagulation therapy with warfarin. This therapy is monitored in the usual fashion: Prothrombin levels should be kept about one and a half times normal, or the International Normalization Ratio should be between 1.5 and 2 to avoid the risk of bleeding in older adults. In addition, the person should be taught appropriate use of compression stockings to aid venous return.

PREVENTION AND HEALTH PROMOTION

Throughout this chapter, examples have been provided of ways to prevent disease and to prevent complications once a condition is present. This section discusses more specific ways to plan and help the patient with prevention techniques. Although the ability to conceptualize treatment in prevention terms is not a new phenomenon, it has not been emphasized throughout nursing education, practice, and research (McCance & Reiber, 1982). The guidelines in *Healthy People 2000* (USDHHS, 1988) have presented a challenge to all healthcare providers to practice according to a health promotion and disease prevention paradigm based on objectives for change. Prevention can be divided into primary, secondary, and tertiary components; each level has a different goal and activities.

Primary Prevention

The goal of primary prevention is to provide information about preventing the appearance of specific problems. This level of prevention is needed for the physically and emotionally healthy population—those who are functionally capable and active. The essential components of this level include education and information about the causes of specific conditions and ways to avoid these conditions. Both emotional and decisional support are provided to assist the client in following the prevention guidelines.

Because age is already a risk factor for the development of cardiovascular problems, one might reason that primary prevention does not apply to older adults. However, even people who have had bypass surgery can benefit from knowledge about the risks for other noncardiac conditions (e.g., accidents) that can interfere with the maintenance of a healthy cardiovascular system. Therefore, primary prevention should still be a focus with older adults. This level of prevention should include both assessment and education for the individual. Assessment includes a baseline of data pertinent to the individual's readiness to learn. It requires that the advanced practice nurse be attuned to that person's learning style, literacy level, socioeconomic and cultural factors, and physical or emotional impediments to learning; the potential for that person to accept responsibility for self-care; and areas requiring support and assistance with decision making. The support needed, for example, may be periodic visits to review the patient's understanding of self-care as well as any changes in lifestyle or habits such as diet plan or activity. Educational activities include presenting topics about the risks for developing hypertension; the risks associated with tobacco use, a lack of aerobic physical activity, being overweight, and high LDL and triglyceride levels; and the effects of stress. Primary prevention can be a family affair: Older family members can engage the adult children and grandchildren in the process by teaching them about risk factors, especially if the family history includes cardiovascular risk factors.

Secondary Prevention

This level of prevention, characterized by early diagnosis and intervention, must focus on a periodic evaluation of the older person's health status. If educational materials and a follow-up evaluation of the patient's understanding of that material have been instituted, the advanced practice nurse has a base for determining the needed frequency of periodic assessments (e.g., once a year or every 3 to 6 months).

This level of prevention requires the involvement of the patient and family members and their responsibility to report changes. In addition, the advanced practice nurse must be aware of risk factors for the early detection of complications. The specific interventions used depend on the person, his or her diagnosis, and available resources. Ettinger and associates (1994) reported that the specifics of disability in functional status depend on the specific pathology. Self-reports from people 65 years and older revealed increased difficulty with aerobic work such as walking or heavy housework. Two thirds of the difficulty with physical functioning in these community dwellers was associated with arthritis, cardiac and pulmonary disorders, and stroke.

Secondary prevention provides an opportunity to involve other providers, such as a dietitian or a social worker, whether they are part of an interdisciplinary team or are community practitioners. Additional educational materials may be needed, such as information about drugs, the need to report specific symptoms, and caution about self-treatment, especially the use of over-the-counter systemic or topical medications that could interfere with other drugs or exacerbate a condition such as PVD. The instructions provided should focus on making gradual changes and should not encourage patients to try to alter their habits immediately. For example, the length of exercise should be increased gradually, beginning with 5 minutes and advancing to 30 minutes. Ten-minute warm-up and cool-down periods may be needed. A periodic review of food and fluid intake with the patient, including a 3-day diet history, is helpful to point out both positive and negative aspects of the diet. If advance directives or a treatment plan have not been introduced, discussion should be initiated with client and family when appropriate. Each state varies in the specific format developed, but advanced planning is the essential issue (see Chapter 3).

Tertiary Prevention

This is the most intensive level of intervention. It is focused on *rehabilitation* and restoration of the person to the highest level of function possible. At this level of prevention, the pathology is either fixed, stable, or irreversible, and the goal is to enable the individual to incorporate the condition into his or her life. This level of prevention often presents the most problems for older people owing to patterns of living that have persisted over many years. By this time, the pathological process has interfered with normal functioning. The extent of restorative therapy needed may be stressful for the older person as well as the caregiver. The extent of loss of function and the costs (financial, emotional, and physical) may compromise the person's incentive and ability to be an active participant in rehabilitation. Both patient and caregiver may require counseling. Other special therapies, home health care, or transfer to a nursing care facility may also be needed. Teaching continues during this level, but the spacing of information, level of instruction, and methods used may need to be changed depending on the patient's cognitive ability, functional status, and energy level. Continued focus on diet, with reductions in salt and fat intake, and the use of exercise at a level appropriate to cardiac functioning are still beneficial.

Prevention also means being alert to situations (other than risk factors such as elevated LDL or lack of exercise) that may precipitate a cardiovascular problem or exacerbate an already established condition. Examples of these situations include hypothyroidism or hyperthyroidism, low vitamin C intake, bereavement, tooth decay, depression, and untoward effects of drugs, such as acute confusion.

Working with Older Adults and Caregivers

To achieve the goals of disease prevention, enhance communication, foster independence and self-care, and promote effective outcomes, the advanced practice nurse cannot function alone. Active collaboration between the advanced practice nurse and the patient can be achieved with the use of teaching guides and flow sheets maintained by both individuals. The type of record keeping used should fit the individual's routine. Record keeping should

not be considered a punishment, and cooperation with this task will be improved if it is approached as a team effort. When appropriate, the use of a contract with the patient or family member may also help delineate each person's responsibility in managing care and records. Written information and repetition are essential for patients to retain and incorporate that information into self-care. Older adults are of course capable of learning, but the teaching must be meaningful to them and have some application to present life. By relating present instructions to past experiences, the older adult tends to conceptualize the meaning rather than try to remember only facts. Therefore, it may be useful, for example, to compare the time and level of exercise needed for cardiac rehabilitation with the recuperation time required for a fractured arm as a youngster or following abdominal surgery 30 or 40 years ago. Sharing information about practice protocols with the patient and his or her family is another way of letting them become active participants in care.

The possibility exists that older adults with severe cardiovascular problems may need 24-hour care in a nursing care facility or extensive home health care. Families and older adults tend to understand less about these methods of care than they do about acute care. Therefore, all individuals involved need to be educated about the extent of involvement of the patient and his or her family members in both situations. Most patients and family members experience loss when a person needs extensive care, especially when the older person is admitted to a nursing facility. Acknowledging that loss and helping the older adult express feelings continues to be part of tertiary prevention. For example, the anxiety experienced by the older person who has been admitted to a nursing facility with diagnoses of hypertension and CHF and a history of two myocardial infarctions can create a potentially serious situation. To maintain function and prevent further complications, it may help to engage in anticipatory planning with the patient and family, share data collected by and about the patient with nursing home staff members, and maintain contact with the patient and family after admission.

SUMMARY

This chapter has presented an overview of age-related changes in the cardiovascular system and the risk factors associated with the development of cardiovascular pathology. The diagnosis and management of specific conditions may be problematic owing to the interaction of age, risk factors, and environmental influences. Specific guidelines were presented for the detection, diagnosis, and treatment of three common conditions: hypertension, CHF, and ischemic cardiovascular conditions. The interaction of these three conditions as well as the influence of other chronic cardiac and noncardiac problems was noted as a factor contributing to the complexity of necessary care. The major role of the advanced practice nurse in all levels of prevention and management of these conditions was addressed. Appendix 21–4 is a brief list of resources that can provide information related to common cardiovascular conditions of older adults; the information provided may also be useful for teaching clients about their condition.

REFERENCES

Ambepitiya, G., Roberts, M., Ranjadayalan, K., & Tallis, R. (1994). Silent exertional myocardial ischemia in the elderly: A quantitative analysis of anginal perceptual threshold and the influence of autonomic function. *Journal of the American Geriatrics Society, 42,* 732–737.

Applegate, W. B. (1994). Hypertension. In W. R. Hazzard, E. L. Bierman, J. P. Blass, et al. (Eds.), *Principles of geriatric medicine and gerontology* (3rd ed., pp. 541–554). New York: McGraw-Hill.

Applegate, W. B., & Rutan, G. H. (1992). Advances in management of hypertension in older persons. *Journal of the American Geriatrics Society, 40,* 1164–1174.

Barkis, G. L. (1993). Hypertension. In J. H. Stein (Ed.), *Internal medicine* (3rd ed., pp. 171–187). Norwalk, CT: Appleton & Lange.

Benfante, R., Reed, D., & Frank, J. (1991). Does cigarette smoking have an independent effect on coronary heart disease incidence in the elderly? *American Journal of Public Health, 81,* 897–899.

Benfante, R., Reed, D., & Frank, J. (1992). Do coronary heart disease risk factors measured in the elderly have the same predictive roles as in the middle aged: Comparisons of relative and attributable risks. *Annals of Epidemiology, 2,* 273–282.

Bittner, V., Weiner, D. H., Yusuf, S., et al. (1993). Prediction of mortality and morbidity with a 6-minute walk test in patients with left ventricular dysfunction. *Journal of the American Medical Association, 270,* 1702–1707.

Diamond, G. A., & Forrester, J. S. (1979). Analysis of probability as an aid in the clinical diagnosis of coronary artery disease. *New England Journal of Medicine, 300,* 1350–1358.

Ettinger, W. H., Fried, L. P., Harris, T., et al. (1994). Self-reported causes of physical disability in older people: The Cardiovascular Health Study. *Journal of the American Geriatrics Society, 42,* 1035–1044.

Flack, J. M., Ensrud, K. E., Mascioli, S., et al. (1991). Racial and ethnic modifiers of the salt-blood pressure response. *Hypertension, 17*(suppl. 1), 115–121.

Fleury, J. (1992). Long-term management of the patient with stable angina. *Nursing Clinics of North America, 27,* 205–230.

Gambert, S. R. (1987). *Handbook of geriatrics* (pp. 17–50). New York: Plenum Medical Book Company.

Gardner, A. W., & Poehlman, E. T. (1995). Predictors of the age-related increase in blood pressure in men and women. *Journal of Gerontology, 50A,* M1–M6.

Gerstenblith, G. (1995). Coronary artery disease. In W. B. Abrams, M. H. Beers & R. Berkow (Eds.), *The Merck manual of geriatrics* (pp. 474–481). Whitehouse Station, NJ: Merck & Co., Inc.

Gillett, P., Johnson, M. A., Juretich, M., et al. (1993). The nurse as exercise leader. *Geriatric Nursing, 14,* 133–137.

Gilligan, D. M., Quyyumi, A. A., & Cannon, R. O. (1994). Effects of physiological levels of estrogen on coronary vasomotor function in postmenopausal women. *Circulation, 89,* 2545–2551.

Grady, D., Rubin, S. M., Petitti, D. B., et al. (1992). Hormone therapy to prevent disease and prolong life in postmenopausal women. *Annals of Internal Medicine, 117,* 1016–1037.

Greendale, G. A., & Judd, H. L. (1993). The menopause: Health implications and clinical management. *Journal of the American Geriatrics Society, 41,* 426–436.

Grobbee, D. E. (1991). Methodology of sodium sensitivity assessment: The example of age and sex. *Hypertension, 17*(suppl. 1), 1-109–1-114.

Hausdorff, J. M., Forman, D. E., Ladin, Z., et al. (1994). Increased walking variability in elderly persons with congestive heart failure. *Journal of the American Geriatrics Society, 42,* 1056–1061.

Hopkins, P. N., & Williams, R. R. (1986), Identification and relative weight of cardiovascular risk factors. *Cardiology Clinics, 4,* 3–31.

Joint National Committee on Prevention, Detection, Evaluation, and Treatment of High Blood Pressure (1997). The sixth report of the Joint National Committee on Prevention, Detection, Evaluation, and Treatment of High Blood Pressure. *Archives of Internal Medicine, 157,* 2413–2446.

Jones, W. W., & Fagan, T. C. (1993). Hypertension. In R. Bressler & M. D. Katz (Eds.), *Geriatric pharmacology* (pp. 79–103). New York: McGraw-Hill.

Kane, R. L., Ouslander, J. G., & Abrass, I. B. (1994). *Essentials of clinical geriatrics.* (3rd ed., pp. 256–279). New York: McGraw-Hill.

Kannel, W. B., & Abbott, R. D. (1984). Incidence and prognosis of unrecognized myocardial infarction. *New England Journal of Medicine, 311,* 1144–1147.

Kannel, W. B., Dawber, T. R., Sorlie, P., & Wolf, P. A. (1976).

Components of blood pressure and risks of atherothrombotic brain infarction: The Framingham Study. *Stroke, 7,* 327–330.

Konstam, M., Dracup, K., Baker, D., et al. (1994). *Heart failure: Management of patients with left-ventricular systolic dysfunction. Quick reference guide for clinicians, no. 11.* Agency for Health Care Policy and Research Publication No. 94-0613. Rockville, MD: U.S. Department of Health and Human Services, Public Health Service, Agency for Health Care Policy and Research.

Lakatta, E. G. (1995). Normal changes of aging. In W. B. Abrams, M. H. Beers & R. Berkow (Eds.), *The Merck manual of geriatrics* (pp. 425–441). Whitehouse Station, NJ: Merck & Co., Inc.

Lindenfeld, J. (1990). Congestive heart failure. In R. W. Schrier (Ed.). *Geriatric medicine* (pp. 251–264). Philadelphia: W. B. Saunders.

Mayo, F. (1956). *Care of the long-term patient, vol. 2.* New York: National Health Council.

McCance, K. L., & Reiber, G. E. (1982). Prevention: Implications for nursing research. *Advances in Nursing Science, 4,* 79–87.

Mittelmark, M. B. (1993). Prevalence of cardiovascular diseases among older adults: The cardiovascular health study. *American Journal of Epidemiology, 137,* 311–317.

National Institutes of Health (1993). *The fifth report of the joint national committee on detection, evaluation, and treatment of high blood pressure.* NIH Publication No. 93: 1088. Bethesda, MD: National Institutes of Health, National Heart, Lung, and Blood Institute.

Naunheim, K. S., Kern, M. J., McBride, L. R., et al. (1987). Coronary artery bypass surgery in patients aged 80 years and older. *American Journal of Cardiology, 59,* 804–807.

Pham, H., & Robinson, B. E. (1993). Peripheral vascular disease. In T. Yoshikawa, E. L. Cobbs & K. Brummel-Smith (Eds.), *Ambulatory geriatric care* (pp. 528–536). St. Louis, MO: Mosby-Year Book.

Phillips, A. N., Neaton, J. D., Cook, D. G., et al. (1992). Leukocyte count and risk of major coronary heart disease events. *American Journal of Epidemiology, 136,* 59–70.

Phillips, S. J., Whisnant, J. P., O'Fallon, W. M., & Frye, R. L. (1990). Prevalence of cardiovascular disease and diabetes mellitus in residents of Rochester, Minnesota. *Mayo Clinical Proceedings, 65,* 344–354.

Rich, M. W., Bosner, M. S., Chung, M. K., et al. (1992). Is age an independent predictor of early and late mortality in patients with acute myocardial infarction? *American Journal of Medicine, 92,* 7–13.

Rocella, E. J., Bowler, A. E., & Horan, M. (1987). Epidemiolgic considerations in defining hypertension. *Medical Clinics of North America, 71,* 785–789.

Rosenthal, G. E., & Fortinsky, R. H. (1994). Differences in the treatment of patients with acute myocardial infarction according to patient age. *Journal of the American Geriatrics Society, 42,* 826–832.

Schechter, B. M., Erwin, W. G., & Gerbino, P. P. (1990). The role of the pharmacist. In W. B. Abrams & R. Berkow (Eds.) *The Merck manual of geriatrics* (pp. 193–199). Rahway, NJ: Merck Sharp & Dohme Research Laboratories.

Secretary's Task Force on Black and Minority Health (1985). *Report of the secretary's task force on black and minority health, vol. 1: Executive summary.* Washington, D.C.: U.S. Department of Health and Human Services.

Selma, T. P., Beizer, J. L., & Higbee, M. D. (1997). *Geriatric dosage handbook* (3rd ed.). Cleveland, OH: Lexi-Comp, Inc.

Sempos, C., Cooper, R., Kovar, M. G., & McMillen, M. (1988). Divergence of the recent trends in coronary mortality for the four major race-sex groups in the United States. *American Journal of Public Health, 78,* 1422–1427.

SHEP Cooperative Research Group (1991). Prevention of stroke by antihypertensive drug treatment in older persons with isolated systolic hypertension: Final results of the systolic hypertension in the elderly program (SHEP). *Journal of the American Medical Association, 265,* 3255–3264.

Simonsick, E. M., Guralnik, J. M., Hennekens, C. H., et al. (1995). Intermittent claudication and subsequent cardiovascular disease in the elderly. *Journal of Gerontology: Medical Sciences, 50A,* M17–M22.

Sorkin, J. D., Andres, R., Muller, D. C., et al. (1992). Cholesterol as a risk factor for coronary heart disease in elderly men: The Baltimore Longitudinal Study of Aging. *Annals of Epidemiology, 1,* 59–67.

Tjoa, H. I., & Kaplan, N. M. (1990). Treatment of hypertension in the elderly. *Journal of the American Medical Association, 264,* 1015–1018.

U.S. Department of Health and Human Services (1988). *Healthy People 2000: National health promotion and disease prevention objectives.* Washington, D.C.: U.S. Department of Health and Human Services.

Udvarhelyi, I. S., Gatsonis, C., Epstein, A. M., et al. (1992). Acute myocardial infarction in the Medicare population. *Journal of the American Medical Association, 268,* 2530–2536.

Vokonas, P. S., Kannel, W. B., & Cupples, L. A. (1988). Epidemiology and risk of hypertension in the elderly: The Framingham Study. *Journal of Hypertension, 6*(suppl. 1), S3–S9.

Wolfel, E. E. (1990). Coronary artery disease. In R. W. Schrier (Ed.), *Geriatric medicine* (pp. 237–250). Philadelphia: W. B. Saunders.

Wong, N. D., Wilson, P. W. F., & Kannel, W. B. (1991). Serum cholesterol as a prognostic factor after myocardial infarction: The Framingham Study. *Annals of Internal Medicine, 115,* 687–693.

Discharge Instructions for Patients with Congestive Heart Failure

SELF-CARE

If you take your medications exactly as ordered, weigh daily, and avoid too much fluid intake, your symptoms of congestive heart failure should improve or disappear. Weigh daily (first thing in the morning, after urinating but before having a bowel movement, and with the same clothing). (*A weight gain of 3 to 4 lb in 1 to 2 days necessitates prompt action—the extra fluid causes your heart to work harder! Your physician will advise you if extra diuretic is needed.*)

ACTIVITIES, LIMITATIONS, EXERCISES, AND SEXUAL ACTIVITY

Most patients with heart failure have to space out their activities, taking rest periods in between. Avoiding strenuous exercise, extreme temperatures, or heavy lifting (>10–30 lb) reduces the workload for your heart. You are the best judge of what activities are right for you. Generally, walking is a good form of exercise. Sexual intercourse takes about the same energy as climbing a flight of stairs. As with any other activity, stop if you get symptoms—shortness of breath, chest pressure, or unusual fatigue.

DIET AND FLUIDS

Restricting sodium and fluid intake is perhaps the most important thing you can do to prevent symptoms of heart failure. Because your body saves sodium and fluid when heart failure occurs, you must limit your intake of sodium to less than 2 g (or _____) per day! Avoid cooking with or adding salt to your foods. Use the written materials on sodium restriction as you plan your meals. Also, if you drink a lot of fluid, your body will retain it and make your symptoms of heart failure worse. (See the Fluid Exchange Sheet for details about fluid restriction if your physician advises this.) Alcohol has a slight "weakening" effect on the heart muscle. Limit any alcoholic beverages to two a week.

PROBLEMS TO REPORT TO YOUR PHYSICIAN

Call your physician if you experience any signs that your heart failure is not in good control, such as the following:

- Weight gain of 3 to 4 lb within 1 to 2 days
- Persistent cough or shortness of breath
- Swelling of feet or hands

Also let your physician know of any (1) chest pain or pressure, (2) nausea or vomiting, (3) abdominal pain or bloating, (4) bleeding or bruising, (5) fast heartbeat, (6) dizziness or fainting, or (7) increased fatigue or weakness. If you are on a blood thinner (e.g., warfarin), you will need to have your prothrombin level checked once a month or as your physician instructs.

EQUIPMENT, SUPPLIES, AND SAFETY AIDS

You need your own set of bathroom scales—inexpensive scales are fine, be sure you don't move them around and check the zero point each time before you weigh.

COMMUNITY RESOURCES (AGENCY AND PHONE NUMBER)

Most patients with heart failure can be managed by their primary or local physician. When needed, your physician can call the Center for Heart Failure at Emory (404-712-4460) or the Emory Heart Center (1-800-43 HEART).

Adapted from Emory University Hospital Center for Heart Failure, Atlanta, GA.

Fluid Exchange Sheet (Required for All Center for Heart Failure Patients)

Some physicians ask their patients to limit fluids to 8 cups (64 oz) per day (including all fluids taken with meals or medications). As you plan your 8 cups per day fluid intake, be sure to include all of the following:

| water | juice | yogurt | pudding | ice cubes | ice cream |
| coffee | milk | soup | jello | tea | soda |

Example: The juice of 1 orange or 1/2 grapefruit counts as 4 oz of fluid.

Measurements you may find helpful:

1 cup = 8 oz
4 cups = 32 oz = 1 qt = 1000 cc = 1 L
8 cups = 64 oz = 2 qt = 2000 cc = 2 L

If you drink 4 oz of juice, this equals 120 cc of fluid. Since each ounce is 30 cc, 4 ounces × 30 cc = 120 cc.

Ice cubes do count as fluid. Melt a few of your ice cubes to see how much fluid they equal.

You may use moderate amounts of sugar-free candy to help with a dry mouth.

Adapted from Emory University Hospital Center for Heart Failure, Atlanta, GA.

Congestive Heart Failure Teaching Plan

Purpose: To assist the patient or significant other in understanding the recommendations to maintain optimal heart function.

LEARNER OBJECTIVES	CONTENT
State the cause of congestive heart failure or dilated cardiomyopathy.	Congestive heart failure (CHF) occurs when the heart muscle is weakened in its pumping action. The cause of CHF may be related to valvular disease, cardiomyopathy, coronary artery disease, chronic lung disease, hypertension, congenital lung disease, anemia or hyperthyroidism. (Discuss with the patient likely cause of heart failure for his/her situation.) The cause of dilated cardiomyopathy is usually unknown but may be related, for example, to virus infection, coronary artery disease, pregnancy, and labor.
Identify the signs and symptoms requiring physician notification or change in medications.	Signs and symptoms for which you should notify your physician include the following: 1. 3–4 lb weight gain within 1–2 d 2. Persistent cough or shortness of breath 3. Swelling of feet or hands 4. Chest pain or pressure 5. Nausea or vomiting 6. Abdominal pain or bloating 7. Bleeding or bruising 8. Fast heart beat 9. Dizziness or fainting
Discuss process for daily weight and the relationship between daily diuretic dosage and morning weight.	Weigh daily (at the same time each morning wearing the same clothing). *A weight gain of 3 to 4 lb in 1 to 2 days necessitates prompt*

action—the extra fluid causes your heart to work harder! Your physician will advise you if extra diuretic is needed.

Identify the importance of consistent daily medication regimen and indications to vary dosage, if any.

Emphasize the relationship of diuretic and daily weight and the importance of all medications in maintaining optimum cardiac function. Refer to medication cards or schedule.

Identify the expected fluid restrictions, diet, and activity required for management of heart failure.

Emphasize the effect of sodium on fluid retention with heart failure and the need to limit sodium to a specific number of g per day, using written material on sodium restriction and amount of fluid recommended by physician. Review instructions about limiting alcoholic drinks. Because caffeine is a stimulant and can cause more work for the heart by making it beat faster, it is best to limit intake of caffeinated beverages to two servings per day (i.e., one serving is equal to an 8-oz cup of coffee or a 12-oz beverage can). Review the handout instructions about activity.

Note: Documentation is used to ensure coverage of all these areas and the ability of patient or caregiver to demonstrate knowledge of each area.

Adapted from Emory University Hospital Center for Heart Failure, Atlanta, GA.

APPENDIX | 21-4 |

Resources

American Heart Association
7320 Greenville Avenue
Dallas, TX 75231
Telephone 800-242-8721
Each state also has local affiliates.

County or regional Agency on Aging and State Division of Aging can
provide information about healthy aging or Elder Care Locator
Telephone: 800-677-1116

Emory University Hospital Center for Heart Failure Therapy
1364 Clifton Road N.E.
Atlanta, GA 30322
Telephone: 404-712-4460

National Institute on Aging
P.O. Box 8057
Gaithersburg, MD 20892-8057
Telephone 301-496-1752
Provides consumer information on various topics though publication
of free *Age page.*

U.S. Department of Health and Human Services
Public Health Service
Agency for Health Care Policy and Research
Executive Office Center, Suite 501
2101 East Jefferson Street
Rockville, MD 20852
Telephone 800-358-9295

Sensory Disorders

Barbara A. Brant

Sensory-perceptual alteration is a phenomenon produced by a change in the amount and intensity of sensory input or stimulation in the environment. *Perception* is the process of integrating, classifying, discriminating, and assigning meaning to sensory stimuli. Perceptions change with experience as the meaning of signals become internalized; conversely, learned perceptions may become increasingly pivotal in guiding individuals as sensory receptors decline in function with aging (Hooper, 1994). Central to the understanding of sensory-perceptual alterations is the concept of individual differences in optimum levels of stimulation.

Optimal adaptation in a constantly changing environment occurs through sensory-neural processes. Both the internal and external environments of the individual play an important role in these processes and in the manner in which the messages are sent and received. Barriers to receiving and perceiving stimuli through the senses (i.e., vision, hearing, taste, smell, and touch) can seriously affect adaptation and appropriate interaction with the environment (Carp, 1991). Because communication occurs through the senses, the need to keep in touch with reality and the environment through normal sensory stimulation is vital. This need is seriously hampered when diminished sensory input interferes with that vital connection.

This chapter discusses sensory-perceptual alterations related to the aging process; disorders associated with sensory-perceptual alterations; assessment factors pertinent to vision, hearing, taste, and smell; emergency conditions; and the management of common sensory-perceptual disorders in the older adult.

VISION

Age-Related Changes in the Eye

Sensory changes occur with extreme variability throughout the aging process, and similar to other physical changes, not all sensory changes impair function in the older person. The incidence and prevalence of normal and abnormal vision changes increase with aging (Table 22–1).

Visual changes occurring gradually over time often impede daily functioning and can reduce the quality of life for older people. These changes may be readily compensated for by minor changes in lifestyle, or they may significantly reduce the efficiency with which day-to-day functions are carried out.

The visual system comprises numerous ocular structures necessary for vision function. Structures and age-related changes of the eye are presented Table 22–2. In the absence of pathological changes, prominent changes in

TABLE 22-1

Epidemiology of Normal and Abnormal Visual Changes with Aging

Normal	Abnormal
Nearly 65% will be presbyopic	>15% will have cataracts
65–70% will be astigmatic	9% will have related maculopathy
60% will be hyperopic	3% will have diabetic retinopathy
20% will be myopic	2% will have glaucoma

Adapted from The American Optometric Association (1995). St. Louis: MO.

the eye common to nearly all older people are lens growth, loss of accommodation, and miosis. The cornea, normally spherical in structure, becomes curved as it ages, leading to what Ludlam and Freid (1993) referred to as "against-the-rule" astigmatism.

Arcus senilis, a deposit of calcium and cholesterol salts, appears as a gray-white ring at the edge of the iris; however, this is not usually linked to systemic disease. Miosis is a reduction in pupillary size attributed to atrophy of the smooth muscles of the iris. This reduction is caused by a decrease in the sympathetic tone of the autonomic nervous system, resulting in a decrease in the amount of light entering the retinal chamber (Ludlam & Freid, 1993). The reduction in both pupil size and the amount of light reaching the retina makes visability difficult for older people, especially in dimly-lit or darkened areas. Because the pupil reacts more slowly to light changes, the aging eye needs additional time to adjust when going from a brightly lit area to a darker one. Examination of the fundus or other structures of the eye through the undilated pupil is difficult.

With aging, the lens becomes rigid, discolored, flat, and sclerotic (Michaels, 1994). These structural changes occurring on the anterior surface of the lens reduce the functional ability for accommodation (focusing). *Presbyopia* (loss of accommodation for near vision), the most common of the sensory changes, usually occurs between 40 and 50 years of age, requiring corrective lenses for close work.

As the aging lens yellows, the discoloration filters out both short- and long-wavelength lights; however, the greatest sensitivity in color vision occurs in the blue and green end of the spectrum, where colors appear darker to older people. The key to enhancing color discrimination is to maximize luminance contrast. Color contrasts for people with low color vision have been developed by the Lighthouse Center for Vision and Aging (see Appendix 22–1). Because subtle changes in color vision may be indicative of a developing disease or a drug toxicity, such as with digoxin, color vision should be evaluated regularly.

Lens opacities increase the scattering of light passing through the lens. Problems with glare

TABLE 22-2

Schematic Section and Age-Related Changes of the Eye

Eyelid flaccidity

Lacrimal gland atrophy

Conjunctiva thinning

Scleral yellowing and thinning

Arcus senilis

Pupil miosis

Decreased iris pigment

Cilial muscle atrophy

Corneal flattening and opacity

Lens rigidity, yellowing, and opacity

Vitreous shrinking and liquefaction

Loss of neurons in retina

Thinning of blood vessels

Increase in drusen bodies

Figure redrawn with permission of The American Optometric Association, St. Louis, MO.

can occur, particularly in bright light or with oncoming car headlights while driving at night. Lens opacities also decrease the amount of light reaching the retina. Older adults require at least three times the illumination as do younger people.

The retina, the central nervous system link to the brain, becomes thinner with increasing age, owing to the loss of neural cells. Arterioles become smaller secondary to atherosclerotic changes. The veins have fibrotic narrowing and may show marked venous indentation (nicking) at the arteriovenous crossings. The optic nerve tends to have less distinct margins and may be slightly paler because of capillary reduction in this area. Yellowish-white spots (drusen) may be present in the macular area, which may also show pigmentation changes. These changes are usually not significant unless accompanied by changes in visual acuity or a distortion of objects. Because the retina is unable to regenerate itself, the occurrence of retinal disorders does threaten sight. Retinal tears may occur from the detachment of the vitreous in advanced age. Floaters (opacities)

and flashes of light, relatively common with vitreous detachment, may cause annoyance and anxiety. A vitreous detachment must always be differentiated from a serious retinal detachment, as the vasculature is usually involved with the latter.

Flaccidity and ptosis of the eyelids occur from shrinking orbital fat and weakening levator muscles, which control the opening and closing of the lids. Two conditions associated with lid changes are entropion and ectropion. With *entropion*, there is increased flaccidity of the lower lid and an inward rotation of the lashes, which can seriously mar the intactness of the corneal surface. Irritation, discomfort, pain, and scarring may occur. *Ectropion* results from a flaccidity and outward prominence of the upper lid and lashes, causing the punctum to fall away from the conjunctiva. Inflammation and tearing often result. Surgical intervention is usually indicated in both conditions before permanent damage occurs.

Failure of the lacrimal pump results in diminished tear secretion in many older people, particularly older postmenopausal women

(Kane et al., 1994). Decreased tear secretion is often accompanied by dryness of the eyes, irritation, and discomfort. Because tear production decreases with aging, the older eye cries less but waters more. Untreated, this condition may jeopardize the intactness of the corneal surface, already compromised by a loss of integrity with aging. The use of artificial tears can relieve *dry eye syndrome* unless a serious malfunction of the lacrimal duct itself exists.

ASSESSMENT FACTORS

- Assess visual acuity at least annually for any change. Distance visual acuity while the patient is wearing corrective lenses should be screened in each eye separately using the Snellen eye chart set at a distance of 20 feet. A tumbling "E" chart can be used with patients who do not understand the English alphabet. Patients demonstrating either significant changes in visual acuity, a visual acuity of 20/40 or less using corrective lenses, or a difference between the two eyes of at least one line on the eye chart should be referred to an eye care specialist for additional testing (Castor & Carter, 1995; Office of Disease Prevention and Health Promotion, 1994). Near visual acuity can be assessed by having the individual read ordinary newsprint or by using the Rosenbaum eye card held at a distance of 14 inches.

  Note: The Snellen eye chart alone does not necessarily evaluate the visual acuity required in everyday life. Self-administered instruments such as the Visual Impairment Questionnaire (Rubenstein & Lohr, 1982) and the longer, standardized Activities of Daily Vision Scale (Mangione et al., 1992) that assess the individual's perception of his or her visual functional impairment may be useful in identifying patients who need referral to an eye care specialist.

- Assess the visual acuity of older people in their home environment, whenever possible, to determine functional ability in a more familiar environment.
- Observe the older adult as he or she performs the instrumental activities of daily living (IADL), as new decrements in vision more often manifest themselves in IADL than in the personal care activities of daily living (ADL).
- Perform a fundoscopic assessment of the disk, vascularity, and macular area.
- Assess the older adult's ability for upward range of ocular movements and sustaining convergence. Refer for a neurological examination if these ocular limitations are found.
- Assess visual fields by using the confrontational method: Face the patient, and bring a moving object such as a pencil from the periphery into the patient's visual field from different directions while covering one eye. The examiner compares his or her own visual fields against those of the patients. Complete the same procedure for both eyes. Refer for an ophthalmological examination if significant visual field deficits are found.
- Assess the older person's understanding of changes in the aging eye.

EMERGENCY CONDITIONS

- Abrupt changes in visual acuity, an interruption of blood supply to the visual system, temporal pain or observed macular edema, and scratching and irritation of the cornea constitute emergency conditions.

MANAGEMENT PRIORITIES

- Reinforce with asymptomatic older adults the importance of scheduling periodic eye examinations with an eye specialist.
- Educate clients and their families at their level of understanding regarding normal age-related visual changes.
- Provide educational material (e.g., videotapes, large charts, or large print brochures) for office reading or reading at home.
- Teach the following strategies to minimize the effects of age-related visual alterations:
  ○ Use good illumination, with incandescent rather than fluorescent lighting
  ○ Use increased color contrast to amplify color identification and depth perception

- Regularly use eyeglasses, if prescribed; special tinted or coated lenses may help decrease glare problems
- Use sunglasses and a hat on sunny days to decrease glare problems
- Caution the older driver to practice defensive driving. Instruct him or her to avoid looking directly into the beams of oncoming cars at night to decrease problems with glare and dark adaptation.
- Consult with the pharmacist regarding the use of large print labels on prescription bottles.
- Be aware that Medicare and most third-party insurance carriers do not reimburse for routine eye examinations or corrective lenses; however, they do cover eye specialist costs associated with the diagnosis and treatment of eye diseases. Eyeglasses and contact lenses are covered by Medicare only after cataract surgery.
- For patients who cannot afford to pay for corrective lenses, contact the State Department for the Visually Impaired, the local Society for the Prevention of Blindness, and other organizational resources to see what assistance they might provide (see Appendix 22–1).

Heckheimer (1989) provides a comprehensive list of other nursing and environmental interventions to manage visual changes associated with aging.

Common Disorders Affecting the Aging Eye

Detecting disorders of the aging eye is increasingly important owing to (1) the increased longevity of the elderly, resulting in greater numbers of the population affected; (2) the risk of functional alterations, injuries associated with falls, other types of accidents, and depression related to visual impairment (see Table 22–3 for definitions); and (3) new technologies and insights resulting from research that can extend today's knowledge and change approaches to the management of visual disorders. Most people with visual disorders enter their retirement

TABLE 22-3

Definitions of Visual Impairment

Vision impairment	Inability to read newsprint with best eyeglass correction
Low vision	Decreased visual performance that prevents performance to a full capacity compared with a normal person of the same age and gender; may be a consequence of reduced visual acuity, abnormal visual field, reduced contract sensitivity, or other ocular dysfunction
Legally blind	Best corrected visual acuity is ≤20/200 in the better eye or the visual field is ≤20°
Partially sighted	Best visual acuity is ≤20/70 in the better eye or the visual field is ≤30°
Functional visual impairment	Visual acuity is ≤20/50; affects everyday activities such as ability to read a newspaper with corrective lenses

Data from Castor & Carter (1995).

years with what could be considered "normal" sight for older adults; however, many disorders that compromise sight occur during middle age and often go unnoticed until later life. Most visual disorders are progressive and require intervention to prevent further deterioration. The most common disorders of the aging eye—cataracts, glaucoma, macular degeneration, diabetic retinopathies, and temporal arteritis—are discussed in this section. The systemic medications with ocular side effects are also discussed (Table 22–4).

CATARACTS

Cataracts are the leading cause of visual disorders in older adults. A cataract, defined as a loss of transparency of the lens or its capsule, constitutes the most frequently observed alteration of the crystalline lens in the aging eye (Cataract Management Guideline Panel, 1993). Cataract symptoms, which are generally progressive, include an increased sensitivity to glare (most common), a blurring of vision, halo images, cloudiness, decreased visual acuity, and decreased contrast sensitivity. In early cataract formation, the refractive power of the lens increases, shifting toward myopia. This

TABLE 22-4

Ocular Side Effects of Systemic Medications

Drug	Effect
Antiarthritics	
Corticosteroids	Cataract; increased intraocular pressure; impaired corneal wound healing; increased risk of viral, fungal, and bacterial infections
Antidepressants	
Lithium	Severe loss of central acuity
Tricyclic antidepressants	Increase in intraocular pressure; ocular muscle imbalances; amitriptyline and imipramine can result in visual hallucinations
Antiepileptics	
Barbiturates	Sluggish pupillary response; miosis or mydriasis; transient nystagmus; motility disturbance
Carbamazepine	Diplopia; impaired accommodation; nystagmus
Diphenylhydantoin	Nystagmus; conjunctivitis; mydriasis; ptosis; Stevens-Johnson syndrome
Primidone	Ptosis
Trimethadione	Glare in bright light; slowed dark adaptation
Antihistamines	
	Mydriasis; impaired accommodation; decreased tear production
Antineoplastics	
Chlorambucil	Keratopathy
Vincristine	Ocular motility disturbances; ptosis
Antipsychotics	
Chlorpromazine	Fine pigmentation on anterior lens capsule and back of cornea
Haloperidol	Cataract
Thioridazine	Pigmentary retinopathy without bull's eye pattern; decreased vision
Trifluoperazine	Miosis; blurred vision
Antituberculosis Agents	
Aminosalicylic acid	Blepharitis; superficial punctate keratopathy; corneal ulcerations; dry eye; central scotoma with coadministration of thiacetazone
Ethambutol	Retrobulbar neuritis
Isoniazid	Optic neuritis; optic atrophy; keratitis with coadministration of pyridine-3-aldehydethiose micarbazone; impaired accommodation
Streptomycin	Nystagmus; motility disturbances; impaired acuity during head movement; impaired accommodation
Cardiac Medications	
Digitalis	Flickering vision; dazzling lights; color illusions; impaired visual acuity
Propranolol	Mild decrease in intraocular pressure
Quinidine	Decreased visual field
Verapamil	Blurred vision
Diuretics and Antihypertensive Agents	
Alpha-methyldopa	Small subclinical decrease in intraocular pressure
Chlorothiazide	Xanthopsia; acute myopia; cortical blindness
Hydralazine	Lid edema; lacrimation
Hydrochlorothiazide	Acute bilateral myopia with perimacular edema
Spironolactone	Small subclinical decrease in intraocular pressure

TABLE 22-4

Ocular Side Effects of Systemic Medications *Continued*

Drug	Effect
Nonsteroidal Antiinflammatory Agents	
Ibuprofen	Reduced central acuity; optic neuritis; eye pain; diplopia; hallucinations; uveitis; keratoconjunctivitis
Salicylates	Nystagmus; retinal hemorrhage
Indomethacin	Corneal deposits
Naproxen	Corneal opacity
Phenylbutazone	Stevens-Johnson mucositis; severe keratitis; optic neuritis; palsy of nerve IV
Oral Hypoglycemics	
Chlorpropamide	Optic neuropathy; keratoconjunctivitis; acute transient myopia
Tolbutamide	Optic neuritis
Miscellaneous	
Aminophylline	Rapid decrease in intraocular pressure
Dicumarol, heparin, and warfarin	Spontaneous intraocular hemorrhages
Ergotamine	Miosis
Quinine	Decreased central acuity with blindness; pupillary dilatation; optic atrophy; narrowing of retinal vessels
Allopurinol	Cataract; retinopathy
Morphine	Optic neuritis
Vitamin A	Conjunctival deposits; papilledema
Vitamin D	Conjunctival deposits; corneal opacity

Adapted from Brady, K. D., & Ellis, P. P. (1985). Ocular pharmacology. In M. C. Kwitco & F. J. Weinstock (Eds.), *Geriatric ophthalmology.* Orlando, FL: Grune & Stratton; additional data from Vaughan, D., Asbury, T., & Riordan-Eva, P. (1992). *General ophthalmology* (13th ed.). Norwalk, CT: Appleton & Lange.

increased refractive power, known as *second sight,* can temporarily correct presbyopia, thus allowing a person aged 60 to 70 years to read again without glasses (Kupfer, 1995). With more advanced cataract formation, the lens may become so totally opaque and swollen that it creates pressure on the anterior chamber angle, causing angle-closure glaucoma to occur.

Risk factors for cataract formation include diabetes mellitus, heredity, ultraviolet-B radiation exposure, smoking, corticosteroid drugs, alcohol use, and insufficient ingestion of antioxidant vitamins (Cataract Management Guideline Panel, 1993; Weinreb et al., 1990). Although research has been inconclusive, other drugs implicated as being cataractogenic include thiazide diuretics and major tranquilizers such as phenothiazine. Different risk factors are associated with different types of lens opacities. Although no longitudinal studies are available on prevention, it seems prudent to recommend decreasing sun exposure by wearing a hat and sunglasses, increasing the intake of antioxidant vitamins, and undergoing smoking cessation (Cataract Management Guideline Panel, 1993).

When cataract symptoms interfere with daily functioning, surgical intervention is recommended (Cataract Management Guideline Panel, 1993). The severity of the interference can range from simple symptoms of glare disability to more severe symptoms of difficulty reading, driving, and performing daily activities. Surgery should be considered only when optical, medical, and environmental interventions have been ineffective in helping the person maintain his or her activities.

An ocular implant is the most commonly used procedure for optical correction after cataract extraction. Other approaches for optical correction may involve the use of contact lenses or cataract glasses, depending on the type and outcome of the surgery and the client's visual needs. In the absence of other ocular disorders, vision should improve with surgical intervention.

Assessment Factors

- A cataract evaluation must include the older client's (1) perception of visual change and its effect on functional status; (2) best corrected near and distance visual acuity; (3) ability to read normal print; (4) glare disability; and (5) other causes of decreased visual function (Harkins, 1993).
- Diagnostic indicators of a cataract are the direct visualization of the lens opacity and an inability to visualize the details of the fundus.

Emergency Conditions

- In most cases, preoperative and postoperative complications are minimal. The presence of inflammation, infection, wound leakage, or corneal or macular edema requires immediate referral to an ophthalmologist. Prolonged macular edema can lead to permanent loss of central vision (Michaels, 1994).

Management Priorities

According to the recommendations of the Cataract Management Guideline Panel (1993), treatment should be determined by the degree of visual comfort or discomfort of the older client and the degree of cataract development (Cataract Management Guideline Panel, 1993).

- During early cataract formation, clients should be educated and reassured about the cause of visual problems, its treatment, and the prognosis. At early stages, visual impairment can often be reduced by non-surgical means such as a change in eyeglass prescriptions for both distance and bifocal lenses, the use of magnification or other visual aids, and appropriate lighting.
- When cataract symptoms begin to interfere with activities, educate the client regarding the benefits and the risks of cataract surgery.
- Factors such as concomitant ocular disease, the ability of the older client to tolerate the stress of surgical intervention, and the ability to tolerate a contact lens necessitate consideration and intervention. The insertion of an intraocular lens in people with known diabetes may pose a risk for ocular damage (Kupfer, 1995).

GLAUCOMA

Glaucoma is the second leading cause of blindness in the United States and is a major cause of blindness in African Americans. This disorder is defined by a slowly progressing loss of vision with characteristic signs of damage to the optic nerve (U.S. Preventive Services Task Force, 1996). Although increased intraocular pressure is common in patients with glaucoma and contributes to optic nerve damage, it is no longer considered a diagnostic criterion for glaucoma.

All forms of glaucoma are caused by an increased resistance to aqueous outflow rather than to an increase in aqueous secretion (Heath, 1992). The visual loss associated with glaucoma is principally the loss of peripheral vision caused by ocular pressure exerted on the retina and the optic nerve fibers, which, if left untreated, can cause permanent damage.

Risk factors for glaucoma include race, family history, ocular hypertension, advanced age, myopia, retinal vascular disturbance, corticosteroid drug use, diabetes mellitus, postoperative complications such as vitreous loss, and vascular crises (e.g., changes in blood pressure or blood volume) (Michaels, 1994; U.S. Preventive Services Task Force, 1996). Glaucoma is classified based on whether the angle of the anterior chamber is open or narrow and whether the glaucoma is primary or secondary.

The most common type of glaucoma, accounting for 80 to 90% of cases in the United States, is *primary, open-angle glaucoma* (POAG) (U.S. Preventive Services Task Force, 1996). POAG is found more commonly in blacks, who also tend to have more severe disease than whites, and in diabetics (Kupfer, 1995). POAG progresses slowly and insidiously until an irreversible loss of visual field occurs. Other symptoms, when they become apparent, include decreased contrast sensitivity, decreased dark adaptation, decreased central visual acuity, and glare disability. POAG is usually discovered on routine eye examination and tonometry testing by an eye specialist. Although it cannot be cured, it can usually be controlled with topical and/or systemic medication.

The other type of primary glaucoma, *narrow-angle closure*, accounts for approximately 10%

of glaucomas in the United States. It occurs most frequently in Asians, especially Native Alaskans and Chinese, and in far-sighted individuals (Kupfer, 1995). Narrow-angle glaucoma is characterized by a sudden and marked increase in intraocular pressure, with accompanying redness and pain in the eye, headache, nausea or vomiting, corneal edema, and decreased vision at the onset. These acute attacks may be precipitated by an obstruction of the vitreous outflow track, by a foreign substance, or during dilation of the pupil. Narrow-angle glaucoma is usually more responsive to corrective treatment.

Secondary glaucomas, which account for approximately 10% of glaucomas in the United States, result from prior or concurrent ocular disease or trauma (Kupfer, 1995) These glaucomas are characterized by an anatomical or functional blockage of the outflow channels. They may be open-angle (e.g., with corticosteroid-induced pressure increase) or closed-angle (e.g., induced by a swollen cataractous lens). Because secondary glaucoma can persist for many years in the absence of clinical pathology or visual loss, a gradual loss of visual fields often goes unnoticed by the older person. Patients usually present with a red, painful eye, which is usually accompanied by decreased vision. Even with eventual destruction of the optic nerve, 20/20 vision can still exist in the presence of destroyed extramacular visual fields. Treatment is directed toward eliminating the underlying cause of the glaucoma—for example, by removing an ocular tumor, using antiinflammatory drugs to treat uveitis, or changing antiglaucoma medications. If these measures are unsuccessful, surgery should be used to create a new outflow path for the aqueous humor to leave the eye (Kupfer, 1995).

Assessment Factors
- Accurate glaucoma screening is best performed by eye specialists with access to specialized equipment to evaluate the optic disc and measure visual fields (U.S. Preventive Services Task Force, 1996).
- There is currently no efficient and reliable method for glaucoma screening by primary care providers. Observe for visual field deficits and cupping of the optic nerve.

Emergency Conditions
- Severe eye pain associated with acute narrow-angle glaucoma may be precipitated by mydriatic eye drops such as pilocarpine or systemic anticholinergic drugs (Heath, 1992). An immediate ophthalmological evaluation is indicated to determine medical intervention.

Management Priorities
Early diagnosis and treatment are key to preventing the visual impairment associated with glaucoma.

- The definitive diagnosis regarding the type of glaucoma and its treatment rests with the ophthalmologist.
- In primary open-angle glaucoma, pharmacological intervention is indicated to lower the intraocular pressure. The most commonly used drugs are topical beta-blockers such as timolol (Timoptic), betaxolol (Betoptic), or levobunolol (Betagan Liquifilm). Other agents used are systemic carbonic anhydrase inhibitors such as acetazolamide (Diamox) or methazolamide (Neptazane), topical carbonic anhydrase inhibitors such as dorzolamide (Trusopt), topical miotics such as pilocarpine (e.g., Pilocar, Isopto Carpine, Pilostat, Piloptic), and topical alpha-adrenergic agents such as apraclonidine (Iopidine) (Kupfer, 1995).
- Closely monitor the side effects of ophthalmological drugs for potential systemic absorption. Although rare, timolol has been associated with fatal reactions. Its been estimated that 80% of a timolol eye drop is absorbed directly into the vascular system if the lacrimal system is not closed during its administration. Because the drug can reach target organs before it is detoxified in the liver, the blood level following improper ophthalmic administration is proportionately higher than when the drug is given orally (Vaughan et al., 1992). Depression and significant weight loss associated with nausea and anorexia can occur with the use of systemic carbonic anhydrase in-

hibitors, particularly acetazolamide. Beta-blockers can also cause depression and aggravate marginal congestive heart failure, asthma, and chronic obstructive lung disease. Confusion and disorientation may occur with several of these drugs.

- To minimize the systemic effects of topical eye medications, teach clients the proper method of administering eyedrops.
- In patients with acute narrow-angle glaucoma, immediate ophthalmological referral is required to control intraocular pressure medically prior to surgical intervention with laser iridotomy.
- Recognize that, in treating systemic disorders, medications such as corticosteroids can raise intraocular pressure and precipitate glaucoma.
- Note that package inserts for anticholinergic drugs such as oxybutynin (Ditropan) often contain warning labels regarding their use in glaucoma patients. These warnings are frequently misleading. Clients with open-angle glaucoma and those with narrow-angle glaucoma treated with iridotomy are not at risk for an increase in intraocular pressure from these drugs. These drugs should not be used in patients with untreated narrow-angle glaucoma who, unfortunately, are usually undiagnosed.
- Counsel clients with open-angle glaucoma about the importance of taking their medication indefinitely to control the disease, even if symptoms are not present. Advise them to have eye examinations every 6 months to check the effectiveness of treatment.
- Counsel the older person with compromised vision about the importance of maximizing independence through low vision (use of partial sight or vision) rehabilitation by personnel trained in the use of optical devices such as high-powered spectacles, magnifiers, and nonoptical aids (e.g., large print reading materials, telephone dials, taking books, and writing guides). These products are available from the Lighthouse National Center for Vision and Aging or the American Foundation for the Blind (see Appendix 22–1).

MACULAR DEGENERATION

Age-related macular degeneration (ARMD), often referred to as *senile macular degeneration,* is one of the most common and progressive causes of low vision in older people and the leading cause of untreatable legal blindness in the United States in this age group. The prevalence of ARMD is approximately 30% between the ages of 75 and 81 years; however, only one third of those people diagnosed with ARMD are projected to have functional visual loss (Heath, 1992). Those people at risk for ARMD are whites, cigarette smokers, and people with hypertension (Weinreb et al., 1990). The cause of macular degeneration is not clearly understood, and the prognosis is poor.

The macular area—the area of central vision with the highest degree of visual resolution—is located approximately 3 mm temporal to the optic disk and is clearly visible on ophthalmological examination. During the aging process, the macula may undergo a degenerative process resulting in loss of central vision; however, peripheral or side vision remains unaffected (Weinreb et al., 1990). Rarely do people with ARMD experience complete blindness. Other signs and symptoms include difficulty reading or identifying faces, distortion of objects, increased glare sensitivity, and decreased color vision.

ARMD presents in two forms: (1) atrophic or *dry,* characterized by slow, progressive, and painless visual loss; and (2) neovascular or *wet,* characterized by an acute abnormal subretinal neovascularization and irreversible scarring in the macular area (Weinreb et al., 1990). There is no known treatment for the dry type of ARMD. Neovascular ARMD is often treatable with laser therapy in its early stages. Both forms may be present in the older adult at the same time.

Assessment Factors
- Observe for signs and symptoms of central vision distortion, such as objects increasing or decreasing in size and/or straight lines appearing bent or missing a segment.
- Observe for hemorrhage and edema on ophthalmological examination.

- Evaluate the client's perception and information about sensory/perceptual disorders or alterations.
- Determine the older person's motivation for low vision intervention.
- Refer to an ophthalmologist for a thorough evaluation of the macula and retinal structures.

Emergency Conditions

- Macular edema and neovascular hemorrhage into the subretinal space, damaging the rods and cones, result in irreversible visual loss. Damage can occur within days after symptom onset.

Management Priorities

Early detection, referral, and intervention are critical in patients with subretinal ARMD.

- Symptom management is crucial to reduce the potential for subretinal bleeding and other complications of ARMD.
- Closely monitor the subretinal and macular areas and vasculature.
- Promptly evaluate any symptoms occurring in the unaffected eye.
- Instruct high-risk patients (e.g. those with age-related maculopathy in one eye or a family history) in the use of an Amsler test grid (Fig. 22–1) to detect early distortion in central vision that could benefit from laser treatment.
- Counsel the client in the use of magnifying lenses and high-intensity lighting for use in near vision tasks (e.g., reading and watching television). A telescopic lens may help the person identify street signs and perform other visual tasks to facilitate travel. If available, contact the State Department for the Visually Impaired to provide magnification instruments and educational materials. The Lighthouse National Center for Vision and Aging can also provide visual aids (see Appendix 22–1).
- Urge clients who have difficulty in coping with visual impairments to seek counseling.
- Refer to a vision rehabilitation specialist to evaluate and enhance remaining visual function.

DIABETIC RETINOPATHY

Retinal vascular disease is one of the major causes of retinal function compromise (Kupfer, 1995). The most common, disabling, and life-threatening of these retinopathies is associated with complications secondary to diabetes mellitus. Diabetic eye changes are currently the leading cause of blindness in the adult population and generally occur in long-standing ($\geq$15 years) disease (Castor & Carter, 1995). Diabetic retinopathy may affect the macula only or the entire retina. Symptoms include decreased visual acuity, decreased contrast sensitivity, decreased color perception, decreased dark/light adaptation, scotomas, and glare disability. Laser photocoagulation is used to treat severe diabetic retinopathy.

Assessment Factors

Conditions affecting the retina, optic nerve, disk, and the arterial/venous blood supply in the aging eye are often time specific and sudden. Skilled ophthalmological assessment is required to quickly identify these often minute changes. Prompt ophthalmological referral is necessary to ensure optimal visual function.

- Because the time frame for signs and symptoms of vascular changes varies with the onset of diabetes mellitus, a thorough ophthalmological assessment must become part of the comprehensive health assessment of older people
- Obtain a thorough diabetic history, including a family history and vision history.
- Assess for loss of visual function, visual field deficit, and central visual impairment.
- Observe for signs of leaking, hemorrhage, and macular edema on funduscopic examination. The hallmark of macular edema is retinal thickening.

Emergency Conditions

- Vitreous hemorrhage, and the size, location, and severity of new and often fragile vessel growth constitute emergency conditions.

Management Priorities

- Prompt intervention is pivotal to the prevention of maculoneovascular hemorrhages in diabetic retinopathy.

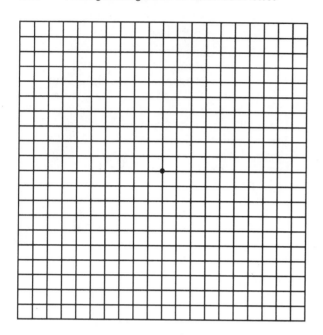

FIGURE 22–1. Amsler grid. (Reproduced with permission of Prevent Blindness America, Schaumberg, IL.)

- Impress on the older person that diabetic control is essential to minimize or reduce the potential for serious visual impairment, particularly in the later years of the disease.
- Stress the importance of an annual ophthalmological examination.

TEMPORAL ARTERITIS

Temporal arteritis (giant cell arteritis) is a form of central retinal artery occlusion. The condition is described as an idiopathic, atheromatous, vascular inflammatory process involving the temporal arterial blood supply to the optic nerve, often resulting in prolonged ischemia of the optic nerve and sudden visual loss on the affected side (Heath, 1992). Temporal arteritis is usually accompanied by head and neck pain, pain in the jaw on chewing, fever, generalized fatigue, and apprehension. These symptoms are always accompanied by an elevated erythrocyte sedimentation rate (Kupfer, 1995). In ischemic optic neuropathy associated with atheromatosis, however, pain is usually not present. Diminished visual loss with resultant pallor of the optic disk ensues. Early recognition of the signs and symptoms of temporal arteritis and prompt long-term intervention can reduce the

risk of visual loss in either eye, as the opposite eye is at risk within months to years of the episode.

Assessment Factors
- Assess for symptoms of arthritis, polymyalgia rheumatica, and other rheumatoid involvement.
- Observe for temporal artery enlargement.
- In the funduscopic examination, observe for disc edema and pallor of the optic nerve. The hallmark of primary optic atrophy is the white appearance of the optic nerve.
- Obtain an erythrocyte sedimentation rate.

Emergency Conditions
- Immediate attention to a positive diagnosis can delay the threat of involvement of the opposite eye. Once the ischemic episode has occurred, however, treatment is of no avail (Kupfer, 1995). Permanent and total blindness can result from ischemic optic neuropathy.

Management Priorities
- Refer immediately to an ophthalmologist, who will usually confirm the diagnosis with a biopsy of the temporal artery.

- Initiate corticosteroid therapy (e.g., prednisone) to reduce the inflammatory process.
- Try to allay the older person's anxiety and fear.
- Reduce pain associated with temporal arteritis using nonsteroidal antiinflammatory agents.
- Relieve associated systemic symptoms.

HEARING

Hearing loss, the third most prevalent chronic condition of aging, affects more than 28 million older people (National Institute for Deafness and Communication Disorders, 1992). The prevalence of hearing loss increases significantly with aging (Table 22–5). As with most changes in the sensory system of older people, the loss of hearing is gradual and insidious.

Hearing impairment can directly affect older adults' quality of life, placing them at risk for further disability and impingement on their safety. In many instances, ADL, and especially IADL, are affected by a hearing deficit. The inability to communicate effectively with another human being may lead to depression and isolation (Chen, 1994).

Age-Related Changes in the Ear

The auditory system comprises the external, middle, and internal ear structures; the eighth cranial nerve; and the auditory system, inclusive of the auditory brain stem and auditory cortex. The auditory cortex is located in the temporal lobe of the brain. Within the inner ear are housed the cochlea and the vestibular

TABLE 22-5

Prevalence of Hearing Loss in Older People

>30% between ages 65 and 74 years
>45% beyond age 75 years
>85% of elderly people in institutions

Data from Glass (1990); National Institute for Deafness and Other Communication Disorders (1992).

systems; the eighth cranial nerve is innervated by the vestibular and cochlear nerve branches. Table 22–6 presents structures and age-related changes of the ear.

Auditory perception is concerned with how sound patterns are converted by the auditory system and experienced by the listener. In the normal inner ear, the sensory cells of the auditory system lie in the organ of Corti, closely aligned with the cochlea and in contact with fibers of the eighth cranial nerve. The motility of the outer hair cells of the cochlea is influenced by nerves from the central nervous system. The inner cells, known as the mechanoreceptors, transmit the auditory information from the cochlea to the brain stem and the central nervous system via the eighth cranial nerve. Within this complex auditory system, multiple age-related changes can occur (see Table 22–6). Hearing loss may result from the dysfunction of any component of the auditory system. In older people, hearing loss is primarily caused by senescent changes in the outer hair cells of the cochlea (Bamford & Saunders, 1991; Soucek & Michaels, 1990).

Functionally, many older people lose hearing for pure tones; experience difficulty in hearing and understanding speech, a hallmark of age-related hearing impairment (peripheral pathology); experience difficulty in localizing sound and in binaural listening (brain stem pathology); and have problems with difficult speech and language difficulties (cortical pathology). Speech discrimination performance is a good indicator of the cause and degree of sensorineural hearing loss (Rees et al., 1994). Research can neither confirm nor deny that these auditory changes are related purely to the aging process in the auditory system (Soucek & Michaels, 1990). Current research on the complex mechanisms of normal hearing and aural rehabilitation at the National Institute for Deafness and Other Communication Disorders may yield a greater understanding of the cause and treatment of changes in the auditory system.

Common Disorders Affecting the Ear

CONDUCTIVE HEARING LOSS

Conductive hearing loss is caused by a defect or disease of the external or middle ear or

TABLE 22-6
Sensorineural Apparatus of the Inner Ear and Age-Related Changes in the Auditory System

Excessive hair growth on the pinna

Loss of elasticity and increase in size of pinna

Loss of elasticity and narrowing of external meatus

Stiffened and more translucent tympanic membrane

Stiffening of the ossicular chain

Degeneration of cells in the inner ear

Degeneration and loss of ganglion cells and eighth cranial nerve fibers

Calcification of inner ear membranes

Reduced cochlear blood supply

Reduced number of functional neurons in the central auditory system

Atrophy and cell loss in auditory areas of the cortex

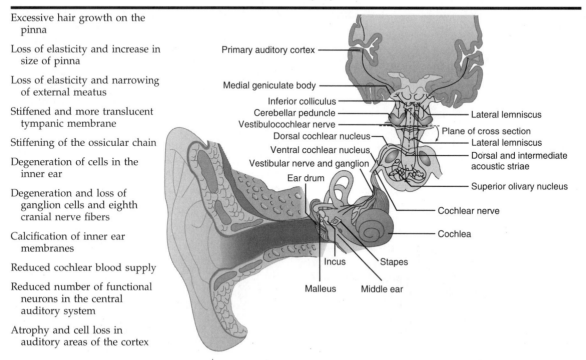

Figure redrawn from Weinstein, B. E. (1989). Geriatric hearing loss: Myths, realities, and resources for the physician. *Geriatrics, 44,* 42.

both that adversely affects the transmission of sound to the inner ear from the external environment (Gulya, 1995). A conductive hearing loss is confirmed when air conduction results demonstrate a hearing deficit but bone conduction results remain normal (Rees et al., 1994). A common contributor to conductive hearing loss is the accumulation of cerumen in the external ear canal. Dry, hard cerumen results from a decrease in the number of ceruminal glands as well as atrophying of the sebaceous glands, producing dry, scaly tissue and itching in the external ear canal. Tumors, perforations, and a history of ear disease also contribute to hearing loss. Conductive hearing loss is generally correctable, depending on the severity of the occlusion.

Otosclerosis. Otosclerosis is one of the most common of the conductive disorders affecting the middle ear, particularly the stapes; it interferes with the interpretation of sound. Otosclerosis, which affects approximately one of 100 older people, is usually bilateral and is believed to be more common in older women than in older men (National Institute on Deafness and Other Communication Disorders, 1992). The condition has been linked with childhood otitis media, measles, and other viral infections of the middle ear. Recent research has resulted in significant progress in the development of implants for the replacement of middle ear ossicles. Surgical intervention in the conductive portion of the ear may be indicated to enhance hearing aid usage.

SENSORINEURAL HEARING LOSS

Sensorineural hearing loss results from changes in the sensorineural mechanism and hair cells or fibers of the cochlear nerve (Gulya, 1995). When a hearing deficit is present, sensorineural hearing loss can be confirmed by both air condition and bone conduction (Rees et al., 1994). Damage to or degeneration of inner ear structures, particularly the cochlea, can cause sensorineural hearing loss, which is an irreversible condition usually not alleviated by medical or surgical intervention. Cochlear transplant research, however, has provided some encouraging results for sensorineural hearing impairment.

Sensorineural auditory dysfunction can also occur from the use of systemic drugs that may induce an ototoxic effect on the auditory system. Such drugs include aminoglycoside antibiotics (e.g., gentamicin, streptomycin, and other broad-spectrum "mycins"); diuretics (e.g., ethacrynic acid and furosemide), which may adversely affect speech discrimination; salicylates (e.g., aspirin); and antiinflammatory agents (e.g., ibuprofen), which may provoke high-frequency tinnitus (Kane et al., 1994).

Presbycusis. The most prevalent and least studied auditory disorder of older adults is presbycusis, which is caused by inner ear degeneration and manifested by a reduction in hearing acuity (Rees et al., 1994). In presbycusis, high-pitched sounds such as g, t, f, and s are affected, as is speech discrimination. Older people tend to be able to hear human voices but have great difficulty in understanding speech communication. These symptoms of hearing loss are not usually recognized before one reaches middle age. Factors contributing to presbycusis include noise overload or exposure, genetic predisposition to early hearing loss, arteriosclerosis, Meniere's syndrome, systemic diseases such as diabetes mellitus, and ototoxic drugs.

Tinnitus. Tinnitus is a high- or low-pitched buzzing or tingling in the ears that often accompanies hearing loss. It tends to affect the left ear more than the right and is more prevalent in men than in women (Hazell, 1987). Tinnitus can be disruptive, especially at night. Vertigo may or may not accompany auditory

alterations caused by tinnitus. Although vertigo has many causes, vertigo with tinnitus may be suggestive of involvement of the vestibular apparatus, thus requiring further investigation (Shulman, 1991). Tinnitus maskers and a soft noise environment may be helpful in controlling the disorder.

MIXED AUDITORY LOSS

Mixed auditory loss involving both conductive and sensorineural hearing loss is more commonly found in older than in younger adults. It can be easily detected when there is a loss of auditory sensitivity for bone conduction in combination with an increased loss of air conduction. One common example of mixed auditory loss is a sensorineural hearing deficit compounded by a cerumen impaction.

ASSESSMENT FACTORS

- Obtain a complete auditory history.
- Assess the appropriateness of responses when eliciting the auditory history and in communicating with the older person.
- Assess hearing acuity in a normal but nondistracting environment.
- Assess the effect of hearing loss on the person's ability to carry out normal activities. The Hearing Handicap Inventory (Ventry & Weinstein, 1992) is useful in screening for auditory disability.
- Observe closely for signs and symptoms of depression, isolation, and/or hostility.
- Assess the client's motivational level for auditory intervention.
- Examine *both* ears with an otoscope to observe for cerumen accumulation and impaction and the presence of otalgia, otitis media, perforation or tympanic membrane perforation or bulging.
- Employ screening tests such as the Weber and the Rinne for air and bone conduction, using a 512-Hz tuning fork held at the base of the instrument, or an audioscope. Rees and colleagues (1994) cautioned that tuning forks, although used frequently in assessing air and bone conduction, may not accurately identify hearing loss in older

people, as hearing loss is primarily in the higher frequencies.

- If it is available, perform an assessment with a screening audiometer, a built-in component of the otoscope, or a portable audiometer (40 dB); these instruments have been effective in audiologic screening programs and evaluations performed in the practitioner's office (Rees et al., 1994).
- Recognize that altered speech discrimination and tinnitus may be initial clues to hearing impairment.
- Safety is a priority, and a home assessment is strongly recommended. A home visit can identify areas for intervention and teaching. Hearing acuity in the office or in a confined quiet space can be entirely different from hearing in one's home, where environmental noises can be distracting to people with hearing disorders.

EMERGENCY CONDITIONS

- Otalgia, bleeding, suppurative drainage, and postoperative complications all constitute an auditory emergency; these patients should be referred to an otolaryngologist.

MANAGEMENT PRIORITIES

- Use strategies to improve communication by first getting the client's attention; then, face to face, speak clearly, distinctly, and unhurriedly.
- Discuss important matters with the older person when he or she is fresh, alert, and able to communicate attentively. Fatigue may hamper the person's ability to hear.
- Allow the older adult ample time to respond to questions. Rephrase the statement if the communication is distorted, unclear, or misunderstood.
- Do *not* shout when speaking to the older person. Use a clear, lower voice modulation.
- Reduce sensory overload in the environment.
- Involve the family and/or staff members in implementing communication strategies.

- For cerumen accumulation, recommend the use of carbamide (Debrox) drops or mineral oil drops at bedtime can aid in softening ear wax. Instruct clients that cotton-tipped applicators should be used only to remove cerumen in the outer portion of the ear canal. A warm-water irrigation may be used if the ear drops fail to remove the impaction. However, irrigation is contraindicated in patients with Meniere's disease and tympanic membrane perforation (Stabb & Lyles, 1990). If an ear spoon is used to remove the impaction, special care must be given to the tympanic membrane to prevent otalgia and bleeding (Yoder, 1995).
- Clients with a known tympanic membrane perforation, a history of mastoidectomy, or a severely occluded ear canal(s) should be referred to an otolaryngologist for cerumen removal (Stabb & Lyles, 1990).
- If a hearing deficit exists, refer elderly patients for audiologic or audiometric testing by a qualified specialist, *prior to* the purchase of hearing devices. Request that hearing aids be brought with the client at the time of his or her next visit. Instruct the client and the family in the operation and control of the hearing device.
- Refer older people diagnosed with sensorineural hearing disorders for aural rehabilitation and orientation, including amplification.
- Keep attuned to new audiologic technologies that can improve the quality of life of older people. Use resources!

GUSTATION AND OLFACTION

The biochemistry of gustation (taste) and olfaction (smell) is considered a young branch of chemosensory science. Much of the work of researchers in the chemical senses has focused on gustation and the taste buds (the chemoreceptors in the oral cavity that serve to stimulate taste associated with sensory and nerve innervation) and with olfactory bulb chemosensation (Wiffenbach, 1991).

Gustation

Taste buds in the oral cavity are enervated by sensory axons from either the facial (VII), glossopharyngeal (IX), or vagal (X) nerves; hence, the posterior tongue, roof of the oral cavity, pharynx, and epiglottis all are involved in the sensation of taste. The presence of an intact nerve supply is essential for taste bud maintenance. Taste transduction occurs on the microvilli of the taste cells; these cells undergo constant processes of birth, differentiation, and replacement, which are poorly understood.

Although gustation may normally be well preserved in older people, alterations may occur through neural changes within the oral cavity, environmental factors, diseases, and medications that affect taste and/or smell (Schiffman, 1997). In the oral cavity, lingual papillae are reduced, and taste buds may be reduced approximately 30% by 70 years of age (Abbey, 1991). Diminished activity of the salivary glands results in diminished production of mucin, leading to mouth dryness (xerostosis). Medications and gingival conditions can also contribute to xerostosis. As a result of these changes, thresholds for the identification of substances (e.g., sweet, sour, salty, bitter) tend to decline. One common contributor to gustatory alteration is smoking. Upper oral prosthetics may also contribute to a decrease in gustatory acuity.

Older people often express concern over unpleasant taste sensations in the mouth, a loss of taste (dysgeusia), the sensation of an unpleasant smell (dysomnia), or a combination of these. An investigation of these alterations may reveal an undiagnosed pharyngeal or esophageal cancer or, more rarely, a central nervous system disorder (Wilson, 1995). Undernutrition can be a significant outcome of normal and pathological changes in taste and smell. A variety of diseases, nutritional deficiencies, and drugs contributing to alterations in gustation and olfaction have been reported. Some diseases and drugs that have contributed to altered gustatory disturbances are shown in Table 22–7.

Olfaction

The sense of smell derives from an elaborate and complex chemosensory system. The olfactory system tends to rely on what Price (1987) described as "parallel activation of its neural machinery" to encode an odor stimulus (p. 81). The retrieval and transfer of information are achieved through the cortical region. This region receives direct information from the main olfactory bulb, which is believed to be directly involved in processing olfactory stimuli and information to the frontal cortex and the hypo-

---

TABLE 22-7

Conditions and Drugs Affecting Taste and Smell

Diseases
Allergies
Alzheimer's disease
Bronchial asthma
Cancer
Epilepsy
Diabetes mellitus
Hypothyroidism
Korsakoff's syndrome
Liver disease
Parkinson's disease
Renal failure or insufficiency
Viral infections
Nutrition
Vitamin deficiencies (vitamins B_3 and B_{12})
Zinc deficiency
Other
Radiation therapy (head)
Drugs
Angiotensin-converting enzyme inhibitors
Anesthetics
Antibiotics
Anticonvulsants
Antidepressants
Antihistamines
Antihypertensives
Antiinflammatories
Antineoplastics
Beta-blockers (selected)
Bronchodilators
Calcium channel blockers
Lipid-lowering agents
Vasodilators

Data from Lawless (1987) and Schiffman (1997).

thalamus. With aging, the olfactory system decreases its sensitivity to odorants. The significance of these chemosensory deficits in older people is the deprivation of their "built-in" warning systems.

The senses of gustation and olfaction significantly affect nutritional patterns. In older people, a greatly diminished atrophy of the bulbs of olfaction and a declining supersensitivity for odor, combined with decreased gustatory acuity, can lead to a reduction in the desire for food (Friedman & Mattes, 1991). Many deficits in primary and cortical sensation continue to go undetected, posing safety hazards in daily living as well as functional alterations.

ASSESSMENT FACTORS

- Assess the oral cavity, noting the use and fit of dental prostheses and the ability to chew. Upper dentures and problems in chewing may alter taste function.
- Assess gustatory nerve function (cranial nerves VII and IX). Test the tongue's ability to taste sweet, sour, salt, and bitter substances. Note the pattern of the papillae and the size of the tongue. Changes in pattern may be indicative of vitamin deficiencies.
- Examine the buccal cavity visually and digitally for evidence of gingivitis, stomatitis, lesions, dental caries, hydration of the mucous membranes, and leukoplakia; this should be done with the dental prosthesis removed, if worn.
- Explore with the older person the possibility of esophageal reflux or regurgitation, a gastric condition that may interfere with or contribute to alterations in taste and appetite. If the condition is present, medical intervention is indicated.
- Assess olfactory nerve function (cranial nerve I) using such products as coffee, lemon juice, cloves, and vanilla to determine the patient's ability to smell. Ammonia, perfumes, and alcohol should be avoided in testing.
- Examine the nasal passages for patency and any evidence of discharge, which may interfere with the ability to smell. Smoking

may reduce the sensations of both smell and taste.

EMERGENCY CONDITIONS

- Age-related changes in gustation and olfaction per se seldom constitute emergency conditions. Nevertheless, alterations in the buccal or nasal cavities may be indicative of serious conditions that require immediate attention. Malnutrition, vitamin deficiencies, and lesions are among these conditions.

MANAGEMENT PRIORITIES

- Maximize gustatory function by pleasantly enhancing nutritious foods using a variety of flavors to improve the taste, such as adding bacon or cheese flavors to soups and vegetables or marinades to meat and poultry (Schiffman, 1997). Add some texture to the food to make it less bland.
- Introduce smaller portions of food to stimulate the appetite. Large portions at mealtime tend to reduce the desire to eat. Offer smaller portions more frequently.
- Introduce pleasant and familiar smells to stimulate taste.
- Encourage meticulous oral hygiene to reduce gingival disorders and improve the sensation of taste. Proper care of dental prosthetics is a must.
- Review medications used by the older adult that may interfere with taste or smell.
- Safety, health, and quality of life can be threatened by changes in olfaction and gustation that directly affect dietary intake, food enjoyment, and the ability to detect harmful odors. Monitor the home environment regularly for evidence of contaminated food, faulty heaters, defective smoke and carbon monoxide detectors, and gas or other noxious odors.

SUMMARY

Sensory-perceptual changes in vision, hearing, taste, and smell are natural concomitants of the aging process. However, pathological changes can occur in the aging sensory system that are quite serious and can threaten the quality of life and safety of the elderly. The advanced practice nurse has a critical role in health promotion, disease detection, and the management of sensory-perceptual alterations. A variety of resources are available locally, statewide, and nationally to assist in sensory rehabilitation. In gerontological nursing, there is no "typical" older person, but a total, complex individual who has unique needs.

REFERENCES

Abbey, J. C. (1991). Physiological illness in aging. In E. M. Baines (Ed.), *Perspectives on gerontological nursing* (pp. 292–293). Newbury Park, CA: Sage.

Bamford, J., & Saunders, E. (1991). *Hearing disorders. Hearing impairment, auditory perception and language disability: Studies of disorders of communication* (pp. 71–75). San Diego, CA: Singular.

Carp, F. M. (1991). Living environments of older adults. In E. M. Baines (Ed.), *Perspectives on gerontological nursing.* (pp. 185–197). Newbury Park, CA: Sage.

Castor, T. D., & Carter, T. L. (1995). Low vision: Physician screening helps to improve patient function. *Geriatrics, 50*(12), 51–57.

Cataract Management Guideline Panel (1993). *Cataracts in adults: Management of functional impairment.* Agency for Health Care Policy and Research Publication No. 93-0542. Rockville, MD: U. S. Department of Health and Human Services, Public Health Service, Agency for Health Care Policy and Research.

Chen, H. (1994). Hearing in the elderly: Relation of hearing loss, loneliness, and self-esteem. *Journal of Gerontological Nursing, 20*(6), 22–28.

Friedman, M. I., & Mattes, R. D. (1991). Chemical senses and nutrition. In T. V. Getchell, L. M. Bartoshuk, R. L. Doty & J. B. Snow (Eds.), *Smell and taste in health and disease* (pp. 391–404). New York: Raven.

Glass, L. E. (1990). Hearing impairment in geriatrics. In B. Kemp, K. Brummel-Smith & J. W. Ramsdell (Eds.), *Geriatric rehabilitation* (pp. 235–253). Boston: Little, Brown.

Gulya, A. J. (1995). Ear Disorders. In W. B. Abrams, M. H. Beers, R. Berkow & A. J. Fletcher (Eds.), *The Merck manual of geriatrics.* (2nd ed., pp. 1315–1342). Whitehouse Station, NJ: Merck & Co., Inc.

Harkins, T. (1993). Geriatric ocular disease. In S. J. Aston & J. H. Maino (Eds.), *Clinical geriatric eye care* (pp. 65–86). Boston: Butterworth-Heinemann.

Hazell, J. (1987). *Tinnitus* (pp. 96–118; 195–197). New York: Churchill-Livingstone.

Heath, J. M. (1992). Vision. In R. J. Ham & P. D. Sloane (Eds.), *Primary care geriatrics: A case-based approach* (2nd ed., pp. 482–497). St. Louis, MO: Mosby–Year Book.

Heckheimer, E. F. (1989). *Health promotion of the elderly in the community.* Philadelphia: W. B. Saunders.

Hooper, C. R. (1994). Sensory and sensory integrative development. In B. R. Bonder & M. B. Wagner (Eds.), *Functional performance in older adults.* (pp. 93–106). Philadelphia: F. A. Davis.

Kane, R. L., Ouslander, J. G., & Abrass, I. B. (1994). Sensory impairment. *Essentials of clinical geriatrics.* (3rd ed., pp. 309–328). New York: McGraw-Hill.

Kupfer, C. (1995). Ophthalmologic disorders. In W. B. Abrams, M. H. Beers, R. Berkow & A. J. Fletcher (Eds.), *The Merck manual of geriatrics* (2nd ed., pp. 1289–1314). Whitehouse Station, NJ: Merck & Co., Inc.

Lawless, H. T. (1987). Gustatory psychophysics. In T. E. Finger & W. L. Silver (Eds.), *Neurobiology of taste and smell.* New York: John Wiley & Sons.

Ludlum, W. M., & Freid, A. N. (1993). A review of non-pathological and pathological changes in the aging eye. In F. Liberman & M. F. Collen (Eds.), *Aging in good health: A quality lifestyle for the later years.* (pp. 91–105). New York: Insight Books.

Mangione, C. M., Phillips, R. S., Seddon, J. M., et al. (1992). Development of the "Activities of Daily Vision Scale". A measure of visual functional status. *Medical Care, 30,* 1111–1126.

Michaels, D. D. (1994). The eye. In W. R. Hazzard, E. L. Bierman, J. P. Blass, et al. (Eds.), *Principles of geriatric medicine and gerontology* (3rd ed., pp. 441–456). New York: McGraw-Hill.

National Institute for Deafness and Other Communication Disorders (1992). *National strategic research plan for hearing and hearing impairment and voice disorders.* National Institutes of Health Publication No. 93-3443. Washington, D.C.: National Institutes of Health Clearinghouse.

Office of Disease Prevention and Health Promotion (1994). *Clinician's handbook of preventive services.* Washington, D.C.: U.S. Department of Health and Human Services, Public Health Service.

Price, J. L. (1987). The central and accessory olfactory systems. In T. E. Finger & W. L. Silver (Eds.), *Neurobiology of taste and smell* (pp. 179–205). New York: Wiley.

Rees, T. S., Duckert, L. G., & Milczuk, H. A. (1994). Auditory & vestibular function. In W. R. Hazzard, E. L. Bierman, J. P. Blass, et al. (Eds.), *Principles of geriatric medicine & gerontology.* (3rd ed., pp. 457–472). New York: McGraw-Hill.

Rubenstein, L. Z., & Lohr, K. N. (1982). Visual impairments. *Conceptualization and measurement of physiologic health for adults. Vol. 12.* Santa Monica, CA: Rand Corporation.

Schiffman, S. S. (1997). Taste and smell losses in normal aging and disease. *Journal of the American Medical Association, 278,* 1357–1362.

Soucek, S., & Michaels, L. (1990). Clinical diagnosis and audiometric studies. *Hearing loss in the elderly.* (pp. 21–28; 103). New York: Springer-Verlag.

Stabb, A. S., & Lyles, M. F. (1990). *Manual of geriatric nursing.* Glenview, IL: Scott Foresman/Little Brown Higher Education.

U. S. Preventive Services Task Force. (1996). *A guide to clinical preventive services.* (2nd ed.). Baltimore: Williams & Wilkins.

Vaughan, D., Asbury, T., & Riordan-Eva, P. (1992). *General ophthalmology* (13th ed.). Norwalk, CT: Appleton and Lange.

Ventry, I., & Weinstein, B. (1992). The hearing handicap for the elderly. *Ear and Hearing, 3,* 128–134.

Weinreb, R. N., Freeman, W. R., & Selezinca, W. (1990). Vision impairment in geriatrics. In B. Kemp, K. Brummel-Smith & J. W. Ramsdell (Eds.), *Geriatric rehabilitation* (pp. 223–251). Boston: Little, Brown.

Wiffenbach, J. M. (1991). Chemical senses in aging. In T. V. Getchell, L. M. Bartoshuk, R. L. Doty & J. B. Snow (Eds.), *Smell and taste in health and disease* (pp. 369–389). New York: Raven.

Wilson, W. R. (1995). Nose and throat disorders. In W. B. Abrams, R. Berkow, M. H. Beers & A. J. Fletcher (Eds.), *The Merck manual of geriatrics* (2nd ed., pp. 1343–1347). Whitehouse Station, NJ: Merck & Co., Inc.

Yoder, M. G. (1995). Geriatric ear, nose and throat problems. In W. Reichel, (Ed.), *Clinical aspects of aging* (4th ed, pp. 441–450). Baltimore: Williams & Wilkins.

APPENDIX 22-1

Resources

VISION

American Council of the Blind
1155 15th Street, N.W.
Suite 720
Washington, D.C. 20005
800-424-8666

American Foundation for the Blind
11 Penn Plaza, Suite 300
New York, NY 10001
212-502-7600
Information Line 800-232-5463

Better Vision Institute
1655 N. Fort Myer Drive
Suite 200
Roslyn, VA 22209
800-424-8422

Lighthouse National Center for Vision & Aging
111 East 59th Street
New York, NY 10022
800-334-5497

National Library Service for the Blind and Physically Handicapped
Talking Books Hotline
Library of Congress
1291 Taylor Street, N.W.
Washington, D.C. 20542
800-424-8567

Prevent Blindness America
500 East Remington Road
Schaumberg, IL 60173
847-843-2020

HEARING

American Academy of Audiology
8201 Greensboro Drive, Suite 300
McLean, VA 22102
703-610-9022

American Speech, Language & Hearing Association
10801 Rockville Pike
Rockville, MD 20852
800-498-2071

American Tinnitus Association
P.O. Box 5
Portland, OR 97207
800-634-8978

Better Hearing Institute
P.O. Box 1840
Washington, DC 20013
800-327-9355

National Association For the Deaf
814 Thayer Avenue
Silver Spring, MD 20910-4500
301-587-1788

National Information Center on Deafness
Gallaudet University
800 Florida Avenue, N.E.
Washington, D.C. 20002
202-651-5051

*National Institute on Deafness and Other
Communication Disorders*
Information Clearinghouse
1 Communication Avenue
Bethesda, MD 20892-3456
800-241-1044

Self-Help For Hard of Hearing People, Inc.
7910 Woodmont Avenue, Suite 1200
Bethesda, MD 20814
301-457-2248

TASTE / VESTIBULAR SENSATION

*National Institute on Deafness and Other
Communication Disorders*
Information Clearinghouse
1 Communication Avenue
Bethesda, MD 20892-3456
800-241-1044

Vestibular Disorders Association
P.O. Box 4467
Portland, OR 97208-4467
503-229-7705

Compiled with the assistance of Lori Shiffman, M.S., O.T.R., and the Virginia Geriatric Education Center, Virginia Commonwealth University, Richmond, VA.

Alcoholism

Sally A. Salisbury

Alcoholism is a chronic, progressive, primary, and fatal disease that afflicts an estimated 10% of the population. Among those older than 65 years, conservative estimates are that 2 to 10% of community-dwelling people, 7% to 22% of those hospitalized for medical problems, and 40% of those residing in nursing homes suffer significant alcohol-related problems (Fink et al., 1996; National Institute on Alcohol Abuse and Alcoholism, 1995; Wartenberg & Nirenberg, 1995). The elderly alcoholic is often undiagnosed, yet consequences of continued drinking may include the unsuccessful treatment of concomitant diseases, loss of cognitive and motor ability, and failure to thrive. This chapter defines the disease of alcoholism and describes the clinical presentation of the elderly alcoholic. The section on clinical consequences of alcoholism in the elderly addresses common

psychiatric and medical problems related to continued alcohol abuse. The section on assessment presents guidelines for diagnosing the disease of alcoholism. The final sections on treatment provide information for clinicians on various treatment approaches and also address the issue of codependency in professional healthcare providers.

THE DISEASE OF ALCOHOLISM

There are many different definitions of an alcoholic and alcoholism. Most concisely, an *alcoholic* is a person who is addicted to alcohol. The Joint Committee of the National Council on Alcoholism and Drug Dependency and the American Society of Addiction Medicine define alcoholism as follows:

The revision of this chapter was built on the work of Carole Chenitz, RN, EdD.

a primary, chronic disease with genetic, psychosocial, and environmental factors influencing its development and manifestations. The disease is often progressive and fatal. It is characterized by impaired control over drinking, preoccupation with the drug alcohol, use of alcohol despite adverse consequences and distortion in thinking, most notably denial.

MORSE & FLAVIN, 1992, pp. 1012–1014

Alcoholics Anonymous (AA) defines an alcoholic as a person who has lost control. According to AA, alcoholism is a chronic progressive illness characterized by a physical sensitivity (allergy) to alcohol and a mental obsession with drinking that cannot be stopped by the use of willpower (AA, 1976). Forrest (1994) identified four characteristics that define an alcoholic: the drinking is compulsive, is of long duration, and results in intoxication; and the drinking behavior patterns interfere with interpersonal function.

The American Psychiatric Association (APA) defines alcohol abuse, alcohol intoxication, and alcohol dependence separately. *Alcohol abuse* is the recurrent use of alcohol that results in clinically significant impairment or distress as manifested by one or more of the following: (1) a failure to fulfill obligations at home or work, (2) legal problems, (3) social and interpersonal problems, and (4) the use of alcohol in physically hazardous situations (APA, 1994). *Alcohol intoxication* is determined if the patient has recently ingested alcohol and displays significant maladaptive behaviors, such as inappropriate sexual or aggressive behavior and poor judgment. In addition, the patient has one or more of the following signs that cannot be explained by a general medical condition or mental disorder: slurred speech, incoordination, unsteady gait, nystagmus, impairment in attention or memory, or stupor (APA, 1994). A clinical diagnosis of alcohol intoxication does not alone preclude a diagnosis of alcoholism. Addiction in the elderly is defined as the frequent use of a potentially addictive substance that is associated with biomedical, psychological, or social consequences or that puts the person at risk for developing symptoms of withdrawal (Solomon et al., 1993). *Alcohol dependence* is characterized by tolerance, withdrawal symptoms,

and a pattern of compulsive use (APA, 1994). The criteria for dependence as they relate to the elderly are discussed in greater detail later in the chapter. Forrest chronicled the developmental stages of the disease of alcoholism, as shown in Table 23–1.

The disease of alcoholism typically has periods of remission and relapse. The individual may achieve sobriety for brief or long periods, sometimes many years, and then relapse into active drinking and alcoholic behavior until treatment is resumed. It is important that healthcare providers understand relapse as a part of the disease and not give up or fail to offer treatment options. The causes of alcoholism are still not clearly defined. Relevant theories of the cause of alcoholism are summarized in Table 23–2.

ALCOHOLISM IN THE ELDERLY

Advanced practice nurses may encounter older people with alcohol-related problems across a variety of clinical settings; these may include the elderly alcoholic's own home or apartment or a retirement or life care facility. Nurses in acute care, particularly those practicing in an emergency department, are likely to encounter elderly alcoholics (Tabisz et al., 1991).

Elderly alcoholics, like their younger counterparts, show great variations in physical and psychosocial characteristics; the process of identifying the older alcoholic, the older alcoholic's patterns of life problems and physical complaints associated with alcoholism, and the assessment and treatment of alcoholism all show similarities to those in younger age groups (Schuckit, 1990). However, some factors and differences need to be considered. Studies have indicated that determinants specifically

TABLE 23-1
Developmental Stages of Alcoholism

Stage 1: Experimental and Social Drinking

The potential alcoholic experiences different
reinforcement from drinking and intoxication than the
nonalcoholic during initial contacts with alcohol
consumption. Alcohol helps the person feel better, and
he or she learns that drinking can bring relief from
anxiety and depression. The potential alcoholic
indulges in periods of relief drinking that are usually
well controlled and free of long-lasting consequences
during this stage.

Stage 2: Excessive Drinking

Considerably more time is spent drinking; the individual
begins to minimize the amount of drinking he or she
tells others about and now drinks to prepare himself or
herself before anticipated stressful occasions. In this
stage, relationships become primarily those associated
with drinking, and increased tolerance for alcohol
develops.

Stage 3: Alcohol Addiction

The alcoholic's drinking is out of control, and the
individual is unable to stop drinking until he or she
loses consciousness or becomes too ill to continue
drinking. Amnesia for periods of drinking may
develop. The individual becomes progressively more
isolated, and family, peer relationships, and work life
are adversely affected. Increasing feelings of remorse
and self-hatred may lead to suicide.

Stage 4: Chronic Alcoholism

The drinker may drink continually and, if alcohol is not
available, may substitute substances containing alcohol
(e.g., mouthwash). As a result of years of continuous
drinking, tolerance often diminishes. Continued drinking no longer brings pleasure or relief, but not drinking
leads to withdrawal. In this stage, medical
complications, cirrhosis, peripheral neuropathy,
gastrointestinal illness, cognitive impairment, and
pancreatitis may be present.

Data from Forrest (1994).

related to alcohol problems in the elderly include a history of alcohol use and abuse, social
isolation, reduced mobility, and being male,
single, and relatively well educated (Fink et
al., 1996).

For several reasons, the unique manifestations of alcoholism in the elderly may make its
recognition and diagnosis difficult (Marion &
Stefanik-Campisi, 1990). Medical- or alcohol-

related cognitive loss may invalidate self-report, families themselves may be in denial or
may minimize the amount of drinking to protect the elderly family member, and the symptoms of prolonged drinking may be subtle and

TABLE 23-2
Theories of the Cause of Alcoholism

Genetic Theory

Inherited genetic personality traits influence the
susceptibility to and control over the addictive process,
protective factors, psychiatric disorders that may lead
to alcoholism, and the predisposition toward medical
complications.
Research includes efforts to isolate genetic components
related to the inheritance of alcohol metabolism as well
as linkage studies to identify genetic components in
behavioral characteristics.

Personality Theory

Characteristics or clusters of traits predispose an
individual to alcoholism. Traits include exaggerated
sensitivities, poor impulse control, low tolerance to
frustration, dependency, weak ego, emotional and
sexual immaturity, inability to delay gratification, and
feelings of powerlessness.
Research cannot document a causal relationship between
personality traits and alcoholism. No single trait or
cluster has been established for all alcoholics.

Behavioral Learning Theory

Drinking is a learned behavior that produces
psychological rewards for the individual. Rewards
perpetuate the drinking, and addiction follows.

Cultural Theory

Certain cultural groups have a lower incidence of
alcoholism and may define specific ways in which
alcohol can be used in limited amounts.

Social Theory

Alcoholism is the result of social deprivation,
hopelessness, poverty, feelings of anomie, and
powerlessness. Alcohol is used as an antidote to
negative social forces.

Multifocal/Multicausal Theory

No single theory explains alcoholism. The interaction
among personality, genetics, and social and cultural
forces produces alcoholism.

Data from Anthenelli & Schuckit (1992); Denzin (1987a,
1987b); Goldman (1987–1988); Kaplan et al. (1994); and
Reich (1987–1988).

less obvious than in the younger drinker (Adams et al., 1992). The elderly may present with medical problems or signs of alcohol abuse that may be confused with signs associated with aging, such as changes in appetite or in the sleep-wake cycle (Krach, 1990).

The APA's criteria for substance dependence are presented here with modifications to describe the elderly alcoholic. According to the APA, substance dependence is "a maladaptive pattern of substance use, leading to clinically significant impairment or distress, as manifested by three [or more] of the following, occurring at any time in the same 12-month period" (APA, 1994, p. 181).

1. *Tolerance* is defined as a need for increased amounts of the substance to achieve the desired effect, or a decreased effect with the same amount of substance. The elderly may experience intoxication and problems with lower consumption owing to age-related changes, which include increased brain susceptibility to the depressant effects of alcohol, a decreased rate of liver metabolism, and a decline in total body water content (APA, 1994). The relatively complete absorption of alcohol and smaller volume in which alcohol is distributed may cause the elderly to attain higher blood levels than a young, robust person drinking the same amount (Blazer, 1995; Solomon et al., 1993).

2. *Withdrawal* occurs when alcohol intake is substantially decreased or stopped without the substitution of other forms of sedation. The severity of withdrawal depends on the individual's general health, quantity of alcohol consumed, duration of last drinking episode, and history of severe withdrawal. Minor manifestations of withdrawal appear within 36 hours after drinking has stopped. Alcohol withdrawal seizures occur most frequently within 2 days of cessation, and delirium tremens occurs within 5 days of abstinence (Greenberg, 1993). Symptoms of withdrawal are summarized in Table 23–3. It is possible that the elderly alcoholic will not be identified; when drinking is suddenly interrupted by hospitalization

TABLE 23-3

Symptoms of Withdrawal

Minor	Severe
Tremor, insomnia	Gross tremor, insomnia
Diaphoresis	Profuse diaphoresis
Anxiety	Extreme restlessness
Agitation	Agitation
Loss of appetite	
Alcohol withdrawal seizures	
Disturbed perception; benign hallucinations	Delusions
	Frightening hallucinations
Brief minimal disorientation	Profound disorientation
Tachycardia	Tachycardia
Elevated blood pressure	Elevated blood pressure
Nausea and vomiting	Fever

Data from Eisendrath (1997); and Greenberg (1993).

for an acute illness, for example, sudden-onset withdrawal may occur but may be undiagnosed. The consequences may be life-threatening tachycardia, seizures, or extreme agitation.

3. Larger amounts of alcohol are consumed and over a longer period than was intended. The elderly alcoholic is often an isolated individual, and data about the amount and duration of drinking often are not available.

4. There is a persistent desire to drink; attempts to cut down or control alcohol use are unsuccessful.

5. An extensive amount of time is spent in activities necessary to obtain and use alcohol and to recover from its effects. Many elderly become very efficient in obtaining alcohol; for example, local markets or friendly neighbors may deliver alcohol daily. Many drinkers find residences close to stores or taverns. In some long-term care institutions, personnel may become willing providers of contraband substances in exchange for money.

6. "Important social, occupational or recreational activities are given up or reduced because of substance abuse" (APA, 1994, p. 181). The elderly alcoholic is usually retired. He or she may have outlived many colleagues and cohorts. Often, the elderly alcoholic has another valid physi-

cal rationalization for giving up hobbies or activities, and drinking is not suspected.

7. The drinking of alcohol continues "despite knowledge of having a persistent or recurrent physical or psychological problem that is likely to have been caused by or exacerbated by" drinking (APA, 1994, p. 181). The elderly alcoholic may intellectually understand the physical consequences of continued drinking but still choose to remain in the disease, rationalizing that the effects of prolonged drinking are already irremediable. One elderly patient clearly stated this when he said, "My legs are already shot. I need one of these contraptions to get around. I have nothing to look forward to so I'll just stay drunk."

It is now widely accepted that there are two types of elderly alcoholics: the chronic long-standing alcoholic and the late-onset alcoholic (Gambert, 1992). The majority are chronic long-standing alcoholics whose drinking has persisted over time and into old age (American Medical Association [AMA] Council on Scientific Affairs, 1996; Blazer, 1995); they are young alcoholics grown old. These elderly alcoholics are considered survivors, as there is a high mortality rate among alcoholics as a group. One study found a 24% mortality rate of alcoholics aged 55 years and older (N = 21,139) during the 4 years after an index episode of care—a mortality rate 2.64 times higher than expected (Moos et al., 1994). The older chronic alcoholic typically has multiple concomitant diagnoses: coronary artery disease; pulmonary disease; cirrhosis; gastric, pancreatic, endocrine, and blood system disorders; and organic psychosis (AMA Council on Scientific Affairs, 1996; APA, 1994; Fink et al., 1996). The combination of multiple medical problems, social isolation, scant resources, and substance abuse often make these patients outliers in a system of managed care. Continued drinking, noncompliance with treatment, and poor outcomes all contribute to the negative stereotyping many healthcare professionals carry for the older alcoholic.

A late-onset alcoholic is a person whose pattern of moderate drinking changed during old age. This change is often the result of or response to specific stressors such as the losses associated with aging (Schuckit, 1990). There is some evidence that common conditions in later life make the elderly susceptible to alcoholism. These conditions are (1) retirement, which can produce boredom, loss of income, low self-esteem, and a change in role status; (2) the death of family and friends; (3) poor health, decreased mobility, pain, and distress; and (4) loneliness (Brody, 1982; Wartenberg & Nirenberg, 1995). When confronted with the inevitable stressor of increasing age, problem drinkers are more likely to use cognitive avoidance responses to negative life events (Moos et al., 1990). Women with late-life drinking problems differ from men with similar problems in that they tend to consume less alcohol, have a later onset of drinking problems, and experience stressors more related to their family and spouse than to financial problems (Brennan et al., 1993).

Although any alcoholic may be a candidate for rehabilitation, the late-onset alcoholic whose drinking is a reaction to a traumatic loss is the most responsive to treatment (Forrest, 1994). These patients often respond very positively to alcohol recovery programs, especially if they are accompanied by environmental interventions. It is worthwhile to take a careful alcohol history and perform a physical assessment to distinguish late-onset from chronic alcoholism. The onset of dementia may be accompanied by an increase in problem drinking. Associated anxiety, depression, and a feeling of loss of control may precipitate excessive drinking. The cognitive loss associated with intoxication may cause the dementia to seem more severe than it is and may exacerbate behavior and management problems. In summary, the late-onset elderly alcoholic may not present with the constellation of medical complications of long-term alcoholism but nevertheless challenges the clinician with a different set of psychiatric and psychosocial problems.

CLINICAL CONSEQUENCES OF ALCOHOLISM

Alcoholism threatens the independent living status of those affected with the disease

(Pizzi & Mion, 1993). The advanced practice nurse who has an understanding of the clinical consequences of alcoholism is in an excellent position to address the physical, social, and psychological needs of this challenging group of patients. One study of an academic general medicine clinic found that by adding a two-item alcoholism screening instrument to the intake process, nursing staff members were successful in screening 90.4% of the 1328 patients needing alcoholism counseling (Goldberg et al., 1991). Nurses are also in a powerful advocacy and education position and can be instrumental in establishing programs and protocols for the provision of services in a variety of other healthcare settings (Parette et al., 1990). The consequences of alcoholism for the elderly are multifactorial and interrelated and are roughly classified as psychiatric and medical.

Psychiatric Consequences

Depression. Patterns of comorbidity of alcoholism, anxiety, and depression are well established (Merikangas et al., 1994; Solomon et al., 1993). Alcoholism and depression have been associated with suicide attempts and suicides in the elderly (AMA Council on Scientific Affairs, 1996). As the alcoholic inevitably experiences depression, shame, hopelessness, guilt, and low self-esteem during the course of the disease, the risk of suicide increases. Twenty percent of female alcoholics and 5% of male alcoholics have reported suicide attempts (Fulop et al., 1993). Screening for depression and suicidal ideation should be done early in treatment (i.e., as soon as sobriety is achieved) and can be conducted in any inpatient or outpatient setting. This topic is discussed further in the chapter on depression (see Chapter 17). Treatment for depression can be undertaken early in recovery, once drinking is controlled, but active drinking delays any psychotherapeutic treatment. Pharmacological treatment of depression should not be undertaken with a patient who is actively drinking; such treatment is dangerous because of the potentiating effect of alcohol.

Cognitive Loss. Chronic alcohol use can cause a wide range of cognitive deficits as well as memory loss related to vitamin deficiencies (particularly of the B vitamins), neurotoxicity, or repeated head trauma (Solomon et al., 1993; Victor, 1993). Cognitive losses associated with chronic alcoholism are described in Chapter 18 on dementia. Although sobriety, good nutrition, and hydration can partially reverse these neuropathological changes and improve performance, some cognitive deficits may be permanent (Feldman & Plum, 1993; Parsons & Nixon, 1993). The nurse or other members of the healthcare team will then need to assist the family or patient in determining an appropriate level of care at which the patient's function can be supplemented by environmental supports.

Common Medical Consequences

Malnutrition. Regular alcohol use by elderly individuals has been shown to decrease total caloric and protein intake and cause lower serum albumin levels in patients, even when food intake is adequate (Solomon et al., 1993). Chronic alcoholism produces delayed gastric emptying (Sankaran et al., 1994), malabsorption, and an increased excretion of nutrients. Alcoholic gastritis and esophageal inflammation may hinder the intake and absorption of food. Pancreatitis, an uncommon but serious complication of ingesting large quantities of alcohol, is another factor in malnutrition. Multiple pancreatic cysts may form but are amenable to surgical intervention (Fedorak et al., 1994). Nutritional support is an important part of treatment. Many chronic alcoholics have developed very poor eating habits. They may have lost the taste for food, and attempts to eat may be followed by nausea, vomiting, and abdominal pain. Nutritional support is an important adjunct to treatment. Simple but nourishing, easily digested foods in small, frequent meals should be supplemented with thiamine and additional feedings, if needed. The recovering alcoholic needs to relearn or learn good nutritional habits and to rediscover the pleasure and nurture of eating good food.

Cirrhosis of the Liver. Since the 1970s, there has been a substantial decline in deaths caused by liver cirrhosis in this country (Smart & Mann, 1991). Nevertheless, chronic alcoholics are highly susceptible to liver cirrhosis because the long-term ingestion of alcohol produces nutritional deficits and an increased susceptibility to industrial toxins, both of which are correlated with liver disease (Lieber, 1994). Liver pathology may result in hepatic encephalopathy, causing sudden-onset confusion, hallucinosis, and a fluctuating mental state that may be mistaken for a brain syndrome. Cirrhosis is a progressive and eventually fatal disease, but much can be done to delay the progress of the disease and to alleviate symptoms such as confusion, edema, or ascites. The medical management of cirrhosis is complex and requires close collaboration among the patient, physician, and nurse. Treatment is aimed at reducing the workload of the incompetent liver and reducing toxicity levels by curtailing dietary protein during acute episodes, administering lactulose to prevent toxins from being absorbed by the bowel, and administering neomycin to control the intestinal flora of the bowel. Ascites can be treated with dietary sodium and fluid restrictions, diuretics, and/or paracentesis. Coagulation abnormalities can result from a failure to synthesize clotting constituents in the liver. Bleeding that tends to occur is treated with vitamin K preparations, and transfusions may be necessary (Friedman, 1997). The disease has a fluctuating course and progressively worsens over time. Alcoholics are not considered liver transplant candidates in most transplant centers. However, their quality of life can be enhanced and their life prolonged with close monitoring and aggressive symptom management.

Seizures. It has long been assumed that seizures occur in chronic alcoholics as a result of alcohol withdrawal and ethanol toxicity. Recent studies have shown a correlation between the number of times a person has undergone detoxification and the probability that that person will have a seizure disorder (Lechtenberg & Horner, 1992). It is now thought that seizures occur in alcoholics because of the short-term kindling effect of recurrent detoxifications as well as the short-term effects of alcohol exposure (McCowen & Breese, 1990). Most emergency department personnel are familiar with the alcoholic who has a seizure disorder. However, it was the summary opinion of the First International Symposium on Alcohol and Seizures (held in 1988 in Washing-

ton, D.C.) that a significant number of these patients would have comorbidity and/or an underlying process that might cause mortality. Patients with status epilepticus should be given a workup and treated regardless of whether it is caused by alcoholism; hospitalization, a computed tomography scan, and the use of sedatives and anticonvulsants are required. Patients need a quiet protected environment, skilled nursing care, and frequent close observation until seizures are controlled, regardless of the cause of the seizures.

Infections. When alcoholics present with fever, the cause is often assumed to be related to alcohol withdrawal. Given the general poor health and poor living situations of many elderly alcoholics, all fevers require a workup. Pneumonia and occult urinary tract infections were seen surprisingly often in one study (Wrenn & Larson, 1991). Also of interest in this study was the number of noninfectious causes of fever, existing alone or coexisting with an infectious cause; subarachnoid hemorrhage and a postictal state were the most common of these (Wrenn & Larson, 1991). Although Wrenn and Larson advocated hospitalization for all alcoholics presenting with fever of unknown origin, this may not always be possible. However, active outreach programs, case finding, and an assertive home nursing program may successfully treat at least the infectious causes with outpatient care.

Gait Disorders. Gait and balance disorders are among the most disabling effects of long-term alcohol use seen in the elderly. The potential causes are numerous: cerebellar degeneration; neuropathies resulting from vitamin deficiencies and ethanol toxicity; and muscle weakness caused by myopathy, peripheral neuropathy, hypokalemia, and deconditioning. Orthostatic hypotension can result from peripheral or autonomic neuropathy (Solomon et al., 1993). Although recent studies question whether falls are increasingly associated with alcohol use in the elderly (Nelson et al., 1992), gait disorders are known to severely limit mobility and decrease independence. The older alcoholic patient often walks with a hesitant, wide-based gait, rigid arms, and a forward-leaning stance. Turning balance is often poor, and proprioceptor sense is decreased. Typically the feet do not pass each other in stride, and the feet may not raise or show ventral flexion, causing the person to walk with a low slapping step.

With sobriety, the gait disorder may cease to worsen but may also show little improvement. However, mobility can be increased with vigorous physical therapy and rehabilitation nursing. The use of walking aids, walkers, or canes as well as wheelchairs for long trips can increase independence and mobility. Before the patient returns home, it is essential to conduct a home visit to assess for safety; suggest which hazards should be removed; and determine the need for restorative equipment such as hand rails, raised commode chairs, and shower benches. Physical or occupational therapy in extended care or in the home can do much to teach adaptive techniques. Most important, the patient must be motivated and sober before rehabilitation can be undertaken. Peripheral neuropathies are often very painful, and the pain can become as disabling as the neuromuscular degeneration. Regular dosing with nonsteroidal antiinflammatory agents is effective if there are no concurrent gastrointestinal illnesses. Topical application of capsaicin (Zostrix), an antiirritant that gradually saturates peripheral nerve endings and blocks the transmission of pain impulses, has been shown to be very effective if used regularly.

Cardiovascular. Although current studies show that light to moderate alcohol consumption can be correlated with improved health, the persistent abuse of alcohol has a negative effect on the cardiovascular system (Klatsky et al., 1992; Iso et al., 1995; Ridker et al., 1994). Cardiomegaly; cardiac fibroses; microvascular infarcts and swelling; and altered subcellular myocardial components, glycogen, and lipid deposition are seen with chronic alcohol ingestion (Gambert, 1992). Myocardial contractility and output are reduced, and tachycardia can occur (Gambert, 1992). Sudden death, stroke, hypertension, and heart failure all have been associated with chronic heavy drinking (Ahlawat & Siwach, 1994).

ASSESSMENT

The first step in treatment is to discover and uncover the often hidden signs of alcoholism (Goodman, 1988). Several instruments are available to screen older people for alcohol problems (Buchsbaum et al., 1992; Fink et al., 1996; Willenbring et al., 1987). The patient history should include questions about the pattern of life problems to assess if alcohol may be a contributory factor.

The American Geriatrics Society (AGS) has developed clinical guidelines to assist clinicians with the assessment and management of alcohol use disorders in older adults (AGS, 1997). The guidelines recommend that all people older than 65 years be asked at least annually about their alcohol use. Specific questions should be asked about drinking behavior and drinking patterns, such as the kind and amount of alcohol consumed as well as the frequency of such drinking. If possible, additional information should be obtained from family members or a friend (Blazer, 1995; Schuckit, 1990). Following the inquiry on the type, frequency, and quantity of alcohol use, the AGS guidelines recommend that the CAGE screening questionnaire be used with people who indicate any use of alcohol. The CAGE instrument consists of four questions (AGS, 1997):

C: Have you ever felt you should *cut down* on your drinking?
A: Have people *annoyed* you by criticizing your drinking?
G: Have you ever felt bad or *guilty* about your drinking?
E: Have you ever had a drink (*eye opener*) first thing in the morning to steady your nerves or to get rid of a hangover?

Based on the assessment findings, drinking is classified as light, safe, or heavy and/or risky (Table 23–4).

The CAGE questionnaire has been found to effectively discriminate between elderly people with and without a history of a drinking problem; it also discriminates between elderly people with and without alcohol abuse and dependence. However, this questionnaire does not distinguish active from inactive drinkers (Buchsbaum et al., 1992; Fink et al., 1996).

Mental status should be assessed for possible cognitive deficits and for a baseline value to monitor changes that may occur over time (Blazer, 1995). The physical assessment may

TABLE 23-4
Classification of Drinking

Classification	Amount/Frequency	CAGE Score		Dysfunction Related to Drinking		Use of Medications
Light, safe drinking	On average, ≤1 drink/day, or ≤7 drinks/week, or ≤3 drinks on heavy drinking occasion	0	*and*	No evidence of physical, psychological, or social dysfunction related to drinking	*and*	Not using medications that interact adversely with alcohol
Heavy and/or risky drinking	On average, >1 drink/day, or >7 drinks/week, or >3 drinks on heavy drinking occasion	Any drinking and ≥1 on the CAGE	*or*	Evidence of drinking-related dysfunction	*or*	Using medications that may interact adversely with alcohol

Adapted from American Geriatrics Society (1997). *Clinical guidelines on alcohol use disorders in older adults,* New York: American Geriatrics Society.

uncover signs and symptoms of intoxication or withdrawal. Signs and symptoms of the clinical consequences of long-term drinking described in the previous section should alert the clinician to active or remittent alcoholism. Most practitioners are familiar with the classic signs of the alcoholic: spider hemangiomas on the face, ecchymoses, palmar erythema, an enlarged liver, unsteady gait, muscle wasting, hand tremors, and cognitive losses. However, these signs may be mistakenly attributed to other disorders or advanced age (Gambert, 1992).

Relevant laboratory abnormalities may provide clues to alcoholism (AGS, 1997; Blazer, 1995). An elevated gamma-glutamyltransferase level is a sensitive indicator of heavy drinking, as 70% of individuals with a high level (>30 units) are persistent heavy drinkers (APA, 1994). Deficiencies of B vitamins and toxic effects of alcohol on erythropoiesis may cause an elevation of the mean corpuscular volume. Liver function tests (e.g., lactase dehydrogenase, aspartate aminotransferase or serum glutamic-oxaloacetic transaminase, alanine aminotransferase or serum glutamate pyruvate transaminase, and alkaline phosphatase) may reveal liver damage that can be a consequence of heavy long-term drinking. A stool guaiac test should be done (Blazer, 1995). Blood alco-

hol levels can be used to assess tolerance to alcohol. A concentration of 100 mg of ethanol per dL of blood in an individual who does not show intoxication may indicate the development of some degree of tolerance (AGS, 1997; APA, 1994). However, the elderly do not maintain tolerance to alcohol as they age, so this test may give false negatives with older patients.

Once an alcohol problem has been identified, further exploration is needed to determine the older person's perception of the problem, the readiness to accept treatment, and the type of treatment needed. Brief intervention approaches that provide counseling and education can be effective as the first step toward preventing progression of the problem (AGS, 1997; AMA Council on Scientific Affairs, 1996; Samet et al., 1996).

TREATMENT ISSUES FOR THE PROFESSIONAL

Countertransference and Codependency

This section of the chapter deals with issues that may decrease the effectiveness of the practitioner, particularly in settings in which contacts with the patient are usually more protracted than those in an acute care setting. Countertransference and codependency issues must be recognized and processed if therapeutic effectiveness is to be maintained. This brief discussion is presented only to bring the issues into awareness and to suggest some avenues that can provide help and resources.

Countertransference refers to the totality of feelings that nurses experience toward the patient, whether these feelings are conscious or unconscious and whether they relate to the patient or to significant others in their life (Katz, 1990). This process is natural and unavoidable and can be helpful in fostering empathy for the patient and a deeper understanding of self and patient (Katz, 1990). Melody Beattie defined codependency as follows: "A codependent person is one who has let another person's behavior affect him or her, and who is obsessed with controlling that person's behavior" (Beattie, 1992, p. 36). Codependent people tend to appear as if others depend on them, often to an extensive degree; but in reality, they depend on others, needing others' well-being and gratitude to feel good about themselves.

Although codependent people appear to be controlling, they actually feel helpless and experience feelings that are controlled by the people they appear to serve (Beattie, 1992). Codependent people often become overextended and then experience feelings of anger, resentment, and exhaustion—feelings that are often referred to as *burnout* among professionals. Codependent professionals have difficulty setting boundaries and tend to relate to patients as if they were friends. As friends, they may participate in the denial of the disease of alcoholism, make excuses for the patient, not confront the patient, and take over functions and tasks that the patient should do for himself or herself. The codependent nurse often experiences shame at being unable to cure the patient or stop the patient's drinking. As a result, the nurse may blame himself or herself for the patient's continued substance abuse.

The cycle of shame and blame is central to the relationship between the codependent nurse and the alcoholic patient (Robinson, 1990). One of the basic tenets of Al-Anon for families of alcoholics is that another individual is not responsible for the alcoholic or his or her disease. This is expressed in the statement, "You didn't cause it, you can't cure it, and you can't control it." Only the alcoholic can deal with his or her disease. This realization can help bring about needed detachment in the helping person, professional, or family. Detachment is the only way to cease the cycle of shame and blame, overhelping, and rejecting that characterizes a codependent relationship (Robinson, 1990).

Time and effort spent attempting to control a patient are time and effort taken away from providing the help that can actually be given: interventions aimed at education, reasonable support, and managing those medical and functional problems that can be addressed. Self-monitoring by care providers is essential to maintain objectivity and detachment (Robinson, 1990).

Supervision, consultation, and education all are helpful in detaching from codependent nurse-patient relationships. Supervision and consultation may be obtained from professionals in the field of substance abuse. Attending Al-Anon meetings can also be helpful. The time and location of local meetings can be obtained by calling the county Alcohol Services Center. Al-Anon also publishes a newsletter for professionals.

TREATMENT OF ALCOHOLISM IN THE ELDERLY

The goal of treatment for alcoholism is recovery. *Recovery* is a state in which addicted individuals are at peace with themselves and others and experience a sense of an ever-improving quality of life. *Sobriety,* defined as complete abstinence from alcohol and mood-altering chemicals, is basic to recovery (AMA Council on Scientific Affairs, 1996; Eisendrath, 1997; Gambert, 1992). Complete abstinence is necessary because there is a cross-tolerance between alcohol and other mood-altering drugs, such as barbiturates and anxiolytics. It is not uncommon for an alcoholic to stop drinking and to use other mood-altering drugs, both legal and illegal, to replace the alcohol. In this way, the individual stops the recovery process, which requires that the patient be willing to experience reality and discontinue the pattern of altering it with chemicals.

Detoxification

The first steps in treatment are abstinence, detoxification, and treatment of the minor symptoms of withdrawal. Withdrawal from alcohol must be carefully executed, particularly in the elderly. Alcohol withdrawal includes symptoms such as anxiety; irritability; an increase in heart rate, blood pressure, and temperature; and diaphoresis. Serious symptoms include hallucinations, convulsions, and delirium (Eisendrath, 1997; Greenberg, 1993). The symptoms associated with delirium tremens can be avoided by the use of medications specific for detoxification. Medications should be carefully titrated according to the severity of symptoms to assist the individual in withdrawing smoothly from alcohol. Benzodiazepines remain the medication of choice for treating withdrawal (Schuckit, 1990; Wartenberg & Nirenberg, 1995). One standard method is to prescribe the equivalent daily dose of benzodiazepine that would correspond to the patient's average daily alcohol ingestion and to then decrease this dose by 10% every other day. Adrenergic agents such as clonidine and atenolol are useful adjuncts in the treatment of withdrawal symptoms (Bohn, 1993). In the older patient, however, careful monitoring of vital signs and the level of alertness are needed to prevent drug toxicity and overdose of benzodiazepines. Benzodiazepine toxicity may significantly prolong hospitalization, and the use of the shorter-acting benzodiazepines, although less likely to cause toxicity, may not be effective in preventing seizure (Hill & Williams, 1993).

During detoxification, elderly patients have more withdrawal symptoms for a longer period than do younger patients; they also require medication over a longer period. The elderly have been shown to experience more symptoms of cognitive impairment, daytime sleepiness, weakness, and elevated blood pressure (Brower et al., 1994). Other aspects of treatment include restoring fluid and electrolyte balance by slow hydration of 500 to 1000 mL of 0.45% NaCl and the use of dietary supplements, especially the B vitamins and magnesium (Blazer, 1995; Wartenberg & Nirenberg, 1995).

Barriers to Treatment

Once detoxification is complete and abstinence has been achieved, the next step—one that is crucial for recovery—is for the alcoholic to admit that he or she has a disease that is out of control and to express a sincere wish to achieve lasting recovery. The following step is referral and admission to an alcohol treatment program. It is at this critical juncture that barriers may present themselves. Barriers may come from the patient in the form of denial or from the treatment personnel themselves in their attitudes toward alcoholism and aging (AMA Council on Scientific Affairs, 1996). Entrenched denial on the part of the patient may be confronted by marshaling the patient's family, medical personnel, community workers, neighbors, or friends to express their concern to the patient and to verbally acknowledge how the alcoholic's disease and its behavioral consequences are affecting his or her relationships. Creating a unified and informed intervention team that is sensitive to aging issues can be effective in leading the elderly alcoholic to a desire to change. All elderly people have a network that can be employed or created to move the client to an acceptance of the need for help (Lindblom et al., 1992).

A barrier to treatment for the older alcoholic may be an unrecognized ageism on the part of alcohol treatment staff members. The operating myth may be, "So what if they drink; if I were that age, I would too." Ageism may create therapeutic nihilism concerning the older client, as reflected in attitudes such as, "They aren't going to change now; they are too old to change" (Walker & Kelly, 1981). Nurses' attitudes toward alcoholics are marked by ambivalence and negativity (Naegle, 1983). Research into nurses' attitudes has found that although nurses accept the disease concept, they also believe that the alcoholic can stop drinking if he or she really wants to. Some reasons for nurses attitudes are feelings of frustration and discouragement during their first experiences with alcoholic clients; nurses' expectations of treatment; and nurses' personal values and beliefs combined with the chronic relapsing nature of the disease and its behavioral manifestations (Burkhalter, 1975).

The older alcoholic may not enter treatment until he or she has serious medical problems. Often the elderly alcoholic enters an alcohol treatment program from a general hospital or is referred by a primary care physician. Acute medical problems will of course have to be assessed, diagnosed, and treated; medical problems that are nonacute or of long-standing duration, however, can be controlled but should not be the focus of treatment. Once a patient is in a treatment program, medical problems can interfere with the treatment of alcoholism in two ways. First, the problem can interfere with the elderly alcoholic's ability to participate in the program. Second, the elderly alcoholic may focus on a medical problem and view alcoholism as only a secondary problem. Because the elderly as a group have many chronic medical problems, staff members expert in alcohol treatment but not familiar with gerontology may feel overwhelmed by medical problems and may focus on these instead of the alcoholism, unwittingly supporting the alcoholic's denial that alcoholism is his or her primary problem. On the other hand, medical problems that potentially interfere with treatment cannot be ignored.

Types of Treatment

The various treatment approaches for alcoholism in the elderly are summarized in Table 23–5. After inpatient detoxification, the treatment of choice for the frail elderly alcoholic is a residential program. Over the past few years, many inpatient treatment programs have relaxed their admission criteria to remain competitive and garner a market share of clients. It is now less difficult to find a program that accepts a person who is taking medication. Many programs accept cross-addicted patients (those addicted to alcohol and/or opioid analgesics or mood-altering drugs) and those with active, even terminal, medical problems. As the population ages, so does the client base in recovery programs. Funding remains a problem, however, because many insurance programs and Medicare do not cover inpatient recovery.

Outpatient programs may vary in philosophy, treatment modality, and cost. The local National Council on Alcoholism affiliate can provide the clinician or client with area resources. Some programs use a psychotherapeutic model with adjunctive pharmacological interventions. Private psychiatric day hospitals in some areas provide substance abuse treatment. However, one of the most effective and accessible programs remains AA (Blazer, 1995).

ALCOHOLICS ANONYMOUS

The advantages of AA are its ready availability, no-charge policy, peer support, program for recovery, and high rate of success. AA has an adjunct, Al-Anon, for families and significant others of alcoholics. Many residential treatment centers offer 12-step programs based on the AA philosophy of recovery. The advantage of this type of residential program is that it bonds the patient to the AA community during the critical stage of early sobriety and also provides the patient with a ready-made peer support group and ongoing treatment when he or she leaves.

Many professional healthcare providers do not have an understanding of AA and may feel threatened or resentful of a program that is staffed not by professional caregivers but by recovered alcoholics themselves. Peers or colleagues of AA members may be critical of the amount of time AA members devote to "living the AA program."

As an AA member once said, "AA is not about staying sober; it is a plan for life." From the time the alcoholic publicly acknowledges his or her illness in an AA meeting, that person experiences a level of human relatedness, acceptance, and compassion that he or she has not known before. Many alcoholics attend daily meetings for a year and, once in the program, commonly attend one or more meetings a week for years. Working the 12 steps of the program, an individual lives a lifestyle that is antithetical to many dynamisms that serve

TABLE 23-5
Treatment Approaches for Alcoholism

Prevention

Identifies risk factors.
Provides education and counseling on the following:
  1. Coping with age-related changes
  2. Adverse medical, psychological, and social consequences of prolonged or heavy drinking

Detoxification

Assists clients in recovering from acute alcohol intoxication and withdrawal and is usually a precursor to other
  treatments. Detoxification provides around-the-clock supervised treatment, which includes the following:
  1. Assessment of acute medical problems
  2. Close supervision and monitoring of treatment
  3. Assessment of psychosocial needs and development of a plan for continuing treatment
  4. Referral for medical and continuing alcoholism treatment; may be part of a hospital, an outpatient program, or
     another community treatment setting

Traditional Psychiatric Programs

May be the most common form of treatment for alcoholics, because alcohol can mimic psychopathology. Drinking is
  viewed as a symptom of a primary psychiatric condition and as evidence of maladaptation. Treatment focuses on the
  underlying sources of the emotional problem or personality defect. The patient may use mood-altering drugs to relieve
  symptoms and produce another dependence. It is difficult to keep the alcoholic in treatment.

Behavior Modification Therapy

Based on learning theory that drinking is a learned behavior, this therapy tries to reverse the learned drinking pattern
  with nondrinking or controlled drinking rather than uncontrolled drinking. Treatment involves the programmed
  manipulation of rewards or punishments associated with drinking. It includes aversion therapy drugs, such as
  disulfiram (generally not recommended for use in the elderly, owing to possible cardiovascular effects).

Psychosocial Therapy Programs

May be age-specific inpatient or outpatient programs. Includes one-to-one therapy, group therapy, and family therapy. The
  following psychosocial issues are addressed:
  1. Focus is on improving social support network
  2. Referral to resources such as Alcoholics Anonymous, religious counseling, other community social programs
Newer approaches include brief intervention in the clinical setting:
  1. Consists of short, patient-centered counseling/advise sessions
  2. Focus on motivation to change behavior, developing coping strategies
Pharmacological adjunct to psychosocial therapy:
  1. Use of naltrexone, an opioid antagonist, to reduce alcohol craving and drinking

The Comprehensive Alcoholism Treatment Model

Alcoholism is viewed as a chronic, progressive, multiphasic illness that can be arrested. Treatment is focused on providing
  the essential needs (medical, psychological, and social) of the alcoholic and developing a comprehensive care plan; it
  may include other approaches as needed, such as psychiatric treatment.

Data from American Geriatrics Society (1997); American Medical Association Council on Scientific Affairs (1996); Anderson
(1981); Eisendrath (1997); O'Brien et al. (1996); Samet et al. (1996); and Wartenberg & Nirenberg (1995).

to maintain the process of alcohol addiction. The fellowship of AA, in reality a therapeutic community, assists in personal growth and empowers the person to perform many behaviors that would have been insurmountable tasks before (Forrest, 1994). Many communities have elderly meetings and active outreach. AA members may go to residential care homes or nursing homes to hold AA meetings, or they may provide transportation for those who are too frail to go to meetings. The locations and types of meetings can be obtained by calling the local AA chapter or county alcoholism services number (Appendix 23–1).

Recovery is possible at any age. The advanced practice nurse who is not a specialist in substance abuse can be a key player in helping the alcoholic patient recognize the disease and choose to seek treatment. Detached, empathetic, and realistic diagnosis and treatment of alcohol-related problems can best prepare the patient to enter treatment. The first step in the recovery process can be initiated by informing a person about local resources for the alcoholic elderly and facilitating his or her access to these services. Understanding relapse, maintaining a caring, nonjudgmental attitude, and treating medical complications promptly can be instrumental in maintaining recovery.

SUMMARY

Alcoholism is a devastating, progressive, and fatal disease that can fill the last stage of life with despair, isolation, and loneliness. In recent years, the growing number of aged people as well as society's heightened awareness of the problem of alcohol and chemical dependency has brought attention to the special needs and problems associated with alcoholism in the elderly. With the early recognition and appropriate treatment of alcoholism, many elderly alcoholics are able to live out their lives in the peace and happiness that freedom from alcohol addiction can bring.

REFERENCES

Adams, W. L., Magruder-Habib, K., Trued, S., & Broome, M. L. (1992). Alcohol abuse in elderly emergency department patients. *Journal of the American Geriatrics Society, 40,* 1236–1240.

Ahlawat, S. K., & Siwach, S. B. (1994). Alcohol and coronary artery disease. *International Journal of Cardiology, 44,* 157–162.

Alcoholic Anonymous (1976). *Alcoholics anonymous* (3rd ed.). New York: Alcoholics Anonymous World Services.

American Geriatrics Society (1997). *Clinical guidelines: Alcohol use disorders in older adults* [Brochure]. New York: American Geriatrics Society.

American Medical Association Council on Scientific Affairs (1996). Alcoholism in the elderly. *Journal of the American Medical Association, 275,* 797–801.

American Psychiatric Association (1994). *Diagnostic and statistical manual of mental disorders* (4th ed.). Washington, D.C.: American Psychiatric Association.

Anderson, D. J. (1981). *Perspectives on treatment: The Minnesota experience.* Center City, MN: Hazelden Educational Materials.

Anthenelli, R. M., & Schuckit, M. A. (1992). Genetics. In J. H. Lowinson, P. Ruiz & R. B. Millman (Eds.), *Substance abuse: A comprehensive textbook* (2nd ed., pp. 39–50). Baltimore: Williams & Wilkins.

Beattie, M. (1992). *Codependent no more* (2nd ed.). San Francisco: Harper.

Blazer, D. G. (1995). Alcohol abuse and dependence. In W. B. Abrams, M. H. Beers & R. Berkow (Eds.), *The Merck manual of geriatrics* (2nd ed., pp. 1245–1248). Whitehouse Station, NJ: Merck & Co., Inc.

Bohn, M. J. (1993). Alcoholism. *Psychiatric Clinics of North America, 16,* 679–692.

Brennan, P. L., Moos, R. H., & Kim, J. Y. (1993). Gender differences in the individual characteristics and life contexts of late middle aged and older problem drinkers. *Addiction, 88,* 781–790.

Brody, J. A. (1982). Aging and alcohol abuse. *Journal of the American Geriatrics Society, 30,* 123–126.

Brower, K. J., Mudd, S., Blow, F. C., et al. (1994). Severity and treatment of alcohol withdrawal in elderly vs. younger patients. *Alcoholism, Clinical and Experimental Research, 18,* 196–201.

Buchsbaum, D. G., Buchanan, R. G., Welsh, J., et al. (1992). Screening for drinking disorders in the elderly using the CAGE questionnaire. *Journal of the American Geriatrics Society, 40,* 662–665.

Burkhalter, P. K. (1975). *Nursing care of the alcoholic and drug abuser.* New York: McGraw-Hill.

Denzin, N. K. (1987a). *The alcoholic self.* Newbury Park, CA: Sage.

Denzin, N. K. (1987b). *Treating alcoholism.* Newbury Park, CA: Sage.

Eisendrath, S. (1997). Psychiatric disorders. In L. M. Tierney Jr., S. J. McPhee & M. A. Papadakis (Eds.), *Current medical diagnosis and treatment* (36th ed., pp. 949–1006). Stamford, CT: Appleton & Lange.

Fedorak, I. J., Rao, R., & Prinz, R. A. (1994). The clinical challenge of multiple pancreatic cysts. *American Journal of Surgery, 168,* 22–28.

Feldman, E., & Plum, F. (1993). Metabolic dementia. In P. J. Whitehouse (Ed.), *Dementia* (pp. 307–336). Philadelphia: F. A. Davis.

Fink, A., Hays, R. D., Moore, A. A., & Beck, J. C. (1996). Alcohol-related problems in older persons: Determinants, consequences, and screening. *Archives of Internal Medicine, 156,* 1150–1156.

Forrest, G. G. (1994). *The diagnosis and treatment of alcoholism* (2nd ed.). Northvale, NJ: Jason Aronson.

Friedman, L. S. (1997). Liver, biliary tract, and pancreas. In L. M. Tierney Jr., S. J. McPhee & M. A. Papadakis (Eds.), *Current medical diagnosis and treatment* (36th ed., pp. 607–643). Stamford, CT: Appleton & Lange.

Fulop, G. I., Reinhardt, T., Strain, J. J., et al. (1993). Identification of alcoholism and depression in a geriatric medicine outpatient clinic. *Journal of the American Geriatrics Society, 41,* 737–741.

Gambert, S. R. (1992). Substance abuse in the elderly. In J. H. Lowinson, P. Ruiz & R. B. Millman (Eds.), *Substance abuse. A comprehensive textbook* (2nd ed., pp. 843–851). Baltimore: William & Wilkins.

Goldberg, H. I., Mullen, M., Ries, R. K., et al. (1991). Alcohol counseling in a general medical clinic. A randomized controlled trail of strategies to improve referral and show rates. *Medical Care, 29*(7), JS49–JS56.

Goldman, D. (1987–1988). Genetic studies on alcoholism at NIAAA Intramural Laboratories. *Alcohol Health Research World, 12*(2), 102–103.

Goodman, L. (1988). Would your assessment spot a hidden alcoholic? *RN, 51*(8), 56–60.

Greenberg, D. A. (1993). Ethanol and sedatives. *Neurologic Clinics, 3*, 523–534.

Hill, A., & Williams, D. (1993). Hazards associated with the use of benzodiazepines in alcohol detoxification. *Journal of Substance Abuse Treatment, 10*, 449–451.

Iso, H., Kitamura, A., Shimamoto, T., et al. (1995). Alcohol intake and the risk of cardiovascular disease in middle-aged Japanese men. *Stroke, 26*, 767–773.

Kaplan, H. I., Sadock, B. J., & Grebb, J. A. (1994). Alcohol-related disorders. In *Kaplan and Sadock's synopsis of psychiatry: Behavioral sciences, clinical psychiatry* (7th ed., pp. 396–411). Baltimore: Williams & Wilkins.

Katz, R. S. (1990). Using our emotional reactions to older clients. In B. Genevay & R. S. Katz (Eds.), *Countertransference and older clients* (pp. 17–26). Newbury Park, CA: Sage.

Klatsky, A. L., Armstrong, M. A., & Friedman, G. D. (1992). Alcohol and mortality. *Annals of Internal Medicine, 117*, 646–654.

Krach, P. (1990). Discovering the secret: Nursing assessment of elderly alcoholics in the home. *Journal of Gerontological Nursing, 16*(11), 32–38.

Lechtenberg, R., & Horner, T. M. (1992). Total ethanol consumption as a seizure risk factor in alcoholics. *Acta Neurologica Scandinavica, 85*(2), 90–94.

Lieber, C. S. (1994). Alcohol and the liver: 1994 update. *Gastroenterology, 106*, 1085–1105.

Lindblom, L., Kostyk, D., Tabisz, E., et al. (1992). Chemical abuse, an intervention program for the elderly. *Journal of Gerontological Nursing, 18*(6), 6–14.

Marion, T. R., & Stefanik-Campisi, C. (1990). The elderly alcoholic: Identification of factors that influence the giving and receiving of help. *Perspectives in Psychiatric Care, 25*, 32–35.

McCowen, T. J., & Breese, G. R. (1990). Multiple withdrawals from chronic ethanol "kindles" inferior collicular seizure activity: Evidence for kindling of seizures associated with alcoholism. *Alcoholism, Clinical and Experimental Research, 14*, 394–399.

Merikangas, K. R., Risch, N. J., & Weissman, M. M. (1994). Comorbidity and co-transmission of alcoholism, anxiety and depression. *Psychological Medicine, 24*, 69–80.

Moos, R. H., Brennan, P. L., Fondacaro, R. R., & Moos, B. S. (1990). Approach and avoidance coping responses among older problem and non–problem drinkers. *Psychology and Aging, 5*, 31–40.

Moos, R. H., Brennan, P. L., & Mertens, J. R. (1994). Mortality rates and predictors of mortality among late-middle aged and older substance abuse patients. *Alcoholism, Clinical and Experimental Research, 18*, 187–195.

Morse, R. M., & Flavin, D. K. (1992). The definition of alcoholism. The Joint Committee of the National Council on Alcoholism and Drug Dependence and the American Society of Addiction Medicine to study the definition and criteria for the diagnosis of alcoholism. *Journal of the American Medical Association, 268*, 1012–1014.

Naegle, M. A. (1983). The nurse and the alcoholic: Redefining an historically ambivalent relationship. *Journal of Psychosocial Nursing and Mental Health Services, 21*(6), 17–23.

National Institute on Alcohol Abuse and Alcoholism (1995). *Alcohol Alert, 27*, 1–4. Washington, D.C.: National Institute on Alcohol Abuse and Alcoholism.

Nelson, D. E., Sattin, R. W., Langlois, J. A., et al. (1992). Alcohol as a risk factor for fall injury events among elderly persons living in the community. *Journal of the American Geriatrics Society, 40*, 658–661.

O'Brien, C. P., Volpicelli, J. R., & Volpicelli, L. A. (1996). Naltrexone in the treatment of alcoholism: A clinical review. *Alcohol, 13*(1), 35–39.

Parette, H. P., Jr., Hourcade, J. J., & Parette, P. C. (1990). Nursing attitudes toward geriatric alcoholism. *Journal of Gerontological Nursing, 16*(1), 26–31.

Parsons, O. A., & Nixon, S. J. (1993). Neurobehavioral sequelae of alcoholism. *Neurologic Clinics, 11*, 205–218.

Pizzi, C. H., & Mion, L. C. (1993). Alcoholism in the elderly: Implications for hospital nurses. *Med Surg Nursing, 6*, 453–458.

Reich, T. (1987–1988). Beyond the gene: Research directions in family transmission of susceptibility to alcoholism. *Alcohol, Health Research World, 12*(2), 104–107.

Ridker, P. M., Vaughn, D. E., Stamfer, M. J., et al. (1994). Association of moderate alcohol consumption and plasma concentration of endogenous tissue-type plasminogen activator. *Journal of the American Medical Association, 272*, 929–933.

Robinson, J. (1990). Unhooking: Co-dependence, substance abuse and countertransference. In B. Genevay & R. S. Katz (Eds.), *Countertransference and older clients* (pp. 94–109). Newbury Park, CA: Sage.

Samet, J. H., Rollnick, S., & Barnes, H. (1996). Beyond CAGE: A brief clinical approach after detection of substance abuse. *Archives of Internal Medicine, 156*, 2287–2293.

Sankaran, M., Larkin, E. C., & Rao, G. A. (1994). Induction of malnutrition in chronic alcoholism: Role of gastric emptying. *Medical Hypotheses, 42*, 124–128.

Schuckit, M. A. (1990). Assessment and treatment strategies with late life alcoholics. *Journal of Geriatric Psychiatry, 23*(2), 83–89.

Smart, R. G., & Mann, R. E. (1991). Factors in recent reductions in liver cirrhosis deaths. *Journal of Studies on Alcohol, 52*, 232–240.

Solomon, K., Manepalli, J., Ireland, G., & Mahon, J. (1993). Alcoholism and prescription drug abuse in the elderly: St. Louis University Grand Rounds. *Journal of the American Geriatrics Society, 41*, 57–69.

Tabisz, E., Badger, M., & Meatherall, R., (1991). Identification of chemical abuse in the elderly admitted to emergency. *Clinical Gerontology, 11*, 27–39.

Victor, M. (1993). Persistent altered mentation due to ethanol. *Neurologic Clinics, 11*, 639–661.

Walker, B, & Kelly, P. (1981). *The elderly: A guide for counselors.* Center City, MN: Hazelden Educational Materials.

Wartenberg, A. A., & Nirenberg, T. D. (1995). Alcohol and other drug abuse in older patients. In W. Reichel (Ed.), *Care of the elderly. Clinical aspects of aging* (4th ed., pp. 133–141). Baltimore: Williams & Wilkins.

Willenbring, M. L., Christensen, K. J., Spring, W. D., Jr., & Rassmussen, R. (1987). Alcoholism screening in the elderly. *Journal of the American Geriatrics Society, 35,* 864–869.

Wrenn, K. D., & Larson, S. (1991). The febrile alcoholic in the emergency department. *American Journal of Emergency Medicine, 9,* 57–60.

APPENDIX 23-1

Resources

Several resources are available to provide healthcare professionals with information on alcohol use disorders (AGS, 1997).

Alcoholics Anonymous (AA)
P.O. Box 459
Grand Central Station
New York, NY 10163
212-870-3400; or visit: www.alcoholics-anonymous.org; or check phone book listing for local AA

National Clearinghouse for Alcohol and Drug Information
P.O. Box 2345
Rockville, MD 20847-2345
800-729-6686; or e-mail: info@prevline.health.org; or visit: www.health.org/index.htm

National Council on Alcoholism and Drug Dependence (NCADD)
12 West 21st Street
New York, NY 10010
212-206-6770; or e-mail: ncadd _ web@ncadd.org; or visit: www.ncadd.org

The National Institute on Alcohol Abuse and Alcoholism (NIAAA)
Office of Scientific Affairs, Willco Building
6000 Executive Boulevard, Suite 409
Bethesda, MD 20892-7003
301-443-3860; or visit: www.niaaa.nih.gov

Special Concerns

Intimacy and Sexuality

Amie Modigh

Sexuality is part of a larger concept known as intimacy. Although sexuality is a difficult topic for many clinicians to discuss, intimacy is a subject that most people can discuss fairly comfortably, even as it relates to the elderly. Thus, by presenting sexuality as an important component of intimacy, it is hoped that clinicians as well as patients will be able to adopt a more positive and realistic approach to sexuality. The advanced practice nurse should envision the total circle of intimacy needs and how he or she can assist patients in meeting these needs (Fig. 24–1).

The word *intimacy* comes from the Greek word *intima*, meaning "closest to; inner lining of blood vessels." Intimate restaurants, friends, and atmosphere all denote a pleasurable meaning. Intimacy is a warm, meaningful feeling of joy that has many components. The more completely the intimacy needs are met, the higher the quality of life. When one need is unmet, other needs become more important. For example, if the physical need of the sexual kind is not met, physical needs of the nonsexual kind such as hugging from close friends or relatives become more important.

This chapter describes several different intimacy needs. Sexuality as a component of inti-

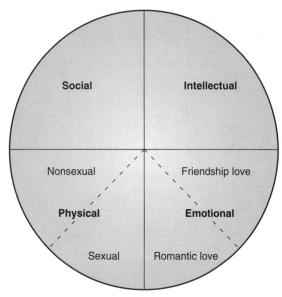

FIGURE 24–1. The circle of intimacy, illustrating four major components and two subcomponents.

macy is elaborated on to provide factual information for advanced practice nurses. The assessment of intimacy needs and sexual function are discussed, along with practical suggestions for how clinicians can assist clients in understanding intimacy and sexuality and how these concepts change with aging. Specific interventions are presented for managing normal age-related changes and changes caused by illness and medications.

TYPES OF INTIMACY

Intimacy is joy that has many levels. Much can be done to assist elderly clients in enjoying these riches. *Social intimacy* is the joy of experiencing fellowship with friends and relatives on a deep level. It involves relationships of real caring and sharing and much self-revelation. This type of intimacy may occur between individuals who are single or among couples. It is, however, an intimacy in which many losses can occur, especially if all friends are in the same age group. It is therefore wise for individuals to cultivate friends of different age groups.

Intellectual intimacy is a unique joy. It crosses

all ordinary barriers and can develop suddenly when two people discover a common interest. It is a mind-sharing intimacy that can involve such activities as sports, music, historical events, bridge, and bird watching. Colleagues at work may experience an intellectual intimacy as they work together on a research project. Having satisfying intellectual intimacy can certainly enrich a person's life. However, this intimacy can also be a source of friction in a relationship if, for example, a spouse is insecure or threatened by his or her spouse's enthusiasm over a golf game or concert and the person with whom this interest is shared.

Emotional intimacy is popularly called love. There are two distinct parts to love. Friendship love is the caring and deep feelings one has for parents, siblings, or friends, usually of same sex but also of the opposite sex. This intimacy usually involves a small number of people, as opposed to social intimacy, which can involve many people and groups. Romantic love is the intimacy feeling one experiences with a spouse or lover.

Physical intimacy also has two distinct parts. The nonsexual part is the hugging and touching done with parents, grandparents, children, friends, and pets. The sexual part of physical intimacy involves sexual behaviors such as sexual intercourse and masturbation. All these intimacy needs are important and contribute to quality of life. Depending on circumstances, some may be more important at one time than others. A study conducted at a Department of Veterans Affairs Nursing Home (Bullard-Poe et al., 1994) examined definitions of intimacy in 68 male veterans aged 70 to 80 years. Subjects were asked to rank the different types of intimacies in their order of importance to them. By far, the most important intimacy need was social intimacy, followed closely by nonsexual physical intimacy. Although a similar questionnaire given to the same age group of healthy community-dwelling adults might reveal very different results, these findings are important because nursing home staff members can do much to help residents meet these two identified intimacy needs and thus increase the residents' quality of life in an institutional environment. The focus of this chapter is on the sexual type of physical intimacy—an area full of myths in which both healthcare professionals and elderly people lack knowledge.

Human sexuality, particularly as it relates to the elderly, is minimally included in the curricula of most nursing schools and is almost non-existent in medical school curricula. Curriculum changes are needed so that healthcare providers can assist and guide older adults with their questions and concerns about sexual functioning.

SEXUALITY FROM DIFFERENT PERSPECTIVES

Historical Background

In biblical times, sexual activity was portrayed in two ways—enjoyable, healthy, natural, and God-given; or sinful and a threat to piety and a healthy society. St. Augustine (354–430) lived a frivolous life as a young man and was often unable to control his sexual desires. Convinced that the only way to return to God was to avoid giving into bodily desires such as sex, he converted to Catholicism and later became a Bishop, a great scholar, and a prolific writer. His staunch teachings had and still have far-reaching effects, such as celibacy for priests. He strongly advocated that although sexual intercourse must occur for the purpose of procreation, it should take place only for this purpose, and "the act should be completed as quickly as possible" (Brasch, 1973).

Sigmund Freud (1856–1939) developed the theory that libido and instinct for self-preservation were the driving force behind all human activity. He described the normal male as having an insatiable sexual drive. Freud's theory—that the female was a passive participant in sexual intercourse and was sexually immature if she did not experience vaginal orgasm—had negative consequences on sexual satisfaction for women who believed this.

Research

There has been a paucity of research on human sexuality. Studies of older individuals have been especially limited. Because the topic of sexuality was not previously considered proper or important for research, much of what has been written is based on philosophical beliefs rather than on empirical evidence. The Rockefeller Foundation was the only supporter of sex research between 1913 and 1954. Alfred Kinsey was the first recipient of this funding for sex research. Kinsey and colleagues' reports, *Sexual behavior in the human male* (1948) and *Sexual behavior in the human female* (1953), were a major breakthrough in this area, bringing the topic of sex into U.S. homes. Their work, however, was not representative of the elderly population. Men and women older than 60 years were represented by 2.4% and 0.9% of the subjects, respectively.

Masters and Johnson's *Human sexual response* (1968) measured physiological events that occurred during sexual intercourse in a laboratory setting. Their findings proved to be an important point for women—namely, that there is no physiological difference between orgasm resulting from vaginal versus clitoral stimulation. Although their research significantly increased knowledge regarding sexual intercourse, the number of people in the study older than 60 years was only 31 (11 women and 20 men) out of 694 participants. Sex therapy became increasingly prevalent after Masters and Johnson's published works and has continued to be popular.

Sexuality is no longer a taboo subject in the United States. It is discussed on many talk shows, and movies and magazines are inundated with the topic. In October 1994, both *Time* and *U.S. News and World Report* published the results of the "most important survey since the Kinsey report" (Elmer-Dewitt, 1994; Schrof & Wagner, 1994). However, even this study applied mostly to the young. As Robert Butler (1994, p. 8) pointed out in the editorial response, "It is disturbing that an otherwise excellent survey on sex in America excluded people 60 years of age and older. This perpetuates the myth that sexual desires capacity and satisfaction are extinct in later years." With very few exceptions, such as *The Cosby Show, The Golden Girls, Empty Nest*, and the movies *On Golden Pond* and *Cocoon*, mature individuals have rarely been depicted as romantically or intimately involved, much less sexually interested or active (Solomon & Salend, 1992).

Longitudinal studies conducted by Duke University's Center for the Study of Aging and Human Development (Busse & Maddox, 1985) followed the cases of a large number of older individuals over many years. Conclusions from this study finally dispelled multiple myths related to sexual functioning in the elderly. Results indicated that sexual activity and interest decline to some degree in both men and women as they age. However, a significant number of healthy elderly remain both interested and active until very advanced age. The findings of these studies were supported by later studies (Brecher, 1984; Butler & Lewis, 1976; Starr & Weiner, 1981).

Research is currently being conducted on erectile dysfunction and its various treatments such as medications and surgical implants. Studies are needed on the emotional intimacy aspect of sexuality, which is discussed later in the chapter.

Sexuality in the United States

Why is sexuality in the elderly still "in the closet" today? Many negative stereotypes about aging persist in U.S. society. Even birthday cards depict depressing scenes such as being "over the hill" at ages 30 and 40 years and in a rocking chair at the age of 50 years. Advertisements of most products portray young women. The elderly person is usually seen in advertising for dentures or laxatives. Love, sex, and romance are almost always associated with the very young. A young man turning around to look at an attractive woman is described as sexy, virile, and macho; an older man doing the very same thing is labeled a "dirty old man."

Today's octogenarians received their sex education soon after the Victorian era; sex was still not discussed at all in "proper circles." The general message was that sex occurred among the young and married couples and generally ceased after menopause. Because elderly individuals are assumed not to be interested in sex, they are seldom asked about their sexuality by anyone, including healthcare providers. Older adults, in turn, do not want to raise the topic of sex; because no one ever asks them about it, they think they should not be

interested (Butler & Lewis, 1993). Brecher's 1984 study indicated that 86% of more than 4000 individuals older than 50 years believed that "society thinks of older people as nonsexual." The religious impact may be very strong. Some religions hold firmly that sexual activity is for procreation only and not for recreation. This may have a negative and conflicting effect on those elderly people who enjoy continued sexual activity long past childbearing age. Finally, it should be remembered that the large number of healthy active elderly people aged 70, 80, and even 90 years is a relatively new phenomenon in society. In 1900, 4.1% of the population was older than 65 years; in 1991, 12.6%, or 31.8 million people, were of the same age (American Association of Retired Persons, 1994).

Demographics

As people live and remain healthier longer, future studies will likely show an increase in the number of elderly people who continue to be sexually active. In an early study (Pfeiffer et al., 1968), researchers found that sexual interest remained high in 37% of men aged 78 years and in 43% of women in the same age group. Women's sexual activity is strongly influenced by marital status, whereas their sexual interest is not. Duke University's longitudinal studies (Busse & Maddox, 1985) indicated that 68% of men older than 65 years and 25% of those older than 75 years were still sexually active. Corresponding figures for women were 55% and 22%, respectively.

Brecher (1984) reported that 95% of women were sexually active in their 50s, 89% in their 60s, and 81% in their 70s. The proportions of sexually active men in the same age groups were 98%, 91%, and 79%, respectively. Starr and Weiner's (1981) report on sexually active individuals (800 subjects between the ages of 60 and 91 years) showed a gradual decrease in activity with age. However, in the age group of 80 to 91 years, 60% of men and 43% of women were still active.

Stages of Sexuality

In very young children, sex is polymorphous. The child explores his or her body more out of curiosity than either release or pleasure seeking. In the young adult, sexual activity is directed toward relief, particularly in the young male, who reaches his height of sexual activity between 18 and 20 years. Women reach their peak of sexual activity in their mid-30s. The mature age of sexual activity takes on a broader aspect for both the man and the woman; the romance, the foreplay, and the caring, hugging, and kissing become as enjoyable as sexual intercourse itself. In fact, according to Starr (1985), those who do not broaden their sexuality during maturity become fixated with "completing the act" instead of experiencing it. To those who have had a satisfying sexual life, older age becomes a continuation of the mature stage of sexuality. The focus is often more on the partner's satisfaction than on one's own (Renshaw, 1983). The multiple aspects of sexual activity in the older individual are described by some as deeper and more satisfying because of knowing the partner better, having intimate communication, and having more experience.

Types of Sexual Activity

Research indicates that heterosexuality is by far the predominant sexual orientation in today's society. The exact percentages are difficult to establish because of differing methodologies across studies. Kinsey and colleagues (1948, 1953) reported that 50% of men were exclusively heterosexual throughout their adult life, 4% were exclusively gay and 46% were bisexual. For women, the figures were 72%, 3%, and 25%, respectively. A recent survey (Elmer-Dewitt, 1994) suggested that 10% of the U.S. population is homosexual. More important than the exact percentages and numbers, however, is the fact that different sexual orientations exist. The advanced practice nurse concerned with holistic care and quality of life for older adults must be knowledgeable about all aspects of sexuality.

Limited research has been conducted in the areas of homosexuality and bisexuality. Berger's (1982) book *Gay and gray: The older homosexual man*, is considered an excellent resource for understanding many aspects of the aging gay man. The acquired immunodeficiency syndrome (AIDS) crisis has had a major impact on all types of sexual activity. Initially, AIDS was predominantly associated with gay men and intravenous drug users. As this dreadful disease has spread to others, however, one effect has been an increase in monogamous relationships in all types of sexual orientation, which should decrease the spread of AIDS.

The number of elderly gays and lesbians is expected to increase (Starr, 1985). Future generations of elderly people who have experienced the gay rights movement are likely to have a greater proportion of individuals coming "out of the closet." Many authors have speculated that homosexual relationships will increase in elderly women for three reasons: (1) women tend to take a more assertive role in sexual activity as they mature; (2) the gay liberation movement has led to a slight increase in society's acceptance of homosexuals; and (3) a demographic dilemma exists: women outnumber men about seven to one after the age of 65 years (Kassel, 1983). The sexual problems that elderly gays and lesbians face are similar to those of heterosexual elderly people. However, the stigma attached to homosexuality often prevents these individuals from voicing their concerns (Hammond, 1987). Several organizations are available to assist gays and lesbians as they age.

Of all sexual issues, masturbation is the one that still evokes the highest amount of defensiveness, guilt, and discomfort. Most religions scorn masturbation. Publications in the early 1920s advised parents to stop at almost nothing "to prevent their children from touching their sex organs" (Butler & Lewis, 1993). Masturbation was also said to cause every terrible curse from warts to epilepsy and insanity. Butler and Lewis (1993), however, stated unequivocally that "masturbation is a common and healthy practice, a source of pleasure to be learned and enjoyed"; it "resolves sexual tension and helps preserve sexual function" (p. 243). It is the key element in every therapy program for developing sexual response (Comfort, 1976; Kaplan, 1974). Although in one study, 85% of women and 76% of men thought that masturbation was normal and acceptable for those who chose to masturbate, when asked the question "Do you masturbate?," the affirmative answers dropped to 47% of women and 45% of men

(Starr & Weiner, 1981). These findings emphasize the fact that a very sensitive and understanding approach to this subject is of utmost importance.

FACTORS AFFECTING SEXUALITY AND PRACTICE IMPLICATIONS

Physical and Psychosocial Changes with Aging

Age-related changes in sexual responses in men and women complement each other in many ways; that is, both sexes need increased time in precoital stimulation, even though it is for different reasons (Table 24–1). None of the normal age-related changes in either men or women preclude the continuation of a happy, healthy sexual life.

NORMAL CHANGES IN MEN

Men experience a gradual decrease in the testicular secretion of testosterone. Although it is no longer believed to have any significant effect on erection, testosterone does affect the libido. The decrease in testosterone contributes to the other age-related changes in the sexual response cycle in men. The testes become smaller and the scrotum more flaccid, and the excitement and stimulation phase show a need for increased direct penile stimulation to achieve an erection. However, once erection is

achieved, the man is often able to maintain this much longer before ejaculation, thus allowing more time to stimulate his partner as well as himself. The penis may not enlarge as much as in younger years and may not be as rigid. However, if the penis is not rigid enough for vaginal penetration, the partner can facilitate penetration by easing the penis in and holding it in her vagina for a short time. Sexual excitement usually occurs, resulting in an erection adequate to complete intercourse. The orgasmic phase continues to be very enjoyable, although slightly less explosive and of shorter duration. Seminal fluid is not expelled with the same force, and sperm count decreases; however, most healthy older men remain fertile into very old age. The resolution phase is rapid, and the penis becomes limp almost immediately after orgasm. One of the most significant changes for the man is the increased refractory time with age. The time between orgasm and the next erection may be several hours to several days; this varies greatly among individuals (Masters & Johnson, 1981). Brecher (1984) found that 35% of men in his study did not have an increased refractory period by the age of 60 years.

ERECTILE DYSFUNCTION

Impotence, or erectile dysfunction, as it is more accurately named, is the inability to obtain and maintain an erection firm enough and long enough to complete satisfactory sexual inter-

---

TABLE 24–1

Age-Related Changes in the Sexual Response Cycle

Phase	Male	Female
Excitement (Young age, 15–30 sec; elderly, 5–10 min)	Increased time needed for penile erection Direct stimulation often needed	Increased time needed for vaginal lubrication
Plateau (Changes are accommodating)	Penis may not enlarge as much in length or breadth	Vaginal barrel expansion reduced
Orgasmic (Does not interfere with enjoyment)	Increased time before ejaculation and decreased amount of fluid ejaculated Slight decrease in force and duration of orgasm	Decreased number of contractions Decreased force of contractions Remains capable of multiple orgasms
Resolution (Important for both partners to know that there is a normal difference here)	Penis reduces in size immediately May not be able to have another erection for several hours or up to 2 days (great individual variation here)	Slight decrease, but can usually be aroused again after a short rest (minutes)

course. Most men experience an occasional episode of erectile failure, but 1 in 10 (i.e., more than 10 million) men in America experience chronic impotence (Krane et al., 1989). Impotence is *not* a normal part of aging. It does occur more frequently in the elderly, however, partly owing to normal physiological changes that are usually modifiable as well as disease processes associated with aging (Feldman et al., 1994). Causes of erectile dysfunction include vascular disease, radical surgery, endocrine disorders, traumas, multiple sclerosis, medications, and psychological disorders (National Institutes of Health [NIH] Consensus Statement Online 1992; available at http://text.nlm.nih.gov/nih/cdc/www/91txt.html). If nocturnal erection is present, psychogenic causes may be present and should be explored (Whitehead & Nagler, 1994).

Erectile dysfunction can be a devastating situation for the man. Today, however, most cases of erectile dysfunction can be treated successfully. If a detailed patient history and physical examination indicate the need for further diagnostic workup and treatment, a urologist or other physician with expertise in erectile failure should be consulted.

Treatment of erectile dysfunction is initially directed toward correcting any reversible medical problem that may be contributory. This includes eliminating or substituting those medications that may be inducing the erectile failure (Butler et al., 1994a).

If testosterone levels are decreased, testosterone injections may be useful to increase libido and decrease hypogonadism; however, these injections do not improve erectile function (Mulligan & Modigh, 1992). As a precautionary measure, the prostate-specific antigen (PSA) level should be measured prior to testosterone injections. If it is elevated, testosterone should not be given, as it could increase the risk for testicular cancer.

Several interventions are used to manage erectile dysfunction; these include (1) drug therapy, (2) vacuum constriction devices, (3) penile prostheses, and (4) vascular surgery (NIH Consensus Statement, 1992). Drug therapy includes intracavernosal injection drugs, urethral suppositories, and oral medication. Self-injection of vasodilator drugs into the corpora of the penis has had excellent success in producing penile erections within minutes. The most effective and well-studied of these agents are papaverine, phentolamine (Regitine), and alprostadil (Caverject), which have been used singly or in combination (NIH Consensus Statement, 1992). These drugs, especially papaverine, may cause priapism (inappropriate persistent erection), and they should not be used in patients with severe psychiatric illness, liver dysfunction, poor manual dexterity, or poor vision or in patients who are receiving anticoagulant therapy or are unable to tolerate transient hypotension. These injections appear to be most successful in men with mild to moderate vascular disease.

Alprostadil, recently released in a urethral suppository form (Muse), is similar to naturally occurring prostaglandin E_1, which causes smooth muscle relaxation and allows vasodilatation in the corpus cavernosum of the penis. Effects generally occur within 5 to 10 minutes, with erections lasting up to 30 to 60 minutes. Common side effects include aching in the penis, testicles, legs, and perineum; warmth or burning sensation in the urethra; penile redness due to increased blood flow; and minor urethral bleeding or spotting due to improper administration.

The most exciting development in erectile dysfunction treatment is the recent release of sildenafil (Viagra), the first oral medication that causes erections within 20 minutes of ingestion. Sildenafil works by blocking an enzyme found mainly in the penis that breaks down cyclic guanosine monophosphate (GMP), a chemical produced during sexual stimulation. An erection is more likely to occur the longer cyclic GMP is present. Unlike intracavernosal injection therapy, sildenafil does not cause an erection unless the man is sexually stimulated. Contraindications include the use of nitrates, erythromycin, ketoconazole, and cimetidine.

Vacuum constriction devices such as Erec-Aid are available (Fig. 24–2). These devices are applied to the penis externally and draw blood into the penis with a pumping action. The blood is kept in the penis with the use of a constriction band placed at the base of the penis. Vacuum constriction devices have been successful in as many as 80% of users and have minimal side effects (Butler & Lewis, 1993). These devices should not be used if a man is

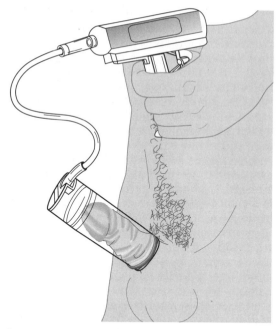

FIGURE 24–2. Vacuum constriction device.

on anticoagulant therapy or suffers from any blood abnormalities.

Penile prostheses are also widely used. Although there is a high satisfaction rate in male users, limited research has indicated a considerably lower satisfaction rate of the partner (Kramarsky-Binkhorst, 1978). Penile prostheses are used when the impotence is chronic, when external devices do not work, and when drug therapy is not an option or is no longer effective. A surgical implant should be mutually desired by both partners.

The malleable prostheses are relatively inexpensive (>$5000), can be bent to improve concealment, and are inserted under local anesthesia. The disadvantage is that the penis is always rigid and may not feel as natural as with other devices. With the self-contained inflatable prosthesis, the penis is semiflaccid until an erection is desired. At this time, the front of each of the two cylinders implanted within the corpora cavernosa must be squeezed and released in a pumping action to make the penis erect. The three-piece inflatable prosthesis consists of fluid-filled cylinders in the corpora cavernosa, a scrotal pump, and an abdominal reservoir. To achieve an erection, the bulb portion

of the pump is squeezed several times, releasing fluid out of the reservoir and into the cylinders. To relax the penis, a deflation site is pressed, which moves the fluid back to the reservoir. This type of device most closely approximates the process of natural erection and offers a softer, flaccid state. It is the most expensive ($10,000), however, and mechanical failure is fairly common. These types of devices are constantly being improved, and new devices will soon be on the market.

Vascular surgery to repair venous leakage within the penis as well as arterial revascularization procedures may be performed in selected cases within medical centers by experienced personnel. Because these procedures are still considered investigative, additional research is needed to clarify their indications and role in erectile dysfunction.

NORMAL CHANGES IN WOMEN

Women experience certain physiological and psychological changes before, during, and after menopause. Seventy million women in the United States will be menopausal by the year 2000. Menopause is a normal and natural transition for women as they come to the end of the childbearing years and enter a new phase in life. To many, because pregnancy is no longer possible, it is a time of relief and a new opportunity to explore life with a spouse or significant other. To others, it causes feelings of gloom and sadness and a loss of self-worth and self-esteem. Menopause may be difficult psychologically for some women because it signifies the end of reproductive life. Women who have placed great emphasis on reproduction may experience a threat to their feminine identity (Neugarten, 1970). Certain cultures place a lower value on women after menopause (Friedan 1993; Lock, 1986). The vast majority of women (75–85%) have minimal or no symptoms during menopause (Friedan, 1993; Weg, 1983).

Common pathologies at this stage in life such as vaginitis, urological disorders, osteoporosis, depression, and an increase in cardiovascular disease are partially caused by sex steroid depletion. Many of these conditions respond well to estrogen replacement therapy (ERT), which gained enormous popularity throughout the 1960s and early 1970s after Wilson (1966) published the book *Feminine forever*. However, ERT declined drastically after studies showed its association with endometrial and breast cancer. Subsequently, multiple studies (e.g., Dawber, 1980; Lobo, 1990) have demonstrated that estrogen has preventive effects against both cardiac disease and osteoporosis. Furthermore, by adding progestin, research has found that cancer risks are greatly decreased, although cardiovascular benefits are also reduced (Falkeborn et al., 1992). The controversy continues. Women should be provided with information on all the known risks and benefits of combination hormone replacement therapy (HRT). Each woman can then make an informed choice that is best for her regarding whether to undergo short-term, long-term, or no treatment with HRT. Because there is no single therapy that suits everyone, the wisest option for patients and their practitioners is to "resist irrational fear of estrogen as well as estrogen evangelism" (Friedan, 1993).

The woman experiences most of her physical changes during and after menopause because of the decrease in estrogen. The breasts are less full and tend to sag, which may have a negative effect on body image. The vaginal walls become less elastic and thinner, and thus the vagina becomes less capable of expanding in both length and width. As estrogen levels decrease, the Bartholin glands that lubricate the vagina during the excitement phase respond more slowly (Masters & Johnson, 1981). In young women, stimulation for 15 to 20 seconds is often enough to produce adequate lubrications for penile penetration. Three to 5 minutes of stimulation may be required for older women.

Lack of lubrication is the most common cause of dyspareunia, but it is also one of the easiest problems to correct. The use of a water-soluble lubricant is a simple cure (Butler et al., 1994b). Glycerin (K-Y jelly) is very satisfactory and inexpensive. Replens, a glycerin vaginal suppository that is effective for 3 days, not only moistens the vagina but also keeps acidity in proper balance to prevent infection. It is more expensive, however. An oil-based lubricant such as Vaseline should be avoided because it can be a medium for bacteria. Lubricants should be kept at room temperature and easily accessible (e.g., in a bedside drawer). Vaginal estrogen creams are preferred by some women; in addition to counteracting the dryness, these creams may help improve the elasticity of vaginal walls. These creams should be applied at least 1 hour prior to intercourse to take effect and decrease exposure to the partner.

The pubic area loses much of the fatty deposits, making both the labia majora and minora thinner. The clitoris may not be as protected and may become irritated as a result, especially if prolonged thrusting occurs during intercourse. The clitoris may diminish in size, but this varies with individuals. However, it remains extremely sensitive to sexual stimulation.

The orgasmic stage remains very enjoyable although slightly shorter for the older woman, and she remains capable of multiple orgasms. On occasion, she may experience excessive uterine contraction mimicking severe menstrual cramps. This can be relieved by estrogen and sometimes by just changing position. There is no increase in the refractory period for women (Masters & Johnson, 1981).

Especially if she is regularly sexually active, the aging woman is fully capable of sexual performance, including orgasm, until very late in life. Any decrease in activity is generally caused by the lack of a functional partner.

Health Conditions Affecting Sexuality

Acute and chronic illnesses can be a serious deterrent to sexual activity. Although acute illnesses are not common in the elderly, they do occur. Urinary tract infection (UTI) in women can result from sexual activity. In elderly women, "honeymoon cystitis" is common. This occurs owing to fragile urethral walls and the decreased protection of the urinary meatus that results from the loss of fatty tissue in the labia minora and majora. Irritation of the urinary meatus may result from intercourse, particularly with prolonged penile thrusting. Thus, a change of position may be helpful in preventing UTIs. If a UTI does develop, appropriate antibiotic treatment should be implemented.

Urinary incontinence can be a serious deterrent to sexual activity. In Mooradian and Greiff's (1990) study of 125 elderly women attending an incontinence clinic, 46% of women stated that incontinence had seriously affected their sexual life. Every effort should be made to deal with this often solvable condition (see Chapter 10). If the woman experiences dyspareunia for any length of time, she may develop involuntary vaginal muscle contraction (vaginismus). The degree can vary from mild to so severe that penile penetration is impossible. The cause of dyspareunia will determine the treatment and its success. If there is a significant psychological component, sex therapy should be included. Milder cases of dyspareunia may be relieved if the patient practices contracting and relaxing of the vaginal introitus. The woman may apply gentle pressure with one or two fingers as she tries to contract and relax. When gently done by the partner, this can also be successful. Using the side-by-side or crosswise position may be the next step to gradually eliminate this problem (Modigh & Mulligan, 1992). Masters and Johnson's three-stage method is also recommended for these conditions and has had much success. In this method, partners are taught to progress from nongenital touching to genital touching and then to intercourse; pleasure is the focus—not performance (Masters & Johnson, 1970).

Peyronie's disease, the cause of which is unknown, produces an upward turn of the tip of the penis. There is fibrous thickening of the walls of the blood vessels of the corpora cavernosa of penis, causing pain with erection. If the penis is angled too far, painful intercourse can result. The disease, which occurs most frequently in men between 40 and 60 years of age, disappears in weeks or months without treatment. Although the use of aminobenzoate potassium (Potaba Plus) for 6 months is often recommended, it is not known whether this treatment is effective. If there is no improvement and sexual intercourse is difficult or painful, surgery is recommended to remove the fibrous area. Peyronie's disease is believed to be greatly underreported. Unless it causes a great deal of discomfort, men tend to not bring it to a practitioner's attention.

Benign prostatic hypertrophy, a normal result of aging, does not interfere with sexual activity but should be followed for signs of urinary obstruction and to rule out cancer. If surgery becomes necessary, a small number (10%) of men may be unable to have an erection. Fortunately, successful treatments as previously described are available.

Chronic conditions are more common in the elderly, some of which may cause sexual activity to decrease or cease altogether (Shover, 1988). More than 50% of men with diabetes mellitus experience impotence by the age of 60 years (Brecher, 1984). The effect on women is minimal but may contribute to a further decrease in vaginal lubrication and a possible decrease in clitoral sensation because of decreased blood supply. Arthritis may lead to a decrease in sexual activity because of painful joints. Positional changes may be needed, and it may help to schedule medications to have their maximum effect in time for sexual activity. Rheumatoid arthritis tends to cause increased joint stiffness and more pain in the morning; thus, sexual activity may be more pleasurable later in the day. For people with osteoarthritis, the best time for sexual intercourse tends to be in the morning. Couples should be instructed that during sexual intercourse, cortisone released from adrenal glands acts as a natural endorphin and can relieve pain (Weg, 1975).

Heart disease of any kind does not need to interfere with sexual activity. However, much reassurance is needed for cardiac patients, especially those who have had a myocardial infarction (MI). The suggested waiting period for sexual activity after a MI can vary from 8 to 14 weeks, depending on the general fitness and conditioning of the individual. Several studies have shown that sexual intercourse is no more stressful to the heart than is climbing two flights of stairs or walking briskly for 10 minutes (Butler & Lewis, 1993). Self-stimulation and mutual masturbation can often be started earlier. Much love and affection at this time can aid the person in maintaining self-worth and can prevent the fear and depression that often follow an MI. This is an excellent example of when other intimacy needs predominate; being able to satisfy these needs increases quality of life. When the individual does resume sexual activity, he or she should note and consult a healthcare provider if anginal pain occurs during or after intercourse, if severe palpitations occur lasting more than 15 minutes, or if marked fatigue persists.

Mental health influences sexual activity. If an individual is depressed, sexual desires tend to decrease or cease. Depression is a common problem in the elderly and can be easily treated with both therapy and medications (see Chapter 17).

In the past, sexually transmitted diseases were not much of a concern in the elderly. Today, however, primarily because of the AIDS epidemic, caution is a must. Eleven to 12% of new AIDS cases a year fall in the age group of 50 years and older (Butler & Lewis, 1993). Honest and open discussion of the new partner's past sexual activity and history should be strongly encouraged.

Multiple medications may have major effects on sexual activity in both men and women. For men, the inability to obtain or maintain an erection is often the most devastating side effect. Other side effects in men may decrease libido, delay or stop the ability to ejaculate, cause engorged breasts, and cause priapism (prolonged painful erection). Women report symptoms such as engorged breasts and decreased vaginal lubrication. The most common drugs affecting sexual activity are antihypertensives, cardiovascular drugs, antidepressants, tranquilizers, antiulcer medications, and certain chemotherapy drugs. At present, the only drug category that does not have any reported effect on sexual activity is nonsteroidal antiinflammatory medications. It is important to take a thorough drug history and check the side effects of all drugs the patient is taking. Consider alternate drugs if there are problems. It is not uncommon for men to discontinue their antihypertensive medication if it causes impotence. If a sexual history is not taken, erectile difficulties may not be known until severe damage has occurred.

Because many medications can affect erectile function and/or libido, every drug should be suspected until proved otherwise. A number of studies have demonstrated that most antihypertensive medications interfere with both erections and libido in men. Angiotensin-converting enzyme inhibitors and some calcium channel blockers such as felodipine (Plendil) seem to have the least offensive effect. However, these are newer medications whose side effects may not have been reported as yet. Nicotine, like other drugs that affect circulation, may contribute to erectile failure. Women appear to be less affected by medications; however, few studies have investigated the effects of drugs on sexual function in women.

Drugs reported to have aphrodisiac effect often have the opposite effect on both sexual interest and function when used in high doses or for long periods (Butler & Lewis, 1993). Alcohol is frequently considered an aphrodisiac because it may loosen inhibitions and in small amounts may increase libido. However, in larger amounts, alcohol has a negative effect on sexual performance; it is a depressant and slows down the physical processes necessary for sexual arousal and orgasm.

Other Factors Affecting Sexuality

The most reliable predictor for an active, fulfilling sex life in very old age is an active, fulfilling sex life in younger life. The Duke University longitudinal studies (Busse & Maddox, 1985) found that couples who had received much pleasure from hugging, kissing, and being close during younger years adjusted far better to normal age-related changes than those who received pleasure only from sexual intercourse. Pfeiffer and colleagues (1972) found that 78% of women attributed the cessation of sexual activity to their spouse's death, illness, loss of interest, or inability to perform. Seventy-one percent of men stated their reasons for cessation to be illness, a loss of interest, or an inability to perform. Thus, it is apparent that most reasons for sexual inactivity are related to events surrounding the man. Marital status is very important for today's elderly, especially to the woman who still prefers a socially sanctioned partner. Thus, even though an older woman may be interested in sexual activity, she is less likely to be sexually active.

There is a strong double standard operating in the United States regarding male and female aging. The older man displaying gray or white hair is considered distinguished, his wrinkles serving as evidence of character and wisdom. These same changes are not viewed as positively in women, who often feel that they are losing their sexual appeal as a result of these same changes. Being able to discuss this and being offered reassurance can do much to improve these feelings. Boredom is a common reason for couples to decrease or stop sexual activity. Consistent use of the same pattern can lead to the activity becoming routine and meaningless. Being able to communicate and trying new methods or a new environment, even as minor as changing the room or position, can be enough to enhance lovemaking. It is never too late to add romance to the environment. That may be as simple as a candle and flowers on the dinner table or a favorite, meaningful piece of music. It may be as extravagant as a cruise or as inexpensive as browsing through a bookstore together looking at books on sex or reading Alex Comfort's books *The joy of sex: A cordon bleu guide to lovemaking* (1972), *The more joy of sex* (1975), or *A good age* (1976).

Family members can have major negative effects on older people's sexual activities. Grown children tend to think, "my parents never had sex" and "they certainly don't now" (Hammond, 1987). If parents live with one of their children, it is vital that privacy be honored and respected. This issue may need to be explored by the advanced practitioner. Even more likely to present a problem is a situation in which a widowed or divorced parent lives with an adult child. In many instances, it does not occur to the son or daughter that the parent may be interested in a romantic or sexual relationship. The parent in turn is very hesitant to say anything for fear of criticism (Mulligan & Modigh, 1991). The following vignette demonstrates some of these concerns.

Case Study

A 76-year-old widow lived with her daughter and son-in-law for 5 years. She met several people with whom she socialized at a senior center. She became very attracted to a 72-year-old widower who lived with his daughter. It was a mutually growing romance. One weekend when Mrs. X.'s daughter was supposed to be away, Mr. Q. stayed overnight. The daughter found out and became upset; she angrily asked her mother what she thought the neighbors would think and made her promise to not ever do that again. Many sad and painful months

followed, but fortunately the older couple's relationship was strong enough that they managed to not only survive the criticism but also find an apartment and move in together. They married a year later at a ceremony attended by both sets of children.

Unfortunately, all situations of this kind do not have such a happy ending. Older adults and their adult children need more education and open discussion on the intimacy needs of elderly people. A sensitive nurse can often elicit pertinent data, offer helpful suggestions, and bring in other family members as needed or refer them to appropriate resources.

ASSESSMENT OF SEXUAL FUNCTION

History

The advanced practice nurse should take a sexual history as part of the routine patient history. Studies reveal that although the physician rarely takes a sexual history and the nurse practitioner only occasionally does (Butler & Lewis, 1993; Ende et al., 1984; Ross & Landis, 1994), the vast majority of patients appreciate the opportunity to be asked questions about their sexuality. In the many years of this author's experience, only one patient stated emphatically that it was not an important issue to him and he did not want to talk about it further. If the patient appears uncomfortable when the sexual questions are asked, inquire whether he or she would prefer to discuss this with a clinician of the same gender.

There are several instruments that may be useful in evaluating sexual concepts. The Aging Sexuality Knowledge and Attitude Scales (ASKAS) (White, 1982) has been used extensively with staff members and residents in nursing homes as well as with older adults and their families in the community. It is a 61-item questionnaire consisting of true or false questions in the knowledge section and 7-point Likert scales in the attitudes section. It can be self-administered or completed in an interview format; the interview format requires 30 to 40 minutes. If the patient is willing to take it home to complete, the ASKAS can serve as a beginning tool for assisting him or her with sexual questions. The Personal Assessment of Intimacy in Relationships (PAIR Inventory) (Schaefer & Olson, 1981) measures five types of intimacy and can serve as a helpful instrument in determining the need for intervention.

Each clinician will find his or her own best approach for introducing the subject of sexuality. A natural opening may occur during the review of systems, when asking questions about the genitourinary system. Another opening might be when discussing the older adult's relationship with the spouse while taking the family or psychosocial history. Clinicians should remember that not all people have a spouse, and they should be prepared for a variety of responses. Problems, concerns, or even questions may not surface during the first visit, but the fact that the subject has been brought up gives "permission" for the patient to bring it up again. With experience, the clinician will learn to recognize when it is beneficial to pursue questioning or when he or she should wait for a more suitable time to conduct a more detailed history.

In the primary care setting, when time is usually limited, a simpler approach may be helpful. This author has found the 10 questions listed in Table 24–2 to be useful in eliciting information and leading to more in-depth discussions when needed. In addition, the circle of intimacy has often been used successfully as an introduction to the sexual history (see Fig. 24–1).

If the patient is not currently sexually active, the clinician may want to explore whether that status is satisfactory to the patient. If the decrease in sexual activity occurred by both partners' mutual agreement or a gradual decrease in interest and activity, it may be appropriate to ask about the importance of intimacy and its expression in the patient's relationship (question #7). Asking patients about their knowledge of normal age-related changes that can affect sexuality (question #9) will almost always lead to further discussions and offers an excellent opportunity for teaching at subse-

TABLE 24-2
Brief Questionnaire to Assess Intimacy and Sexuality

1. How would you describe your relationship with your spouse or partner?
2. Are you sexually active now?
3. Is there any difference in your sexual enjoyment from earlier times? Do you think there is for your partner?
4. If yes, how is your sexual enjoyment different?
5. Do you have any idea why it is different?
6. Do you and your partner discuss sex and intimacy?
7. How important is intimacy in your relationship? Are activities such as hugging, kissing, and just being close important parts of your relationship?
8. Are you satisfied with the kind and amount of intimacy you receive?
9. Do you understand the normal age-related changes that might affect your sexual activity?
10. Would your spouse come in with you to discuss these items?

quent visits. Often, it is helpful to include the spouse or partner in these questions.

If the patient's sexual functioning is satisfactory, these questions will take approximately 2 minutes to complete. Even then, it is common that the query on normal age-related changes will stimulate questions either then or during a later visit. If both partners are interested, a session should be scheduled to provide factual information. If only one partner is present, the clinician can still accomplish much by listening, talking, and teaching. There may be problems more appropriately solved by someone else. For example, a patient with chronic impotence should be referred to a urologist who specializes in erectile failure and/or a sex therapist. Dyspareunia due to uterine contraction or vaginismus may require referral to a gynecologist and/or a sex therapist.

Physical Examination

The physical examination must be conducted with sensitivity and professionalism. The examination of the man must include careful observation as well as palpation for any abnormalities. This time can offer an excellent opportunity for questions and teaching. Examine the penis for signs of Peyronie's disease, observing the angle of the penis. If an angle is observed when the penis is in the flaccid state with the foreskin retracted, it is highly probable that the disease is severe enough that it interferes with sexual intercourse. Observe the foreskin and see how well it retracts; look for signs of discharge, irritation, or infections. A gentle, thorough testicular examination palpating for nodules is important to rule out cancer. While examining the scrotum, check for evidence of inguinal hernias. Observe the rectum for lesions, fistulas, or trauma; these are more commonly found in gay men owing to anal intercourse. Gently insert a finger into the rectum and examine the prostate gland. It should be firm and smooth with a palpable groove. Slight enlargement is normal in the elderly man, and the groove may then disappear. Only the posterior part of prostate gland can be palpated; thus, nodules could be present on anterior aspect of the gland. A manual examination and a PSA blood test are considered the best available methods of screening for prostate cancer. A hard nodule is highly suspicious of cancer. A soft, boggy prostate is indicative of prostatitis. A PSA level from 0 to 4 ng/L is considered normal; however, in the elderly, it is not uncommon for the PSA to be evaluated to 10 ng/L without concern. The most important factor in evaluating the PSA level is a sudden increase from a baseline PSA.

The physical examination of the woman should include both a pelvic and rectal examination. The pubic area should be inspected for any skin lesions and palpated for masses. Observe the labia majora and minora to determine if there is decreased fat; also note whether the clitoris is exposed and irritated. Touching gently to assess tenderness is useful. Also, observe the urinary meatus for irritation and or leakage. Inspect the vagina for dryness, discharge, odor, redness, or any signs of infection. Vaginal secretions become less acidic and may even become alkaline. This in turn alters the bacterial flora, causing the woman to become more susceptible to bacterial vaginitis. Before inserting a warm, moist speculum, gently exert pressure on the posterior part of the introitus. Be sure that the speculum size is appropriate for the size of the vagina. A 70-year-old woman who has not been sexually active for 10 years and has narrowing of the vaginal vault cannot tolerate a large speculum. If a smaller speculum is not available, postpone that part of the pelvic examination until a suitable speculum is available. The cervix may be more gray than pink in the older woman, but it should be smooth and free from lesions. As the cervix is swabbed, a small amount of bleeding may occur. If it does, the patient should be instructed that she may note a small amount of bleeding later at home. Reassurance is important, as is telling her to call if she observes a large amount of bleeding that lasts for several days. The woman should have a careful rectal examination as well, especially if she practices anal intercourse.

Always ask the patient at the end of a physical examination if he or she has any questions. Sometimes it is easier for patients to ask questions once the examination has been completed.

ROLE OF THE ADVANCED PRACTICE NURSE

The most important behaviors that describe the role of the advanced practice nurse are being nonjudgmental and accepting. The purpose of accepting sexuality in the elderly is not to force sexual activity or values on them or to say that nonsexuality is a less valued lifestyle. Rather, the purpose is to allow older adults to determine their own mode and frequency of sexual expression.

First, nurses must understand their own sexuality (Smook, 1992). How does one feel when picturing an elderly couple making love, or two men, or two women? Open discussions with colleagues can be useful in desensitizing oneself to the subject. It is especially helpful to discuss sexuality issues with colleagues who have expertise and knowledge on the subject. Although nurses may not agree with the type of sexual activity the patient prefers, they should accept the patient, be nonjudgmental, offer whatever knowledge is available, and know where to refer the patient for more indepth information if needed.

Nurses who have more knowledge on human sexuality will find it easier to approach the topic in a professional and helpful manner with patients. They are also less likely to be shocked or uncomfortable with anything the patient may want to discuss. Education is important for healthcare providers as well as for patients and their partners. This education should include information on intimacy needs, normal psychosocial and physical changes that affect sexual functioning, and helpful measures to alleviate simple problems.

Advanced practice nurses should offer to conduct educational workshops on sexuality and intimacy at senior centers, adult daycare centers, hospitals, community colleges, and universities. By involving these latter institutions, another group in dire need of education might be reached—the adult children of older people.

Nursing home administrators and staff members also need education on sexuality. Even today, many nursing home staff members discourage, sometimes punish, and often ridicule any form of sexual activity between residents. In one instance of this, a caring and unique administrator of a Midwest nursing home had the perfect answer. The nurse in charge came to the administrator's office horrified, asking what she should do, as she had seen Mr. Smith, aged 90 years, go into his wife's room and "now they were in bed having intercourse." He replied that she should close the door and make sure that they were not disturbed. Attitude and knowledge workshops on human sexuality often result in a positive change in attitudes among personnel. It is vital that upper-level administration also be involved in these sessions (Lyder, 1992).

SUMMARY

Intimacy and sexuality are part of normal healthy living from birth to death. The importance of various aspects of intimacy and sexuality fluctuate across the life span. Intimacy needs are vitally important throughout life. The more fully that intimacy needs are met, the higher the quality of life. When some intimacy needs cannot or are not met, other intimacy needs become more important. Sexual activity is one small part of the circle of intimacy. To some people, either by choice or because of circumstances, sexual activity has never been important. However, for those whose sexual activity has always been a source of joy and fulfillment, it can continue to be so into very old age. Advanced practice nurses should provide factual information on sexuality in a professional, nonjudgmental, and sensitive manner.

REFERENCES

American Association of Retired Persons (1994). *Facts on aging.* Washington, D.C.: American Association of Retired Persons.

Berger, R. M. (1982). *Gay and gray: The older homosexual man.* Urbana, IL: University of Illinois Press.

Brasch, R. (1973). How did sex begin? *Library of Congress Catalog Card Number: 72– 92655.*

Brecher, E. M. (1984). *Love, sex & aging.* Boston: Little, Brown & Co.

Bullard-Poe, L., Powell, C., & Mulligan, T. M. (1994). The importance of intimacy to men living in a nursing home. *Archives of Sexual Behavior, 23*(2), 231–236.

Busse, E. W., & Maddox, G. L. (1985). *The Duke longitudinal studies of normal aging (1955–1980).* New York: Springer.

Butler, R. N. (1994). Sex in America (Letter to the editor). *U.S. News and World Report, October,* p. 8.

Butler, R. N., & Lewis, M. I. (1976). *Love and sex after 60.* New York: Ballantine Books.

Butler, R. N., & Lewis, M. I. (1993). *Love and sex after 60* (2nd ed.). New York: Ballantine Books.

Butler, R. N., Lewis, M. I., Hoffman, E., et al. (1994a). Love & sex after 60: How to evaluate and treat the impotent older man. A roundtable discussion: Part 2. *Geriatrics, 49*(10), 27–32.

Butler, R. N., Lewis, M. I., Hoffman, E., et al. (1994b). Love & sex after 60: How to evaluate and treat the sexually-active woman. A roundtable discussion: Part 3. *Geriatrics, 49*(11), 33–42.

Comfort, A. (1972). *The joy of sex: A cordon bleu guide to lovemaking.* New York: Crown.

Comfort, A. (1975). *The more joy of sex.* New York: Crown.

Comfort, A. (1976). *A good age.* New York: Crown.

Dawber, T. (1980). *The Framingham Study: The epidemiology of atherosclerotic disease.* Boston: Harvard University Press.

Elmer-Dewitt, P. (1994). Now the truth about Americans and sex. *Time Magazine, 144*(16), 62–71.

Ende, J., Rockwell, S., & Glasgow, M. (1984). The sexual history in general medicine practice. *Archives of Internal Medicine, 144,* 558–561.

Falkeborn, M., Persson, I., Adami, H. O., et al. (1992). The risk of acute myocardial infarction after estrogen and estrogen-progestin replacement. *British Journal of Obstetrics and Gynaecology, 99*(10), 821–828.

Feldman, H. A., Goldstein, I., Hatzichristou, D. G., et al. (1994). Impotence and its medical and psychosocial correlates: Results of the Massachusetts Male Aging Study. *Journal of Urology, 151,* 54–61.

Friedan, B. (1993). *The fountain of age*. New York: Simon & Shuster.

Hammond, D. H. (1987). *My parents never had sex*. New York: Prometheus Books.

Kaplan, H. S. (1974). *The new sex therapy: Active treatment of sexual dysfunction*. New York: Brunner Mazel in cooperation with Quadrangle.

Kasempfer, S. H., & Fisher, S. G. (1992). Measuring sexuality: Physiologic, psychologic and relationship dimensions. In M. Frank-Stromberg (Ed.), *Instruments for clinical nursing research* (pp. 205–236). Boston: Jones & Barlett.

Kassel, V. (1983). Long-term care institutions. In R. B. Weg (Ed.), *Sexuality in later years: Roles and behavior* (pp. 167–182). New York: Academic Press.

Kinsey, A. C., Pomeroy, B., & Martin, E. (1948). *Sexual behavior in the human male*. Philadelphia: W. B. Saunders.

Kinsey, A. C., Pomeroy, B., & Martin, E. (1953). *Sexual behavior in the human female*. Philadelphia: W. B. Saunders.

Kramarsky-Binkhorst, S. (1978). Female partner perception of Small-Carrion implant. *Urology, 12*(5), 545–548.

Krane, R., Goldstein, I., & DeTejada, I. S. (1989). Impotence. *New England Journal of Medicine, 321*(24), 1648–1659.

Lobo, R. (1990). Estrogen and cardiovascular disease. *Annals of the New York Academy of Sciences, 592*, 286–294.

Lock, M. (1986). Ambiguities of aging: Japanese experience and perceptions of menopause. *Culture, Medicine and Psychiatry, 10*(1), 23–46.

Lyder, C. (1992). NPs play major role in promoting sexuality among institutionalized elderly. *Nurse Practitioner, 17*(9), 10, 13.

Masters, W. H., & Johnson, V. E. (1968). *Human sexual response*. Boston: Little, Brown & Company.

Masters, W. H., & Johnson, V. E. (1970). *Human sexual inadequacy*. Boston: Little, Brown & Company.

Masters, W. H., & Johnson, V. E. (1981). Sex and the aging process. *Journal of the American Geriatrics Society, 29*(9), 385–390.

Modigh, A., & Mulligan, T. M. (1992). Sexual dysfunction in the aging woman. *Geriatric Medicine, News & Reports, 1*(2), 10–11.

Mooradian, A., & Greiff, V. (1990). Sexuality in older women. *Archives of Internal Medicine, 150*, 1033–1038.

Mulligan, T. M., & Modigh, A. (1991). Sexuality in dependent living situations. *Clinics in Geriatric Medicine, 7*(1), 153–160.

Mulligan, T. M., & Modigh, A. (1992). Sexual dysfunction in the aging man. *Geriatric Medicine, News & Reports, 1*(2), 8–10, 21.

National Institutes of Health Consensus Statement Online (1992). Dec. 7–9; *10*, 1–31.

Neugarten, B. L. (1970). Dynamics of transition of middle age to old age. *Journal of Geriatric Psychiatry, 4*(1), 82.

Pfeiffer, E., Verwoerdt, A., & Davis, G. C. (1972). Sexual behavior in middle life. *Archives of the American Journal of Psychiatry, 128*(10), 82–84.

Pfeiffer, E., Verwoerdt, A., & Wang, H. (1968). Sexual behavior in aged men and women. Observations on 254 community volunteers. *Archives of General Psychiatry, 19*, 253.

Renshaw, D. C. (1983). Sex, intimacy and the older woman. *Women & Health, 8*(4), 43–53.

Ross, P. E., & Landis, S. E. (1994). Development and evaluation of a sexual history-taking curriculum for first- and second-year family practice residents. *Family Medicine, 26*(5), 293–298.

Schaefer, M. T., & Olson, D. H. (1981). Assessing intimacy: The PAIR Inventory. *Journal of Marital Family Therapy, 7*(1), 47–60.

Schrof, J. M., & Wagner, B. (1994). Sex in America. *U. S. News and World Report, 117*(15), 74–81.

Shover, L. (1988). *Sexuality and chronic illness*. New York: Guilford.

Smook, K. (1992). Nurses' attitudes towards the sexuality of older people: An investigative study. *Nursing Practice, 6*(1), 15–17.

Solomon, D., & Salend, E. (1992). *A consumer's guide to aging*. Baltimore: Johns Hopkins University Press.

Starr, B. D. (1985). Sexuality in aging. *Annual review of gerontology and geriatrics, 5*, 97–126.

Starr, B. D., & Weiner, M. G. (1981). *The Starr-Weiner report on sex and sexuality in the mature years*. New York: Stein & Day.

Walz, T. H., & Blum, N. S. (1987). *Sexual health in later years*. Lexington, MA: D. C. Health and Company.

Weg, R. B. (1975). Physiology & sexuality in aging. In I. M. Burnside (Ed.), *Sexuality and aging* (pp. 7–17). Los Angeles: University of Southern California University Press.

Weg, R. B. (1983). *Sexuality in the later years*. New York: Academic Press.

White, C. B. (1982). A scale for the assessment of attitudes & knowledge regarding sexuality in the aged. *Archives of Sexual Behavior, 11*(6), 491.

Whitehead, E. D., & Nagler, H. M. (Eds.) (1994). *Management of impotence and infertility*. Philadelphia: J. B. Lippincott.

Wilson, R. A. (1966). *Feminine forever*. New York: M. Evans.

Restraint-Free Care

Eileen M. Sullivan-Marx
Neville E. Strumpf
Lois K. Evans

In 1989, it was estimated that in the United States more than 500,000 older adults in institutional care were tied daily to beds or chairs (Evans & Strumpf, 1989). Evidence of the negative effects and limited efficacy of physical restraints, coupled with nursing home legislation aimed at reducing or eliminating restraints, has driven advocates and clinicians to change practice. Although physical restraints continue to be used, a growing number of nursing homes have demonstrated that support and security for older adults can be provided in a restraint-free environment (Blakeslee et al., 1990; Rader, 1991).

Restraint-free care (as contrasted with restraint reduction) is now the standard of care for older adults, although transition to that standard is still in progress. Despite policy change aimed at restraint elimination as well as repeated demonstrations that restraint-free care is beneficial to older adults, debate continues. Lobbying efforts by the nursing home industry for the use of restraints in special circumstances, conflicting policy by the federal government regarding use of restraints (Weick, 1992), and a lack of state support for federal regulations certainly contribute to this ongoing debate. Legal and policy mandates, along with education and other efforts to alter practice, have failed to eliminate the use of physical restraints. In 1992, the prevalence of physical restraints in nursing homes in the United States still far exceeded that of several other western countries (Strumpf & Evans, 1992).

Restraint-free care is not only possible and beneficial, as shown by demonstration projects and research, but also is the appropriate standard of care for older adults. In this chapter, the current status of restraint-free care of older adults is discussed. Appropriate interventions aimed at individualizing care for patients who are at high risk for restraint use are presented.

HISTORICAL BACKGROUND

Although Gerdes (1968) and Cubbin (1970) questioned the use of mechanical restraints with confused elderly patients, it was not until 1987 that U.S. consumers and professionals shifted their views on physical restraints. What were once considered a routine and effective part of care came to be viewed as ineffective, potentially harmful, and an assault on the dignity of older adults (Strumpf & Tomes, 1993). Indeed, in the 19th and early 20th centuries, restraints were considered deleterious for the patient.

Clara Weeks' *Textbook for nursing* (1885, cited in Strumpf & Tomes, 1993, p. 21) stressed that restraints worsened delirium and instead suggested the use of alternatives such as diversion and freedom. In 1908, Emma Hawley noted in the *American Journal of Nursing* that the nurse is often "compelled to fasten [a delirious patient] under a fastening sheet, which many times will seem to infuriate her patient" (Hawley, 1908, p. 758). The first geriatric nursing text (Newton, 1950) made no mention of restraint use, even in the section on care of senile patients.

The term *protector* (Strumpf & Tomes, 1993, p. 12) was used first in 1941 to describe the purpose of restraints, connoting a belief that such devices provided safety for the patient. At that time, the nursing literature suggested using physical restraints with aged individuals to prevent falls. In the 1950s, an emphasis on patient safety coalesced with increasing concerns about liability in cases of injury. Advertisements by manufacturers of restraints increasingly appeared in nursing journals, along with recommendations for the use of side rails and physical restraints. By the 1970s, a subtle yet steady process of more "entrenched views on the necessity of restraint in certain circumstances, a deliberate pattern of educating nurses about the types and uses of such devices, and limited debate concerning the efficacy of physical restraint" (Strumpf & Tomes, 1993, p. 13) had formed the foundation for extensive and unregulated use of restraints with the elderly.

By the mid-1980s, efforts to reform the use of physical restraints in older adults came to the forefront in several ways. Doris Schwartz, an esteemed leader in community health and gerontological nursing, put out a "Call for Help" (Schwartz, 1985, p. 9) that challenged nurses and consumers to reevaluate what she considered a disturbing prevalence of routine physical restraint. At the time of Schwartz's letter, however, the use of restraints was not considered a research priority in long-term care (Brower & Crist, 1985). Clinical issues identified as research priorities were the treatment of urinary tract infections and pressure ulcers.

The years following Schwartz's letter were marked by increased attention and research on physical restraints in the elderly (Strumpf & Evans, 1992) and the related issues of falls, confusion, and incontinence (Funk et al., 1992). In December 1989, the United States Senate Special Committee on Aging sponsored a symposium, "Untie the Elderly: Quality Care Without Restraints," to explore restraint-free care.

The Nursing Home Reform Law, which was included in the Omnibus Budget Reconciliation Act of 1987 (OBRA, 1987), set new standards for the use of restraints in care facilities. In response, consultation services and educational programs expanded to assist nursing homes in meeting these regulations. Accounts of restraint-free facilities (Mion & Mercurio, 1992), including an exemplary restraint-free nursing care facility at Kendal-Crosslands in Kennett Square, Pennsylvania (Blakeslee, 1988), illustrated that restraint-free care was possible and preferable for both staff members and residents.

To date, efforts to promote restraint reduction have included a newsletter, *Untie the elderly,* first published by the Kendal Corporation in 1989 (What is the law?, 1989); a regular series on restraints in *Geriatric Nursing* in 1990 and 1991 (Blakeslee et al., 1990; Bloom & Braun, 1991; Suprock, 1990); and other publications such as *A practical guide to reducing restraints in nursing homes* (cited in Cutchins, 1991) and *Toward a restraint-free environment* (Braun & Lipson, 1993). An editorial in the *New York Times* in March 1992 affirmed the notion of freedom from restraint as an issue of quality of life for nursing home residents. A year later, a feature article on restraint removal in nursing homes was published by the *New York Times* ("Free Nursing Home Patients," 1993).

At the University of Pennsylvania School of Nursing, the Gerontological Nursing Consultation Service has developed an education and consultation service in restraint reduction that was based on guidelines now available in *Restraint free care: Individualized approaches for frail elders* (Strumpf et al., 1998). Most recently, audio and video technologies have been used to market environmental modifications as part of restraint-free care (Middleton & Williams, 1993; Dveirin, 1992). The combination of these preceding events—legislation, consumer advocacy, and research—has helped focus attention on physical restraints.

The profound influence of OBRA '87 also has been felt by acute care hospitals, where policies on the use of physical restraints are beginning to change. The 1991 restraint and seclusion guidelines of the Joint Commission on Accreditation of Health Care Organizations (JCAHO) (Joint Commission Perspectives Insert, MA 1.4-MS 2.5) require that hospitals specify time frames in which to complete medical orders and use restraints; conduct periodic observations of each patient; and, if restraint use is to be continued, reevaluate the patient's condition and write new medical orders as needed. In 1992, the U.S. Food and Drug Administration responded to reports of restraint-related deaths and other known risks of physical restraints by mandating that all devices carry a warning label concerning potential hazards (Department of Health and Human Services, 1992).

Recent changes in JCAHO guidelines have moved further toward restraint-free care by setting new standards that support restraint reduction in policies, assess the human resources needed to meet this goal, and educate staff members. Further reductions are expected with the use of assessments that identify patient behavior and environmental risk factors. After assessment, a process that addresses approaches to care other than the use of physical restraints is identified and reflects underlying causes of patient problems (JCAHO, 1996).

As debate and ambivalence about restraint use continue, research regarding restraint-free care in hospital settings is sorely needed (Hibbs, 1992; Phillips et al., 1993; Sullivan-Marx, 1994). Indeed, whether in hospitals or nursing homes, the "reduction or elimination of restraints has not yet fully taken hold in the minds of all who deliver services to the elderly" (Strumpf & Evans, 1992, p. 4).

PREVALENCE OF PHYSICAL RESTRAINTS

Restraint Use Prior to the Omnibus Budget Reconciliation Act

Prior to the implementation of the Nursing Home Reform Law in 1990, uniform definitions of physical restraint did not exist, and the use of restraint was therefore difficult to estimate. In 1977, a national survey of nursing homes in the United States indicated that 25% of 1,303,000 residents were regularly restrained (geriatric chairs were not included as restraints in the survey). By 1988, based on self-reports from nursing homes, it was estimated that 41.3% of residents in skilled care and 31.7% in intermediate care were restrained (Health Care Financing Administration, 1988). Prevalence rates of physical restraint ranged from 7 to 22% in acute care hospitals (Frengley & Mion, 1986; Mion et al., 1986; Robbins et al., 1987). A study conducted on an acute rehabilitation unit found that 34% of patients were restrained (Mion et al., 1989). For hospitalized older adults, the prevalence of physical restraints apparently increases with age, ranging from 18 to 20% in those 65 years and older to 22% in those 75 years and older (Frengley & Mion, 1986; Lofgren et al., 1989; Robbins et al., 1987).

In instances in which hospitalized elderly patients are deemed confused or at risk of falling, the likelihood of physical restraint exceeds 50% (Appelbaum & Roth, 1984; Gillick et al., 1982; Innes & Turman, 1983). During hospital stays, restraints are used with patients who have been diagnosed with dementia or delirium, who have a severe illness, or who reside in a long-term care facility (Berland et al., 1990; Lofgren et al., 1989; Robbins et al., 1987); this pattern of use suggests that the most frail elderly are at risk of being restrained.

In sharp contrast to the prevalence of physical restraint in the United States, a descriptive study of acute, long-stay, and psychogeriatric units in Scotland found that only 3.8% of frail elderly patients were restrained (Evans & Strumpf, 1987). In this study, observations of 826 patients in 9 geriatric facilities (4 general hospitals, 4 psychiatric hospitals with psychogeriatric services, and a free-standing geriatric hospital) revealed no hand, mitt, vest, wrist, or ankle restraints. Restraints noted for the entire sample included only 1 bed rail in an intensive care unit, 2 seat belts, 10 geriatric chairs, and 19 tilting chairs.

Restraint Use After the Omnibus Budget Reconciliation Act

Following the passage of the 1987 Nursing Home Reform Law (OBRA, 1987) and enactment of the regulations in October of 1990, the Health Care Financing Administration in 1991 nevertheless reported a 22.5% prevalence of restraints in nursing homes nationally. As in past surveys, this figure was based on self-reports and may represent underreporting.

More recently, a number of facilities have reported successes in restraint reduction (less than 7% prevalence of restraint use) or elimination (Mion & Mercurio, 1992). Werner and colleagues (1994) reported a drop in the prevalence of physical restraints from 31 to 2% following efforts to remove restraints in a long-term care facility. A descriptive study of a facility restraint reduction team showed reductions from 67.5 to 36.7% (Sundel et al., 1994).

EFFECTS OF PHYSICAL RESTRAINTS

The assumed benefits of restraint use include reduced injuries from falls or wandering, the provision of security, improved positioning and posture, the accomplishment of treatment, and the facilitation of institutional schedules and efficiency (Evans & Strumpf, 1990). To date, there has been no evidence in the literature documenting the efficacy of physical restraints in facilitating treatment or in controlling behavior in older people. Paradoxically, "protective devices" such as side rails or physical restraints may actually exacerbate many of the problems for which the devices are customarily applied. Among older adults who fall, serious injuries from falls are greater when physical restraints are in use (Capezuti et al., 1996, 1998; Mion et al., 1989; Tinetti et al., 1992; Walshe & Rosen, 1979). That no increase in serious falls occurred in a nursing home study (Ejaz et al., 1994) and that fall-related injuries did not significantly increase during the 4 years following a restraint reduction program in a hospital setting (Powell et al., 1989) further support restraint-free care as the standard for practice.

Mounting evidence of the untoward effects of physical restraints with older adults outweighs any nonvalidated benefits for the use of these devices. Among the known detrimental effects are pressure ulcers, infections, incontinence, loss of functional capacity, cardiac stress, and altered nutrition (Lofgren et al., 1989; Mion et al., 1989; Strumpf et al., 1997). Agitated behaviors; emotional desolation; and feelings of anger, discomfort, resistance, and fear are consequences of enforced immobility and social isolation during periods of physical restraint (Evans & Strumpf, 1989). Reports of accidental death by strangulation or asphyxiation and other serious injuries from physical restraints add to the argument that physical restraints do more harm than good (DiMaio et al., 1986; Dube & Mitchell, 1986; Miles & Irvine, 1992; Ney, 1993; Scott & Gross, 1989).

When restraints are applied to older adults, their use is likely to be prolonged, resulting in increased disability and frailty. Unfortunately, the most physically dependent and least mobile elderly people are the most likely to be restrained, leading to a vicious cycle of increasing frailty and prolonged restraint. The use of restraints has also been challenged on ethical grounds, because of the negative impact on quality of care (Strumpf & Evans, 1991). From an ethical perspective, Moss & LaPuma (1991) noted that the therapeutic benefits of physical restraint have never been established.

Although limited in number, studies of restraint-free care do show improved outcomes, including decreased resident agitation (Suprock, 1990), shortened hospital stays (English, 1989), reduced pressure ulcers and sleep disturbances (Bloom & Braun, 1991), and the use of fewer psychotropic drugs (Powell et al., 1989; Rose, 1987; Siegler et al., 1997). Restraint reduction, moreover, has been successful without increases in staff (Bloom & Braun, 1991; Evans et al., 1997). In a multistate study of 276 nursing homes, costs did not increase following restraint reduction (Phillips et al., 1993) (Table 25-1).

REASONS FOR RESTRAINT USE

Physical restraints are generally applied to address three care problems: (1) the risk of falling,

TABLE 25-1
Effects of Restraint Use and Restraint-Free Care

Restraint Use	Restraint-Free Care
Serious injuries from falls	No increase in falls
Pressure ulcers	Less agitation
Infections	Fewer pressure ulcers
Incontinence	Decreased hospital stay
Loss of functional capacity	Less sleep disturbance
Altered nutrition	Fewer psychotropic drugs
Emotional desolation	No increase in staffing
Agitation	No increase in cost
Discomfort	
Fear	
Accidental death	

(2) interference with treatment, and (3) disturbing behaviors (Dunbar et al., 1996; Evans, Strumpf & Williams, 1991; Rader et al., 1992). As noted earlier, however, the discontinuation of restraints has not led to an increase in falls or fall-related serious injuries; on the contrary, restraint use has been linked to a greater risk of serious injury.

Restraints that prevent the disruption of treatment devices can be avoided by reevaluating the need for specific treatments (e.g., nasogastric tubes, indwelling urinary catheters) that may also be noxious to the individual. Disguising treatment devices with padding, relieving pain, or providing distraction during necessary treatment can often prevent the need for restraint.

Physical restraint is commonly viewed as the only reasonable method for protecting a patient from harm when agitated behaviors and impairments in judgment develop. Physical restraints, however, often increase agitation and confusion in the older individual (Evans, Strumpf & Williams, 1991).

Fear of litigation is often cited as a significant reason for the use of physical restraints, despite knowledge of the negative effects of restraints, including serious injuries and deaths. Kapp (1994) pointed out that successful litigation in restraint cases occurs most often when there is evidence of "inappropriate ordering of restraints, failure to monitor and correct their adverse effects on the patient, or errors in the mechanical application of the restraint" (p. 4).

Despite their known negative consequences and limited efficacy, physical restraints continue to be used for controlling behavior and maintaining safety. Staff beliefs about the efficacy of physical restraints and limited knowledge of other interventions contribute to the high prevalence of restraint use with older adults.

Concerns for patient safety as well as the desire to control patient behavior undergird a cultural environment (largely based on habit) that further contributes to restraint use. Circumstances in which restraints are tolerated, if not openly sought, are created by a need to control patient behavior (Evans & Strumpf, 1990), a lack of knowledge of interventions (Evans, Strumpf & Williams, 1991), a limited assessment of behavior (Francis, 1989), a belief in a principle of safety above all (Evans & Strumpf, 1990; Yarmesch & Sheafor, 1984), and a lack of awareness of the negative consequences associated with restraint use (Evans & Strumpf, 1990; MacPherson et al., 1990; Yarmesch & Sheafor, 1984). The perceptions of staff members that cognitively impaired individuals lack judgment to consent or participate in treatment decisions may also create an attitude of paternalism that supports restraint use (Evans & Strumpf, 1990).

Family and friends concerned about loved ones in institutional settings may contribute to a need to "do something" about problems such as wandering or falling, thereby leading to unwarranted restraint use. Quinn (1993) found that even when nurses felt that restraint use was not indicated, they nevertheless applied restraints to older adults if the family requested their use. The ambivalence of family members about the use of physical restraints (Hardin et al., 1993) suggests that these individuals need to be included in efforts to establish restraint-free care.

Concerns about patient safety, especially in the face of actual or perceived administrative pressures to minimize any risks that might precipitate legal action, compete with concerns for patient autonomy, ethical practice, and professional integrity. The best protection for patient, caregiver, and agency is care delivered with dignity and humanity, using the most current knowledge available.

Individual Factors Associated with Restraint Use

To develop interventions aimed at restraint-free care, it is useful to understand the characteristics of restrained residents. The following conditions increase the likelihood of being restrained: advanced age, physical dependence, cognitive impairment, experiencing mental health disorders, and exhibiting behaviors that are disturbing to others. Some of these characteristics have been statistically associated with restraint use only in studies using univariate statistical analysis, whereas other analyses have found that other characteristics remain risk factors even when items such as age or physical function are controlled (Table 25–2). Such characteristic risk factors, however, almost exclusively involve individuals who are also vulnerable to the detrimental effects of physical restraints.

Social Policy

OMNIBUS BUDGET RECONCILIATION ACT OF 1987

Although the prevalence of physical restraints reportedly declined following the enactment of OBRA '87 legislation, one study showed few changes during the first 6 months following implementation (Evans, Strumpf, Capezuti, et al., 1992). Worries persist among regulators, advocates, and clinicians that many of the so-called successes in reducing restraints have occurred by substituting less restrictive devices. Nevertheless, the legislation has over time certainly affected the use of physical restraints. Surveyors of long-term care facilities are now expected to monitor all restraint use according to guidelines; these guidelines require that clinical assessment and comprehensive care planning weigh the risks of using restraint against any potential benefits and also inform residents or their representatives of these risks.

Institutional Influences

ORGANIZATIONAL ISSUES

From an organizational perspective, the following factors have been associated with restraint use: administrative commitment (Robbins, 1986), fear of litigation (Evans & Strumpf, 1990; Quinn, 1993), high patient-to-staff ratios (Scherer et al., 1993), and minimal interdisciplinary collaboration (Frengley & Mion, 1986; MacPherson et al., 1990; Strumpf & Evans, 1988).

To implement a restraint-free policy in nursing homes, the Kendal Corporation (Blakeslee et al., 1990) has recommended targeting efforts at the board of directors, administrators, physicians, nursing home staff members, residents, and family and friends. System-wide efforts,

TABLE 25-2
Individual Risk Factors for Physical Restraint Use in Older Adults

Study	Age	Physical Dependence	Limited Health Status	Cognitive Impairment	Mental Disorders	Adverse Behaviors
Frengley & Mion (1986)*	√‡		√‡			
Robbins et al. (1987)*	√‡		√‡	√‡		
Berland et al. (1990)*	√‡			√‡	√‡	√‡
Sloane et al. (1991)†	√§	√§	√§	√§		
Tinetti et al. (1991)†		√‡		√‡		
Burton et al. (1992a)†		√‡		√‡		
Mion et al. (1989)*		√§	√§	√§	√§	
Gillick et al. (1982)*				√§		
Burton et al. (1992b)†		√§		√§	√§	√§
Evans, Strumpf, Taylor, et al. (1991)†		√‡		√‡	√‡	√‡

Key
*Hospital
†Nursing home
‡Univariate analysis
§Multivariate analysis

involving all people with any relationship to the facility or its residents, are needed if physical restraints are to be reduced (Kallman et al., 1992; Martin & Hughes, 1993; Powell et al., 1989; Suprock, 1990).

The Restraint Minimization Project, a 2-year effort involving 16 nursing homes in 4 states, employed a combination of approaches, including multidisciplinary teams, staff incentives, and various interventions to reduce physical restraints (e.g., exercise programs, postural supports, rest, assistance with elimination) (Dunbar et al, 1996). At the end of 2 years, restraint use had declined by 90%, and serious injuries had not increased. The participation of board members, administrators, and all employees was considered essential to the success of the project.

STAFFING

Sloane and colleagues (1991) conducted a case control study of restraint use on dementia units in nursing homes. They reported that a high patient-to-staff ratio was an independent predictor of restraint use. The myth, "We have to restrain because of inadequate staffing" (Evans & Strumpf, 1990, p. 126), has contributed to restraint use and stems from a limited awareness of more appropriate interventions. Indeed, studies suggest that caring for restrained individuals requires more rather than less time (Morse & McHutchion, 1991; Phillips et al., 1993; "What Is the Law?," 1989). A study of nursing home costs and efficiency suggested that the presence of residents in restraints had negative effects on these economic measures (Sexton et al., 1989).

RESTRAINT-FREE CARE

Change Process

TRANSITION THEORY

Restraint-free care is achieved through a transitional process involving commitment from everyone associated with a facility. The transition toward restraint-free care is exemplified at the organizational level by changes in structure, function, or interpersonal dynamics; individuals undergoing transition experience changes in "identity, roles, relationships, abilities, and patterns of behavior" (Schumacher & Meleis, 1994, p. 121). Restraint-free care requires the development of new facility policies, procedures, and practices by staff members at all levels as well as key multidisciplinary and administrative leaders (Blakeslee et al., 1990; Strumpf et al., 1998). Transition at the organizational level is facilitated by effective communication, teamwork, trust, and cooperation among staff members (Schumacher & Meleis, 1994). If the goal of restraint-free care is to be reached, administrators, board members, nursing and medical staff members, families, friends, and clients involved in an organizational community must be educated regarding the lack of efficacy and potential harm of physical restraints as well as the benefits of nonrestraint.

Evidence of an ineffective transition toward restraint-free care might include a lack of cohesion among staff members, increased absenteeism and turnover, the presence of rumors and suspicions, decreased cooperation, resignations, and a failure to recruit new personnel (Schumacher & Meleis, 1994). Conditions supporting a transition toward restraint-free care include meaningfulness of the transition for staff members, a desire for change, expectations concerning a realistically obtainable goal, sufficient knowledge and skill of staff members in applying interventions, and an environment supported by appropriate planning to achieve the goal (Schumacher & Meleis, 1994).

CHANGE THEORY

To avoid an ineffective transition and to promote restraint-free care, it is useful to think of change as occurring in three phases: unfreezing, moving, and refreezing (Lewin, 1947). Table 25–3 lists actions that should occur during each of these phases.

During *unfreezing*, a philosophy is set, leaders are identified, and clear goals are established (Strumpf et al., 1998). Educational programs are initiated, and dialogue is begun and incorporated into staff meetings and team rounds. In the *moving* phase, people who are restrained are assessed, and interventions to discontinue physical restraints are implemented. Successful outcomes that build staff confidence can be promoted by starting this process with new admissions and/or specific units in the facility. For example, restraints are most easily discontinued in situations in which a more appropriate intervention is fairly obvi-

TABLE 25-3
Implementing a Process of Change

Unfreezing

Develop a philosophy of restraint-free care
Identify leaders responsible for implementing restraint-free care
Set clear goals
Provide fundamental education regarding restraint-free care
Facilitate open communication and dialogue regarding restraint-free care

Moving

Become aware of people who are restrained
Determine the reason(s) for each restraint
Eliminate restraints on the easiest cases first
Except in an emergency, prohibit the application of restraints once they have been eliminated
Develop a *restraint-free* protocol for new admissions
Establish a protocol for emergency response to specific behaviors
Create an evaluation for feedback system: track medications, falls, and injuries and progress toward goal
Provide ongoing education
Celebrate successes

Refreezing

Develop and refine policies and procedures to reflect changes
Enforce policies and procedures in a consistent manner

From Strumpf, N. E., Robinson, J. P., Wagner, J. S., & Evans, L. K. (1998). *Restraint-free care: Individualized approaches for frail elders.* New York: Springer.

ous (e.g., a positioning problem solved by support wedges). Feedback and evaluation are critical in this phase and can be integrated into ongoing educational efforts and celebrations of success. During the *refreezing* phase, policies and procedures can be refined. It is important to enforce policies in a consistent manner.

IMPLICATIONS FOR NURSING PRACTICE

Goals for establishing restraint-free care include the following: (1) facility compliance with OBRA '87 mandates and institutional policy, (2) an environmental design that facilitates restraint reduction, and (3) the implementation of individualized approaches to care.

Policy and facility initiatives were discussed earlier in the chapter. Redesigning the physical environment to reflect home-like settings has been associated with low restraint use (Middleton, 1993). Case studies suggest that environmental adjustments aimed at facilitating function, providing security, and promoting freedom also contribute to restraint reduction in nursing homes (Cutchins, 1991; Middleton, 1993; Rader, 1991).

Individualized Approaches to Care—Methods

Individualized care is a philosophical approach based on the following principles: (1) all behavior is meaningful; (2) systematic approaches are required to assess behavior; and (3) once behavior is understood, underlying needs can be addressed (Strumpf et al., 1998). These principles should guide the selection of interventions other than physical restraints; these interventions have been categorized as physiological, psychosocial, activity related, or environmental (see Appendix 25–1) (Evans, Strumpf & Williams, 1991). It is generally felt that changing the traditional, and even habitual, practice of physical restraint depends on altering beliefs and increasing knowledge about appropriate practices and standards of care.

Continuing Education

The education of staff members is frequently described in the literature as a method of promoting restraint reduction (Blakeslee et al., 1990; Kallman et al., 1992; Martin & Hughes, 1993; Suprock, 1990). Yarmesch and Sheafor (1984) investigated decisions in restraint application and found that nurses with continuing education in geriatrics had greater knowledge of alternatives than those without geriatric education. Two nursing home studies using one-group pretest-posttest designs have shown that a restraint reduction program may positively influence the attitudes and knowledge of staff

members; restraint use increased in one of these studies, however (Evans & Strumpf, 1992), and decreased in the other (Sundel et al., 1994).

The authors have used a series of 10 education classes to promote clinical staff members' knowledge of restraint-free care (Strumpf et al., 1998). The following topics are covered:

- Use of physical restraints
- Implementing a process of change
- Making sense of behavior
- Facts about falls
- Caring for persons at risk for falling
- Caring for the person who interferes with treatment
- Caring for the person with agitated/restless behavior
- Responding to behaviors perceived as disturbing
- Maintaining a process of change

It is critical to include every member of the clinical team in any educational effort. Each staff member has a contribution to make based on knowledge and clinical experience. Nursing assistants, intimately aware of resident daily routines, often provide keen insights about behavioral symptoms such as agitation or wandering. Other team members such as physicians or physical therapists may facilitate the least restrictive treatment for a given condition or suggest other creative interventions.

In continuing education, the teacher must engage learners in a problem-solving process and promote the testing of new ideas. To overcome resistance, celebrating early successes can empower staff members to continue the momentum of individualized, restraint-free care.

Consultation

The use of advanced practice nurses with expertise in geriatric care (e.g., clinical nurse specialists and nurse practitioners) has been particularly valuable in complex situations, such as the care of ambulatory elderly patients with severe cognitive impairment. Based on change theory and principles of consultation, Evans, Strumpf, Allen-Taylor, and colleagues (1997) investigated the effects of two experimental interventions designed to reduce restraint use in nursing homes. One intervention consisted of a structured program of education for staff members over a 6-month period; the second intervention consisted of the same educational program plus consultation from a clinical nurse specialist; a control nursing home received neither intervention. All three nursing homes were affected by mandated regulatory change aimed at restraint reduction (OBRA, 1987). The consultation with education intervention was associated with a statistically significant reduction in the use of restraints as compared with the "education only" or control groups.

Other studies have reported reductions, but not the total elimination, of physical restraints following consultative nursing interventions. In a cohort of 121 restrained nursing home residents, restraint use was reduced from 67.5 to 36.7% following a team effort to eliminate restraints; the team included a clinical nurse specialist (Sundel et al., 1994).

In another descriptive survey, 57 of 63 residents remained restrained following an institutional policy to remove restraints. A geriatric clinical nurse specialist then initiated an intervention using an individualized approach to care, with discontinuation of restraints in all but six residents (Werner et al., 1994).

Individualized Approaches to Care—Interventions

Rigorous clinical assessment precedes interventions aimed at individualizing care. A behavior log (Appendix 25–2) is essential for identifying and specifying care problems. The log can be used over several days or weeks, depending on the type of problem being assessed. By noting the "when, what, where, and who" of a particular problem, staff members can demystify it and try various solutions. The log promotes communication among staff members caring for an older adult and facilitates problem solving among all caregivers. The following is an example of how a behavior log might be used.

The presence of agitated, anxious behavior in a nursing home resident with moderate dementia of the Alzheimer's type is noted each weekday at 4:00 P.M. by staff members. The weekend staff members note on the behavior log that the resident's daughter visits on Saturday and Sunday at 4:00 P.M. and that agitated, anxious behaviors do not occur on those days. The staff members conclude that the resident becomes agitated and anxious when his daughter does not arrive for the 4:00 P.M. visit. An individualized approach might be to arrange for the daughter to call her father on the telephone at 4:00 P.M. each weekday to reassure him that all is well.

The literature is resplendent with examples of restraint-free care based on the use of physiological, psychosocial, activity-related, or environmental measures. Appendix 25–1 outlines a matrix of behaviors (fall risk, treatment interference, and other behaviors) and types of interventions that can be used as part of an individualized plan of care (see also Chapters 15 and 27).

SUMMARY

Review of the literature and recent research indicates that the application of a physical restraint is far from a benign procedure, especially owing to its physical and psychological impact on older people. It poses a critical ethical dilemma for all providers of healthcare. The foregoing discussion demonstrates the need for interventions that are consistent with standards of professional practice and that guarantee individualized, dignified care for frail, institutionalized older adults. It is our belief that restraint-free care has emerged as the standard of practice. Interventions exist and are known to succeed in other countries and at restraint-free facilities in the United States. Full achievement of the standard must now be accomplished if advanced practice nurses are to be true to their responsibilities for patient autonomy, personal safety, and quality of life. The transition to restraint-free care remains one of the great challenges for those who nurse and care deeply about older people in our society.

REFERENCES

Appelbaum, P. S., & Roth, L. H. (1984). Involuntary treatment in medicine and psychiatry. *American Journal of Psychiatry, 141*(2), 202–205.

Berland, B., Wachtel, T. J., Kiel, D. P., et al. (1990). Patient characteristics associated with the use of mechanical restraints. *Journal of General Internal Medicine, 5,* 480–485.

Blakeslee, J. A. (1988). Untie the elderly. *American Journal of Nursing, 88,* 833–834.

Blakeslee, J. A., Goldman, B. D., Papougenis, D., & Torell, C. A. (1990). Debunking the myths. *Geriatric Nursing, 11,* 290.

Bloom, C., & Braun, J. V. (1991). Restraints in the 90s: Success with wanderers. *Geriatric Nursing, 12,* 20.

Braun, J. V., & Lipson, S. (1993). *Toward a restraint-free environment.* Baltimore: Health Professions Press.

Brower, H. T., & Crist, M. A. (1985). Research priorities in gerontologic nursing for long-term care. *Image: The Journal of Nursing Scholarship, 17,* 22–27.

Burton, L. C., German, P. S., Rovner, B. W., et al. (1992a). Physical restraint use and cognitive decline among nursing home residents. *Journal of the American Geriatrics Society, 40,* 811–816.

Burton, L. C., German, P. S., Rovner, B. W., et al. (1992b). Mental illness and the use of restraints in nursing homes. *Gerontologist, 32,* 164–170.

Capezuti, E., Evans, L., Strumpf, N., et al. (1996). Physical restraint use and falls in nursing home residents. *Journal of the American Geriatrics Society, 44,* 627–633.

Capezuti, E., Strumpf, N., Evans, L., et al. (1998). The relationship between physical restraint removal and falls and injuries among nursing home residents. *Journal of Gerontology: Medical Sciences, 53A*(1), M47–M52.

Cubbin, J. K. (1970). Mechanical restraints: To use or not to use? *Nursing Times, 6,* 752.

Cutchins, C. H. (1991). Blueprint for restraint-free care. *American Journal of Nursing, 91*(7), 36–44.

Department of Health and Human Services (1992). *Food and Drug Administration: Medical devices; protective restraints; revocation of exemptions from 510(K) premarket notification procedures and current manufacturing resolutions.* 21 CFR 880, 890 (Docket No. 91N-0487). Federal Register 7(119), 27397.

DiMaio, J. M., Dana, S. E., & Bux, R. C. (1986). Deaths caused by restraint vests [Letter to the editor]. *New England Journal of Medicine, 255,* 905.

Dube, A. H., & Mitchell, E. K. (1986). Accidental strangulation from vest restraints. *Journal of the American Medical Association, 256,* 2725–2726.

Dunbar, J. M., Neufeld, R. R., White, J. C., & Libow, L. S. (1996). Retrain, don't restrain: The educational intervention of the national nursing home restraint removal project. *Gerontologist, 36*(4), 539–542.

Dveirin, G. (1992). *Mastering fall prevention, issues and answers: A guide for nurses.* Boulder, CO: Tactilitics.

Ejaz, F. K., Jones, J. A., & Rose, M. S. (1994). Falls among nursing home residents: An examination of incident reports before and after restraint reduction programs. *Journal of the American Geriatrics Society, 42,* 960–964.

English, R. A. (1989). Implementing a non-restraint philosophy. *Canadian Nurse, 85*(3), 52–55.

Evans, L. K., & Strumpf, N. E. (1987, November). *Patterns of Restraint: A Cross-Cultural View.* Paper presented at the meeting of the Gerontological Society of America, Washington, D.C.

Evans, L. K., & Strumpf, N. E. (1989). Tying down the elderly: A review of the literature on physical restraint. *Journal of the American Geriatrics Society, 37,* 65–74.

Evans, L. K., & Strumpf, N. E. (1990). Myths about elder restraint. *Image: Journal of Nursing Scholarship, 22,* 124–128.

Evans, L. K., & Strumpf, N. E. (1992). Reducing restraint: One nursing home's story. In S. G. Funk, E. M. Tornquist, M. T. Champagne & R. A. Wise (Eds.), *Key aspects of elder care: Managing falls, incontinence, and cognitive impairment.* New York: Springer.

Evans, L. K., Strumpf, N. E., Allen-Taylor, L., et al. (1997). A clinical trial to reduce restraints in nursing homes. *Journal of the American Geriatrics Society, 45,* 675–681.

Evans, L. K., Strumpf, N. E., Capezuti, E., et al. (1992). Shortterm effects of regulatory change on nursing home practice: The case of physical restraints [Abstract No. 64]. *Gerontologist, 32*(special issue II), 60.

Evans, L. K., Strumpf, N. E., Taylor, L., et al. (1991, November). *Characteristics of Restrained Older Nursing Home Residents.* Paper presented at the meeting of the Gerontological Society of America, San Francisco, CA.

Evans, L. K., Strumpf, N. E., & Williams, C. (1991). Redefining a standard of care for frail older people: Alternatives to routine physical restraint. In P. Katz, R. Kane & M. Mezey (Eds.), *Advances in long-term care, vol. 1.* New York: Springer.

Francis, J. (1992). Delirium in older patients. *Journal of the American Geriatrics Society, 40,* 829–838.

Free nursing home patients [Editorial]. (1992, March 7). *New York Times,* pp. xx.

Frengley, J. D., & Mion, L. C. (1986). Incidence of physical restraints on acute general medical wards. *Journal of the American Geriatrics Society, 34,* 565–568.

Funk, S. G., Tornquist, E. M., Champagne, M. T., & Wiese, R. A. (Eds.). (1992). *Key aspects of elder care: Managing falls, incontinence, and cognitive impairment.* New York: Springer.

Gerdes, L. (1968). The confused or delirious patient. *American Journal of Nursing, 6,* 1228–1233.

Gillick, M. R., Serrell, N. A., & Gillick, L. S. (1982). Adverse consequences of hospitalization in the elderly. *Social Science and Medicine, 16,* 1033–1038.

Hardin, S. B., Magee, R., Vinson, M. H., et al. (1993). Patient and family perceptions of restraints. *Journal of Holistic Nursing, 11,* 383–397.

Hawley, E. A. (1908). Manifestations of delirium in the night-time. *American Journal of Nursing, 8,* 757–761.

Health Care Financing Administration (1988). *Medicare/Medicaid nursing home information: 1987–1988.* Washington, D.C.: U.S. Government Printing Office.

Hibbs, P. J. (1992). Risks, dignity, and responsibility in residential homes for the elderly: Freedom or restraint. *Journal of the Royal Society of Health, 112,* 199–201.

Innes, E. M., & Turman, W. G. (1983). Evolution of patient falls. *Quality Review Bulletin, 9*(2), 30–35.

Joint Commission on Accreditation of Healthcare Organizations (1991). Restraint and seclusion guidelines. *Joint Commission Perspectives,* January/February(insert), D1–5.

Joint Commission on Accreditation of Healthcare Organizations (1996). Restraint and seclusion standards plus scoring. *1996 comprehensive accreditation manual for hospitals, standards TX7.1–TX7.1.3.3* (pp. 191–193). Oakbrook

Terrace, IL: Joint Commission on Accreditation of Healthcare Organizations.

Kallman, S. L., Denine-Flynn, M., & Blackburn, D. M. (1992). Comfort, safety, and independence: Restraint release and its challenges. *Geriatric Nursing, 13*(3), 142–148.

Kapp, M. B. (1994, Winter). Physical restraints in hospitals: Risk management's reduction role. *Journal of Healthcare Risk Management,* 3–8.

Lewin, K. (1947). Frontiers in group dynamics: Concept, method and reality in social science. *Human Relations, 1,* 5–42.

Lofgren, R. P., MacPherson, D. S., Granieri, R., et al. (1989). Mechanical restraints on the medical wards: Are protective devices safe? *American Journal of Public Health, 79,* 735–738.

MacPherson, D. S., Lofgren, R. P., Granieri, R., & Myllenbeck, S. (1990). Deciding to restrain medical patients. *Journal of the American Geriatrics Society, 38,* 516–520.

Martin, L. S., & Hughes, S. R. (1993). Using the mission statement to craft a least-restraint policy. *Nursing Management, 24*(3), 65–66.

Middleton, W. G. (1993, May). Homelike settings aid in creation of restraint-free environment. *Provider,* 45–46.

Middleton, W. G., & Williams, C. C. (1993). *Restraint-free care and the environment.* Philadelphia: University of Pennsylvania Press.

Miles, S., & Irvine, P. (1992). Deaths caused by physical restraints. *Gerontologist, 32,* 762–766.

Mion, L. C., Frengley, J. D., & Adams, M. (1986). Nursing patients 75 years and older. *Nursing Management, 17*(9), 24–28.

Mion, L. C., Frengley, J. D., Jakovcic, C. A., & Marino, J. A. (1989). A further exploration of the use of physical restraints in hospitalized patients. *Journal of the American Geriatrics Society, 37,* 949–956.

Mion, L. C., & Mercurio, A. T. (1992). Methods to reduce restraints: Process, outcomes, and future directions. *Journal of Gerontological Nursing, 18*(11), 5–11.

Morse, J. M., & McHutchion, E. (1991). Releasing restraints: Providing safe care for the elderly. *Research in Nursing & Health, 14,* 187–196.

Moss, R. J., & LaPuma, J. (1991). The ethics of mechanical restraints. *Hastings Center Report,* January/February, 22–25.

Newton, K. (1950). *Geriatric nursing.* St. Louis: C. V. Mosby.

Ney, A. (1993, April 27). Death in personal care home ruled an accident. *Citizen Voice,* pp. 4, 24.

Omnibus Budget Reconciliation Act (1987). *Subtitle C, nursing home reform.* Publication No. PL 100-203. Washington, D.C.: U.S. Government Printing Office.

Phillips, C. D., Hawes, C., & Fries, B. E. (1993). Reducing the use of physical restraints in nursing homes: Will it increase costs? *American Journal of Public Health, 83,* 342–348.

Powell, C., Mitchell-Pedersen, L., Fingerote, E., & Edmund, L. (1989). Freedom from restraint: Consequences of reducing physical restraints in the management of the elderly. *Canadian Medical Association Journal, 141,* 561–563.

Quinn, C. A. (1993). Nurses' perception about physical restraints. *Western Journal of Nursing Research, 15,* 148–162.

Rader, J. (1991). Modifying the environment to decrease

use of restraints. *Journal of Gerontological Nursing, 17*(2), 9–13.

Rader, J., Semradek, J., McKenzie, D., & McMahon, M. (1992). Restraint strategies: Reducing restraints in Oregon's long-term care facilities. *Journal of Gerontological Nursing, 18*(11), 49–56.

Robbins, L. J. (1986). Restraining the elderly patient. *Clinics in Geriatric Medicine, 2*(3), 591–599.

Robbins, L. J., Boyko, E., Lane, J., et al. (1987). Binding the elderly: A prospective study of the use of mechanical restraints in an acute care hospital. *Journal of the American Geriatrics Society, 35,* 290–296.

Rose, J. (1987). When the care plan says restrain. *Geriatric Nursing, 8,* 20–21.

Scherer, Y. K., Janelli, L. M., Wu, Y. B., & Kuhn, M. M. (1993). Restrained patients: An important issue for critical care nursing. *Heart and Lung, 22*(1), 77–83.

Schumacher, K. L., & Meleis, A. I. (1994). Transitions: A central concept in nursing. *Image: The Journal of Nursing Scholarship, 26,* 119–127.

Schwartz, D. (1985). Call for help [Letter to the editor]. *Geriatric Nursing, 6,* 9.

Scott, T. F., & Gross, J. A. (1989). Brachial plexus injury due to vest restraints [Letter to the editor]. *New England Journal of Medicine, 320,* 598.

Sexton, T. R., Leiken, A. M., Sleeper, S., & Coburn, A. F. (1989). The impact of prospective reimbursement on nursing home efficiency. *Medical Care, 27*(2), 154–163.

Siegler, E., Capezuti, E., Maislin, G., et al. (1997). Effects of a restraint reduction intervention and OBRA, '87 regulations on psychoactive drug use in nursing homes. *Journal of the American Geriatrics Society, 47,* 791–796.

Sloane, P. D., Mathew, L. J., Scarborough, M., et al. (1991). Physical and pharmacologic restraint of nursing home patients with dementia. *Journal of the American Medical Association, 265,* 1278–1282.

Strumpf, N. E., & Evans, L. K. (1988). Physical restraint of the hospitalized elderly: Perceptions of patients and nurses. *Nursing Research, 37,* 132–137.

Strumpf, N. E., & Evans, L. K. (1991). The ethical problems of prolonged physical restraint. *Journal of Gerontological Nursing, 17*(2), 27–30.

Strumpf, N. E., & Evans, L. K. (1992). Alternatives to physical restraints. *Journal of Gerontological Nursing, 18*(2), 4.

Strumpf, N., Evans, L., Capezuti, E., & Maislin, G. (1997). Consequences of hospital restraint use for older nursing home residents. *Gerontologist, 37*(special issue 1), 252.

Strumpf, N. E., & Tomes, N. (1993). Restraining the troublesome patient: A historical perspective on the contemporary debate. *Nursing History Review, 1,* 3–24.

Strumpf, N., Robinson, J. P., Wagner, J. S., & Evans, L. K. (1998). *Restraint-free care: Individualized approaches for frail elders.* New York: Springer Publishing Company.

Sullivan-Marx, E. M. (1994). Physical and chemical restraints: Meeting the challenge. *Dimensions of Critical Care Nursing, 13,* 58–59.

Sundel, M., Garrett, R. M., & Horn, R. D. (1994). Restraint reduction in a nursing home and its impact on employee attitudes. *Journal of the American Geriatrics Society, 42,* 381–387.

Suprock, L. A. (1990). Changing the rules. *Geriatric Nursing, 11,* 288.

Tinetti, M. E., Liu, W.-L., & Ginter, S. F. (1992). Mechanical restraint use and fall-related injuries among residents of skilled nursing facilities. *Annals of Internal Medicine, 116,* 369–374.

Tinetti, M. E., Liu, W.-L., Marottoli, R. A., & Ginter, S. F. (1991). Mechanical restraint use among residents of skilled nursing facilities: Prevalence, patterns, and predictors. *Journal of the American Medical Association, 265,* 468–471.

Walshe, A., & Rosen, H. (1979). A study of patient falls from bed. *Journal of Nursing Administration, 9*(5), 31–35.

Weick, M. D. (1992). Physical restraints: An FDA update. *American Journal of Nursing, 92*(11), 74–80.

Werner, P., Koroknay, V., Braun, J., & Cohen-Mansfield, J. (1994). Individualized care alternatives used in the process of removing physical restraints in the nursing home. *Journal of the American Geriatrics Society, 42,* 321–325.

What is the law? (1989). *Untie the Elderly, 1*(1), 1.

Yarmesch, M., & Sheafor, M. (1984). The decision to restrain. *Geriatric Nursing, 5,* 242–244.

25-1

Matrix of Behaviors and Interventions

Types of Interventions	Fall Risk	Treatment Interference	Other Behaviors
Physiological	• Identification of reasons for falling and comprehensive assessment • Medication review/elimination of troublesome drugs • Evaluation and prescription for physical or occupational therapy, etc. • Rest • Elimination schedule	• Comfort • Pain relief • Assistance with elimination • Evaluation of need for change in treatment (e.g., remove intravenous or nasogastric tubes, catheters)	• Comfort • Pain relief • Correction of underlying problem (e.g., dehydration) • Positioning • Attention to or assistance with elimination • Sensory aids • Massage or aroma therapy
Psychosocial	• Supervision • Authorization of "no restraint" from resident/family • Fall-risk program • Anticipation of needs	• Companionship and supervision • Authorization of "no restraint" from resident/family • Encouragement of appropriate advance directive • Reassurance • Maintenance of communication with family/resident • Ethics consultation as indicated	• Companionship • Therapeutic touch • Active listening • Calm approach • Provision of sense of safety and security; validation of concerns • "Timeout" as needed • Caregiver consistency • Supervision • Promotion of trust and sense of purpose/mastery • Attention to resident's agenda • Reality orientation (if appropriate) • Remotivation • Attention to feelings and concerns • Facilitation of resident control over activities of daily living • Pastoral/spiritual counseling • Family visits and information sharing • Communications that are calm, sensitive to cues, and use simple statements or instructions

Types of Interventions	Fall Risk	Treatment Interference	Other Behaviors
Activities	• Daily physical therapy, ambulation, or weight bearing • Gait training • Fall prevention program • Transfer assistance • Restorative program • Meaningful activity	• Distraction • Television, radio, music • Something to hold	• Distraction • Planned recreation (consistent with interest and abilities) • Exercise • Physical or occupational therapy; training in activities of daily living • Social activity • Outlets for anxious behavior, especially structured activity • Nighttime activities as needed • Redirection toward unit • Pet therapy • Structured routines • Spiritual activities and outlets
Environmental	• Chairs that slant or fit body, wedge cushions, abductor pillow or other customized seating • Low beds, bed rails, down or single side rails, pads, accessible call light, mattress on floor, bedside commode, table placed in front of chair • Mobility aids and supportive shoes • Safety awareness training, fall-safe environment, alarm signal system, assistive devices, elevated toilet seat • Varied sitting locations • Optimal lighting	• Placement near nursing station • Accessible call light • Camouflaged or padded treatment site • Protective sleeves, garments, etc.	• Decreased use of intercom • Decreased or increased light as appropriate • Quiet room or soothing background music and rocking chair • Personalized area; homelike environment with familiar objects • Camouflaged doors, exits, elevators • Floor tape (grids) or planters to signal end of hall • Special locks • Alarm systems • Velcro "doors" • Contained areas that are safe and interesting • Special clothing • Varied seating and furnishings • Personal space • Structured environment • Room changes as appropriate

Adapted from Strumpf, N. E., Robinson, J. P., Wagner, J. S., & Evans, L. K. (1998). *Restraint-free care: Individualized approaches for frail elders.* New York: Springer.

Behavior Log

Specific Behavior: _____

_____

Client's Name: _____ Room # _____

Date	Exact time	What happened?	Where?	Who else was present?	What could be happening internally (*inside* client) to cause behavior?	What could be happening externally (*outside* client) to cause behavior?	What interventions help (or could help) client?

From Strumpf, N. E., & Evans, L. K. (1994–1998). *Maintaining restraint reduction in nursing homes* (1 RO1 AGO 8324). Bethesda, MD: National Institute on Aging.

Drug Use and Misuse

Ginette A. Pepper

Appropriate drug use is one of the most important determinants of quality of life in the geriatric population. Medications are not only the most common therapeutic intervention for diseases in the elderly (Avorn & Gurwitz, 1997), but medication use is also increasingly common as a component of health promotion and disease prevention. Drugs have the capacity for great benefit, as well as for significant harm, for the elderly. Skilled and knowledgeable nursing care is essential to ensure that elderly patients enjoy the greatest advantage possible from pharmacotherapy. Requisite knowledge and skills for providing optimal pharmacotherapeutic care are listed in Table 26–1. In addition to this extensive knowledge base, in the majority of states where nurses in advanced practice roles have prescriptive authority (Pearson, 1998), additional knowledge is required for differential diagnosis and drug selection. Yet it is the fundamentals of nursing care—knowing the patient as a unique biopsychosocial being, informed observation, patient education, and individualization of care in concert with the client—that are most important in realizing optimal outcomes in gerontologic drug therapy.

SCOPE OF THE PROBLEM: DRUG USE AND MISUSE

Prevalence of Drug Use

Inappropriate drug use is a particular problem for the elderly, mainly because of greater

TABLE 26-1

Essential Knowledge for Appropriate Drug Therapy

Pharmacology of Medications

Clinical indications
Pharmacodynamics (mechanism of action)
Pharmacokinetics (especially route of elimination)
Adverse drug effects
Dosage, strength, form, and route

Physiology of Aging

How physiology of normal aging affects pharmacological mechanisms
How pathophysiology of age-related illnesses affects pharmacological mechanisms
Drug-induced diseases

Clinically Significant Drug Interactions

Drug-drug interactions
Drug-disease interactions (contraindications)
Drug-test interactions (laboratory and other diagnostic tests)
Drug-nutrient interactions

Monitoring Drug Effects (Adverse and Therapeutic)

History-taking
Physical assessment
Selection and interpretation of diagnostic tests

Medication Counseling and Teaching

Age-appropriate educational strategies
Cognitive, psychosocial, environmental, cultural assessment
Assessment of compliance
Promoting patient participation in decision-making

Drug Administration

Five Rights: right drug, right patient, right dosage, right route, right time
Selection and operation of administration devices
Dosage calculation

Measures to Promote Drug Outcome

Nonpharmacological and complementary therapies
Techniques to prevent and ameliorate adverse effects

Ethical, Legal, Social, and Economic Factors

Costs of medication
Ethical decision-making
Health policy and health care financing

prevalence of chronic disease resulting in more medication use, which also increases the probability of drug error, drug interaction, and adverse drug effects. Although constituting less than 12% of the population in the United States, adults over 65 years of age use 31% of prescription drugs. Eighty-five percent of community-dwelling elderly and ninety-five percent of elderly living in nursing homes take prescription drugs (Lamy, 1986a). During hospitalization, elderly patients also receive more prescriptions than younger adults (Nolan & O'Malley, 1988b). The average number of prescribed medicines increases consistently with age, with elderly individuals filling an average of 7.5 to 17.9 prescriptions per year (Jinks & Fuerst, 1992). The mean number of prescription drugs taken concurrently by the elderly ranged from 1.5 to 6.1 in various studies (Darnell et al., 1986; Helling et al., 1987; Pollow et al., 1994; Stoller, 1988). Characteristics associated with highest use of medication are being white, female, poor, and less educated (National Center for Health Statistics, 1983b). The number of

drugs used determines the risk for adverse effects due to drug interaction: when two drugs are taken the potential for interaction is 6%, but with five drugs the risk increases to 50% and the risk is 100% with eight or more concurrent drugs (Cadieux, 1989; Stein, 1994). Elderly patients are more likely than other adults to receive drugs commonly implicated in drug interactions (Castleden & George, 1984; Murdoch, 1980).

PRESCRIPTION PATTERNS

Based on a study of community-dwelling elderly people, Wilcox and associates (1994) judged that nearly one quarter (23.5%) of older Americans receive inappropriate prescriptions. Studies of nurse practitioners have concluded that the prescriptions of advanced practice nurses were appropriate for the medical diagnosis and that advanced practice nurses with prescriptive authority order fewer drugs than physicians (Avorn, 1991; Brown, 1993; Bupert, 1995; Holland et al., 1985; Safriet, 1992).

A survey of 380 million patient visits to physicians showed that the drugs most commonly prescribed for the elderly were cardiovascular agents (21% of prescriptions), central nervous system medications (18%), and agents to promote electrolyte balance (14%) (National Center for Health Statistics, 1982). Most likely to take more than two prescription drugs concurrently are patients with ischemic heart disease (52.4%), diabetes (36.1%), depressive/neurotic disorders (32.2%), and hypertension (28.1%), all of which are conditions prevalent in the elderly population (National Center for Health Statistics, 1983a).

Most studies of drug use among the elderly are conducted in long-term care settings where problems are even more conspicuous than in ambulatory and hospital settings. Not only do elderly patients in long-term care settings receive more prescriptions than other older patients, but also the pattern of prescribing differs, with greater use of drugs that are commonly associated with adverse effects and drug interactions: psychotropic drugs, cardiovascular drugs, analgesics, laxatives, and antibiotics (Nolan & O'Malley, 1988b; Vestal, 1985). Numerous authors have criticized prescription practices in long-term care, which include frequent selection of inappropriate agents and excessive ordering of "as needed" drugs, placing responsibility to diagnose and treat on the nursing staff (Ayd, 1985; Dawson, 1984; Nolan & O'Malley, 1988b). Although there are preliminary indications that federal legislation limiting the use of psychotropic drugs among institutionalized elderly has improved prescription practices in long-term care, the long-term impact of health policy initiatives on prescriptive practice remains to be determined (Kane & Garrand, 1994; Zullich et al., 1993).

OVER-THE-COUNTER SELF-MEDICATION

In addition to prescription drug usage, 70 to 89% of elderly people self-medicate with over-the-counter drugs without consulting a health-care professional (Pollow et al., 1994). Concurrent use of several over-the-counter medications is common, with the average number of medications per person ranging from 1.3 to 4.6 (Darnell et al., 1986; Helling et al., 1987; Pollow et al., 1994; Stoller, 1988). Categories of over-the-counter drugs that have been linked to adverse effects are analgesics, antacids, cold remedies and decongestants, fluid pills, laxatives, and sleeping aids (Pollow et al., 1994). The potential role of alcohol in adverse drug reactions is often overlooked as a problem in the elderly; even moderate use can cause deleterious drug interactions (Atkinson, 1984; Kofoed, 1985). In a survey of community-dwelling elderly, Forster and associates (1993) concluded that 24.9% of respondents were at risk for one or more adverse effects due to the combination of alcohol and prescription or over-the-counter medications. Herbal remedies are increasingly used by the elderly. Erroneously considered safe by consumers and innocuous by prescribers, herbal preparations are another overlooked source of adverse effects and drug interactions (D'Arcy, 1991, 1993; Haak & Hardon, 1988).

Adverse Drug Responses

RATE OF ADVERSE EFFECTS

An adverse effect or adverse drug response is any unintended or undesirable drug effect, including side effects, toxicity, or allergic reaction. Both initiation and discontinuation of drugs can trigger adverse drug reactions. Although elderly people may not report adverse effects unless specifically questioned, studies indicate they are two to seven times more likely to experience adverse drug effects than are younger adults (Hutchinson et al., 1986; Macisaac et al., 1989). A survey of the American Association of Retired Persons (1982) suggested that 40% of elderly community-dwelling Americans taking prescription medications experience adverse drug effects. Similar rates of adverse events have been noted in hospitals and nursing homes (Gerety et al., 1993; van Kraaij et al., 1994).

Although there is a dearth of recent, properly controlled, epidemiological studies on the incidence and cause of adverse drug effects, research indicates that multiple pathology and the associated high rate of prescribing is more important than the biological effects of aging in determining prevalence of adverse drug reactions among the elderly (Borchelt & Horgas, 1994; Chrischilles et al., 1992; Gurwitz & Avorn, 1991; Nolan & O'Malley, 1988a, 1988b; Solomon & Gurwitz, 1997). Factors that contribute to a high incidence of adverse effects in the elderly are (1) inadequate clinical assessment, (2) excessive prescribing of drugs, (3) inadequate supervision, (4) altered pharmacokinetics and pharmacodynamics, and (5) lack of compliance (Roberts & Tumer, 1988). Decreasing adverse drug effects among the elderly has been identified as a priority public health goal for this decade (USDHHS, 1991).

DRUG-INDUCED ILLNESS REQUIRING HOSPITALIZATION

Adverse drug reactions range from minor inconveniences to serious illnesses requiring hospitalization. Elderly people are more likely than younger people to be hospitalized for drug-induced illness. Individuals over 60 years of age account for nearly 30% of drug-related hospitalizations and more than half the deaths from adverse drug reactions (Kimelblatt et al., 1988). Adverse drug reactions are responsible for 2 to 15% of hospital admissions among the elderly, and inappropriate prescribing is often a contributing factor (Jankel & Fitterman, 1993; Lin & Lin, 1993; Lindley et al., 1992; Mannesse et al., 1997; van Kraaij et al., 1994). It was estimated that in 1985, drug-induced illnesses nationwide included 163,000 cases of cognitive impairment, 32,000 hip fractures, and 61,000 cases of parkinsonism (Surgeon General's Workshop, 1989). Drugs historically associated with hospitalization include digoxin, diuretics, aspirin, corticosteroids, psychotropics, and cytotoxics; recently, nonsteroidal anti-inflammatory drugs have become a leading cause of drug-induced hospitalization of elderly patients (Beard, 1992; Gerety et al., 1993; Lin & Lin, 1993). In some immigrant and indigenous populations, herbal remedies are a significant contributor to drug-induced hospitalization (Huxtable, 1990; Lin & Lin, 1993). With the recent changes that liberalized laws governing herbal products in the United States (Herbal Roulette, 1995), herbal toxicity may increase

in this country. Table 26–2 outlines concerns around use of "problem" drug groups, which have been implicated in studies of drug-induced hospitalization or identified by a consensus panel as inappropriate for elderly people (Beers, 1997; Beers et al., 1991; Wilcox et al., 1994).

COST AND BENEFIT

All drug therapy is based on consideration of the balance of risk and benefit, or the *cost-benefit ratio*. This means that healthcare providers must weigh the potential improvement from a particular prescription or dose of medication against the hazards that may accrue and, ideally in collaboration with the client, select the course that has greatest overall advantage for the patient. The risks of drug therapy range from minor discomfort to death. How much risk of adverse effects is acceptable depends on the degree of benefit to be gained. For example, although cytotoxic drugs used to treat cancer are among the most common causes of drug-induced hospitalization in the elderly, these chemotherapy drugs are used to treat a life-threatening disease for which a high degree of risk is acceptable.

In addition to the "costs" associated with adverse outcomes of drugs, the actual cost in terms of purchase price of medications and follow-up tests is increasingly considered to be one critical factor in the evaluation of cost-benefit ratio and in drug selection. Unfortunately, research indicates that many prescribers have little notion of the costs of drugs (Glickman et al., 1994). Prescription drug prices rose 88% between 1981 to 1988, more than three times more than the increase in the Consumer Price Index (Jinks & Fuerst, 1992). Although third-party funding may relieve the financial burden to individuals, health policy experts have suggested that increased prescription benefits may actually increase the problems of medication mismanagement, since cost will no longer constrain the number of prescriptions written or filled for an elderly person (Manasse, 1989).

TABLE 26-2

Drugs that Commonly Cause Problems for Elderly Patients

Group/Examples	Drug-Related Problems	Predisposing Factors
Nonsteroidal Antiinflammatory Drugs (NSAIDs) Aspirin Indomethacin (Indocin)* Phenylbutazone*	Acute renal failure, hyperkalemia	Preexisting renal impairment, volume depletion, salt depletion, CHF, cirrhosis, nephrosis, diabetes mellitus, concurrent triamterene (Dyrenium; in Dyazide, Maxzide)
Ibuprofen (Motrin, Advil) Naproxen (Anaprox, Aleve) Piroxicam (Feldene) Sulindac (Clinoril)	Peptic ulcer, gastrointestinal hemorrhage	Prior history of peptic ulcer, corticosteroid or anticoagulant use, NSAIDs with long half-life, first weeks of therapy
Ketoprofen (Orudis) Ketorolac (Toradol)	Allergy	Asthma, nasal polyps, cross allergy to another NSAID
	Depression, confusion	CHF, renal insufficiency, preexisting cognitive deficit
Benzodiazepines Chlordiazepoxide (Librium)* Diazepam (Valium)* Flurazepam (Dalmane)* Temazepam (Restoril) Midazolam (Versed) Lorazepam (Ativan)	Daytime sedation Increased risk of falls Driving impairment Withdrawal (taper slowly) Delirium, confusion	Benzodiazepines with long half-life and active metabolites, hepatic insufficiency, cognitive or neurological deficit, prior fall history, dementia, concurrent use of enzyme inhibitors, such as cimetidine (Tagamet; see Table 26–7).
Oral Hypoglycemics Chlorpropamide (Diabinese)* Tolbutamide (Orinase) Glipizide (Glucotrol) Glyburide (DiaBeta, Micronase)	Hypoglycemia Driving impairment (?) *Chlorpropamide:* hyponatremia; syndrome of inappropriate antidiuretic hormone; disulfiram reaction with alcohol	Concurrent salicylates, alcohol, disopyramide (Norpace), beta-blockers; hepatic or renal insufficiency; hepatic enzyme inhibitors such as cimetidine (Tagamet; see Table 26–7); highly albumin-bound drugs like phenytoin (Dilantin).
Cyclic Antidepressants Amitriptyline (Elavil)* Doxepin (Sinequan)*	CNS: sedation, increased falls, lower seizure threshold	Darkness, frailty, seizure disorder; concurrent use of other sedating drugs
Imipramine (Tofranil) Desipramine (Norpramin) Trazodone (Desyrel)	Cardiac: hypotension, dysrhythmia	Other hypotensive drugs, impaired left ventricular function, cardiac conduction abnormalities
	Anticholinergic: urine retention, constipation, dry mouth, confusion	Concurrent use of other anticholinergics or hepatic enzyme inhibitors such as cimetidine (Tagamet; see Tables 26–5, 26–6, and 26–7), prostatic hypertrophy, other constipating drugs, dementia, delirium.
Antipsychotic Drugs Chlorpromazine (Thorazine)* Thioridazine (Mellaril) Fluphenazine (Prolixin)	CNS: sedation, increased falls, extrapyramidal (parkinsonism, tardive dyskinesia), lowered seizure threshhold	Seizure disorder, darkness, dementia, high potency (low dose) antipsychotics (e.g., haloperidol)
Thiothixene (Navane) Haloperidol (Haldol)	Cardiac: hypotension, conduction disturbance	Low potency agents (e.g., thioridazine); see antidepressants above
	Anticholinergic: urine retention, constipation, dry mouth, confusion	Low potency agents (e.g., thioridazine); see antidepressants above

Table continued on following page

TABLE 26-2

Drugs that Commonly Cause Problems for Elderly Patients *Continued*

Group/Examples	Drug-Related Problems	Predisposing Factors
Sedative-Hypnotics Pentobarbital (Nembutal)* Secobarbital (Seconal)* Meprobamate (Equanil, Miltown)* Phenobarbital	Morning hangover, confusion, delirium, decreased effects of concurrent drugs due to hepatic enzyme induction, physical dependence, withdrawal (taper slowly)	Drugs susceptible to induction of metabolism (e.g., theophylline, phenytoin), sedatives with long half-lives and active metabolites, cognitive impairment
Over-the-Counter Sleep Aids Diphenhydramine (Benadryl, Nytol, Sominex, others)* Pyrilamine (Dormarex, others)	Morning hangover, anticholinergic effects (urine retention, dry mouth, constipation, confusion)	Dementia, prostatic hypertrophy, other constipating drugs (e.g., verapamil), other anticholinergic agents, dentures (dry mouth)
Antihypertensive Drugs Propranolol (Inderal) Reserpine* Methyldopa (Aldomet)* Clonidine (Catapres) Hydralazine (Apresoline)	*All:* sedation, fatigue, confusion, depression, orthostatic hypotension *Propranolol:* excess bradycardia, prolonged hypoglycemia in diabetic, hyperlipidemia *Clonidine:* dry mouth, sedation *Clonidine and propranolol:* rebound hypertension (withdraw slowly) *Hydralazine:* lupus-like syndrome	Other hypotensive drugs, personal or family history of depression, dementia, drugs with overlapping effects (e.g., sedation and dry mouth from clonidine increased by anticholinergics)
Antiarrhythmic Drugs Lidocaine (Xylocaine) Quinidine Disopyramide (Norpace)* Procainamide (Pronestyl) Mexiletine (Mexitil) Encainide (Enkaid) Flecainide (Tambocor) Propafenone (Rhythmol)	*All:* Protoarrhythmic (cause dysrhythmia), CHF, hypotension *Lidocaine:* seizure, confusion *Disopyramide:* anticholinergic effects	*All:* cardiac structural abnormalities, history of ventricular tachycardia, renal impairment, hepatic impairment; concurrent cardiac depressant drugs *Disopyramide:* concurrent anticholinergic drugs

Diuretics
Thiazides and related:
  hydrochlorothiazide (Esidrex),
  chlorthalidone (Hygroton),
  polythiazide (Renese),
  indapamide (Lozol),
  methyclothiazide (Enduron)
Loop: furosemide (Lasix),
  bumetanide (Bumex), torsemide (Demadex)
Potassium-sparing: amiloride (Midamor), spironolactone, triamterene (Dyrenium)
	Thiazide and loop: orthostatic hypotension, hypovolemia, dehydration, hyponatremia, hypokalemia, glucose intolerance, hypomagnesemia, hyperuricemia, elevated serum cholesterolemia, dry mouth, increased falls, stomach irritation
	Loop: hypocalcemia (see thiazides)
	Potassium-sparing: hyperkalemia
		Longer-acting agents (e.g., chlorthalidone), diabetes mellitus, gout, concurrent hypotensive drugs, concurrent potassium-depleting (e.g., corticosteroids, beta-adrenergic bronchodilators), acute renal insufficiency, bladder problems, nocturia, prostatic hypertrophy
		Loop: osteoporosis
		Potassium-sparing agents: drugs that increase potassium (angiotensin-converting enzyme inhibitors, potassium supplements, salt substitutes)

Cardiotonics Digoxin (Lanoxin, Lanoxicaps)	Toxicity: anorexia, weight loss, restlessness, weakness, syncope, visual disturbances, confusion, arrhythmia Withdrawal reaction: if stable and sinus rhythm, taper slowly and monitor closely	Concurrent magnesium- or potassium-depleting drugs (diuretics, corticosteroids, beta-agonists), hypokalemia, hypomagnesemia, hypercalcemia, renal impairment, recent change to more bioavailable form (liquid, capsules); concurrent drugs that impair elimination (verapamil, quinidine, nifedipine); heart block; doses greater than 0.125 mg daily

TABLE 26-2

Drugs that Commonly Cause Problems for Elderly Patients *Continued*

Group/Examples	Drug-Related Problems	Predisposing Factors
Anticoagulants Warfarin (Coumadin) Heparin	Bleeding, gastrointestinal hemorrhage *Heparin:* osteoporosis	*All:* Hepatic dysfunction, female gender, NSAID or aspirin use, some antibiotics (see below), thrombocytopenia *Warfarin:* hyperthyroidism, hypoalbuminemia, concurrent highly albumin-bound drugs, hepatic enzyme inhibitors *Heparin:* osteoporosis
Corticosteroids Prednisone Prednisolone	Osteoporosis, elevate blood pressure, hyperglycemia, potentiate glaucoma	Osteoporosis, hypertension, diabetes mellitus or prediabetic, glaucoma
Analgesics Meperidine (Demerol)* Pentazocine (Talwin)* Propoxyphene (Darvon)* Morphine Codeine Fentanyl	Dysphoria, irritation, pruritus, constipation, respiratory depression, confusion, seizures	Cognitive impairment, drugs with toxic metabolites (meperidine) or activity at sigma-receptor (normeperidine metabolite, pentazocine, propoxyphene), chronic obstructive pulmonary disease, concurrent sedatives, concurrent constipating drugs (e.g., verapamil)
Laxatives Bulk: psyllium (Metamucil), methylcellulose (Citrucel), polycarbophil (FiberCon) Stimulant/irritant: senna, bisacodyl (Dulcolax), danthron, phenolphthalein	Habituation, hypokalemia, fluid and electrolyte imbalance, withdrawal *Bulk:* esophageal or intestinal obstructions	Inadequate fluid, overdosage, neurological disorder, dementia, lack of knowledge about nonpharmacological methods
Antimicrobials Aminoglycosides: gentamicin, amikacin, kanamycin Amphotericin B Vancomycin Beta-lactams: ticarcillin, cefamandole (Mandole), cefoperazone (Cefobid), moxalactam (Moxam), cefotetan (Cefotan)	*All:* superinfection including pseudomembranous colitis, phlebitis at IV site *Aminoglycosides and vancomycin:* renal damage, hearing damage, muscle weakness, red man syndrome (vancomycin) *Beta-lactams:* hemorrhage and disulfiram reaction	*All:* renal impairment, infused too rapidly, high dosages *Aminoglycosides and vancomycin:* prior hearing impairment *Beta-lactams:* seizure disorder, debilitated state, malnutrition, agents listed in column 1, concurrent anticoagulant therapy, thrombocytopenia

*Drugs that have been identified by consensus of national panels as generally inappropriate for the elderly.
CHF, congestive heart failure; CNS, central nervous system; NSAID, nonsteroidal antiinflammatory drug.

OTHER FACTORS CONTRIBUTING TO DRUG MISUSE

Stereotypes and misconceptions about the aging process contribute to drug mismanagement. For example, clinicians who regard aging as a disease may treat conditions symptomatically, when definitive therapy for the underlying disease condition could cure the problem.

On the other hand, older patients may not receive adequate diagnosis and treatment of diseases if providers assume the symptoms are caused by old age (Hale et al., 1986). One of the most serious problems in drug mismanagement is the treatment of the adverse effect of one drug with the use of another drug. Too often, neither the prescriber nor the patient is aware that a new symptom is an adverse effect of a medication, so a new medication is ordered to manage the symptom. For example, levodopa could be ordered to treat parkinsonism caused by an antipsychotic drug (Avorn, Gurwitz, Bohn, et al., 1995). Adverse effects of the new drug or of the interaction of the new drug with the antecedent drugs may produce new symptoms that are, in turn, treated with medicines, a vicious cycle that leads to polypharmacy, decreased functional status, and decline in quality of life.

AGE-RELATED PHARMACOLOGICAL CHANGES

Aging is associated with physiological changes that alter response to drugs by affecting the pharmacokinetics and pharmacodynamics of drugs. Although the rate of physiological decline can be accelerated by chronic disease and slowed by optimal diet and physical activity, these physiological changes result from decrements in organ function that begin in early adulthood and proceed throughout adult life, as depicted in Figure 26–1 (Cherry & Morton, 1989; Katzung, 1998). At the age of 65 years, which has arbitrarily been defined as the lower limit of old age, healthy individuals without chronic diseases are unlikely to exhibit altered drug response or to require dosage adjustment, except under conditions of extreme physiological stress and homeostatic disruption. On the other hand, by the age of 80 years, most people will have accumulated sufficient degeneration of organ function to exhibit increased sensitivity to drugs and to require dosage modification. Published recommended dosages of drugs are generally determined through research on young or middle-aged adults with no concurrent illnesses or medications. The challenge of geriatric pharmacotherapy is to modify these recommendations to ensure optimal therapy for older clients.

Clinically, the most consistent physiological change is the age-related decline in renal function, which slows the elimination of many drugs, increasing magnitude of effect and duration of action in the majority of elderly patients. However, approximately one third of elderly people have normal creatinine clear-

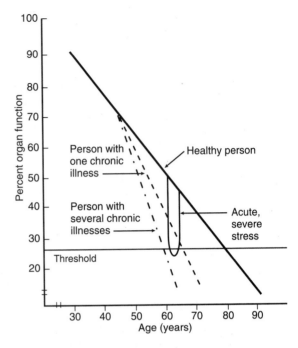

FIGURE 26–1. Schematic representation of the linear decrement of organ function during aging and its effect on drug response. Threshold is the point at which drug response is altered, generally manifested as increased sensitivity to drug effects and toxicity. Chronic diseases accelerate the aging process (dotted lines). Acute illness or other serious stressors can result in reversible, episodic alteration in drug response.

ance, indicating intact renal function (Katzung, 1998). Therefore, chronological age is only one of many determinants of pharmacokinetics and pharmacodynamics. Age-related pharmacokinetic and pharmacodynamic changes are summarized in Table 26–3.

Other age-related physiological changes may also indirectly affect drug response by altering pharmacokinetics and pharmacodynamics. For example, changes in biological rhythms that occur with aging can alter the effectiveness and toxicity of drugs (Fujimura et al., 1992). Gender may also modulate the effects of aging on drug response; certain drugs, such as propranolol (Inderal), ibuprofen (Advil, Motrin), and diazepam (Valium) show a decline in elimination only in men (Cusack, 1988; Greenblatt, 1989).

TABLE 26-3

Summary of Age-Related Changes in Pharmacokinetics and Pharmacodynamics

Process	Changes	Effects
Pharmacokinetics		
Absorption	↓ splanchnic blood flow	Few clinically significant effects
	↓ parietal cells; ↓ acidity	Dosage adjustment not usually required
	↓ motility	Slower absorption; delayed onset
	↓ first pass effect	Greater bioavailability of drugs with
	↓ absorptive surface	high hepatic extraction; first pass
Distribution	↓ body mass	Small elders more sensitive to usual doses
	↓ total body water	
	↑ body fat	Lipophilic drugs have ↑ Vd and ↑ $t_{1/2}$
	↓ lean body mass	Hydrophilic drugs have ↓ Vd, ↑ peak
	↓ binding to albumin	concentrations
	↑ binding to AAG	↑ free drug; drug levels difficult to interpret; effect of AAG unknown
Metabolism	↓ Phase I metabolism	↑ effect and toxicity of drugs
	↓ liver blood flow	metabolized by Phase I or high
	Unchanged Phase II metabolism	hepatic extraction
		No change in drugs metabolized by conjugation
Excretion	↓ glomerular filtration	Accumulation of drug eliminated
	↓ tubular secretion	unchanged
	↓ renal blood flow	Accumulation of metabolites
	Unchanged biliary excretion	Increased effect and toxicity of renally eliminated drugs
Pharmacodynamics		
Receptor binding	Changes in receptor number and affinity	Not known
Receptor coupling	Some second messengers less competent	Decreased beta receptor sensitivity is example
Organ function	Decreased functional capacity	↑ or ↓ response to drugs
Homeostatic mechanisms	Decreased reserve	Greater sensitivity to drug effects

AAG, α_1–acid glycoprotein.

Pharmacokinetic Changes

Pharmacokinetics encompasses all of the physiological processes by which the *body acts on the drug* through absorption, distribution, metabolism, and excretion. Pharmacokinetics determines how much of a drug is at the sites of action and for how long. Thus, the magnitude and duration of drug effect depends on pharmacokinetics. Normal aging affects the pharmacokinetics of each drug differently, owing to the drug's unique chemical and pharmacokinetic properties. For example, a lipid-soluble drug may have a longer half-life ($t_{1/2}$) in the older person, whereas a water-soluble drug could have a shorter half-life in the same person. As a result, an elderly patient may require dosage reductions for some medications and usual adult dosages of other drugs. Individualization of assessment and management is the key to geriatric pharmacotherapeutics, not only because of the diversity of the aging process among the elderly, but also because of the pharmacokinetic heterogeneity among drugs taken by an older individual.

ABSORPTION

Absorption involves all of the processes in the passage of a drug from the site of administration into the systemic circulation. The term *bioavailability* represents the percentage of the administered drug that is absorbed, actually reaching the systemic circulation. Relatively little research on the effects of aging on absorption has been conducted. Theoretically, a number of normal aging processes could alter bioavailability. For example, skin and vascular aging should affect transcutaneous absorption from skin patches (Roskos et al., 1986). In the aging gastrointestinal tract, decreases in motility, surface area, acid production, and blood flow can increase or decrease the bioavailability of various orally administered drugs, depending on each drug's unique pharmacokinetics (Jinks & Fuerst, 1992). As a result of these normal changes of aging, the rate of absorption for most drugs is decreased and the time to peak serum concentrations is increased, but bioavailability is unchanged (Ahronheim, 1992; Avorn & Gurwitz, 1997; Sloan, 1992). Therefore, *drug therapy should not generally require adjustment for age-related changes in absorption* (Katzung, 1998; Montamat et al., 1989; Sloan, 1992).

This does not mean, however, that absorption may not affect drug response in individual elderly patients. In the presence of a malabsorptive disorder, surgical reconstruction, diarrhea, or other gastrointestinal disease, absorption is often impaired (Williams & Lowenthal, 1992). As will be discussed, drug interactions are another common source of variability in drug absorption that can be prevented or minimized by adjusting drug administration. There is evidence that decreased gastric acidity resulting from age-related loss of parietal cells may cause clinically significant alterations in bioavailability of a few drugs. Since as many as 40% of elderly people have achlorhydria, absorption of ketoconazole (Nizoral) could be decreased (Conrad & Bressler, 1982; Sloan, 1992). Calcium carbonate (Tums) is poorly ab-

sorbed in hypochlorhydria, but when taken with meals, absorption is adequate, owing to the stimulation of gastric acid production by food (Ahronheim, 1992). Levodopa (Larodopa) is degraded in acid environments, so elderly people who have less stomach acid may have increased absorption, resulting in greater adverse effects (Ahronheim, 1992). Absorption of prazosin (Minipress) may be decreased in the elderly (Ahronheim, 1992; Jinks & Fuerst, 1992; Williams & Lowenthal, 1992). Dosage forms that require acid environments for proper dissolution, such as enteric-coated and sustained-release products, may also have altered absorption in the elderly (Miller, 1990).

Some drugs are eliminated from the body before they enter the systemic circulation by a process called *first pass metabolism*. Orally administered drugs are first absorbed into the portal circulation, which passes through the liver before entering the systemic circulation. Drugs that are very susceptible to liver metabolism (Table 26–4) are metabolized on this first pass through the liver. Generally, the enzymes responsible for this first pass effect are decreased in the elderly, so bioavailability of the high hepatic extraction drugs could be increased with age. These drugs require dosage reduction for elderly patients because a greater amount of the drug is absorbed and also because what is absorbed will be eliminated slowly by these same impaired enzymes (Cusack, 1988; Kelly & O'Malley, 1992; Williams & Lowenthal, 1992).

Although changes in the gastrointestinal tract have little effect on drug absorption, the gastrointestinal tract is the most common location of mild drug adverse effects, as well as a common site of serious adverse effects leading to hospitalization (Leape et al., 1991; Lin & Lin, 1993). The aging gastrointestinal tract has increased sensitivity to usual concentrations of drugs (Iber et al., 1994). Encouraging patients to take medications with a full glass of water or, when not contraindicated, with food will decrease the concentration of the drug in the gut and prevent some symptoms.

DISTRIBUTION

Distribution includes the processes whereby drugs are stored and transported to the sites

TABLE 26-4
Some Drugs that Have Decreased Elimination in the Elderly

Drugs with High Hepatic Extraction*	Drugs Eliminated by Phase I Metabolism	Drugs Excreted by Kidneys Unchanged
Amitriptyline (Elavil)	Acetaminophen† (Tylenol)	Acetazolamide (Diamox)
Codeine	Alprazolam (Xanax)	Amantadine (Symmetrel)
Desipramine (Norpramin, Pertofrane)	Barbiturates	Amikacin
Imipramine (Tofranil)	Chlordiazepoxide (Librium)	Ampicillin
Labetalol (Normodyne, Trandate)	Diazepam (Valium)	Atenolol (Tenormin)
Lidocaine (Xylocaine)†	Flurazepam (Dalmane)	Cefradine (Velocef)
Meperidine (Demerol)	Ibuprofen (Motrin, Advil)	Cefuroxime (Ceftin, Zinacef)
Metoprolol (Lopressor)	Ketoprofen (Orudis)	Chlorpropamide (Diabinase)
Morphine	Lidocaine (Xylocaine)†	Cimetidine (Tagamet)
Nitroglycerin	Meperidine (Demerol)	Digoxin
Propoxyphene (Darvon)	Naproxen (Anaprox, Aleve)	Disopyramide (Norpace)
Propranolol (Inderal)	Norepinephrine (Levophed)	Doxycycline (Vibramycin)
Tolbutamide (Orinase)	Nortriptyline (Aventyl, Pamelor)	Gentamicin
Verapamil (Isoptin, Calan)	Oxaprozin	Kanamycin
	Phenylbutazone (Butazolidin)	Lithium
	Phenytoin (Dilantin)	Nadolol (Corgard)
	Piroxicam (Feldene)	Pancuronium
	Propranolol (Inderal)	Penicillin
	Quinidine	Tetracycline
	Quinine	
	Theophylline	
	Tolbutamide (Orinase)	

*Drugs with high hepatic extraction undergo first pass metabolism when administered orally.
†Conflicting data have been reported concerning the effect of age on clearance.

of action and organs of elimination. The term *volume of distribution* (Vd) quantifies the distribution characteristics of a drug; drugs with large volumes of distribution are sequestered in peripheral tissues, while those with small volumes of distribution are located primarily in the vasculature. Body mass affects volume of distribution, so small body size, which is common among the very old, requires reduced dosages. In addition, body composition changes as part of the normal aging process. Total body water constitutes about 60% of body weight in young adults, but only 53% of the body weight of an elderly person. Conversely, the proportion of body fat increases with age, from 18% in young males to 36% in elderly males and from 33% in young females to 45% in elderly females (Katzung, 1998). Thus, hydrophilic drugs such as gentamicin and digoxin, which distribute to body water and lean body mass, reach higher peak serum concentrations in elderly people because of de-

creased body water and lean mass. Lipophilic drugs like diazepam (Valium) have increased storage in the expanded body fat of elderly people, causing an increase in the half-life of diazepam from an average of 20 hours in young adults to 80 hours in the elderly (Beers & Ouslander, 1989; Greenblatt et al., 1989; Thornburg, 1998).

Many drugs bind to proteins in plasma. Drugs bound to plasma proteins are pharmacologically inert, unavailable to exit the vasculature to interact with receptor sites or to be eliminated. Only the free drug is pharmacologically active. Changes in the binding of a drug, especially if the drug usually is bound 80% or more, will alter the drug's pharmacological activity. Albumin has several different binding sites and binds many acid drugs such as barbiturates, diazepam (Valium) and other benzodiazepines, furosemide (Lasix), oral hypoglycemics, phenytoin (Dilantin), and warfarin. Elderly people have a lower concentration of albumin, so there are fewer sites to bind drugs and a greater concentration of free drug can result (Greenblatt, 1979). Clinically, this may manifest as increased sensitivity to drugs, especially if age or disease has also compromised drug elimination (Cherry & Morton, 1989; Sloan, 1992; Thornburg, 1998). However, data that suggest a marked drop in albumin levels with aging were based on ill nursing home and hospitalized patients, rather than on healthy elderly people. Therefore, the clinical significance of age on protein binding may be less than originally hypothesized (Beers & Ouslander, 1989; Campion et al., 1988).

Altered albumin binding can confound the interpretation of laboratory results when "blood levels" are ordered (Cherry & Morton, 1989). Since most drug assays report total drug in the plasma (bound drug plus free drug), a reported serum concentration in a patient with hypoalbuminemia may appear below the therapeutic level but actually contain therapeutic amounts of active (unbound) drug. If a prescriber increases the drug dosage based on this laboratory report to achieve therapeutic serum concentrations, the patient could experience toxicity. Because of these limitations, drug assays from the laboratory should not be interpreted in isolation of other data such as results of physical examination and subjective interview; that is, the clinician should *treat the patient, not the laboratory report* (Hayes et al., 1975).

Two other plasma proteins besides albumin that can bind drugs are the lipoproteins and α_1-acid glycoprotein, which binds drugs that are bases like prazosin (Minipress), propranolol (Inderal), lidocaine (Xylocaine), and imipramine (Tofranil). While these two plasma proteins increase in many conditions common in the elderly, the clinical significance of these changes for drug response is not known (Abernathy & Kerzner, 1984; Montamat et al., 1989).

Disease processes can compound normal age changes on drug distribution. Congestive heart failure, nephrosis, weight loss or gain, and dehydration change the fat-to-lean ratio and thereby alter the volume of distribution of medications. Plasma protein binding is also affected by disease; malnutrition and nephrosis decrease albumin concentrations, cancer and inflammatory conditions increase α_1-acid glycoprotein levels, and diabetes mellitus is associated with high lipoprotein concentrations (Montamat et al., 1989).

METABOLISM

Metabolism and excretion are the two modes of drug elimination. Metabolism eliminates the drug by converting the chemical structure into a different molecule, called a metabolite. Most metabolites are inactive, but some are as active or more active at the receptor than the parent drug. *Clearance* is the measurement of drug elimination. Although metabolizing enzymes are found throughout the body, most drug metabolism occurs in the liver. Metabolites are more water soluble than their parent drugs, which facilitates excretion of the metabolites by the kidneys. Drug metabolizing reactions are classified as Phase I reactions, which involve adding or unmasking a polar chemical group to increase water solubility, and Phase II or conjugation reactions, which involve linking the drug to another molecule such as glucose (glucuronidation), acetate (acetylation), or sulfate (sulfonation). In the elderly, Phase I metabolism is often impaired, whereas Phase II metabolism usually is unaffected (Cusack, 1988; Katzung, 1998; Loi & Vestal, 1988; Schmucker, 1985). For this reason benzodiazepines such as lorazepam (Ativan), oxazepam (Serax), and temazepam (Restoril), which are metabolized by Phase II reactions and have no active metabolites, are preferred for elderly patients over drugs like diazepam (Valium), chlordiazepoxide (Librium), and flurazepam (Dalmane), which are cleared by Phase I and have several active metabolites (Cherry & Morton, 1989). Because blood flow to the liver declines by 40% with aging, the metabolism of high hepatic extraction drugs is also impaired in the elderly (Cusack, 1988; Schmucker, 1985). Table 26–4 summarizes the major modes of elimination for common drugs that have decreased elimination in the elderly.

Drug metabolism is a highly variable physiological function that is influenced considerably by genetic inheritance and can be altered by numerous environmental factors such as diet, air pollution, exercise, and, particularly, drug interaction and smoking. Diseases affecting the liver such as hepatitis, cirrhosis, and congestive heart failure can slow hepatic clearance (Catterson et al., 1997). If the drug metabolism of old and young subjects is compared, age explains only a small amount of the variability in hepatic clearance (Montamat et al., 1989; Schmucker, 1985). Although there is little consistency in the effect of aging on drug metabolism among people and across drugs, decreased hepatic clearance is responsible for many adverse drug reactions in the elderly. When selecting drugs eliminated by metabolism for the elderly, *it is best to begin therapy with low doses of agents that are eliminated by Phase II metabolism, have shorter half lives, and/or have no active metabolites.*

EXCRETION

Excretion is the removal of drugs and metabolites from the body. Some excretion occurs from the lungs, saliva, and bile, but most drug excretion occurs via the kidneys. All renal parameters, including kidney mass, renal blood flow, glomerular filtration, and tubular secretion, decline by an average of 35 to 50% between the third and eighth decades (Beers & Ouslander, 1989; German & Burton, 1989). Decline in renal function is the most predictable and important age-related change. *Drugs that are eliminated unchanged by the kidneys or have renally excreted active metabolites require dosage reduction in the elderly to avoid accumulation and toxicity* (Katzung, 1998; Loi & Vestal, 1988). Drug interactions and disease processes further impair drug excretion, intensifying age-related effects. Biliary stasis slows elimination of drugs excreted via bile. Renal insufficiency and renal failure profoundly limit drug excretion.

Estimating Renal Function. Serum creatinine is an unreliable indicator of renal function in the elderly. Creatinine is formed during the metabolism of muscle, and, because muscle mass declines with age, renal function can be significantly impaired despite a serum creatinine level in the normal range (Cherry & Morton, 1989; Gleckman & Czachor, 1989; German & Burton, 1989). Although creatinine clearance is the most reliable indicator of renal function, it is sometimes useful to estimate cre-

atinine clearance using the Cockroft & Gault (1976) formula for men:

$$\text{Creatinine clearance (mL/min)} = \frac{(140 - \text{age}) \times (\text{weight in kg})}{72 \times \text{serum creatinine in mg/dL}}$$

For women the result is multiplied by 0.85 to account for gender differences in muscle mass. This formula can be used to adjust dosage of drugs according to manufacturers' recommendations for patients with decreased renal function. Although decreased renal excretion has long been recognized as the most consistent age-effect on pharmacokinetics and the Cockroft-Gault formula is widely published in literature on geriatric pharmacology, Wells and associates (1996) found that there was little correlation between estimated creatinine clearance and dosages ordered for elderly patients. These researchers also noted clinical evidence of a high prevalence of toxicity of digoxin, a drug predominantly eliminated by the kidneys.

It should be remembered, however, that even renal function varies greatly in the elderly, and the approximately 30 to 35% of elderly people with normal renal function will be undertreated if reduced dosages are used (Katzung, 1998; Loi & Vestal, 1988). Therefore, evaluation of clinical response, and, if available, serum concentrations should be followed to individualize drug dosage. Overall, it is safer to begin with a low dose and titrate the dosage upward until a therapeutic dosage is reached, whether the drug is eliminated by metabolism or excretion.

Pharmacodynamic Changes

Pharmacodynamics includes the processes involved in the interaction of a drug and its effector organ that cause a physiological or biochemical change in the state of the effector organ. Most drugs interact with the effector organ at receptors, although a few have other mechanisms of action. Less research has been conducted on age-related pharmacodynamic changes than on the pharmacokinetic changes, because pharmacodynamics is more difficult to study and the molecular mechanisms are less well understood. Additionally, it is likely that pharmacodynamic changes do not begin to manifest until at least 70 to 75 years of age (Roberts & Tumer, 1988). When the effects of pharmacokinetics are controlled, elders are more sensitive to drugs like anticoagulants, benzodiazepines, barbiturates, neuroleptics, thyroid hormone, and opiates. On the other hand, they are less sensitive to drugs that work at the beta-receptor and to the cardiac effects of calcium channel blockers (German & Burton, 1989; Roberts & Tumer, 1988; Williams & Lowental, 1992). Four possible mechanisms have been proposed to explain pharmacodynamic aging: altered receptor binding, altered postreceptor function, decreased organ capacity, and decreased homeostatic reserve.

Altered Receptor Function. Changes in pharmacodynamic response would occur if aging resulted in an alteration in the number of receptors or the affinity with which the drug binds to the receptor. Although some studies have shown altered number and binding affinity for some alpha- and beta-adrenergic receptors, these changes have not been linked to altered drug sensitivity in the elderly (Williams & Lowental, 1992; Yokoyama et al., 1984).

Altered Receptor Coupling. Binding of a drug with a receptor results in a series of postreceptor chemical events within the cell. This process is called *coupling* because it links receptor activation to the ultimate clinical effect. For example, binding of a beta-agonist like epinephrine to a beta-receptor causes a change in the molecular configuration of the receptor, which, in turn, stimulates the G proteins in the cell membrane, resulting in the activation of an enzyme called adenyl cyclase. This enzyme catalyzes the conversion of adenosine triphosphate (ATP) to cyclic adenosine monophosphate (AMP), a so-called *second messenger*, which stimulates a variety of cellular reactions that increase heart rate, affect glucose metabolism, and dilate the bronchi. Cardiac response to beta-agonists and beta-blockers is blunted in the elderly; heart rate increases less with epinephrine and slows less with propranolol (Inderal). There is also impaired bronchodilator response to albuterol (Connolly et al., 1995). Research indicates that this decreased sensitivity of beta-receptors in the elderly is probably

caused by changes in the activity of the postreceptor processes (Beers & Ouslander, 1989; Williams & Lowenthal, 1992).

Decreased Organ Function. Decreases in organ function with aging alter drug response. Thus, the degree to which an inotropic agent like digoxin will increase the force of cardiac muscle contraction depends on the remaining contractile capacity of the heart muscle. Owing to changes in coronary perfusion, the elderly are less tolerant of drug-induced tachycardia from thyroid hormone, anticholinergics, and vasodilators, which may elicit angina and even myocardial infarction in older persons (Nattel & Watanabe, 1981). Decreased organ reserve also explains the greater incidence of drug-induced parkinsonism among the elderly (Montamat et al., 1989). Parkinson's disease occurs when enough dopamine-producing neurons in the brain degenerate to cause a deficit of dopamine activity in certain parts of the brain. Taking a dopamine blocking agent like the psychotropic haloperidol (Haldol) can illicit drug-induced parkinsonism in an elderly person with little reserve capacity for dopamine production. Recent research suggests that many elderly people are mistakenly being treated for Parkinson's disease when their condition actually is drug-induced parkinsonism from dopamine antagonists like metoclopramide (Reglan) and the antipsychotic drugs (Avorn, Bohn, Mogun, et al., 1995; Avorn, Gurwitz, Bohn, et al., 1995; Kalish et al., 1995).

Decreased Homeostatic Reserve. Much of the increased sensitivity to drugs in aging is caused by a decline in the competence of homeostatic mechanisms (Katzung, 1998). Increased bleeding in elderly persons on anticoagulants has been attributed to age-related impairment of vasospastic response following disruption of the integrity of the vascular system, although there is also evidence of altered receptor activity for warfarin (Crooks, 1983; Gurwitz et al., 1988; Nattel & Watanabe, 1981). Reduction in the competence of baroreceptor reflexes makes elderly people more prone to the orthostatic hypotension when taking antihypertensives, nitrates, antipsychotics, and other drugs that reduce blood pressure (Kelly & O'Malley, 1992; Roberts & Tumer, 1988). Because chemoreceptor function and lung capacities, which normally compensate for respiratory depression, are decreased in the elderly, they have increased susceptibility to the adverse respiratory effects of opioids (Roberts & Tumer, 1988).

DRUG MISADVENTURES

A variety of terms have been used to denote the negative consequences and risks of drug therapy, including side effects, contraindications, adverse drug effects, adverse drug responses, iatrogenic diseases, drug-induced illnesses, and adverse reactions. The term *drug misadventure* is used to indicate in the broadest sense all that can go wrong in the process of using a medication, encompassing errors in prescribing judgment, issues of compliance, proper drug administration, predictable and idiosyncratic responses, and even system errors in the process of bringing drug products to the users (Manasse, 1989). The focus of this section is four areas of drug misadventuring of particular relevance to nursing care of the elderly: polypharmacy, common adverse drug syndromes, drug interactions, and compliance. The final section of this chapter outlines nursing management to limit drug misadventuring.

Polypharmacy

Polypharmacy is the use of excessive or unnecessary medications, which obviously increases the risk of drug interactions and other adverse drug reactions. Simonson (1984) defined the features of polypharmacy as use of medications that have no apparent indication, use of duplicate medications, concurrent use of interacting medications, use of contraindicated medications, use of inappropriate dosage, use of drug therapy to treat the adverse effects of other drugs, and improvement when medications are discontinued. The causes of polypharmacy are

- Lack of adequate diagnosis
- Illogical prescribing due to deficient understanding of pathophysiology and pharmacology

- Failure to establish a therapeutic endpoint
- Inadequate patient education about disease and therapy
- Multiple prescribers with inadequate communication
- Insufficient monitoring of drug response
- Failure to discontinue ineffective or unnecessary drugs

Major Adverse Drug Syndromes

Several adverse drug syndromes are commonly seen in the elderly owing to the accumulated effects of physiological aging, pharmacokinetic and pharmacodynamic changes, age-related pathologies, and the types of drugs commonly used in this age group. The syndromes, common causative agents, predisposing factors, and nursing management are summarized in Table 26–5.

Cognitive Impairment. Medication can contribute to a variety of cognitive dysfunctions, including memory impairment, delirium, and confusion (Oxman, 1996; Palmieri, 1991; Rockwood, 1989; Williams & Caranasos, 1992). Because of increased blood flow distributed to the aging brain, decreased effectiveness of the blood-brain barrier, and increased sensitivity of the central nervous system to drug effects, many drugs have adverse cognitive or affective effects in the elderly. Elderly patients with pre-existing cognitive or neurological deficit will be more prone to manifest cognitive dysfunction. These effects may be masked when these elderly people are in unfamiliar environments and often are not obvious to people who do not know the individual well, so periodic assessment with a standard quantitative scale such as the Mini-Mental State Examination may facilitate detection of this syndrome (Folstein et al., 1975; Palmateer & McCartney, 1985).

Depression. Another drug-induced syndrome common in the elderly is major depression. It has been hypothesized that age-related changes in central neurotransmitter function may predispose elderly people to depression from drugs that further impair cerebral neurotransmitter activity. Patients with a personal or family history of depression or elderly patients

TABLE 26-5

Common Adverse Drug Syndromes in the Elderly

Adverse Drug Syndrome	Associated Drugs*	Predisposing Factors	Nursing Management
Cognitive impairment	*Antiarrhythmics* Lidocaine Procainamide (Pronestyl) Disopyramide (Norpace)† Quinidine *Anticholinergics* (see below) *Anticonvulsants* Phenytoin (Dilantin) Divalproex sodium (Depakote) *Antiparkinsonian* Amantadine (Symmetrel) Levodopa/carbidopa (Sinemet) Bromocriptine *Benzodiazepines* Diazepam (Valium)† Flurazepam (Dalmane)† *Barbiturates*† *Beta-blockers* Propranolol (Inderal) Metoprolol (Lopressor) Digoxin (Lanoxin) Cimetidine (Tagamet) *Corticosteroids* Prednisone Prednisolone *Diuretics* Hydrochlorothiazide Furosemide (Lasix) *Opioids* Meperidine (Demerol)† Pentazocine (Talwin)† Propoxyphene (Darvon)†	Preexisting neurological or cognitive deficit Debilitation Hypertension Pain Immobility Low educational level Lack of environmental cues Excess environmental stimuli Weak social support	Baseline and periodic assessment of cognitive function using standard scale Assess temporal aspects (e.g., "sundowning") Rule out depression ("pseudodementia") Avoid unnecessary medication Discontinue drug(s); changes drug or dose Environmental support: clocks and calendars Avoid excess stimulation Reality orientation Resocialization Use lowest effective doses of drugs
Depression	*Antihypertensives* Reserpine† Clonidine (Catapres) Methyldopa (Aldomet)† *Steroids* Corticosteroids Estrogens Corticotropin	Preexisting neurological disease Family or personal history of depression Concurrent use of >1 depressant drug Poor health status Recent losses Lack of social support	Baseline and regular assessment of depression using standard scale Stop or change drug therapy Suicide precautions Exercise therapy Psychotherapy Family involvement Pet therapy

Problem	Drugs	Risk Factors	Interventions
Falls	*Beta-blockers* Propranolol (Inderal) Metoprolol (Lopressor) *Antiparkinsonian drugs* Amantadine (Symmetrel) Levodopa *Anxiolytics* Diazepam (Valium)† Meprobamate (Equanil)† *Antipsychotics* Thioridazine (Mellaril) Haloperidol (Haldol) Thiothixene (Navane) *Other* Digoxin Procainamide (Pronestyl) Appetite suppressants Antineoplastics Analgesics *Antipsychotics* Chlorpromazine (Thorazine)† Thioridazine (Mellaril) Haloperidol (Haldol) *Antidepressants* Amitriptyline (Elavil)† Doxepin (Sinequan)† Imipramine (Tofranil) *Benzodiazepines/Hypnotics* Diazepam (Valium)† Flurazepam (Dalmane)† Temazepam (Restoril) Alprazolam (Xanax) Chlordiazepoxide (Librium) *Diuretics* Hydrochlorothiazide Furosemide (Lasix) *Antihypertensives* Clonidine (Catapres) Labetalol (Normodyne) Hydralazine (Apresoline) *Anticholinergics* (see below)	Drugs that are sedating, anticholinergic, cause postural hypotension Muscle weakness Female gender Hazardous environment Neurological disease Confused mental state	Assess fall risk Decrease number of drugs; eliminate drugs that cause sedation, hypotension, or anticholinergic effects Provide safe environment Exercise program Visual and auditory prostheses Good lighting Teach safety principles
Anticholinergic syndrome: Sedation Dry mouth Cognitive deficit Confusion	*Antihistamines* Chlorpheniramine† Diphenhydramine† Brompheniramine† Atropine (in Lomotil) Belladonna (in Bellergal)	Confusion Dementia Memory deficit Concurrent sedating drugs Multiple concurrent anticholinergics Prostatic enlargement	Minimize dose: give 2/3 at bedtime and 1/3 in morning Avoid hazardous activities if drowsy Encourage exercise and fluids Good oral hygiene; frequent sips of water Diet high in fruits and vegetables

Table continued on following page

TABLE 26-5

Common Adverse Drug Syndromes in the Elderly Continued

Adverse Drug Syndrome	Associated Drugs*	Predisposing Factors	Nursing Management
Blurred vision Constipation Urinary retention Tachycardia	*Antispasmodics* Clidinium (Quarzan)† Dicyclomine (Bentyl)† Oxybutynin (Ditropan)† *Antidepressants, tricyclic* Amitriptyline (Elavil)† Doxepin (Sinequan)† Imipramine (Tofranil) *Antipsychotics* Chlorpromazine (Thorazine)† Thioridazine (Mellaril) *Antiparkinsonian* Trihexyphenidyl (Artane) Benztropine (Cogentin) *Skeletal muscle relaxants* Methocarbamol (Robaxin)† Carisoprodol (Soma)† Chlorzoxazone (Paraflex)† Metaxalone (Skelaxin)† Cyclobenzaprine (Flexeril)† *Other* Digoxin Pentamidine Quinidine	Renal impairment Hepatic impairment	Avoid excess environmental heat
Movement disorders: Parkinsonism Tardive dyskinesia	*Antipsychotics* Haloperidol (Haldol) Trifluoperazine (Stelazine) Thiothixene (Navane) *Antidepressants* (rare) Metoclopramide (Reglan) Trimethobenzamide (Tigan)†	Female gender Long duration of therapy (tardive dyskinesia) Older Anticholinergic use (tardive dyskinesia) Neurological deficit High-potency antipsychotics	Assess tongue for fasiculations at baseline and every 3 months Lowest effective dose Drug holidays Avoid routine use of antiparkinsonian drugs; use only if parkinsonism appears Use low potency or atypical drugs: risperidone (Risperdal), clozapine (Clozaril)
Postural hypotension	Antihypertensives Antipsychotics Antidepressants Diuretics Dipyridamole (Persantine)†	Anemia Taking several hypotensive drugs Dehydration Heart failure	Postural blood pressures at baseline and every visit Teach activity: rise slowly from supine; don't stand in one place too long

*Associated agents list is not comprehensive but gives examples of agents most likely to cause the syndrome.
†Drugs that have been identified by consensus of national panels as generally inappropriate for the elderly.

on several drugs that can cause depression are at increased risk. Although somatic symptoms associated with medical illness and physical manifestations of adverse drug effects decrease the reliability of screening instruments, periodic use of an assessment such as the Zung Self-Rating Depression Scale may aid detection of drug-induced depression (Ahronheim, 1992; Patten & Love, 1993; Perry & Anderson, 1992; Thornburg, 1998; Zung & Zung, 1986).

Movement Disorders. Elderly people are more susceptible to extrapyramidal symptoms that are caused by dopamine receptor blockers, such as the antipsychotics and metoclopramide (Reglan). Extrapyramidal disorders include akathisia (a feeling of restlessness, tension, or anxiety) and parkinsonism (bradykinesia, gait disturbance, and tremor), which occur in the first days or weeks of therapy. Tardive dyskinesia, involuntary movements (usually of the lips and tongue, less often of the trunk and extremities), manifests after months to years of therapy, often when the drug is discontinued or the dosage is decreased. If the symptoms are not detected early with subsequent discontinuation of the offending drug, tardive dyskinesia is potentially irreversible. Restricting the use of antipsychotic drugs to elderly patients with appropriate target symptoms at the lowest effective dose for the shortest period of time possible is the best way to limit extrapyramidal syndromes (Ahronheim, 1992; Katzung, 1998; Thompson et al., 1983).

Falls. Medications are one of many factors that contribute to falls and resultant injuries. Although results have been inconsistent, research studies have linked the use of benzodiazepines, hypnotics, diuretics, antihypertensives, antipsychotics, and antidepressants to increased incidence of falls and injury (Campbell et al., 1989; Cummings et al., 1991; Monane & Avorn, 1996; Ray, 1992; Ruthazer & Lipsitz, 1993; Tinetti & Speechley, 1989). Mechanisms by which drugs contribute to falls may include orthostatic hypotension, sedation, and anticholinergic activity. A combined intervention of adjustment of number and type of medications, exercise, and patient behavioral instruction can reduce fall incidence among high risk patients (Tinetti et al., 1994). Heparin and corticosteroids increase osteoporosis and risk

for fracture, but thiazide diuretics, which increase reabsorption of calcium by the kidney, actually decrease the incidence of fracture resulting from falls (Felson et al., 1991).

Anticholinergic Syndrome. Many drugs have affinity for the cholinergic receptors of the parasympathetic system, including antihistamines, antipsychotic drugs, antidepressants, some antiarrhythmics and antiparkinsonian drugs, and antispasmodics. These drugs are said to possess anticholinergic, antimuscarinic, or atropine-like properties because they block the cholinergic receptors. Drugs with anticholinergic activity *counter* the effects of parasympathetic stimulation, causing dry mouth, dry eyes, dry skin, tachycardia, hyperpyrexia, constipation, and urine retention. Muscarinic cholinergic receptors are also located in the central nervous system; blockage of these central receptors impairs cognitive function in the elderly, leading to forgetfulness, ataxia, hallucinations, and confusion (Ray et al., 1992). Because of age-related physiological changes, the elderly are particularly sensitive to cholinergic blockade. Tune and associates (1992) found that 10 of the 25 most commonly prescribed drugs have sufficient anticholinergic activity to cause memory and attention impairments in normal elderly people. Many elderly people take two or more drugs with anticholinergic properties (Blazer et al., 1983; Pepper, 1985). Anticholinergic exposure has been correlated with postural instability that is a risk factor for falls and dry mouth, which is usually a minor nuisance, but can lead to serious oral disease (Pepper, 1991; Smith & Burtner, 1994; Thomson et al., 1993). Patients with dementia may be exquisitely susceptible to anticholinergic effects of drugs (Sunderland, 1987).

Orthostatic Hypotension. Decreased competence of baroreceptors plus high usage of antihypertensive drugs and other medications that promote postural hypotension contribute to orthostatic hypotension among the elderly. Alcohol is a significant contributor to postural hypotension. The major danger of orthostatic hypotension is falls and injuries, although precipitous falls in blood pressure can also lead to cardiac and cerebral hypoxia (Ahronheim, 1992; Thornburg, 1998; Tonkin & Wing, 1992).

Pharmacokinetic Drug-Drug Interactions

Although the incidence and severity of drug-drug interactions among the elderly are difficult to quantify, these interactions contribute to altered drug response and development of adverse drug reactions (Hansten, 1998; Jankel & Fitterman, 1993; Lamy, 1986b; Stein, 1994; Tatro, 1988). In this discussion and in Table 26–6, mechanisms of drug interactions are classified by the pharmacokinetic or pharmacodynamic process affected. Pharmacokinetic drug-drug interactions occur when one drug alters the absorption, distribution, metabolism, or excretion of another drug.

Absorption Interactions. Changes in oral absorption can result from formation of drug-drug complexes, altered pH, and altered intestinal motility and gastric emptying. These changes can alter the *rate* of drug absorption, which is seldom clinically significant, or the *extent* of absorption, which can alter drug response. Most common drug interactions decrease the rate of absorption but rarely change bioavailability or response. Interactions affecting oral absorption usually require the simultaneous presence of the interacting drugs in the gastrointestinal tract and can be avoided by administering the medications at least 2 hours apart.

Distribution Interactions. When two drugs that bind to the same site on plasma protein are taken together, one or both may be displaced from the binding site, transiently increasing the proportion of unbound drug. Age-related decreases in albumin increase the susceptibility of elderly people to this drug interaction. Since the unbound drug is the active component, drug effect increases. Because the free (unbound) drug is also more susceptible to metabolism and excretion, the increased drug response is temporary, persisting only until the new steady state develops. As discussed previously, altered protein binding can confound interpretation of drug assay levels.

Metabolism Interactions. The drugs listed in Table 26–7 can alter the elimination of other drugs by stimulating clearance (hepatic enzyme induction) or by decreasing clearance (hepatic enzyme inhibition). Studies indicate that the physiological capacity for hepatic enzyme induction and inhibition is maintained during aging, so these reactions may be common in patients taking numerous drugs (Beers & Ouslander, 1989; Catterson et al., 1997; Loi & Vestal, 1988; Ozdemir et al., 1996). Further, drugs that decrease liver blood flow increase the toxicity of drugs by slowing the first pass effect and elimination of high hepatic extraction drugs.

Excretion Interactions. Drugs that decrease renal blood flow by inhibition of renal prostaglandin synthesis impair the excretion of drugs and metabolites. Additionally, changing urine acidity can alter pH-dependent renal tubular transport mechanisms, thereby decreasing or increasing excretion of acids and bases.

Pharmacodynamic Drug-Drug Interactions

Pharmacodynamic interactions are the most common and clinically significant types of drug-drug interaction. The reactions are caused by the simultaneous use of drugs with overlapping or antagonistic actions. The negative effects of these interactions can be minimized by selecting drugs to avoid the interaction or initiating countermeasures to the anticipated interactions (Hansten, 1998; Tatro, 1988).

Additive or Synergistic Effects. The therapeutic or toxic effects of two coadministered drugs can equal the sum of each drug given alone (additive) or exceed the sum of the two drugs given separately (synergism). These effects often involve drugs acting on the same system, such as two drugs with sedative action on the central nervous system or two hypotensive drugs acting on the cardiovascular system. The herb ginseng has estrogenic effects, which can be enhanced by other drugs with this activity such as phenothiazines, calcium channel blockers, and digoxin, resulting in swollen, painful breasts in women and gynecomastia in men (D'Arcy, 1993).

Antagonistic or Blocker Effects. A drug can counter the effect of another drug by competition at the same receptor, such as when an agonist and an antagonist for the same receptor subtype are given concurrently. An example is

Mechanisms and Examples of Drug-Drug Interactions

Pharmacological Process	Mechanism	Examples
Absorption	Chelation or adsorption of drugs	Antacids, iron, and milk decrease absorption of tetracycline by chelation (chemical reaction between the cation [Ca^{++}, Fe^{+++}, Mg^{++}, Al^{+++}] and the drug molecule). Cholestyramine (Questran) adsorbs digoxin, other drugs, and vitamins.
	Changes in stomach emptying and gastrointestinal motility	Anticholinergics, phenothiazines, and tricyclic antidepressants slow motility and delay gastric emptying, causing delayed drug absorption, but may increase total absorption of drugs like digoxin.
	Changes in gastric pH	Antacids and antiulcer drugs like ranitidine (Zantac), cimetidine (Tagamet), and omeprazole (Prilosec) speed dissolution of enteric coated drugs like bisacodyl (Dulcolax); impair absorption of some acids like ketoconazole (Nizoral); and increase absorption of acid labile drugs like penicillin.
Distribution	Competition for albumin binding	Increased effect of oral anticoagulants, tolbutamide (Orinase), methotrexate, or phenytoin (Dilantin) if taken together or with other highly bound drugs like sulfonamides, sulindac (Clinoril), aspirin, nalidixic acid (NegGram).
Metabolism	Hepatic enzyme induction	Barbiturates, caffeine, smoking, DDT, charcoal broiled foods, and drugs listed in Table 26–7 speed metabolism of oral anticoagulants and theophylline, causing *decreased* effect.
	Hepatic enzyme inhibition	Cimetidine, ciprofloxacin (Cipro), ketoconazole (Nizoral), and inhibitors listed in Table 26–7 slow metabolism of many drugs like theophylline, warfarin (Coumadin), cisapride (Propulsid), terfenadine (Seldane) causing *increased* effect and even death.
	Decreased liver blood flow	Cimetidine (Tagamet) decreases metabolism of propranolol (Inderal) and other high hepatic clearance drugs (see Table 26–4).
Excretion	Competition for renal tubular secretion	Probenecid decreases elimination of penicillins and cephalosporins, increasing peak concentration and duration of action. Aspirin decreases elimination of methotrexate.
	Change in urine pH	Ascorbic acid increases elimination of bases like quinidine. Urine alkalinizers like antacids, acetazolamide (Diamox), and sodium bicarbonate decrease elimination of quinidine, leading to toxicity.
	Altered renal blood flow	Nonsteroidal antiinflammatory drugs decrease blood flow to kidneys and slow elimination of renally excreted drugs (see Table 26–4).
Pharmacodynamics	Altered homeostasis	Altered fluid and electrolyte homeostasis ($\uparrow Ca^{++}$, $\downarrow K^+$, Mg^{++}) increases risk of digoxin toxicity. Elderly are more prone to orthostatic hypotension due to baroreceptor function.
	Additive effects	Warfarin and aspirin together increase bleeding risk by interfering with different clotting pathways. Antihistamines and narcotics both cause sedation and constipation. Alcohol and hypnotics cause excessive sedation together.
	Antagonistic effects	Propranolol (Inderal) blocks bronchodilator response to albuterol (Proventil). Hypoglycemic effects of tolbutamide (Orinase) are decreased by hydrochlorothiazide.

TABLE 26-7
Drugs that Enhance and Inhibit Liver Metabolism

HEPATIC MICROSOMAL ENZYME (CYTOCHROME P-450) INDUCERS

Alcohol (with chronic use)
Barbiturates, especially phenobarbital
Cruciferous vegetables (e.g., broccoli, cauliflower)
Carbamazepine (Tegretol)
Glutethimide
Griseofulvin
Phenylbutazone (mixed inducing and inhibiting effects)
Phenytoin (Dilantin) and other hydantoins
Primidone
Rifampin
Smoking (tobacco, marijuana)

HEPATIC MICROSOMAL ENZYME (CYTOCHROME P-450) INHIBITORS

Alcohol (acute, high dose)
Allopurinol (Zyloprim)
Azithromycin (Zithromax)
Chloramphenicol
Ciprofloxacin (Cipro)
Cimetidine (Tagamet)
Clarithromycin (Biaxin)
Diltiazem (Cardizem)
Disulfiram (Antabuse)
Divalproex (Depakote)
Enoxacin (Penetrex)
Erythromycins
Estrogens (oral contraceptives)
Fluconazole (Diflucan)
Grapefruit juice (inhibits enzymes in intestinal wall)
Isoniazid
Itraconazole (Sporanox)
Ketoconazole (Nizoral)
Lomefloxacin (Maxaquin)
Monoamine oxidase inhibitors
Metoprolol (Lopressor)
Metronidazole (Flagyl)
Miconazole (Monistat)
Nifedipine (Procardia)
Norfloxacin (Noroxin)
Ofloxacin (Floxin)
Omeprazole (Prilosec)
Phenylbutazone (mixed inducing and inhibiting)
Propranolol (Inderal)
Ranitidine (Zantac)
Valproic acid (Depakene)
Verapamil (Isoptin, Calan)

concurrent administration of levodopa, which is converted to dopamine that stimulates dopamine receptors in the brain, and haloperidol (Haldol), which blocks dopamine receptors. Pharmacodynamic antagonism also occurs when drugs act on opposing physiologic systems, such as giving epinephrine, which increases heart rate by stimulating adrenergic receptors, concurrent with bethanechol (Urecholine), which decreases heart rate by stimulating parasympathetic receptors.

Drug-Laboratory Test Interactions

Drugs can interact with diagnostic laboratory tests by two mechanisms (Lamy, 1986b). One is to alter the physiological or pathological processes that are reflected in the laboratory tests. Thus, beta$_2$-adrenergic agonists like terbutaline (Brethine) cause an increase in serum glucose by stimulating gluconeogenesis. The other mechanism is chemical or physical interference of a drug or metabolite with the analytic procedure. For example, some antibiotics cause false-positive readings on tests for urine glucose. Deleterious effects of drug-laboratory test interactions can be minimized by (1) refraining from ordering tests that interact with drugs a patient is using, to decrease the costs of inaccurate tests, (2) informing the laboratory of drugs a patient is taking, and (3) prudence in acting on laboratory results until drug interaction or other source of error has been ruled out.

Drug-Disease Interactions

Although not as well studied as drug-drug interaction, it is likely that drug-disease interactions are a common cause of adverse drug reactions in the elderly (Lindley et al., 1992).

Drug-disease interactions are numerous, reflected in drug references as the contraindications for each drug. One mechanism for drug-disease interaction is alteration of drug pharmacokinetics due to a disease. For example, hepatic dysfunction, congestive heart failure, and acute pulmonary edema decrease the clearance of theophylline, which can result in theophylline toxicity. Another mechanism of drug-disease interaction is overlapping of the drug effects with symptoms of the disease. Elderly people with preexisting hearing impairment are more likely to have hearing loss from ototoxic drugs like furosemide (Lasix), aminoglycosides, or vancomycin (Gleckman & Czachor, 1989). Timolol eyedrops (Timoptic) given for glaucoma contain beta-blockers that can be absorbed and trigger bronchospasm in the patient with asthma (Lamy, 1986b; Stein, 1994).

Drug-Nutrient and Drug-Food Interactions

Drug effects on nutrition range from global, as in the elderly person who is unable to shop for groceries due to postural instability from a sedating or ototoxic drug, to very specific, such as folic acid deficiency that can result from taking phenytoin (Dilantin) or impairment of appetite, taste, or smell (Ackerman & Kasbekar, 1997). Similarly, generalized malnutrition has profound effects on drug pharmacokinetics by decreasing the concentration of albumin and activity of hepatic enzymes (Jorquera et al., 1996). Taking medication with food or meals can increase the extent of absorption, as exemplified by metoprolol (Lopressor), or decrease absorption so much that therapeutic failure results, as with tetracycline (Lamy, 1986b; Roe, 1994; Stein, 1994). Alcohol is another food product commonly used by the elderly that interacts with many drugs, exacerbating drug-induced hypotension or sedation (Forster et al., 1993; Stein, 1994). Acute ethanol ingestion can inhibit drug metabolism by hepatic enzymes, while chronic ingestion can speed the metabolism of many drugs. Because of the wide range of potential drug-nutrition interactions, clinicians need to maintain

a high index of suspicion and assess patients carefully for these effects.

Noncompliance

Because the term *noncompliance* suggests a hierarchical relationship with the powerful prescriber commanding the powerless patient, many clinicians and authors prefer the term *nonadherence*. In this chapter both noncompliance and nonadherence are used to describe patient behaviors that deviate from the recommended drug regimen, whether through intentional decision or unintentional error (Swonger & Burbank, 1995). No matter how comprehensively a patient is assessed, how accurately a diagnosis is made, or how carefully drug therapy is selected, patient behavior in terms of taking the medication is critical to the therapeutic outcome. Research indicates that noncompliance occurs in one third to one half of elderly patients, but that elderly patients are no more likely to be noncompliant than younger patients (Montamet et al., 1989; Morrow et al., 1988). The major causes of noncompliance are attributed to poor prescriber-client communication, deficits in patient cognitive function, and complex drug therapy regimen (Ennis & Reichard, 1997; Williams & Lowenthal, 1992). Other factors in noncompliance include living alone, greater numbers of medications, unpleasant side effects, financial problems, certain types of disease, poor relationship with the provider, lack of understanding of the medication regimen, and dispensing drugs in childproof medicine containers (Sherman, 1985; Swonger & Burbank, 1995). The most common type of noncompliance is taking too little medication. Taking the medication at the wrong time, using medication prescribed for someone else, and saving unused medication are other common errors (German & Burton, 1989). As many as 70% of elderly patients alter their medication intake intentionally, for a variety of reasons including decreasing adverse effects (Cooper et al., 1982). Patient education, clear communication, and inclusion of patient perspectives and concerns in the therapeutic plan are important strategies to improve compliance. Additionally, calendars, medication boxes with separate containers for each dose, electronic bottle caps that signal time for a dose, and supportive caregivers are useful assists to memory (Corlett, 1996; Williams & Lowenthal, 1992).

ADVANCED NURSING PHARMACOTHERAPEUTICS

This chapter has outlined a number of pitfalls in geriatric pharmacotherapy: prevalence of pathology and drug use, inappropriate prescribing practices, excessive incidence of adverse drug reactions and drug-induced diseases, age-related pharmacokinetic and pharmacodynamic changes, and drug misadventuring including polypharmacy, adverse drug syndromes, drug interactions, and noncompliance. These pitfalls can be avoided through comprehensive patient assessment, appropriate selection of therapeutic approach, patient education for self-care, monitoring of drug response, preventing and ameliorating adverse drug effects, and ensuring continuity of care across settings. Recommendations for practice are suggested for each of these functions, totalling 20 guidelines for advanced nursing pharmacotherapeutics.

Patient Assessment

1. *Know all of the patient's health problems.*
Because there are numerous potential drug-disease interactions, effective pharmacotherapeutics requires consideration of all of the health problems of the patient. Comprehensive assessment includes a baseline evaluation of affective and mental status as well as information on the patient's lifestyle and daily activities. For example, drugs like benzodiazepines, antipsychotics, and hypoglycemics should be used with extra caution in the elderly person who drives an automobile, so information on driving status should be assessed (Hemmelgarn et al., 1997; Palmieri, 1991; Ray et al., 1993; Thornburg, 1998).

2. *Obtain a thorough medication history.*
Collecting an initial medication history and updating it at each visit is a time-consuming but essential part of geriatric pharmacotherapeutics. It is important to ensure that information on over-the-counter drugs, herbal remedies and nutritional supplements, social drugs (alcohol, caffeine, nicotine in tobacco), and illicit drugs (marijuana, opiates) is collected. Also specifically question about drugs not taken by the oral route, such as inhaled drugs, topical ointments, or vitamin B_{12} injections, since patients often neglect to list these. Record the drug name, dosage and frequency, prescriber, and patient's view of the purpose and effectiveness of each medication. It is also useful to know the duration of therapy for each drug taken, what medications were used previously, and why each was discontinued or changed. Because aspects of pharmacokinetics and pharmacodynamics are genetically determined, family history, such as a pattern of responsiveness to a particular antidepressant or hyperreactivity to low dosages of medications, should be elicited (Poulsen & Loft, 1994). Allergic reactions and adverse drug effects should be described to ensure proper classification; patients often believe that all adverse effects are allergies (Bernstein, 1995). In a nonjudgmental way, ascertain the degree of compliance with the medication prescriptions. Since compliance is related not only to clinical effectiveness, but also to how the drug affects all aspects of their lives, provide an opportunity for patients to evaluate the drug for impact on overall quality of life (Morris & Schulz, 1993). When drugs are ordered *PRN* (as needed), record frequency of use and efficacy. It is often useful to have patients bring all of the medication bottles with them to the hospital or clinic. However, the patient should be asked to describe how the medication is used, since the prescriber may have changed the dose verbally or by telephone or the patient may use the medication differently than shown on the label.

3. *When there is a new symptom or change in health status, first consider the potential role of current medications.*

Polypharmacy often results when a symptom is not recognized as an adverse drug effect and is treated by another drug. Clinicians should maintain a high index of suspicion that changes in health status are drug-related, especially for cognitive, affective, and behavioral disorders (Gurwirtz & Avorn, 1991; Resnick & Marcantonio, 1997; Sloan, 1992).

Selection of Therapeutic Approach

4. Establish a therapeutic goal.

Drug selection begins with a therapeutic goal, which provides a benchmark for drug selection and for assessing the efficacy of the therapy. Too often, a drug is initiated for an elderly patient because it is the drug of choice for a particular condition, rather than because it will make the patient feel better or have a benefit that can reasonably be expected to manifest during the patient's life span. Drugs selected should be specific and rational based on the therapeutic goal and the pathophysiology of the disease to be treated (Thornburg, 1998). The therapeutic goal is derived from a cost-benefit analysis that reflects the values of the client, prescriber, and caregivers (Morris & Schulz, 1993; Palmieri, 1991; Sloan, 1992). It is important that the therapeutic goal be shared with the entire healthcare team, including the patient and family.

5. Consider nondrug therapy as the sole or complementary prescription.

Many conditions can be managed without drug therapy. For example, behavioral and environmental therapy can often obviate the use of psychotropic medication (Palmieri, 1991). Even if drugs cannot be totally eliminated, use of nondrug therapy such as exercise, diet, physical activity, heat or cold, and rest can often reduce the dose of medication required to attain the therapeutic goal (Sloan, 1992).

6. Know which drugs to avoid and choose the least toxic drug.

Some drug groups, such as benzodiazepines and antiarrhythmic drugs, should be reserved for patients with specific, well-defined indications, because they are commonly associated with adverse effects. Certain agents within a drug group elicit adverse effects at such a high rate that they should virtually never be used for elderly patients. An example is amitriptyline (Elavil), a tricyclic antidepressant that has a very high level of anticholinergic, sedative, and hypotensive activity (Beers, 1997; Beers et al., 1991; French, 1996; Tamblyn, 1996; Wilcox et al., 1994). Alternatives to amitriptyline for the elderly are other cyclic antidepressants with less of these adverse effects, such as desipramine (Norpramin, Pertofrane) and trazodone (Desyrel) or serotonin selective reuptake inhibitors, which are virtually free of these effects, such as fluoxetine (Prozac) and sertraline (Zoloft). Other individual drugs to avoid in the elderly are identified in Table 26–2. Although new federal labeling requirements will increase information available to clinicians, there is usually little prior use of recently released drugs in elderly people with multiple diagnoses and concurrent medications, so it is generally wise to avoid new drugs in the elderly (Beers, 1997; Skolnick, 1997). Other drugs to generally avoid in the elderly are those with long half-lives and active metabolites, because these drugs accumulate and have prolonged duration of adverse effects (Pirmohamed et al., 1994).

7. Prescribe the simplest regimen possible.

Compliance is improved when there are fewer drugs and dosages to be administered. The risk of drug interaction and adverse drug effects are also decreased when a patient takes fewer drugs. Preference should be given to drugs with multiple indications, such as the use of an alpha$_1$-adrenergic blocker, like terazocin (Hytrin) for the elderly male with benign prostatic hypertrophy and hypertension. Combination agents, which have more than one drug in a single tablet or pill, can often simplify a drug regimen, as long as the patient's dosing requirements match an available fixed combination (Stein, 1994).

8. Begin with a low dose and titrate upward slowly.

The aphorism "start low and go slow" is wise advice in geriatric pharmacotherapy. Initial geriatric dosages should be at the lowest levels of published adult dosages; for psychotropic drugs, start dosages are one third to one half recommended adult dosages. Even lower beginning dosages may be required for renally excreted drugs if the estimated creatinine clearance is low (Katzung, 1998). Remembering that most drugs have prolonged half-lives in the elderly, dosage should be advanced no more frequently than every five half-lives. Because homeostatic mechanisms may take more time to readjust, even more gradual dosage titration is justified (Katzung, 1998; Nolan & O'Malley, 1988a; Sloan, 1992; Stein, 1994).

9. Consider cost and convenience.

With the growing number of agents within each drug group, cost and convenience are becoming important determinants of drug selection. Dosages administered once daily are more convenient than drugs requiring multiple doses, but may be more expensive. When comparing cost, consider daily or monthly costs at the probable therapeutic dose, since single tablet comparisons or estimates based on lower dosages may be misleading (Sloan, 1992; Stein, 1994). Generally, generic prescribing is less expensive than using brand name products. However, generic products may vary in color or shape, confusing older patients. In addition, there may be considerable variation in bioavailability among legally equivalent products. If the patient has variable response to different products, the prescriber may request the pharmacist use consistent preparations or require dispensing of the prescribed brand only.

10. Assess drug interactions before selecting drugs.

As more drug products are marketed, the number and complexity of potential drug interactions increase. Often it is possible to select a drug in the same drug group with less risk of interaction or to adjust the therapy to minimize the risk if the drug interaction is identified at the time of drug selection (Pepper, 1997). Even if there are no alternative drugs, monitoring can be established to detect any deleterious effects of the interaction, since interactions usually manifest soon after a change in therapy (Beers & Ouslander, 1989). Encourage patients to use a single pharmacy to fill prescriptions, which increases the likelihood that drug interactions will be detected (Fincham, 1992; Palmieri, 1991; Tamblyn et al., 1996).

Education for Self-Care

11. Educate the patient about the drug and disease.

Although federal law requires pharmacists to provide medication counseling, research indicates that information is most effective if given by the prescriber (German & Burton, 1989). Written information should be provided about the medications, but the clinician should review the handout and emphasize critical points. Understanding on the part of the patient of the correlation between the disease process and the recommended therapy may increase compliance and decrease requests for medication that contribute to polypharmacy (Katzung, 1998; Stewart & Cooper, 1994). Information provided should include the drug names (generic and brand), indications, dosage, how and when to administer the drug, contraindications, adverse effects, drug interactions, and storage. Whenever possible, include a return demonstration where you can observe the patient taking the drug. Memory prosthetics (calendars, pill containers, alarmed medicine bottle caps) are available at pharmacies to promote adherence (Corlett, 1996; Palmieri, 1991).

12. Provide anticipatory counseling about over-the-counter and social drugs.

Patients rarely contact a health care provider before selecting an over-the-counter drug or herbal remedy, but are constantly bombarded with advertisements with recommendations like using histamine blockers as "hors d'oevres" before overeating to avoid heartburn. Recent changes in legislation allow manufacturers of herbal products to promote their products for specific disorders even if adequate scientific evidence of efficacy is lacking. Therefore, counseling about these products should be anticipatory, included in health screening and health promotion visits. For example, patient education might include how to choose over-the-counter treatment for cough and cold and when the physician or nurse should be called for cough and cold. The potential interaction of over-the-counter, herbal, social, or illicit drugs should also be specifically mentioned when a prescription is given (Gurwitz & Avorn, 1991).

Monitoring Drug Response

13. *Proactively plan a focused evaluation of drug response.*

Based on the therapeutic goal and the unique patient characteristics (e.g., concurrent diseases and drugs, age, living situation), a plan for monitoring drug effects should be defined when the drug is prescribed. The monitoring plan includes instructions for patient self-monitoring, proposed laboratory and diagnostic follow-up, and planned focused history and physical examination at the next visit, as well as when the next visit should occur. The monitoring plan also includes assessment of hepatic and renal function, which are critical to drug elimination. Considering shortened appointment times and higher staff-to-patient ratios resulting from managed care and other efforts to decrease health care costs, important information will be overlooked unless the clinician approaches each patient encounter with a focused plan aimed at evaluating the efficacy and adverse effects of drug therapy (Planchock & Slay, 1996; Stewart & Cooper, 1994).

14. *Use serum drug concentrations appropriately.*

Although many drugs lack reliable and valid laboratory tests for serum drug concentrations, serum plasma concentration ("drug level") forms a valuable adjunct to patient monitoring. Drug concentrations should be used to monitor drugs with narrow therapeutic margins (aminoglycosides, digoxin, lithium), dose-dependent elimination (phenytoin), or marked interindividual variability in pharmacokinetics (nortriptyline). Drug concentrations may also be useful in evaluating patient compliance, managing certain drug poisonings, and monitoring at-risk patients. Although some routine testing may be indicated, serum concentrations are most valuable as additional data when the clinical picture is ambiguous (Katzung, 1998; Thornburg, 1998).

Managing Adverse Drug Effects

15. *Prepare the patient to manage adverse drug reactions and noncompliance.*

Many clinicians are hesitant to warn patients about adverse drug effects, fearing it will cause them to develop the adverse effects. However, research indicates that patients who were told about the side effects of a drug are no more likely to develop them than those who were not told (Lamb et al., 1994). Patients often do not connect the adverse effect to the drug and are unlikely to report them to the prescriber (Chrischilles et al., 1992). However, patients who know about adverse effects are able to detect them before they become serious and know which adverse effects are serious enough to require a call to the prescriber. Many adverse effects can be ameliorated by simple measures. For example, good oral hygiene, frequent sips of water, and sucking on sugarless candy markedly decrease the discomfort of dry mouth (Pepper, 1991). A critical component of patient counseling is what to do if a dose is missed, since it is inevitable that this will occur. If the patient reports nonadherence, carefully explore the reasons and offer alternatives and assistance tailored to the problems.

16. *Periodically and prudently "prune" the drug regimen.*

At least every 6 months, the drug regimen of each patient, especially those on several medications, should be critically reviewed. Some clinicians argue that it is risky to discontinue drugs when a patient is stable, but others assert that excessive drugs are "time bombs" waiting to cause serious adverse reactions or drug interactions. Avorn and Gurwitz (1997) suggested that drugs that should be seriously considered for discontinuation are (1) those ordered by another prescriber, (2) those used sporatically, (3) over-the-counter drugs, and (4) those administered by non-oral routes. Have the patient bring all medications to the clinic and offer to safely dispose of old medication, emphasizing the risks of saving and sharing medication. Except for drugs seldom taken, it is wise to taper the elderly person's drugs on discontinuation and to observe for recurrence of disease for at least 4 months after the drug is discontinued. This is critical for drugs like clonidine (Catapres), beta-blockers, and benzodiazepines, but many drugs can cause a rebound effect if abruptly discontinued in the elderly (Gerety et al., 1993; Graves et al., 1997).

17. Use reporting networks for adverse outcomes.

Some of the adverse effects experienced by the elderly can be attributed to the packaging or labeling of drug products. When new products are released, adverse effects and drug interactions that are clinically significant in the elderly population may not have been identified (Waller, 1994). Therefore, it is an important responsibility of clinicians to report adverse events and problems with products to the Food and Drug Administration MedWatch program (5600 Fishers Lane, Rockville, MD 20852-9787) or to the USP Practitioners' Reporting Network (1-800-4-USP PRN).

Promoting Continuity of Care

18. Keep careful patient records.

Research indicates that patients are at higher risk for preventable adverse effects when cared for by providers who do not know them (Petersen et al., 1994; Tamblyn et al., 1996). Transition between health care settings, such as when a patient is transferred from hospital to nursing home or home care is another high risk time for the occurrence of adverse drug effects. Although consistency of provider is preferable, accurate and thorough patient records that document the rationale for care, as well as the care provided, improve continuity of care when the usual provider is unavailable.

19. Provide patient with a portable medication record.

Each elderly client should have a pocket-sized or wallet-sized record of the medications ordered (Stein, 1994). The portable medication record should be updated at each visit and the patient should be encouraged to share the record with other providers. The portable medication record can include a problem list of diagnoses and phone numbers for the clinic and emergency services.

20. Communicate with other providers.

Working with a multidisciplinary team can promote optimal drug therapy (Owens et al., 1990). Direct contact between providers is most effective in assuring continuity of care (Stein, 1994), although increased use of electronic communications such as faxes and electronic mail has expanded the options for communication to modes that are less time-consuming than face-to-face or telephone communication. Clinicians should promote the development of interactive video and other technologies that allow provision of maximally coordinated care to a growing elderly population.

SUMMARY

Because of a high prevalence of chronic disease, elderly people in all settings (community-dwelling, long-term care, and hospital) take more medications than younger adults and, as a result, have a greater incidence of adverse drug effects and drug-induced hospitalizations. Many studies have indicated that inappropriate drug use is common in all settings. Owing to the physiological changes of aging, the elderly have altered pharmacokinetics and pharmacodynamics. Decreased drug elimination, especially of renally eliminated drugs, is the most important change, resulting in prolonged half-life and increased serum concentrations. Polypharmacy, the use of excess medications, is caused by lack of knowledge of providers and patients, inadequate prescriptive practice, and failure to routinely discontinue unneeded medications. Adverse drug syndromes common in the elderly include cognitive dysfunction, depression, extrapyramidal symptoms (parkinsonism and tardive dyskinesia), falls, anticholinergic syndrome, and postural hypotension. Drug interactions that significantly alter drug response in the elderly are drug-drug, drug-disease, drug-nutrient, and drug-laboratory test interactions. The major causes of noncompliance, which occurs in up to half of elderly clients, are poor patient-provider communication, cognitive deficits, and complex drug regimen. Advanced nursing pharmacotherapeutics requires comprehensive patient assessment, careful drug selection, educating patients for self-care, monitoring of drug response, preventing and ameliorating adverse effects, and promoting continuity of care.

REFERENCES

Abernathy, D. R., & Kerzner, L. (1984). Age effects on alpha-1-acid glycoprotein and imipramine plasma protein binding. *Journal of the American Geriatrics Society, 32,* 705–708.

Ackerman, B. H., & Kasbekar, N. (1997). Disturbances of taste and smell induced by drugs. *Pharmacotherapy, 17,* 482–496.

Ahronheim, J. C. (1992). *Handbook of prescribing medications for geriatric patients.* Boston: Little, Brown.

American Association of Retired Persons (1982). *Prescription drugs: A survey of consumer use, attitudes, and behavior.* Washington, D.C.: American Association of Retired Persons.

Atkinson, R. (1984). *Alcohol and drug abuse in old age.* Washington, D.C.: American Psychiatric Press.

Avorn, J. (1991). The neglected medical history and therapeutic choices for abdominal pain: A nationwide study of 799 physicians and nurses. *Archives of Internal Medicine, 151,* 694–698.

Avorn, J., & Gurwitz, J. (1997). Principles of pharmacology. In C. K. Cassel, H. J. Cohen, E. B. Larson, et al. (Eds.), *Textbook of geriatric medicine* (3rd ed., pp. 55–70). New York: Springer.

Avorn, J., Bohn, R. L., Mogun, H., et al. (1995). Neuroleptic drug exposure and treatment of parkinsonism in the elderly: A case control study. *American Journal of Medicine, 99*(1), 48–54.

Avorn, J., Gurwitz, J. H., Bohn, R. L., et al. (1995). Increased incidence of levodopa therapy following metoclopramide use. *Journal of the American Medical Association, 247,* 1780–1782.

Ayd, F. J. (1985). Problems with medications ordered as needed. *American Journal of Psychiatry, 142,* 939–943.

Beard, K. (1992). Adverse drug reactions as a cause of hospital admission in the aged. *Drugs & Aging, 2*(4), 356–367.

Beers, M. H. (1997). Explicit criteria for determining potentially inappropriate medication use by the elderly; an update. *Archives of Internal Medicine, 157,* 1531–1536.

Beers, M. H., & Ouslander, J. G. (1989). Risk factors in geriatric drug prescribing: A practical guide to avoiding problems. *Drugs, 37,* 105–112.

Beers, M. H., Ouslander, J. G., Rollingher, I., et al. (1991). Explicit criteria for determining inappropriate medication use in nursing homes. *Archives of Internal Medicine, 151,* 1825–1832.

Bernstein, J. A. (1995). Nonimmunologic adverse drug reactions: How to recognize and categorize some common adverse drug reactions. *Postgraduate Medicine, 98*(1), 120–122, 125–126.

Blazer, D. G., Federspiel, C. F., Ray, W. A., & Schaffner, W. (1983). The risk of anticholinergic toxicity in the elderly: A study of prescribing practices in two populations. *Journal of Gerontology, 38* (1), 31–35.

Borchelt, M., & Horgas, A. L. (1994). Screening the elderly population for verifiable adverse drug reactions. *Annals of the New York Academy of Sciences, 717,* 270–281.

Brown, S. (1993). *A meta-analysis of process of care, clinical outcomes and cost-effectiveness of nurses in primary care roles: Nurse practitioners and nurse midwives* (Executive Summary). Washington, D.C.: American Nurses Association.

Bupert, C. N. (1995). Justifying nurse practitioner existence: Hard facts to hard figures. *Nurse Practitioner, 20*(8), 43–48.

Cadieux, R. J. (1989). Drug interactions in the elderly: How multiple drug use increases risk exponentially. *Postgraduate Medicine, 86*(8), 179–186.

Campbell, A. J., Borrie, M. J., & Spears, G. F. (1989). Risk factors for falls in a community-based prospective study of people 70 years and older. *Journal of Gerontology, 44*(4), M112–M117.

Campion, E. W., deLabry, L. O., & Glynn, R. J. (1988). The effect of age on serum albumin in healthy males: Report from the Normative Aging Study. *Journal of Gerontology, 43,* M18–M20.

Castleden, C. M., & George, C. F. (1984). Prevalence of adverse drug reactions in the elderly. In K. O'Malley (Ed.), *Clinical pharmacology and drug treatment for the elderly* (pp. 71–72). Edinburgh: Churchill Livingstone.

Catterson, M. L., Preskorn, S. H., & Martin, R. L. (1997). Pharmacodynamic and pharmacokinetic considerations in geriatric psychopharmacology. *Psychiatric Clinics of North America, 20*(1), 205–218.

Cherry, K. E., & Morton, M. R. (1989). Drug sensitivity in older adults: The role of physiologic and pharmacokinetic factors. *International Journal of Aging and Human Development, 28*(3), 159–174.

Chrischilles, E. A., Segar, E. T., & Wallace, R. B. (1992). Self-reported adverse drug reactions and related resource use: A study of community-dwelling persons 65 years of age and older. *Annals of Internal Medicine, 117*(8), 634–640.

Cockroft, D. W., & Gault, M. H. (1976). Prediction of creatinine clearance from serum creatinine. *Nephron, 16,* 31–41.

Connolly, M. J., Crowley, J. J., Charan, N. B., et al. (1995). Impaired bronchodilator response to albuterol in healthy elderly men and women. *Chest, 108*(2), 401–406.

Conrad, K. A., & Bressler, R. (1982). *Drug therapy for the elderly.* St. Louis: C. V. Mosby.

Cooper, J. K., Love, D. W., & Raffoul, P. R. (1982). Intentional prescription nonadherence (noncompliance) by the elderly. *Journal of the American Geriatrics Society, 30,* 329–333.

Corlett, A. J. (1996). Caring for older people: Aids to compliance with medication. *British Medical Journal, 313*(7062), 926–929.

Crooks, J. (1983). Aging and drug disposition: Pharmacodynamics. *Journal of Chronic Diseases, 36,* 85–96.

Cummings, R. G., Miller, J. P., & Kelsey, J. L. (1991). Medications and multiple falls in elderly people: The St. Louis OASI study. *Age and Ageing, 20,* 455–461.

Cusack, B. J. (1988). Drug metabolism in the elderly. *Journal of Clinical Pharmacology, 28,* 571–576.

D'Arcy, P. F. (1991). Adverse reactions and interactions with herbal medicines. Part 1. Adverse reactions. *Adverse Drug Reactions Toxicological Review, 10*(4), 189–208.

D'Arcy, P. F. (1993). Adverse reactions and interactions with herbal medicines. Part 2. Drug interactions. *Adverse Drug Reactions Toxicological Review, 12*(3), 147–162.

Darnell, J., Murray, M., Martz, B., & Weinberger, M. (1986). Medication use by ambulatory elderly: An in-home survey. *Journal of the American Geriatrics Society, 34*(1), 1–4.

Dawson, G. D. (1984). Polypharmacy in long term care. In R. E. Vestal (Ed.), *Drug treatment in the elderly* (pp. 51–58). Sydney: ADIS Health Science Press.

Ennis, K. J., & Reichard, R. A. (1997). Maximizing drug compliance in the elderly. Tips for staying on top of your patients' medication use. *Postgraduate Medicine, 102*(3), 223–224.

Felson, D. T., Sloutskis, D., Anderson, J. J., et al. (1991). Thiazide diuretics and the risk of hip fracture: Results from the Framingham study. *Journal of the American Medical Association, 265*(3), 370–373.

Fincham, J. E. (1992). Monitoring and managing adverse drug reactions. *American Pharmacy, NS32*(2), 74–81.

Folstein, M. F., Folstein, S. E., & McHugh, P. R. (1975). The mini-mental state examination: A practical method of grading cognitive state of patients for the clinician. *Journal of Psychiatric Research, 12,* 189–198.

Forster, L. E., Pollow, R., & Stoller, E. P. (1993). Alcohol use and potential risk for alcohol-related adverse reactions among community-based elderly. *Journal of Community Health, 18*(4), 225–239.

French, D. G. (1996). Avoiding adverse drug reactions in the elderly patient; issues and strategies. *Nurse Practitioner, 21*(9), 90, 96–97, 101–105.

Fujimura, A., Ohira, H., Shiga, T., et al. (1992). Chronopharmacology of furosemide in the elderly. *Journal of Clinical Pharmacology, 32,* 838–842.

Gerety, M. B., Cornell, J. E., Plichta, D. T., & Elmer, M. (1993). Adverse effects related to drugs and drug withdrawal in nursing home residents. *Journal of the American Geriatrics Society, 41,* 1326–1332.

German, P. S., & Burton, L. C. (1989). Medication and the elderly. *Journal of Aging and Health, 1*(1), 4–33.

Gleckman, R. A., & Czachor, J. A. (1989). Reviewing the safe use of antibiotics in the elderly. *Geriatrics, 44*(7), 33–39.

Glickman, L., Bruce, R. A., Caro, F. G., & Avorn, J. (1994). Physicians knowledge of drug costs for the elderly. *Journal of the American Geriatrics Society, 42*(9), 992–996.

Graves, T., Hanlon, J. T., Schmader, K. E., et al. (1997). Adverse events after discontinuing medications in elderly outpatients. *Archives of Internal Medicine, 157,* 2205–2210.

Greenblatt, D. J. (1979). Reduced serum albumin concentration in the elderly: A report from the Boston Collaborative Drug Surveillance Program. *Journal of the American Geriatrics Society, 27,* 20–23.

Greenblatt, D. J. (1989). Disposition of cardiovascular drugs in the elderly. *Medical Clinics of North America, 73*(2), 487–494.

Greenblatt, D. J., Shader, R. I., & Harmatz, J. S. (1989). Implications of altered drug disposition in the elderly: Studies of benzodiazepines. *Journal of Clinical Pharmacology, 29,* 866–872.

Gurwitz, J. H., & Avorn, J. (1991). The ambiguous relation between aging and adverse drug reactions. *Annals of Internal Medicine, 114,* 956–966.

Gurwitz, J. H., Goldenberg, R. J., & Holden, A. (1988). Age related risks of long term oral anticoagulant therapy. *Archives of Internal Medicine, 48,* 1733–1788.

Haak, H., & Hardon, A. P. (1988). Indiginized pharmaceuticals in developing countries: Widely used, widely neglected. *Lancet, 2,* 620–621.

Hale, W. E., Perkins, L. L., & May, F. E. (1986). Symptom prevalence in the elderly. An evaluation of age, sex, disease, and medication use. *Journal of the American Geriatrics Society, 34,* 333–340.

Hansten, P. D. (1998). Appendix II: Important drug interactions and their mechanisms. In B. G. Katzung (Ed.), *Basic and clinical pharmacology* (7th ed.; pp. 1059–1069). Norwalk, CT: Appleton & Lange.

Hayes, M. J., Langman, M. J., & Short, A. H. (1975). Changes in drug metabolism with increasing age. 2. Phenytoin clearance and protein binding. *British Journal of Clinical Pharmacology, 2,* 73–79.

Helling, D., Lemke, J., Semla, T., et al. (1987). Medication use characteristics among the elderly: The Iowa 65+ rural health study. *Journal of the American Geriatrics Society, 35*(1), 4–12.

Hemmelgarn, B., Suissa, S., Huang, A., et al. (1997). Benzodiazepine use and the risk of motor vehicle crash in the elderly. *Journal of the American Medical Association, 278,* 27–31.

Herbal roulette. (1995, November). *Consumer Reports,* 698–705.

Holland, J. M., Batey, M. B., & Dawson, K. (1985). Nurse practitioner prescribing patterns: Drug therapy and client health problems. *Journal of Ambulatory Care Management, 8,* 44–53.

Hutchinson, T. S., Flegel, K. M., & Kramer, M. S. (1986). Frequency, severity and risk factors for adverse drug reactions in adult outpatients: A prospective study. *Journal of Chronic Diseases, 39,* 533–535.

Huxtable, R. J. (1990). The harmful potential of herbal and other plant products. *Drug Safety, 5*(suppl. 1), 126–136.

Iber, F. L., Murphy, P. A., & Connor, E. S. (1994). Age-related changes in the gastrointestinal system: Effects on drug therapy. *Drugs & Aging, 5*(1), 34–48.

Jankel, C. A., & Fitterman, L. K. (1993). Epidemiology of drug-drug interactions as a cause of hospitalizations. *Drug Safety, 9*(1), 51–59.

Jinks, M. J., & Fuerst, R. H. (1992). Geriatric therapy. In M. A. Koda-Kimble & L. Y. Young (Eds.), *Applied therapeutics: The clinical use of drugs* (5th ed.; pp. 79-1–79-17). Vancouver, WA: Applied Therapeutics, Inc.

Jorquera, F., Culebras, J. M., & Gonzalez-Gallego, J. (1996). Influence of nutrition on liver oxidative metabolism. *Nutrition, 12,* 442–447.

Kalish, S. C., Bohn, R. L., Mogun, H., et al. (1995). Antipsychotic prescribing patterns and the treatment of extrapyramidal symptoms in older people. *Journal of the American Geriatrics Society, 43*(9), 767–773.

Kane, R. L., & Garrand, J. (1994). Changing physician prescribing practices: Regulation vs education. *Journal of the American Medical Association, 272*(1), 30–31.

Katzung, B. G. (1998). Special aspects of geriatric pharmacology. In B. G. Katzung (Ed.), *Basic and clinical pharmacology* (7th ed.; pp. 989–997). Norwalk, CT: Appleton & Lange.

Kelly, J. G., & O'Malley, K. (1992). Nitrates in the elderly: Pharmacological considerations. *Drugs & Aging, 1*(1), 14–19.

Kimelblatt, B. J., Young, S. H., & Heywood, P. M. (1988). Improved reporting of adverse drug reactions. *American Journal of Hospital Pharmacy, 45*, 1086–1089.

Kofoed, L. (1985). OTC drug overuse in the elderly: What to watch for. *Geriatrics, 40*(10), 55–59.

Lamb, G. C., Green, S. S., & Heron, J. (1994). Can physicians warn patients of potential side effects without fear of causing those side effects? *Archives of Internal Medicine, 154*, 2753–2756.

Lamy P. P. (1986a). Geriatric drug therapy. *American Family Physician, 34*, 118–124.

Lamy, P. P. (1986b). The elderly and drug interactions. *Journal of the American Geriatrics Society, 34*, 586–592.

Leape, L. L., Brennan, T. A., Laird, N., et al. (1991). The nature of adverse effects in hospitalized patients. Results of the Harvard Medical Practice Study II. *New England Journal of Medicine, 324*, 377–384.

Lin, S. H., & Lin, M. S. (1993). A survey on drug-related hospitalization in a community teaching hospital. *International Journal of Clinical Pharmacology, Therapy, and Toxicology, 31*(2), 66–69.

Lindley, C. M., Tully, M. P., Paramsothy, V., & Tallis, R. C. (1992). Inappropriate medication as a major cause of adverse drug reactions in elderly patients. *Age and Ageing, 21*(4), 294–300.

Loi, C., & Vestal, R. E. (1988). Drug metabolism in the elderly. *Clinical Pharmacology and Therapeutics, 36*, 131–149.

Macisaac, A., Rivers, R., & Adamson, C. (1989). Multiple medications: Is your patient caught in the storm? *Nursing '89, 19*, 60–64.

Manasse, H. R. (1989). *Medication use in an imperfect world: Drug misadventuring as an issue of public policy.* Washington, D.C.: ASHP Research and Education Foundation.

Mannesse, C. K., Derkx, F.H.M., de Ridder, M.A.J., et al. (1997). Adverse drug reactions as a contributing factor for hospital admission; a cross sectional study. *British Medical Journal, 315*(T115), 1057–1068.

Miller, S. W. (1990). Drug product selection: Implications for geriatric patients. *Consulting Pharmacist, 5*, 30–35.

Monane, M., & Avorn, J. (1996). Medications and falls. Causation, correlation, and prevention. *Clinics in Geriatric Medicine, 12*, 847–858.

Montamat, S. C., Cusack, B., & Vestal, R. E. (1989). Management of drug therapy in the elderly. *New England Journal of Medicine, 321*(5), 303–309.

Morris, L. S., & Schulz, R. M. (1993). Medication compliance: The patient's perspective. *Clinical Therapeutics, 15*(3), 593–606.

Morrow, D., Leirer, V., & Skeikh, J. (1988). Adherence and medication instructions: Review and recommendations. *Journal of the American Geriatrics Society, 36*, 1147–1160.

Murdoch, J. C. (1980). The epidemiology of prescribing in an urban general practice. *Journal of the Royal College of General Practitioners, 30*, 593–597.

National Center for Health Statistics, & Cypress, B. K. (1982). Drug utilization in office visits to primary care physicians: The National Ambulatory Care Survey, 1980. *Vital & Health Statistics, 86*, Department of Health and Human Services Publ. No. PHS 82–1250. Hyattsville, MD: Public Health Service.

National Center for Health Statistics, & Cypress, B. K. (1983a). Medication therapy in office visits by selected diagnosis: The National Ambulatory Care Survey, 1980. *Vital & Health Statistics, 86*, Department of Health and Human Services Publ. No. PHS 82–1250. Hyattsville, MD: Public Health Service.

National Center for Health Statistics, & Koch, H. (1983b). Utilization of psychotropic drugs in office-based ambulatory care. The National Ambulatory Care Survey, 1980 and 1981. *Vital & Health Statistics, 90*, Department of Health and Human Services Publ. No. PHS 83–173, Hyattsville, MD: Public Health Service.

Nattel, S., & Watanabe, A. M. (1981). Special considerations in cardiac pharmacology in the elderly. *Cardiovascular Clinics, 12*, 185–194.

Nolan, L., & O'Malley, K. (1988a). Prescribing for the elderly. Part 1: Sensitivity of the elderly to adverse drug reactions. *Journal of the American Geriatrics Society, 36*, 142–149.

Nolan, L., & O'Malley, K. (1988b). Prescribing for the elderly: Part 2: Prescribing patterns: Differences due to age. *Journal of the American Geriatrics Society, 36*, 245–254.

Owens, N. J., Sherburne, N. J., Silliman, R. A., & Fretwell, M. D. (1990). The Senior Care Study: The optimal use of medications in acutely ill older patients. *Journal of the American Geriatrics Society, 38*, 1082–1087.

Oxman, T. E. (1996). Antidepressants and cognitive impairment in the elderly. *Journal of Clinical Psychiatry, 57*(suppl. 5), 38–44.

Ozdemir, V., Fourie, J., Busto, U., & Narajo, C. A. (1996). Pharmacokinetic changes in the elderly. Do they contribute to drug abuse and dependence? *Clinical Pharmacokinetics, 31*, 372–385.

Palmateer, L. M., & McCartney, J. M. (1985). Do nurses know when patients have cognitive deficits? *Journal of the American Geriatrics Society, 11*(2), 6–7, 11–12, 15–16.

Palmieri, D. T. (1991). Clearing up confusion: Adverse clinical effects of medications in the elderly. *Journal of Gerontological Nursing, 17*(10), 32–35.

Patten, S. B., & Love, E. J. (1993). Can drugs cause depression: A review of the evidence. *Journal of Psychiatry & Neuroscience, 18*(3), 92–102.

Pearson, L. J. (1998). Annual update of how each state stands on legislative issues affecting advanced nursing practice. *Nurse Practitioner, 23*(1), 14.

Pepper, G. A. (1985). *Central and peripheral anticholinergic adverse drug effects in the institutionalized elderly.* Unpublished doctoral dissertation, University of Colorado Health Sciences Center, Denver.

Pepper, G. A. (1991). Monitoring the effects of anticholinergic drugs. In W. C. Chenitz, J. T. Stone & S. A. Salisbury (Eds.), *Clinical gerontological nursing: A guide to advanced practice* (pp. 377–389). Philadelphia: W. B. Saunders.

Pepper, G. A. (1997). The perils of P450. *Clinical Letter for Nurse Practitioners, 1*(1), 7–8.

Perry, M. V., & Anderson, G. L. (1992). Assessment and treatment strategies of depressive disorders commonly encountered in primary care settings. *Nurse Practitioner, 17*(6), 25–36.

Petersen, L. A., Brennan, T. A., O'Neil, A. C., et al. (1994).

Does housestaff discontinuity of care increase the risk of preventable adverse events? *Annals of Internal Medicine, 121*(11), 866–872.

Pirmohamed, M., Kitteringham, N. R., & Park, B. K. (1994). The role of active metabolites in drug toxicity. *Drug Safety, 11*(2), 114–144.

Planchock, N. Y., & Slay, L. E. (1996). Pharmacokinetic and pharmacodynamic monitoring of the elderly in critical care. *Critical Care Nursing Clinics of North America, 8*(1), 79–89.

Pollow, R. L., Stoller, E. P., Forster, L. E., & Duniho, T. S. (1994). Drug combinations and potential for risk of adverse drug reaction among community-dwelling elderly. *Nursing Research, 43,* 44–49.

Poulsen, H. E., & Loft, S. (1994). The impact of genetic polymorphisms in risk assessment of drugs. *Archives of Toxicology, 16* (suppl.), 211–222.

Ray, P. G., Meador, K. J., Loring, D. W., et al. (1992). Central anticholinergic hypersensitivity in aging. *Journal of Geriatric Psychiatry and Neurology, 5*(2), 72–77.

Ray, W. A. (1992). Psychotropic drugs and injuries among the elderly: A review. *Journal of Clinical Psychopharmacology, 12,* 386–393.

Ray, W. A., Thapa, P. B., & Shorr, R. I. (1993). Medications and the older driver. *Clinics in Geriatric Medicine, 9*(2), 413–439.

Resnick, N., & Marcantonio, E. R. (1997). How should clinical care of the aged differ? *Lancet, 350,* 1157–1158.

Roberts, J., & Tumer, N. (1988). Pharmacodynamic basis for altered drug action in the elderly. *Clinics in Geriatric Medicine, 4*(1), 127–149.

Rockwood, K. (1989). Acute confusion in elderly medical patients. *Journal of the American Geriatrics Society, 37,* 150–154.

Roe, D. A. (1994). Medications and nutrition in the elderly. *Primary Care, 21*(1), 135–147.

Roskos, K. V., Guy, R. H., & Malibach, H. I. (1986). Percutaneous absorption in the elderly. *Dermatology Clinics, 4,* 455–465.

Ruthazer, R., & Lipsitz, L. (1993). Antidepressants and falls among elderly people in long-term care. *American Journal of Public Health, 83*(5), 746–749.

Safriet, B. (1992). Health care dollars and regulatory sense: The role of advance practice nursing. *Yale Journal on Regulation, 9,* 417–488.

Schmucker, D. L. (1985). Aging and drug disposition: An update. *Pharmacology Reviews, 37,* 133–148.

Sherman, F. T. (1985). Tamper-resistant packaging: Is it elder resistant too? *Journal of the American Geriatrics Society, 33,* 136–141.

Simonson, W. (1984). *Medications and the elderly. A guide for promoting proper drug use.* Rockville, MD: Aspen Systems Publishing.

Skolnick, A. A. (1997). FDA sets geriatric drug use labeling deadlines. *Journal of the American Medical Association, 278,* 1302.

Sloan, R. W. (1992). Principles of drug therapy in geriatric patients. *American Family Physician, 45*(6), 2709–2718.

Smith, R. G., & Burtner, A. P. (1994). Oral side effects of the most frequently prescribed drugs. *Special Care in Dentistry, 14*(3), 96–102.

Solomon, D. H., & Gurwitz, J. H. (1997). Toxicity of nonsteroidal antiinflammatory drugs in the elderly: Is advanced age a risk factor? *American Journal of Medicine, 102,* 208–215.

Stein, B. E. (1994). Avoiding drug reactions: Seven steps to writing safe prescriptions. *Geriatrics, 49*(9), 28–36.

Stewart, R. B., & Cooper, J. W. (1994). Polypharmacy and the aged. Practical solutions. *Drugs and Aging, 4*(6), 449–461.

Stoller, E. (1988). Prescribed and over-the-counter medication use by the ambulatory elderly. *Medical Care, 26,* 1149–1157.

Sunderland, T. (1987). Anticholinergic sensitivity of patients with dementia of the Alzheimer type and age-matched controls: A dose-response study. *Archives of General Psychiatry, 44,* 418.

Surgeon General's Workshop on Health Promotion and Aging. (1989). Summary recommendations of the medications working group. *Journal of the American Medical Association, 262,* 1755–1756.

Swonger, A. K., & Burbank, P. M. (1995). *Drug therapy and the elderly.* Boston: Jones and Bartlett.

Tamblyn, R. (1996). Medication use in seniors. Challenges and solutions. *Therapie, 51,* 269–282.

Tamblyn, R. M., Robyn, M., McLeod, P. J., et al. (1996). Do too many cooks spoil the broth? Multiple physician involvement in medical management of elderly patients and potentially inappropriate drug combinations. *Canadian Medical Association Journal, 1548,* 1177–1184.

Tatro, D. S. (1988). Understanding drug interactions. *Facts and comparisons drug newsletter, 7*(8), 57–59.

Thompson, T. L., Moran, M. G., & Nies, A. S. (1983). Psychotropic drug use in the elderly (Two parts). *New England Journal of Medicine, 308,* 134–138, 194–197.

Thomson, W. M., Brown, R. H., & Williams, S. M. (1993). Medications and perceptions of dry mouth in a population of institutionalized elderly people. *New Zealand Medical Journal, 106*(957), 219–221.

Thornburg, J. E. (1998). Gerontological pharmacology. In T. M. Brody, J. Larner, K. P. Minneman & H. C. Neu (Eds.), *Human pharmacology: Molecular to clinical* (3rd ed.; pp. 885–890). St Louis: Mosby.

Tinetti, M. E., & Speechley, M. (1989). Prevention of falls among the elderly. *New England Journal of Medicine, 320,* 1055–1057.

Tinetti, M. E., Baker, D. I., McAvay, G., et al. (1994). A multifactorial intervention to reduce risk of falling among elderly people living in the community. *New England Journal of Medicine, 331,* 821–827.

Tonkin, A., & Wing, L. (1992). Aging and susceptibility to drug-induced orthostatic hypotension. *Clinical Pharmacology and Therapeutics, 52,* 277–280.

Tune, L., Carr, S., Hoag, E., & Cooper, T. (1992). Anticholinergic effects of drugs commonly prescribed for the elderly: Potential means for assessing risk of delirium. *American Journal of Psychiatry, 149*(10), 1393–1394.

United States Department of Health and Human Services (1991). *Healthy people 2000: National health promotion and disease prevention objectives.* Department of Health and Human Services Publ. No. PHS 91–50213. Washington, D.C.: U.S. Government Printing Office.

van Kraaij, D. J., Haagsma, C. J., Go, I. H., & Gribnau, F. W. (1994, May). Drug use and adverse drug reactions in

105 elderly patients admitted to a general medical ward. *Netherlands Journal of Medicine, 44*(5), 166–173.

Vestal, R. E. (1985). Clinical pharmacology. In R. Andes, E. L. Bierman & W. R. Hazzard (Eds.), *Principles of geriatric medicine* (pp. 424–443). New York: McGraw-Hill.

Waller, P. C. (1994). Dealing with variability: The role of pharmacovigilence. *Journal of Pharmacy and Pharmacology, 46*(suppl. 1), 445–449.

Wells, P., Fastbom, J., Claesson, C. B., et al. (1996). Use of cardiovascular drugs in an older Swedish population. *Journal of the American Geriatrics Society, 44*(1), 54–60.

Wilcox, S. M., Himmelstein, D. U., & Woolhandler, S. (1994). Inappropriate drug prescription for the community dwelling elderly. *Journal of the American Medical Association, 272*, 292–296.

Williams, L., & Caranasos, G. J. (1992). Neuropsychiatric effects of drugs in the elderly. *Journal of the Florida Medical Association, 79*(6), 371–375.

Williams, L., & Lowenthal, D. Y. (1992). Drug therapy in the elderly. *Southern Medical Journal, 85*(2), 127–131.

Yokoyama, M., Kusui, A., & Sakamoto, S. (1984). Age-associated increments in human platelet α-adrenoceptor capacity. Possible mechanism for platelet hyperactivity to epinephrine in aging man. *Thrombosis Research, 34,* 287–291.

Zullich, S. G., Grasela, T. H., Fielder-Kelly, J. B., & Gengo, F. M. (1993). Changes in prescribing patterns in long-term care facilities and impact on incidence of adverse events. *NIDA Research Monograph 131*, 294–308.

Zung, W. K., & Zung, E. M. (1986). The use of the Zung Self-Rating Depression Scale in the elderly. *Clinical Gerontologist, 5*, 137–148.

Managing Problem Behaviors

Geri Richards Hall
Linda A. Gerdner

One of the most common reasons for referrals to advanced practice nurses (APNs) specializing in either gerontology or psychiatry is to assist with care planning for older adults whose behavior does not meet the expectations of care providers. These patients can exhibit a broad range of behaviors that result from secondary symptoms associated with dement-ing illnesses, acute confusional syndrome, psychiatric disorders (e.g., depression or paranoid states), personality disorders, adjustment problems, eccentricities, or lifelong personal coping styles. The challenge to APNs is to determine what constitutes a *problem behavior*, to assess the antecedents and consequences of the problem behavior, and to develop and evaluate interventions using measures that are the least restrictive to the patient.

The primary focus of this chapter is to assist those APNs in consultant or primary care roles with the use of management techniques for common problem behaviors. The relevant research literature is reviewed, and findings are placed into a practical context. A second focus of the chapter is to identify caregiver and staff barriers to recognizing problem behaviors, carrying out recommended interventions, and using nurse-consultants for behavior management.

DEFINITION OF A PROBLEM BEHAVIOR

Although problem behaviors occur in every setting in which older adults are found, they are difficult to define because they are often interpreted subjectively. In the previous edition of this text, Salisbury and Stone provided the following definition of problem behavior:

> Recurring behavior that is deviant from that which is commonly regarded as acceptable by societal norms. These behaviors, while not of the same clinical significance as acute illness or medical diagnostic problems, are a source of consternation and distress to family caregivers and professional health care providers. Their management (or nonmanagement) may have serious financial, legal, and medical consequences for the individual performing the behavior.

A critical component of problem behaviors is their repetitive nature. A single behavioral event, unless it results in injury, rarely requires consultation with an APN. Episodes may be purposeful or not; however, the patient exhibiting problem behaviors often demonstrates a lack of concern for others, threatens their safety, and potentially violates their rights. Behavior problems generally interfere with the outcomes of medical regimens, relationships, and participation in social or recreational activities and may also negatively affect self-esteem. Frequently the patient is fearful and feels a sense of powerlessness or a loss of control over his or her environment.

Problem behaviors should be regarded as symptoms of an unmet need rather than as final diagnoses. The following problem behaviors are addressed in this chapter:

- Disruptive behavior
- Wandering
- Agitation and aggression
- Nocturnal wandering and sundowning
- Hypersexual behavior

These behaviors are defined and their potential causes discussed. Research and specific management strategies are discussed for the APN consulting in a variety of settings. First, however, APNs must understand barriers to referring patients for consultation.

DISRUPTIVE BEHAVIOR

Barriers to the Identification of Disruptive Behavior

Whether they are nursing staff members or in-home family caregivers, care providers often experience difficulty in identifying and seeking help for problem behaviors. They tend to postpone seeking help until the problems become severe enough that relatively simple solutions are impossible. The APN must consider several barriers to consultation.

It has been difficult for nurses to define disruptive behaviors. Three nursing studies have sought to determine which behaviors nurses employed by nursing homes found most disruptive. In a study by Bernier and Small (1988), five behaviors were particularly troubling to staff members: (1) trouble-making behavior, (2) purposely irritating behavior, (3) verbally assaultive behavior, (4) behavior causing destruction to others' property, and (5) threatening behavior in which potential physical harm was perceived. Burgio and colleagues (1988) classified behavior problems into three categories: (1) acting out behaviors such as yelling and slapping, (2) aberrant behaviors, and (3) excess disabilities. In this study, staff members more frequently listed low functioning as a behavior problem than other behaviors such as tantrums or wandering. Kikuta (1991) defined disruptive behavior as yelling and noisiness in patients with organic mental decline. These studies all suggest that problem behaviors are determined by the perceptions of the care provider.

In an institutional setting, nurses are often reticent to diagnose behavior problems, in part because of the potential stigma directed toward nursing staff members. Many nurses have been socialized to believe that their nursing knowledge must be all-encompassing and that they should assume a *therapeutic personality* that meets all patient needs, thereby eliminating conflict and acting out. To admit that a patient's behavior has caused problems severe enough to require a nurse-consultant implies an incapability of meeting patient needs and may give rise to internal conflict about basic competence.

Regulatory agencies and advocates often view aged people as a homogeneous group, hypothesizing that all aged people can integrate appropriately into communal living settings if their individualized needs are met. This approach denies lifelong patterns of dysfunctional coping, mental illness, and unusual presentations of organic decline. As a result, this approach may place nurses in an adversarial position with supervisory agencies that believe behavior problems occur as a matter of nursing mismanagement, uninformed care planning, or a lack of training. Some physicians insist that mood-controlling medications are routinely requested only for nurses' convenience. With messages such as these from the care community, it seems understandable that nurses underreport behavioral issues for fear of sanctions from colleagues and regulatory agencies.

Another reason for underreporting is that some staff members may feel that problem behaviors are a normal part of the aging process. To intervene might challenge the patient's autonomy. Techniques such as behavior modification often raise questions about ethical treatment and patient rights. In the institutional setting, staff members must be encouraged to consider patients' roles within the community of vulnerable adults. Although interventions must not compromise the patient's rights, neither should the disruptive patient compromise the rights of others.

In the home setting, barriers to consultation are equally complex. Families must overcome their denial of conditions, including dementia

and personality disorders. They often fear being forced to make historical disclosures that are required with behavioral assessment, especially when there has been long-standing family dysfunction and conflict. Members of the family's social network may influence the caregiver's decisions to follow through on recommendations, although they may offer few alternatives to remedy problem behavior. Recommendations from the APN may be viewed by the family as an intrusion, a violation of family marital vows, or a possible cause of increased patient anger or family conflict. Intervention strategies must be integrated into the family system to survive criticisms by adult children and other nonparticipant caregivers.

THE PROCESS OF BEHAVIORAL MANAGEMENT

Assessment

The goal of assessing dysfunctional behavior is to gain rapid insight into the causes and effects of the problem behavior. The assessment should lead the APN to select appropriate interventions that can be integrated into the plan of care by all staff and family members.

HISTORY

Assessing the patient's history is critical to determining how past events and coping and behavior patterns contribute to the identified problem. A Lifespan Assessment (Table 27–1) goes beyond the traditional psychosocial assessment by determining the patient's perception of lifestyle choices and sense of mastery (Hall & Buckwalter, 1989). It uses six sets of brief, open-ended questions to determine the patient's lifestyle, perceived choices in major life events, sense of control, coping styles, perceptions of relationships, patterns of socialization, potential for violence, and occasionally undiagnosed mental health problems.

In addition to information gleaned from the Lifespan Assessment, the APN must ascertain the medical and mental health histories, including patterns of substance use. If a patient denies having been hospitalized for mental ill-

---

TABLE 27–1
Lifespan Assessment

---

1. Are you a native of (town currently residing in)? Where were you born and raised? What did your parents do? Tell me about your family while you were growing up.
2. How far did you go in school? Why did you stop? What did you do after school? Why? Did you enjoy it?
3. How did you meet your spouse (partner, significant other)? What made him or her special? How did you decide to marry? Tell me about your early marriage; was it an enjoyable time in your life? When did your children come along? How did that affect your relationship with your spouse? How did it affect your career?
4. What jobs did you hold during your career? Were they rewarding? Did they affect your family or social life? How did you relax?
5. When did you decide to retire? Has that been a difficult adjustment? When you are well, what do you do to keep yourself busy? Does that satisfy you? Has your retirement affected your relationship with your spouse? Family? Friends?
6. Have you had any special problems or losses throughout your life? If so, how have you dealt with them? What have you done to cope during emotional times? When angry?

Adapted from Hall, G., & Buckwalter, K. (1989). Diagnostic clues in the past. *Geriatric Nursing, 10*, 204.

---

ness, try asking if there were periods when he or she "took to his or her bed" for an extended time, was unable to work, had medications prescribed for "nerves," or suffered a "nervous breakdown." The APN should, with the patient's permission, confirm findings with available family members or significant others.

CURRENT STATUS

The evaluation of current status should include physical and functional assessments. Behaviors such as slapping and screaming may be related to painful conditions, local infections such as vaginitis or cystitis, or discomfort from conditions such as constipation. The APN should assess all prescription and nonprescription medications for interactions and potential effects on behavior. Formal mental status testing for cognitive function should be used to determine whether the patient might suffer from delirium or dementia (see Chapter 7).

Depression may result in behavior problems. A formal depression scale such as the Geriatric Depression Scale (Yesavage et al., 1983; Zung, 1965) may be helpful to screen for depressive illness. In addition, the APN should look for a 2- to 3-week pattern of altered sleep patterns, altered eating patterns, low and/or anxious mood, flat affect, slowed responses, morbid ideations, lowered level of function, expressions of sadness or guilt, and feelings of worthlessness. The depressed patient may also appear confused or demented. A good indicator of depression is when the patient answers questions with an apathetic "I don't know."

RELATIONSHIPS WITH SIGNIFICANT PEOPLE

Nonjudgmental observation and evaluation of interactions with family members can provide invaluable information about how patients perceive themselves and their roles within the family structure. Is the patient, previously a dominant figure in the relationship, now relegated to a dependent status? Is the patient able to negotiate with family members to maintain some control over the environment? Is the patient offered choices? Does the patient inflict guilt when family members do not meet his or her expectations? Does the family avoid the patient? These interactions can provide invaluable clues into the meaning of the patient's problem behavior, coping styles, and sense of mastery.

Several anthropological concepts should be considered when observing patient interactions. First, what actions promote patient *autonomy*, which is now considered a primary value in U.S. society. How does the patient express this, and how do the family and staff respond? The second concept is *reciprocity*. To maintain a sense of mastery, older adults need to feel that they can reciprocate for care and favors. How does the patient reciprocate for care provided by family or staff members? Reciprocal gestures may be anything from a smile to money (or promises of an inheritance) to performing a chore such as clearing the table or starting laundry. Do caregivers allow the patient to reciprocate? A third concept is *competitive complaining*, a method used in many cultures whereby elderly people demonstrate autonomy and individuality. Competitive complaining is complaining that resists all solutions. Once the complaint has been resolved, the patient finds the solution ineffective or focuses on another problem to take its place. It can become a problem when people stop listening and miss new problems or when the nurses and family members focus on resolving the complaints. It is important to ask the patient how he or she wants the complaints resolved.

POTENTIAL UNMET NEEDS

Many behavior problems, particularly vocalization, agitation, and aggression, are expressions of unmet needs. The APN needs to consider unmet needs when planning care. Some of the most common needs are listed in Table 27–2.

Assessing and Describing the Identified Disruptive Behavior

Whenever possible, the APN should observe the behavior that staff or family members have identified as a problem. In the previous edition of this text, Salisbury and Stone defined behavior as follows:

> Behavior refers to any observable action or sequence of actions. It does not refer to a description or interpretation. Behaviors are always stated as verbs. . . . A nursing assistant's complaint of "she is just a mean ungrateful person" should be stated specifically, perhaps as "she calls out 'help me, help me' repeatedly every few minutes. This happens when she is tied in her wheelchair in the late afternoon and when she wakes up at night."

Assessing behavior is similar to solving a puzzle. Although the process need not be time consuming, a variety of factors and sources must be considered before determining potentially effective interventions. Only one behavior should be the focus of interventions. Nursing interventions may not make a patient grateful for care but can nevertheless address the problem of throwing food trays at employees, for example. Once the target behavior has been selected, the following issues should be identified.

What does the behavior mean to the individual?

In determining what the behavior means to the patient, the APN should strive to help staff members "reframe" the behavior and place it in another context. Frequently, staff members tend to see their setting as "normal" or "the way things are here" and forget how peculiar the healthcare system is to the general population. In the lay setting, one would never expect to move into a stranger's bedroom, especially when indisposed; yet aged adults are expected to cheerfully share a room and life's most intimate experiences with a person they have never met and likely would never have chosen as a partner.

Look for both internal and external meaning. Although the noise of a roommate's television or snoring might produce agitation, APNs should not overlook internal issues. Pacing might be an indication of back pain, for example. Constipation or a headache might trigger irritability. The patient might be too warm or cold.

Who is involved when the behavior occurs?

Is the patient responding to interactions only with a single person or group of people, or does the behavior occur randomly with anyone? Patients may respond negatively to certain family members or a given staff member, perhaps owing to unresolved family issues, lifelong prejudices, or personality conflicts. In institutional settings, often it is best to accommodate personality conflicts with a given staff member by changing assignments. However, if the patient rejects a staff member from a particular ethnic group, assignment changes may not

---

TABLE 27-2
Unmet Needs Common to Behavior Problems

Personal space	Institutionalization often reduces the person's personal space to a single bed, bedside table, drawers, and small closet. There are few opportunities for individualization or privacy.
Communication	People with impairments that prevent them from expressing themselves or understanding others become frustrated, fearful, and/or demonstrative.
Self-esteem	As people age, they often tend to idealize values of the youth-oriented culture represented in society and the media. As disability increases, self-esteem may be difficult to maintain.
Autonomy and personal identity	As people become more disabled, their choices and options are reduced. They cannot walk away from others and become dependent on the good will and availability of others for assistance. When free choice and individualized environments are limited, frustration may result.
Personal time	Disabled people often cannot choose their time to reflect, be alone, pursue favorite pastimes, or simply watch a favorite program.
Comfort	Disability may limit older people's ability to change positions or may force them to sit for hours. People with limited verbal ability may be unable to express pain and discomfort.
Meaningful activity	The loss of activities, routines, and socialization that provide meaning and quality to life can decrease self-esteem and lead to a sense of hopelessness.
Cognitive understanding	People with dementing illnesses or delirium have an altered ability to perceive environmental stimuli and manage competing stimuli. This can produce ongoing misunderstandings and fear.

---

be possible. Efforts should be made to negotiate with the patient, but if the patient refuses, he or she may have to be relocated to another facility. In either instance, care must be taken to educate and counsel the rejected staff members, avoiding negative feedback whenever possible.

In the home setting, it may not be feasible to change caregivers. Counseling the caregiver and patient may result in small incremental positive changes. In addition, an increased use of supplemental respite and support may enhance the patient's quality of life. Caregiver education—particularly if the patient has suffered cognitive loss—and reframing and suggesting alternative responses to the behavior may make significant improvements in the target behavior. If the target behavior is not modified in any setting, the potential for dependent adult abuse and mistreatment increases.

Where does the behavior occur?

Patients who become combative during bath time are often responding to an extremely frightening and humiliating experience. The following is a typical scenario for patients in an institutional setting when they are bathed: a stranger strips them; wraps them in a blanket; sits them on a wheeled toilet seat; wheels them past crowded areas into a stark, noisy room where frightening medical equipment might be stored; removes the blanket; pushes them into a shower where water is pouring over their head; rapidly washes them, including their most private areas; towels them down; replaces the blanket; and wheels them, while they are cold, wet, and naked, back across the crowded area to a room where only a curtain gives them privacy and protects their dignity. How many staff members would volunteer for this experience?

What is the timing of the behavior? What is the behavioral antecedent, or trigger?

When does the behavior usually occur? Outbursts occurring at mealtime often indicate problems with stimuli in the dining room, whereas late-day agitation may have a component of fatigue. Does the behavior occur every day, or does it cycle every few days? How long does the episode last? Dr. M., for example, failed to sleep for several hours every 3 to 5 nights; his wife complained of fatigue but felt she could manage. Mr. J. became verbally abusive and agitated for 4 hours every evening; his daughter felt this daily assault was more than she could manage.

The frequency and duration of the behavior are good indicators of severity. When developing interventions, projected outcomes should be evaluated by measuring the frequency and duration of the targeted behavior.

What preceded the behavior? In Dr. M.'s case, afternoon visits from colleagues and family members triggered his nocturnal agitation. For Mr. J., late-day activities and dinner with his four young grandchildren served to escalate fatigue and frustration. When placed in a calmer environment, Mr. J.'s behavior became socially acceptable.

How are caregivers or family members currently interpreting the behavior?

Problem behaviors are often interpreted differently by staff and family members and ancillary personnel. It is as important to interview the housekeeping personnel as it is to interview the nursing assistant. When reticent about complaining to the nursing staff, patients frequently communicate with housekeepers, dietary personnel, roommates, and other patients about problems. Clinicians should collect information from as many sources as possible to obtain a balanced view of the target behavior.

What are the consequences of the behavior?

The following case study illustrates how such consequences can affect problem behavior.

Case Study 1

Badly frightened the night before her second mitral valve replacement, Ms. A. fell out of bed. Five nurses raced to her side to check that she was uninjured. Reassuring her and giving her the call bell, they placed her back in bed, raised the side rails, fluffed her pillow, and rubbed her back. Ms. A. did not see another nurse for an hour. Sixty-five minutes later, nurses found her

on the floor again. Staff members repeated the same procedure and applied a chest restraint. Thirty minutes later, Ms. A. was back on the floor. A mental status examination was performed, and Ms. A. was found cognitively intact. Upset by the potential for injury with increased restraint use, the nurses decided to change the consequences of the behavior.

The next time Ms. A. was found on the floor, a single nurse intervened. He calmly assisted her back to bed and sat for a few minutes discussing her fears about surgery. He noted that she was childless and recently widowed. She feared being alone and undergoing the brief rehabilitative nursing home admission following surgery. The nurse then told Ms. A. that he would be back in 20 minutes, timing his return. On his return, he decided that Ms. A. could sit with him at the nursing station while he charted. She did not fall after that. By changing the consequences of the behavior, the staff were able to stop the target behavior.

Planning Interventions for the Target Behavior

There are three ways to plan for behavioral change: (1) change (reframe) the meaning of the behavior for the caregivers, (2) modify the situations that trigger the behavior (the antecedents), or (3) alter the responses (consequences) of the behavior. These techniques can be applied only after the assessment measures just described have been accomplished.

REFRAMING

Once the assessment data have been compiled, new meanings will become apparent to the APN, who then must educate caregivers. Often the problem is one of incomplete understanding of the patient's past as well as any superimposed cognitive deficits.

Case Study 2

Ms. B. was an 85-year-old woman who had spent the last 35 years in a large mental health institute owing to bipolar affective disorder with manic features. She fell, breaking her hip, and was sent to a hospital for orthopedic surgery. Postoperatively, the nursing staff found that she screamed for help night and day despite being given her call bell. Moreover, once standing, she could walk toward the bathroom without difficulty but would not assist in moving to the side of the bed to get to a standing position. Staff labeled her as "willful and attention seeking." When the APN observed Ms. B., she noted a severe motor apraxia and that Ms. B. called out whenever she felt an unmet need such as thirst or a desire to move to the end of a hall. Meeting with staff members, the APN explained that what had appeared as stubbornness was actually motor apraxia. In addition, Ms. B. was used to being housed on large mental health wards where staff members were summoned from glass-enclosed nursing stations.

Once the staff was able to see Ms. B.'s behavior differently, they were able to develop strategies that minimized screaming behaviors and compensatory interventions for the motor apraxia. This also resulted in an easier discharge to a nursing facility.

MODIFYING ANTECEDENTS

The modification of behavioral antecedents or triggers can have a profound impact on disruptive behavior. First, the triggers must be identified. All care personnel and family members should meet and agree on the target behavior. They should describe the triggers of the behavior and set a behavioral goal: "Mr. F. will not kick and strike out while bathing," for example. To modify triggers, staff members might change a routine, eliminate an activity, or add a more pleasant alternative. Instead of taking Mr. F. to the shower while naked on a commode, staff members might try having him bathe at the sink in his bathroom or let him wear underwear while bathing.

CHANGING CONSEQUENCES

Changing the response to a behavior can produce significant improvement if the patient is cognitively intact. Patients with memory loss frequently do not remember the consequences of their behavior and thereby negate the desired effect. The APN should meet with the patient, discuss the problem, outline strategies, and agree on a contract. Common types of reinforcement include the following (Salisbury & Stone, 1991; Smith & Buckwalter, 1991):

- Positive—giving something positive when the goal behavior occurs (e.g., hugs, smiles, or a choice of activities); the reinforcement must be something the patient values
- Negative—removing something negative to produce a positive behavior, for example, "If you eat your lunch, we can postpone your bath until tomorrow night"
- Extinctive—showing no response when the target behavior occurs

When planning to change the consequences of behavior, the rules of reinforcement should be applied. Consequences should have the following characteristics (Smith & Buckwalter, 1991):

- Individualized—something valued by the patient
- Immediate—occurring right after the target behavior
- Contingent—occurring only after the target behavior
- Consistent—occurring every time the target behavior occurs
- Consumable—disposable or temporary (e.g., hugs, smiles, or backrubs)

Staff Preservation

Behavior management programs are often difficult for staff members. It is important to help staff depersonalize the behavior and understand that management techniques are a form of skilled social interaction intended to help the patient cope in a more functional manner. Communications training is essential so that staff members can learn methods for diffusing anger and rising emotions; these methods can include assuming a relaxed dependent body posture, speaking in a lowered tone of voice, and using last names. If patients tend to use physical force, staff members must be trained in defensive maneuvers.

Evaluation

Evaluating the outcomes of behavior management techniques is an ongoing process. The use of an individualized behavioral flow sheet will help staff members (and perhaps the patient) see progress. Recognizing progress is important, as staff or family members may want the target behavior to disappear immediately and thus may not recognize progress toward the goal behavior. The behavior flow sheet will also help with plan modification. Careful documentation is key to the success of the program.

If the target behavior does not change in about 48 hours, the program should be modified but *not discarded*. The failure of behavior management programs is often caused by discarding the entire concept when the first attempts are unsuccessful. Instead, changing to another form of reinforcement or modifying another trigger may prove successful. If the program fails repeatedly, look for a saboteur. Occasionally a staff or family member will receive secondary gain from the disruptive behavior and will provide positive feedback when problems occur. If no saboteur is found, a psychiatric consultation or neuropsychological testing may be warranted.

SPECIFIC PROBLEM BEHAVIORS

Wandering

Wandering is a relatively common occurrence. A national nursing home survey reported that 11.4% of residents are wanderers (Szwabo et al., 1991). Other studies have reported ranges of 4 to 11.4% of residents in nursing homes and 26 to 70% of community-based patients (Teri et al., 1991).

Wandering is one of the few problem behaviors that can pose significant risk to patients in terms of restrictive and/or negative feedback, injury from elopement, excessive caloric use with unremitting pacing, and increased pain

resulting from overusing arthritic and degenerated joints.

Wandering, like other behavioral problems, lacks a clear, concise definition. Martino-Saltzman and colleagues (1991) stated the term as being "so imprecise as to defy definition, having been applied to behavior such as pacing, trying doorknobs, talking about going home, entering other people's rooms, getting lost on a walk, or simply talking in a way that someone considers disoriented" (p. 666). The absence of an operational definition limits studies on wandering and also plagues studies of other problem behaviors.

One of the first nursing studies of wandering was conducted by Monsour and Robb (1982). They defined wandering as engaging in disoriented activities and aimless movements toward indefinable objectives and unobtainable goals. In the study they compared wanderers and nonwanderers to determine any differences in psychosocial lifestyles; all subjects were cognitively impaired and resided in a locked nursing unit. Monsour and Robb reported that wanderers had had higher premorbid levels of social and leisure activities, had experienced a more stressful life, and demonstrated more motoric behavioral styles under stress, including pacing and walking.

Rader and colleagues (1985) described wandering as a form of *agenda behavior*. They hypothesized that wandering occurs from three factors: (1) "the fear engendered by separation from the people and environment with which the person was previously most comfortable and connected; (2) frustration from being stopped in meeting their agenda; and (3) the need to be needed" (Rader et al., 1985, p. 196).

Dawson and Reid (1987) conducted a descriptive study to differentiate wanderers from nonwanderers. Wandering was defined as "frequent and/or unpredictable pacing with no discernible goal." Three major categories of behaviors were identified: cognitive deficits, agitation and aggression, and hyperactivity. Wanderers were more likely to score positively on cognitive impairment and hyperactivity than were nonwanderers; however, agitation and aggression were not found to positively correlate with wandering (Dawson & Reid, 1987).

Algase (1992) studied the cognitive determinants of wandering, defining wanderers as having a "behavior pattern characterized by a high degree of locomotion and gross motor output, a low level of social interaction, and disorientation to person, place, and time" (p. 78). Comparing cognitively impaired subjects who were classified as wanderers or nonwanderers, Algase measured four dimensions of cognitive impairment: abstract thinking, judgment, language, and spatial skills. Findings for wanderers were significant in that their impairment was greater in all these dimensions, but especially for judgment and language skills. In addition, wanderers had more global impairment and complex medical comorbidities. Algase suggested that, with the global impairments seen in the four cognitive dimensions, wanderers are a more heterogeneous group than previously thought and that there may be multiple causes for wandering.

In an intervention study, Szwabo and colleagues (1991) attempted to define behavioral problems associated with wandering by studying the effects of alprazolam (Xanax), a moderate- to long-acting benzodiazepine, on decreasing wandering. Wandering was defined as restless or aimless movement or behavior, and problematic wandering was defined as that which upsets others, such as when a patient gets into the belongings of others, leaves the unit, or becomes verbally or physically threatening to others. Subjects were rated at four intervals: (1) after 2 weeks on the prestudy medication regimen; (2) during a 2-week psychotropic drug holiday; (3) after 4 weeks on alprazolam (minimum dose 0.25 mg twice daily; maximum dose 0.5 mg three times daily); and (4) after 4 weeks without alprazolam (for interventions). Incidents of wandering were recorded during each week and compared for the 4 weeks. No significant differences were found as a result of the treatment; however, there was a slight improvement in speech, decreased irritability, and increased ability to follow a routine. There was a statistically significant increase in drowsiness as a side effect of the alprazolam (Szwabo et al., 1991).

Hussian and Brown (1987) studied the use of two-dimensional tape grids on the floor. After testing, researchers found that eight horizontal tape grids decreased the incidence of wander-

ing from 98 to 42%. Grids with three, four, or six horizontal lines reduced elopement by as much as 55%, but grids with eight lines produced the most clinically significant results. These findings are clinically relevant because tape grids are inexpensive and barrier free, reduce staff time, and allow exits to be kept clear for emergencies.

NURSING MEASURES FOR WANDERING

The most important measure for assessing wanderers is to determine the *agenda* for wandering. Using Rader and colleagues' (1985) theory of agendas for wandering, Hall and colleagues (unpublished) developed a standardized care plan by studying residents who wandered in special care Alzheimer's units (Hall et al., 1995); this care plan is shown in Appendix 27–1.

Agitation and Aggression

Agitation is a common symptom in older adults, interfering with their quality of life and causing frustration and discomfort for patients and their caregivers (Taft, 1989). If allowed to escalate, agitation may develop into aggression or violence, necessitating more invasive treatment options. Most important are the consequences of agitation for the patient, including social isolation, interference with activities, and a decline in health owing to interference with sleep and eating patterns (Taft, 1989). Aggression poses those problems as well as a high potential for injury to the patient, other residents, family members, visitors, and staff members.

In the institutional setting, aggression has serious consequences for staff members and the facility. Of primary concern is staff injury. Although aged patients may appear frail, when frightened or aggressive, many can be quite strong and can cause serious staff injuries. Once injuries have occurred, increased staff turnover often results. Staff members' approaches to the patient change as their perception of danger increases, resulting in increased potential for the mistreatment of elderly patients and avoidance of restorative goals. It is understandable that staff members may not find time to ambulate a patient who spits, slaps, pinches, or pokes them. If the aggression continues, staff members may develop a siege mentality, drawing lots or negotiating to see who cares for the patient each day, or taking two to three staff members into the room each time care must be given, further reducing the patient's sense of control over the environment.

In the long-term care facility, an act of aggression often assumes a life of its own, becoming part of the facility myth. Where a staff member might have suffered a bruise, by the end of the week the "grapevine" will have escalated the injury into a life-threatening injury. Moreover, reports of aggression often leak into the community, giving rise to the perception that it is unsafe for "nice people" to be placed there. In acute settings, patient stays are generally short, and aggressive behaviors may be overlooked. However, the APN must attend to these behaviors for the same reasons just described for long-term care. Acute care nurses cannot expect a family member to be able to manage behavior that could not be managed in the hospital.

As with all problem behaviors, defining agitation is challenging. Most authors agree that agitation involves behavioral disturbance (Struble & Siversten, 1987; Taft, 1989). These disturbances include excessive vocal or motor activity and a degree of inappropriateness of behavior (Cohen-Mansfield & Billig, 1986; Struble & Siversten, 1987; Taft, 1989). Motor activities include restlessness, wandering, irrepressible activity, vocalizations, and excessive motor activity. Inappropriateness includes behaviors such as uttering repetitive unintelligible sounds, nonpurposeful behavior, excessiveness, aberrance, and nonadaptiveness (Cohen-Mansfield & Billig, 1986; Struble & Siversten, 1987; Taft, 1989). One problem with assessing whether behavior is inappropriate is that the determination is based on the perceptions of the caregiver, who may not understand the patient's attempt to express an unmet need (Cohen-Mansfield & Billig, 1986; Hall & Buckwalter, 1987; Taft, 1989).

Aggression arises from the escalation of motor activity. There are two forms of aggressive behavior: a milder form characterized by irritability, excitability, uncooperativeness, or a combination of these; and a stronger form characterized by hostility, assaultiveness, or violence (Taft, 1989). Another characteristic of agitation is strong emotions, characterized by anxiety, tension, urgency, fear, lack of control, and forceful, tumultuous feelings (Taft, 1989).

Struble and Siversten (1987) completed a descriptive study of 23 confused and agitated geriatric patients on a hospital medical unit. Nurses used a behavioral checklist assessment to document episodes of agitation requiring chemical or physical restraint. The checklist allowed behavior to be grouped into four categories: psychomotor behaviors, aggressive or antisocial behaviors, speech patterns, and physiological measures. The nurses also documented the duration of the episode, the intervention selected, and its outcomes. The investigators described *agitation* as a construct indicating a group of behavioral signs and symptoms including excessive (and often purposeless) motor activity and feelings of internal tension, irritability, hostility, and belligerence. In their study they noted that although most health professionals were unable to define agitation, they could identify it (Struble & Siversten, 1987). The number of agitated episodes per patient ranged from 1 to 19, with a mean of 4. Over half (57%) the time, nurses used both restraints and medication; in 4% of the episodes, only restraints were used. Patients exhibited all four types of behaviors (psychomotor behaviors, aggressive or antisocial behaviors, speech patterns, and physiological measures), and increased generalized movement was always present. Also common were refusing to follow directions (82.6%), climbing out of bed (78.3%), and talking loudly (78.3%). The length of an agitated episode ranged from 5 minutes to 3 hours, with a mean of 35 minutes. Other than behavior such as not resting or losing sleep, physiological measures were not indicative of agitation.

Chrisman and colleagues (1991) noted the importance of an objective evaluation of agitation in the clinical setting. Their study defined agitation as "inappropriate verbal, vocal, or motor activity that is not explained by needs or confusion per se" (p. 9). Using Nightingale's theory of environmental management, they compared three assessment tools: the Cohen-Mansfield Agitation Inventory–Second Edition

(CMAI-II), the Confusion Inventory (CI), and the Ward Behavior Inventory (WBI), all of which scored agitation similarly. The CMAI-II documented the most common behaviors to be restlessness, complaining, negativism, cursing, repetitively stating sentences or asking questions, wandering and pacing, and performing repetitive mannerisms. The CI documented the most common behavior as "other restless behavior," followed by complaining, moving extremities randomly or aimlessly, temper outbursts, and muttering or mumbling. Because the most common behavior noted was "other restless behavior," investigators noted the need for increased specificity of behavioral descriptions.

Aggressive behavior is the result of escalated agitation (Taft, 1989). Five nursing studies of aggressive behavior and older adults are summarized in this section. Winger and colleagues (1987) used milieu theory to study aggression in two long-term care units at a Veterans Affairs Hospital. The purpose of the study was to determine the incidence and characteristics of aggression and whether aggressive behavior was correlated with patients' length of stay, level of function, health status, and perceived control over daily life. The sample consisted of 101 subjects from two nursing units. Twenty-three aggressive behaviors were grouped into three categories: endangering to others, endangering to self, and disturbing. Behaviors judged serious enough to endanger self or others were found in 84% of the nursing home residents and 56% of the intermediate care patients. Although no trends for aggression were noted, advanced age, a longer stay, and decreased cognitive function were related to increased aggression (Winger et al., 1987).

Two years later, Winger and Schirm (1989) published an exploratory investigation of the same 101 residents. This study examined the role of additional factors such as perceived health status, functional ability, and perceived control over aggression. The purpose was to develop a causal model of aggressive behavior. However, none of the identified variables had significant direct or indirect effects on aggressive behavior in either intermediate or nursing home residents, and the model was not verified.

Mentes and Ferrario (1989) noted that aggressive incidents often quickly become part of the folklore of the institution and grow with repeated telling. Their study evaluated a staff training program designed to assist nonprofessional staff members in interacting with residents to minimize aggressive episodes. The program included six content areas that focused on three principles: knowing the resident, thinking about prevention, and using protective intervention as a last resort. With the use of the training program, there was a nonsignificant decline in the number of incident reports, and staff members reported a greater sense of satisfaction in their work and understanding of the residents. Supervisors noted increased staff morale and creativity when working with cognitively impaired residents (Mentes & Ferrario, 1989).

Negley and Manley (1990) evaluated the reporting of assaults. In general, staff members do not report assaults because they find it time consuming to fill out forms and also view such assaults as a failure of their performance, an occupational hazard, or just part of the job. The purpose of this clinical study was to evaluate assaultive behavior on a 47-bed Veterans Affairs Alzheimer's unit to determine whether changing the room where patients ate dinner decreased the incidence of assaults and whether staff members would accept a change in their long-standing routine. Two large day rooms on the unit were used for dining, the larger one for patients requiring feeding and the smaller for more independent patients. Prior to the intervention, mealtimes were the peak assault times. After the intervention, a 47.5% overall reduction in assaults was noted, concurring with other reports of dining room environments producing problem behavior (Hall et al., 1986; Van Ort & Phillips, 1992).

In their study on aggression, Beck and colleagues (1992) examined the documentation of physically aggressive acts by geriatric residents in a long-term care facility. The retrospective descriptive study reviewed the charts of 38 residents identified as assaultive. The Ryden Aggression Scale (RAS) and a demographic form were used to evaluate aggression. Licensed practical nurses most commonly reported the incidents. Forty-nine percent of the incidents occurred in the bathroom, 22% in the bedroom, 19% in the day room, and 10% in the dining room. Fifty-five percent of assaultive residents had no visitors. Information in the charts of 45% of the patients suggested cognitive impairment or psychiatric illness. Patterns of aggressive behavior were consistent with the problems that accompany cognitive decline: male residents who are modest, fearing care in the bathroom or bedroom; and residents becoming aggressive in highly stimulating areas such as the dining hall or day rooms. All the investigators noted that staff members underreported assaultive episodes. Additional research is needed to better quantify the incidence of aggressive behaviors, to understand the effects of assault on both staff members and residents, and to break down the barriers to increased reporting of assault.

NURSING MEASURES FOR AGITATION AND AGGRESSION

Physical Safety. To provide a safe environment, anything that is potentially harmful, such as sharp objects or toxic fluids, should be removed (Curl, 1989). Pacing behavior should be contained within a controlled environment that allows patients to pace and wander without excessive risk of injury to self or others (Barnes & Raskind, 1980).

Sense of Control. Patients should be given opportunities to experience a sense of control (Ryden, 1992). Examples include providing consistency in the daily routine (Curl, 1989) and offering choices in terms of food and clothing whenever possible. The use of physical restraints limits mobility and takes away the person's sense of control. Restraints should be used only as a last resort to protect the patient's safety.

Physical Comfort. Nurses should provide ongoing assessment to ensure the patient's physical comfort (Curl, 1989; Ryden, 1992). For example, they should monitor bowel movements to ensure that the patient is maintaining normal elimination patterns (Curl, 1989) and should routinely check for painful developments such as ingrown toenails or adverse medication reactions of which the patient may

not be aware or is unable to report as a source of discomfort.

Basic Health Needs. It is important to ensure that patients' basic health needs are met. Maintaining adequate nutrition, for example, can become a problem when the patient is not able to sit through or ingest an entire meal. Nutritional requirements may be met by serving smaller, more frequent meals; providing finger foods; and offering liquids between meals (Curl, 1989). Nurses should arrange for regular rest periods and adequate sleep in a quiet environment (Hall & Buckwalter, 1987) and reduce the patient's intake of caffeine (Curl, 1989).

Compensate for Sensory Deficits. Several measures can be used to help prevent sensory isolation (Barnes & Raskind, 1980) and the misinterpretation of environmental stimuli. Sensory deficits can be compensated for by providing prosthetic devices such as eye glasses and hearing aids. Appropriate communication techniques (see the following section) can be used to compensate for uncorrected hearing or visual impairment (Curl, 1989). The proper environmental lighting should be used to help compensate for visual impairment.

Compensate for Cognitive Deficits. Complex tasks should be broken down into simple steps. Ensure that activities of daily living do not require motor skills that are beyond the resident's ability. Activities should be adapted to the resident's functional ability and interests and should be culturally sensitive to promote a feeling of success. Activities that are likely to result in failure should be avoided.

Validation therapy can be used when the patient experiences hallucinations and delusions. This approach attempts to understand the patient's underlying feelings and focuses on the "reality" of these feelings (Feil, 1992). Questions that begin with "why," which usually require an intellectual response that the patient is not able to provide, should be avoided (Feil, 1992).

Communication. The patient should be provided with an environment in which he or she feels safe. Such an environment may be conveyed both verbally and nonverbally. Nurses should use a nonthreatening posture and a position that is at eye level with the individual and promotes eye contact. Prior to moving into the patients' personal space to implement care, they should explain in simple terms what is going to be done (Ryden, 1992). They should use a calm, friendly tone of voice (Ryden, 1992), state sentences in a positive manner, and avoid the use of commands including the word "don't." Reassurance should be provided as necessary. Assurance is usually most effective when it comes from a family member or a healthcare provider with whom the patient is familiar and whose role is established (Barnes & Raskind, 1980). Care providers should determine which sense dominates the patient's perception of the world (i.e., auditory, visual, kinesthetic, olfactory, or gustatory). This can be accomplished by listening to the descriptive words used by the patient and communicating with the patient through his or her preferred sense. This type of interaction also promotes a feeling of trust by the patient (Feil, 1992).

When providing care, nurses should use touch in a respectful, careful, unhurried manner (Ryden, 1992). Feil (1992) found that gently stroking the patient from the earlobe to the chin may stimulate the memory of a loved one, such as a mother or spouse, and has a calming effect on the patient. If the resident becomes agitated during a task or procedure, it may be best to stop and try again at a later time when he or she is more calm.

Environmental Modification. Nursing interventions to reduce internal and external stressors can involve modifying and simplifying activities and environmental stimuli (Hall & Buckwalter, 1987). This modification should allow the patient to experience optimal levels of stimuli (Roper et al., 1991; Ryden, 1992). Misleading stimuli, such as television, radios, and mirrors, should be avoided; however, stimuli should not be reduced to the point of creating sensory deprivation, which may make the patient even more agitated and cognitively dysfunctional (Barnes & Raskind, 1980).

Cohen-Mansfield and Werner (1997) found that providing stimulating activities and an enriched environment (e.g., social interaction, videotapes of family members talking to the older person, and music) for the cognitively impaired nursing home residents resulted in reduced verbally disruptive behaviors. In another study on the environmental effects on behavior, they found decreased trespassing, exit seeking, and other agitated behaviors when the nursing home environment was enriched with visual, auditory, and olfactory stimuli that simulated a home environment and an outdoor nature environment (Cohen-Mansfield & Werner, 1998).

Reassuring Therapies. Activities that elicit pleasant memories from an earlier time in the patient's life may produce a soothing effect on an agitated patient. Such activities may be enhanced by the stimulation of multiple senses (i.e., vision, smell, taste, touch, hearing). Examples of sensory cues can include introducing and discussing photo albums and personal memorabilia, providing a favorite food item, playing a musical instrument, or listening to music.

Gerdner (1992) studied the immediate and 1-hour residual effects of individualized music therapy (music that the patient preferred during his or her younger years) on the frequency of agitated behaviors in five elderly patients who were confused and agitated. Findings indicated a reduction in agitated behaviors during the 30-minute implementation of music in four of the five subjects, with a statistically significant reduction in behaviors in the hour immediately following the presentation of music. When using music in this manner, however, care providers should carefully assess patients' personal preferences; specificity is important in regard to preferred song titles, musical instruments, and performers.

Baily and colleagues (1992) have used dolls and stuffed animals in their practice to provide comfort and companionship in a select group of patients with Alzheimer's disease (AD). This technique was particularly effective with a female patient who had regressed to her earlier role as wife and mother. She repeatedly talked about her need to return home to take care of her husband and children and constantly made attempts to elope from the facility in an effort to accomplish these tasks. This behavior warranted the use of physical and chemical restraints. Following the use of doll therapy, the restraints were no longer needed. Dolls and stuffed animals used for this purpose should be constructed safely with nontoxic dyes and nondetachable parts that the patient might swallow.

Pharmaceutical Agents. Nursing considerations are crucial for the safe administration of psychotropic and antianxiety drugs and the ongoing assessment of patients who are receiving them. These medications should be prescribed and administered only if all other methods of managing the agitated behaviors have failed. Mood-controlling medications should be prescribed with a specified dosage range, starting with the lowest possible dose. The administration should be monitored to ensure that the patient has actually received and swallowed the medication. Nurses should be knowledgeable about the desired response to and adverse reactions associated with any medication used. They should monitor the patient's response closely. A realistic expectation for patients is the manifestation of tolerable behavior rather than the elimination of problematic or agitated behavior (Curl, 1989).

Light. Light therapy has been used with some success to treat both agitation and night wakening (Lovell et al., 1995; Satlin et al., 1992). Working with six agitated nursing home residents, Lovell and colleagues administered light therapy for 2 hours each morning and rated the residents' behavior every 15 minutes from 6:00 P.M. to 8:00 P.M.; behavior was evaluated at baseline, during the treatment period, and 5 days afterward. Significant differences from baseline were found on treatment days, suggesting that light therapy should be studied with larger samples as an intervention for agitation (Lovell et al., 1995).

Mixed Therapies. Several authors have agreed that the best intervention strategies are complex, start with behavioral and environmental therapies, and often use adjunct pharmacotherapy when behavioral or environmental therapies prove inadequate or require time-consuming costly institutional interventions (Bakke et al., 1994; Banazak, 1996; Heyman & Lombardo, 1995; Rapp et al., 1992; Tesar, 1993; Weinrich et al., 1995).

Nocturnal Confusion and Sundown Syndrome

Waking at night confused and upset is a common problem in elderly patients, especially those in mid- to late-stage dementias. Three nursing studies have been conducted on night wakening. In a controlled study, Young and colleagues (1988) found that white noise did not significantly affect the occurrence of nocturnal confusion.

Hoch and colleagues (1988) studied sleep patterns of 20 elderly people with AD, 23 depressed elderly people, and 23 normal older adults. Compared with control subjects, alterations in sleep continuity were found in both AD and depressed subjects. AD patients slept better than depressed subjects and chose to go to bed earlier. They also had significantly more rapid eye movement sleep and greater amounts of stage 2 sleep, meaning that people with AD are light sleepers who waken frequently but also return to sleep.

Gall and colleagues (1990) conducted a descriptive observational study of elderly people who were hospitalized for a 3-day study. Thirty-one subjects with varied medical diagnoses were observed. The investigators reported no consistent patterns of sleep but found that it took most subjects about 30 minutes to return to sleep after being awakened.

Closely related to night wakening is *sundown syndrome,* defined as an increase in confusion, restlessness, agitation, and disorientation at the end of the day, or deteriorating behavior in the late afternoon. Alternate descriptions or names for this syndrome include "twilight transient confusional states," "senile nocturne delirium," "acute confusional state," and "nocturnal confusional episodes" (Rindlisbacher & Hopkins, 1991, p. 2). Sundown syndrome is thought to be caused by a number of factors, including alterations in diurnal rhythms, sensory deprivation, decreased ambient light, sleep apnea, alterations in metabolism, medications, neurosis, fatigue, disrupted sleep-wake cycles, and a decreased stress threshold. It can be disabling for the patient and a challenge for nurses (Hall & Buckwalter, 1987; Norton, 1991; Rindlisbacher & Hopkins, 1991). Although not limited to patients with AD, it is strongly associated with severe cognitive decline (Rindlisbacher & Hopkins, 1991).

There are several areas of disagreement about the occurrence of sundown syndrome. One problem is the time of occurrence. Of the

40 articles reviewed by Rindlisbacher and Hopkins (1991), 16 mentioned evening and 24 mentioned nighttime; 3 of these studies compared afternoon behavior with morning behavior. A second controversy regarding this syndrome is its prevalence. Although it is reported as being "common," its exact prevalence is unknown. Estimates range from 15.6% of nondemented frail elderly to 15 to 57% of people with AD (Rindlisbacher & Hopkins, 1991). The relative importance of sundown syndrome is not known, other than that it places burdens on caregivers, and the causes are not understood. Most important, because of the inconsistency of symptoms and its vague conceptualization, sundown syndrome has been difficult to study, and few effective interventions have been developed and tested.

Perhaps the best known nursing study of sundown syndrome was conducted by Evans (1987), who studied 59 randomly selected confused or demented subjects in a long-term care facility. Subjects were divided into two groups, those with afternoon problems and those with morning problems. Eighty-two percent of the sundowners were demented, which was four times the percentage in the confused group; yet only 15% of the demented people suffered from sundown syndrome. Sundowners had a shorter length of stay than did nonsundowners, and 50% of sundowners had been in their present room less than 1 month, suggesting relocation trauma. There were no significant differences in physical factors, except urine odor changes, which were more pronounced in sundowners. Changes in environmental light had no effect. This finding differs slightly from the results of a study by Hopkins and colleagues (1992), in which a positive correlation between light intensity and activity levels was found. Evans found that there were no significant differences in medications, and nonsundowners had had more medical diagnoses. An additional difference was that sundowners had a significantly greater tendency to be wakened by staff members every 2 hours during the night. In this study, it was unclear as to whether this awakening occurred because the residents were toileted by nursing staff or, as demonstrated by Hoch and colleagues (1988), because they were light sleepers.

Beel-Bates and Rogers (1990) conducted an exploratory pilot study of six women (four with dementia) in two nursing homes who regularly experienced an increase in restlessness and verbal behavior as evening approached. They developed an instrument to rate the frequency of verbal behaviors and physical behaviors. Because it was a pilot study and the sample size was small, statistical analyses were not completed. However, demented subjects were found to exhibit increased activity between 4:00 and 6:00 P.M., whereas nondemented subjects decreased their activity during this time.

NURSING MEASURES FOR NOCTURNAL CONFUSION AND SUNDOWN SYNDROME

There are few research-based interventions for nocturnal confusion and sundown syndrome; however, several strategies have been found to be effective in practice. These include regular exercise at least three times a week; rest periods twice daily; limited caffeine intake; lowered light levels at night, especially during bathroom rounds; and, in cognitively impaired patients, decreased stimuli at mealtimes. For unremitting confusion, especially if altered levels of consciousness are present, a physical assessment should be performed, including urine cultures, a creatinine clearance, an electrocardiogram, and checking the patient for mild dependent congestive heart failure.

A study of 10 residents with sundown syndrome or nocturnal wakening hypothesized that bright light therapy might normalize sleep-wake cycles. After a week of baseline data collection, 10 residents were exposed to 2 hours of bright light from 7:00 P.M. to 9:00 P.M. daily for 1 week. Using activity monitors and nursing observation, researchers measured sleep-wake cycles, agitation, restraint use, and the use of any medications required for agitation. They reported increased circadian locomotor activity and decreased nighttime activity during the treatment week. The study also found that those patients with the worst preintervention sundowning benefited the most from the light treatment (Satlin et al., 1992).

Hypersexual or Sexually Aggressive Behaviors

> Humans are sexual beings. Throughout life physiologic, psychological, social and cultural forces affect an individual's expression of sexuality. Because one's self-concept is so closely interwoven with sexual identity, forces which threaten sexual identity also threaten personal identity. The denial of sexuality can have a destructive effect not only on one's sex life, but also on one's image and interpersonal relationships.
>
> Kaas, 1978

Despite the truth of this statement, sexuality is often overlooked in the elderly (Richardson & Lazur, 1995). Some people believe that the main purpose of sexual intercourse is procreation (Smedley, 1991); others are reluctant to acknowledge sexual activity in older people because they may be of the same cohort as their parents or grandparents (Lewis, 1984). These attitudes may explain the myth that sexual activity ceases—or should cease—with advanced age. Elderly people whose lifestyles do not adhere to these beliefs may be labeled as "dirty old men" or "indecent old women" (Kaas, 1978). Likewise, the nurse's attitudes regarding sexuality in the elderly may distort his or her ability to recognize the patient's needs (Kaas, 1978). The nurse should begin by examining personal attitudes and how these have developed (Jacobs & Bobek, 1991).

Elderly people with dementia or chronic mental illness may exhibit sexually inappropriate behaviors. A survey of staff members in one long-term care facility revealed that approximately 25% of the residents exhibited problematic sexual behaviors (Szasz, 1983). These behaviors may include masturbating in public, making sexual advances to others, or disrobing or engaging in other suggestive behaviors. Behavior that appears inappropriate to the healthcare provider may, however, have no sexual content to the patient; for example, a person might disrobe only in response to a desire to go to the bathroom. In these situations it is important to identify the underlying need.

NURSING MEASURES FOR HYPERSEXUAL OR SEXUALLY AGGRESSIVE BEHAVIORS

Assessment. Incorporating the patient's sexual health status into the total nursing assessment may help increase awareness of hypersexual or sexually aggressive behavior. Table 27–3 provides a comprehensive outline for such an assessment, and Chapter 24 provides a more extensive discussion of sexuality in the elderly.

The assessment of a patient's medication regimen is an important part of any sexual function assessment (Richardson & Lazur, 1995), as sexual dysfunction may be associated with prescribed medications. For example, cholinesterase, steroids, and antiparkinsonian medications may cause increased libido (Burnside, 1988). This side effect may be equally or even more problematic than the disorder for which the patient is being treated. Reducing dosage, changing medication, or giving "drug holidays" may be helpful (Jacobs & Bobek, 1991).

Privacy. Kaas (1978) identified a lack of privacy as the most important limitation to sexual expression among the elderly living in nursing homes. Aged people living in institutions are

---

TABLE 27-3
Sexual History

1. Individual's perception of own sexuality and sexual activity prior to illness or disability and after its onset
2. Satisfaction with relationships and sexual function
3. Type of illness or disability:
   a. Level of motor or sensory function
   b. Communication skills
   c. Cognitive function
   d. Related physical problems
4. Presence of other medical problems
5. Medications
6. Current partner's availability and response to illness or disability
7. Individual's and partner's values regarding sexual expression
8. Knowledge level
9. Response to disability that may interfere with sexual relationship

From Smedley, G. (1991). Addressing sexuality in the elderly. *Rehabilitation Nursing, 16*(1), 9–11. Copyright 1991 by the Association of Rehabilitation Nurses.

frequently deprived of their sexual rights and are forced to live in celibacy (Kaas, 1978). Providing privacy when feasible and appropriate can be a means of facilitating sexual expression and identity (Kaas, 1978). Privacy can be achieved by using "do not disturb" signs on closed doors, providing conjugal visits, and arranging home visits (Blackerly, 1988; Kaas, 1978; Richardson & Lazur, 1995; Welch et al., 1991).

Ethical issues can arise when one or both of the parties involved is cognitively impaired. This situation requires careful evaluation of each patient's decision-making capacity. Psychiatric consultation may be helpful in evaluating these patients (Richardson & Lazur, 1995).

Behavioral Approach. Several approaches may be used in managing inappropriate sexual behavior. The first is to gently redirect inappropriate behavior when it occurs (Ballard & Gwyther, 1990). This may be done either verbally or physically, depending on the person's level of cognitive functioning (Blackerly, 1988). A more direct approach includes bringing the behavior to the attention of the individual and stating that this behavior is causing others to feel uncomfortable (Blackerly, 1988). Subsequently, the nurse can assist the patient in managing sexual impulses in a socially acceptable manner (Jacobs & Bobek, 1991).

Basic behavior therapy may also be successful in reducing the frequency of inappropriate behavior. Such therapy involves avoiding any reinforcement of unwanted behavior such as occurs with overreacting, for example (Richardson & Lazur, 1995). Alternatively, care providers can respond in a matter-of-fact fashion. Several approaches can be used to meet the patient's need for affection and attention; for example, clinicians should affirm the inherent dignity of the individual (Ballard & Gwyther, 1990) and treat the person with respect.

Nurses should also work to support the patient and provide situations that maintain and promote the person's self-esteem, for example, by encouraging the patient's involvement in activities and attention to personal appearance. This encouragement should be accompanied by genuine praise for success. Physical appearance is a critical means of sexual expression and identity (Kaas, 1978), and opportunities for

enhancement should be provided. Examples include applying makeup for the patient who prefers to wear it but cannot apply it and providing opportunities for hair styling appointments. Interventions and goals should be agreed on and consistently implemented by all members of the interdisciplinary team (Smedley, 1991).

Medication Therapies. No studies have demonstrated any efficacy of antipsychotics, tranquilizers, antidepressants, or antianxiolytics for controlling hypersexual or sexually aggressive behavior. Although medications with a sedating effect can induce a somnolent state, thereby slowing sexual activity, there are no indications that they reduce sexual desire; they may in fact cause unwanted side effects, including immobility, falls, urinary incontinence, and excess disability. The use of estrogen and other hormonal preparations has been studied with male patients but is controversial.

Medroxyprogesterone Acetate (MPA). MPA is an antilibidinal progesterone whose main hormonal effect is to block testosterone synthesis in the testes. Cooper (1987) studied the effects of MPA on four male subjects with dementia who had exhibited sexual acting out behavior; all previous attempts to manage these behaviors had failed. When administered intramuscularly weekly for 1 year, MPA produced a 90% decrease in testosterone levels. Subjects exhibited a rapid decrease in sexual acting out behavior following 10 to 14 days of treatment. When the MPA was discontinued, however, testosterone levels returned to pretrial levels in all subjects. Three subjects exhibited no sexual acting out behavior for 1 year following treatment, whereas the fourth subject did exhibit a return of sexual acting out behavior, but at reduced levels.

There is much controversy associated with the use of MPA, and additional research is clearly needed. Halleck (1981) posed serious ethical questions regarding the use of pharmacological agents to suppress libido. Some states have even declared the use of MPA unlawful. These issues must be taken into consideration when determining treatment. Informed consent describing the benefits and potential adverse reactions should be obtained from the patient or his or her legal decision maker.

PLISSIT Model. The PLISSIT model (P—permission, LI—limited information, SS—specific suggestions, IT—intensive therapy; Annon, 1976) is a highly versatile model developed to provide a basis for individualized intervention following an assessment of sexual needs. The model is comprised of four levels of descending approach, each requiring increasing degrees of knowledge, training, and skill by the clinician.

Giving Permission. Clinicians should help the patient feel comfortable talking about sex. Providing tactful questioning on matters of sexuality is an integral part of the ongoing nursing assessment and may prompt the elderly patient to express concerns.

Providing Limited Information. By providing the patient with specific factual information directly relevant to his or her particular sexual concerns, clinicians can help the elderly person dispel societal myths and stigmas.

Offering Specific Suggestions. Clinicians should obtain a sexual problem history, which includes the following factors: (1) description of the current problem, (2) onset and course of the problem, (3) patient's perception of cause and maintenance of the problem, (4) past treatments and their outcomes, and (5) current expectations and goals of treatment. Direct attempts should then be made to assist patients in changing their behavior in order to reach their stated goals. All members of the interdisciplinary team should provide specific suggestions and work with the patient and partner to agree on sexual goals.

Providing Intensive Therapy. Intensive sexual therapy should be conducted by professionally trained counselors.

SUMMARY

The care of older adults is never easy because of their altered physiology, loss of homeostatic mechanisms, atypical symptom presentation, and heterogeneity as a population. When aged patients with illness or functional loss present with disruptive behaviors such as wandering, aggressiveness, or hypersexuality, providing care becomes fraught with seemingly insurmountable problems. APNs often are consulted by staff members in all settings to solve the perceived behavioral problems so that therapeutic regimens and programs of care can be implemented with maximum benefit. Challenges facing the consulting APN can include the following:

- Overcoming staff barriers to accepting the nurse-consultant relationship
- Collecting objective data on the target behavior
- Placing these data within a meaningful context for the patient
- Developing interventions that reflect the complexity of the target behavior yet are simple enough for all caregivers to apply consistently
- Evaluating outcomes of the interventions with the goal of modifying unsuccessful components
- Preserving caregiver self-esteem and preventing burnout among staff members

Although caregivers may desire a "recipe" type of approach, the APN should understand that principles of behavior management are generated from knowing what triggers a particular behavior and what response is produced. Once these effects are understood, either can be altered to produce behavior changes. One barrier to a successful consultation on the part of caregivers or staff members is expecting the APN to alter the patient's basic personality structure. Staff training and caregiver counseling must include sensitivity to autonomy and the patient's personality structure, which can be enhanced through an understanding of the Lifespan Assessment.

The APN must keep abreast of research that describes and examines ways to manage problem behaviors as the basis of practice. Studies of problem behaviors are still primarily at a descriptive stage, and research-based interventions are desperately needed to assist caregivers and staff with management issues. The APN with clinical research training is in an ideal situation to add to the knowledge base on interventions for problem behaviors through the conduct of small sample studies.

REFERENCES

Algase, D. (1992). Cognitive discriminants of wandering among nursing home residents. *Nursing Research, 41*(2), 78–81.

Annon, J. (1976). The PLISSIT model: A proposed conceptual scheme for behavioral treatment of sexual problems. *Journal of Sex Education Therapy, 2*(2), 1–15.

Baily, J., Gilbert, E., & Herweyer, S. (1992). To find a soul. *Nursing 92, 22*(7), 63–64.

Bakke, B., Kvale, S., Burns, T., et al. (1994). Multicomponent interventions for agitated behavior in a person with Alzheimer's disease. *Journal of Applied Behavioral Analysis, 27*(7), 175–176.

Ballard, E. L., & Gwyther, L. P. (1990). *Optimum care of the nursing home resident with Alzheimer's disease "giving a little extra."* Durham, NC: Duke University Medical Center.

Banazak, D. A. (1996). Difficult dementia: Six steps in controlling problem behavior. *Geriatrics, 51*(2), 36–42.

Barnes, R., & Raskind, M. (l980). Strategies for diagnosing and treating agitation in the aging. *Geriatrics, 35*(3), 111–119.

Beck, C., Robinson, C., & Baldwin, B. (1992). Improving documentation of aggressive behavior in nursing home residents. *Journal of Gerontological Nursing, 18*(2), 21–24.

Beel-Bates, C., & Rogers, A. (1990). An exploratory study of sundown syndrome. *Journal of Neuroscience Nursing, 22*(1), 51–52.

Bernier, S., & Small, N. (1988). Disruptive behaviors. *Journal of Gerontological Nursing, 14*(2), 8–13.

Blackerly, W. (1988). *Head injury rehabilitation: Sexuality after traumatic brain injury.* Houston: HDL Publishers.

Burgio, L., Jones, L., Butler, F., & Engle, B. (1988). Behavior problems in an urban nursing home. *Journal of Gerontological Nursing, 14*(1), 31–34.

Burnside, I. (1988). Intimacy and sexuality. In *Nursing and the aged—a self-care approach* (3rd ed., pp. 448–483). New York: McGraw-Hill Book Company.

Chrisman, M., Tabar, D., Whall, A., & Booth, D. (1991). Agitated behavior in the cognitively impaired elderly. *Journal of Gerontological Nursing, 17*(12), 9–13.

Cohen-Mansfield, J., & Billig, N. (1986). Agitated behaviors in the elderly: A conceptual review. *Journal of American Geriatrics Society, 34*, 711–721.

Cohen-Mansfield, J., & Werner, P. (1997). Management of verbally disruptive behaviors in nursing home residents. *Journal of Gerontology: Medical Sciences, 52A*, M369–M377.

Cohen-Mansfield, J., & Werner, P. (1998). The effects of an enhanced environment on nursing home residents who pace. *Gerontologist, 38*(2), 199–208.

Cooper, A. J. (1987). Medroxyprogesterone acetate (MPA) treatment of sexual acting out in men suffering from dementia. *Journal of Clinical Psychiatry, 48*(9), 368–370.

Curl, A. (l989). Agitation and the older adult. *Journal of Psychosocial Nursing and Mental Health Services, 27*(12), 12–14.

Dawson, P., & Reid, D. (1987). Behavioral dimensions of patients at risk of wandering. *Gerontologist, 27*(1), 104–107.

Evans, L. (1987). Sundown syndrome in institutionalized elderly. *Journal of the American Geriatrics Society, 35*, 101–108.

Feil, N. (1992). Validation therapy. *Geriatric Nursing, 13*(3), 129–133.

Gall, K., Petersen, T., & Riesch, S. (1990). Night life: Nocturnal behavior patterns among hospitalized elderly. *Journal of Gerontological Nursing, 16*(10), 31–35.

Gerdner, L. A. (1992). *The effects of individualized music on elderly patients who are confused and agitated.* Unpublished master's thesis, University of Iowa, Iowa City.

Hall, G. (unpublished). *Five agendas for wandering: A descriptive study.* Iowa City: The University of Iowa Hospitals and Clinics.

Hall, G., & Buckwalter, K. (1987). Progressively lowered stress threshold: A conceptual model for care of adults with Alzheimer's disease. *Archives of Psychiatric Nursing, 1*(6), 399–406.

Hall, G., & Buckwalter, K. (1989). Diagnostic clues in the past. *Geriatric Nursing, 10*(4), 202–204.

Hall, G., Buckwalter, K., Stolley, J., et al. (1995). Standardized care plan: Managing Alzheimer's patients at home. *Journal of Gerontological Nursing, 21*(1), 37–49.

Hall, G., Kirschling, M., & Todd, S. (1986). Sheltered freedom: An Alzheimer's unit in an ICF. *Geriatric Nursing, 7*(3), 132–136.

Halleck, S. L. (1981). The ethics of antiandrogen therapy. *American Journal of Psychiatry, 138*, 642–643.

Heyman, E., & Lombardo, B. (1995). Managing costs: The confused, agitated, or suicidal patient. *Nursing Economics, 13*(2), 107–111.

Hoch, C., Reynolds, S., & Houck, P. (1988). Sleep patterns in Alzheimer, depressed, and healthy elderly. *Western Journal of Nursing Research, 10*(3), 239–256.

Hopkins, R., Rindlisbacher, P., & Grant, N. (1992). An investigation of sundown syndrome and ambient light. *American Journal of Alzheimer's Care and Related Disorders Research, 7*(2), 22–27.

Hussian, R., & Brown, D. (1987). Use of two-dimensional grid patterns to limit hazardous ambulation in demented patients. *Journal of Gerontology, 42*(5), 558–560.

Jacobs, P., & Bobek, S. (1991). Sexual needs of the schizophrenic client. *Perspectives in Psychiatric Care, 27*(1), 15–20.

Kaas, M. J. (1978). Sexual expression of the elderly in nursing homes. *Gerontologist, 18*(4), 372–378.

Kikuta, S. C. (1991). Clinically managing disruptive behavior on the ward. *Journal of Gerontological Nursing, 17*(8), 4–8.

Lewis, M. (1984). Sexual activity in later life: A challenging issue for nurses. *Imprint, 31*(4), 48–49.

Lovell, D., Ancoli-Israel, S., & Gervitz, R. (1995). Effect of bright light treatment on agitated behavior in institutionalized elderly subjects. *Psychiatry Research, 57*(1), 7–12.

Martino-Saltzman, D., Blasch, B., Morris, R., & McNeal, L. (1991). Travel behavior of nursing home residents perceived as wanderers and non-wanderers. *Gerontologist, 31*(5), 666–672.

Mentes, J., & Ferrario, J. (1989). Calming aggressive reactions—a preventive program. *Journal of Gerontological Nursing, 15*(2), 22–27.

Monsour, N., & Robb, S. (1982). Wandering behavior in old age: A psychosocial study. *Social Work, 27*, 411–416.

Negley, E., & Manley, J. (1990). Environmental interventions in assaultive behavior. *Journal of Gerontological Nursing, 16*(3), 29–33.

Norton, D. (1991). Investigating the sundown syndrome. *Nursing Standard, 5*(47), 26–29.

Rader, J., Doan, J., & Schwab, M. (1985). How to decrease wandering: A form of agenda behavior. *Geriatric Nursing, 6*(4), 196–199.

Rapp, M., Flint, A., Herrmann, N., & Proulx, G. (1992). Behavioral disturbances in the demented elderly: Phenomenology, pharmacotherapy, and behavioral management. *Canadian Journal of Psychiatry, 37*(9), 651–657.

Richardson, J. P., & Lazur, A. (1995). Sexuality in the nursing home patient. *American Family Physician, 51*(1), 121–124.

Rindlisbacher, P., & Hopkins, R. (1991). The sundowning syndrome: A conceptual analysis and review. *American Journal of Alzheimer's Care and Research, 6*(4), 2–9.

Roper, J., Shapira, J., & Chang, B. (1991). Agitation in the demented patient: A framework for management. *Journal of Gerontological Nursing, 17*(3), 17–21.

Ryden, M. B. (1992). Alternatives to restraints and psychotropics in the care of aggressive, cognitively impaired elderly persons. In K. C. Buckwalter (Ed.), *Geriatric mental health nursing: Current and future challenges* (pp. 84–93). Thorofare, NJ: Slack.

Salisbury, S. A., & Stone, J. T. (1991). Managing behavioral problems. In W. C. Chenitz, J. T. Stone & S. A. Salisbury (Eds.), *Clinical gerontological nursing: A guide to advanced practice* (pp. 403–421). Philadelphia: W. B. Saunders.

Satlin, A., Volicer, L., Ross, V., et al. (1992). Bright light treatment of behavioral and sleep disturbances in patients with Alzheimer's disease. *American Journal of Psychiatry, 149*(8), 1028–1032.

Smedley, G. (1991). Addressing sexuality in the elderly. *Rehabilitation Nursing, 16*(1), 9–11.

Smith, M., & Buckwalter, K. (1991). *Geriatric mental health training series.* Cedar Rapids, IA: Abbe Center for Community Mental Health.

Struble, L., & Siversten, L. (1987). Agitated behaviors in confused elderly patients. *Journal of Gerontological Nursing, 13*(11), 40–44.

Szasz, G. (1983). Sexual incidents in an extended care unit for aged men. *Journal of the American Geriatrics Society, 19*, 753–758.

Szwabo, P., Woodward, V., Grossberg, G., & Shen, W. (1991). The use of alprazolam for decreased problem wandering in geriatric patients. *American Journal of Alzheimer's Care and Research, 6*(6), 33–36.

Taft, L. (1989). Conceptual analysis of agitation in the elderly. *Archives of Psychiatric Nursing, 3*(2), 102–107.

Teri, L., Rabins, P., Whitehouse, P., et al. (1991). *Management of behavioral disturbances in Alzheimer's disease: Current status and future directions. Report of an expert panel on problem behavior.* Chicago: Alzheimer's Association.

Tesar, G. (1993). The agitated patient, Part I: Evaluation and behavioral management. *Hospital and Community Psychiatry, 44*(4), 329–331.

Van Ort, S., & Phillips, L. (1992). Feeding nursing home residents with Alzheimer's disease. *Geriatric Nursing, 13*(5), 249–253.

Weinrich, S., Egbert, C., Eleazer, G., & Haddock, K. (1995). Agitation: Measurement, management and intervention research. *Archives of Psychiatric Nursing, 9*(5), 251–260.

Welch, S., Meagher, J., Soos, J., & Phopal, J. (1991). Sexual behavior of hospitalized chronic psychiatric patients. *Hospital and Community Psychiatry, 42*(8), 855–856.

Winger, J., & Schirm, V. (1989). Managing aggressive elderly in long-term care. *Journal of Gerontological Nursing, 15*(2), 28–33.

Winger, J., Schirm, V., & Stewart, D. (1987). Aggressive behavior in long-term care. *Journal of Psychosocial Nursing and Mental Health Services, 25*(4), 28–33.

Yesavage, J., Brink, T., Rose, T., & Adey, M. (1983). The geriatric depression rating scale: Comparison with other self-report and psychiatric rating scales. In T. Crook, S. Ferris & R. Bartus (Eds.), *Assessment in geriatric pharmacology.* New Canaan, CT: Mark Powley Associates, Inc.

Young, S., Muir-Nash, J., & Ninos, M. (1988). Managing nocturnal wandering behavior. *Journal of Gerontological Nursing, 14*(5), 6–12.

Zung, W. (1965). A self-rating depression scale. *Archives of General Psychiatry, 12*, 63–70.

APPENDIX 27-1

Wandering

Type of Wandering	Behavioral Characteristics	Interventions
Tactile wanderings	These patients are nearing the end of the ambulatory dementia phase. They spend their time using their hands to explore the environment. Patients may appear to be blind and unable to interpret visual stimuli consistently. They remain calm and appear to wander by accident as they continue to feel their way through doorways and down halls. These patients often have lost the ability to communicate verbally.	The caregiver should guide or distract the patient from hallways and doors. For chronic wandering, door knobs and locks may be modified and alarm systems used. The patient will typically allow redirection to other tactile objects. The caregiver also can supervise patient walking.
Environmentally cued wandering	These patients appear calm and tend to follow cues within the environment; if they see a window, they look out. A chair may cue them to sit, or a door may indicate an exit. Hallways provide cues to continue walking. These patients wander on a regular basis and may appear to be searching. They respond well to nonrestrictive environmental barriers and concrete indicators of territory. They are usually in the middle to late ambulatory dementia phase, requiring assistance for at least bathing and dressing.	The caregiver should assess the environment for cues of wandering. Doors may be disguised with all coverings that either conceal or divert patients. Windows in doors can be curtained or covered with "mirror plastic" so the patient will try to avoid contact. Special closures can be fitted to the door so the patient is unable to open it. Chairs and other cues to stop should be provided. When no barrier is present, one can be created by adhering a double line of brightly colored tape to the floor. Diversionary activities, such as music therapy, are useful in keeping the patient's attention.

Reminiscent or fantasy wandering	These patients are calm and in the ambulatory phase of the illness. Their desire to wander stems from a delusion or fantasy, usually based in their past (e.g., a person going to work, seeing parents, or doing chores). Frequently, they announce that they are leaving and are reassured that there is a specific place to go.	Depending on the intensity of the patient's mood, the caregiver first may try to gently remind the patient that he or she does not have to go to work, do chores, or see parents at that time. If this results in increased anxiety, a fantasy area might be created, based on experiences or past occupations, such as a desk with papers on it, an area for the housewife to clean up, or stacks of foam for the person to restack. The caregiver also may find that validation of the meaning of the delusion (e.g., the feelings of worth associated with work) will distract the patient. Use of the term "later" and diversional activities also help.
Recreational wandering	These patients may be in the confused or ambulatory dementia phases of the illness. They may have had an active lifestyle prior to becoming ill or may have been taken for walks regularly by a caregiver. The wandering is purposeful, recurs regularly, usually at the same time, and appears to serve a need for exercise. The patients are calm, unless stopped.	The caregiver should plan to take the patient for a walk each day at the same time. Walks should follow exactly the same route each day, beginning and ending at the same place. This will help the caregiver locate the patient, should he or she wander. Walking with the patient is an excellent way for the caregiver to interact on a one-on-one basis and to reminisce with the patient.

| Agitated purposeful wandering | These patients are upset or agitated or exhibit stress-related, problematic behavior such as an angry outburst or increased confusion. They are cognitively and socially inaccessible (lost). Preoccupied with leaving, the patients may pack suitcases to take home. Caregivers are generally unable to reason with these patients and may recognize the patients' fear of them. Caregivers who attempt to remove control from a resident exhibiting this type of behavior may be assaulted as the resident attempts to maintain control by panicking and fleeing. Once recognized, agitated purposeful wandering can be prevented. | *Immediate interventions:* The caregiver should not confront the resident but try to diffuse the situation. Tell the patient about caregiver fears and concerns. Offer suggestions, such as waiting for a glass of juice, that will buy time to allow the patient to regain composure. Use preserved social skills to allow the patient maximum control of the situation. Remove offending stressors.

If the patient leaves, accompany or follow, with a coat when appropriate. Bring the patient back as quickly as possible, providing measures to decrease stress. Assure safety and security.

Prevention of further episodes: Evaluate the cause of the incident. Reduce the amount of stimulus to which the patient is exposed, increase rest periods, or attempt to decrease stressors caused by other individuals, such as negative feedback from others. This patient may benefit from a protected environment in which unconditional positive regard is provided and environmental stimuli are reduced. |

From Hall, G., Buckwalter, K., Stolley, J., et al. (1995). Standardized care plan: Managing Alzheimer's patients at home. *Journal of Gerontological Nursing, 21*(1), 43–44.

Pain and Discomfort

Christine Miaskowski

Pain is a highly subjective yet universal human experience. It may be the most common symptom of disease or injury. Ferrell and colleagues (1990) have noted that pain is an understudied problem in gerontology in both community-based and nursing home residents. Two of the major foci of geriatric nursing practice are the control of symptoms of chronic disease and the restoration of function. The assessment and management of acute and chronic pain are, therefore, a major clinical priority.

PREVALENCE OF PAIN IN THE ELDERLY

The exact prevalence of pain, particularly in the elderly, is unknown. Population-based studies (Brattberg et al., 1989; Crook et al., 1984) have suggested that 25 to 50% of community-dwelling elderly people experience significant pain problems. In a survey of 500 randomly selected households in Ontario, Crook and colleagues (1984) found that 16% of the total population aged 18 to 105 years reported a "significant" pain problem in the preceding 2 weeks. In this study, the incidence of pain was twice as great in individuals older than 60 years than in younger subjects.

The prevalence of pain among nursing home residents may be higher than in community-dwelling elderly populations. Estimates suggest that pain may occur in 45 to 80% of nursing home residents (Ferrell et al., 1990; Lau-Ting & Phoon, 1988; Roy & Michael, 1986). In one study (Ferrell et al., 1990), 97 residents from a 311-bed multilevel teaching nursing home were interviewed, and charts were reviewed for pain problems and management strategies. Results indicated that of the 71% of residents who complained of pain, 34% complained of continuous pain, and 66% described pain of an intermittent nature. Major causes of pain included lower back pain (40%), arthritis (24%), previous fracture sites (14%), and neuropathies (11%). Additional epidemiological studies are warranted to determine the prevalence and severity of pain not only comparing community-based and nursing home residents but also comparing different age groups of elderly (i.e., the young old, middle old, and old old).

AGE-RELATED CHANGES IN PAIN PERCEPTION

Studies of age-related changes in pain perception have produced inconclusive results. The majority of these studies have been done using "normal" volunteers who were subjected to noxious thermal, mechanical, or electrical stimuli. In an excellent review of pain studies, Harkins and colleagues (1984) concluded that no consensus exists in the literature regarding age-associated changes in pain perception, owing to differences in methodology and subject selection. Additional studies are warranted to determine if age-related differences in pain perception and tolerance exist in healthy elderly individuals as well as in elderly individuals experiencing chronic painful disorders.

TYPES OF PAIN IN THE ELDERLY

Pain has been defined as "an unpleasant sensory and emotional experience associated with actual or potential tissue damage, or described in terms of such damage" (Merskey, 1986). Pain can be categorized as either acute or chronic in nature. Acute pain follows tissue injury and abates when the body injury heals. It may be accompanied by sympathetic nervous system activation (e.g., tachycardia, hypertension, diaphoresis). Characteristically acute pain is self-limited; it serves as a warning signal for the body and usually resolves as healing occurs. Chronic pain typically is defined as pain lasting longer than 3 months. With chronic pain, the signs of sympathetic hyperactivity often are absent. In addition, alterations in mood (e.g., depression or anxiety) are common. Chronic pain produces profound disruptions in a patient's functional activities and quality of life.

Pain can be classified by pathophysiological mechanisms as either somatic, visceral, or neuropathic. Somatic pain occurs as a result of nociceptor activation in cutaneous or deep tissues. *Somatic pain* is described as constant and well localized. *Visceral pain* is evoked as a result of injury to sympathetically innervated organs. Depending on the organ or tissue that is injured, pain may be described as deep, dull, and aching sensations or as paroxysmal and colicky. *Neuropathic pain*, also called deafferentation pain, refers to pain evoked by some type of injury to the nervous system and is described as burning, tingling, numbing, pressing, and squeezing, often accompanied by shocklike or lancinating pain. Classification of a patient's pain problem may lead to more appropriate interventions.

Elderly patients can experience either acute or chronic pain or acute pain superimposed on a more chronic pain syndrome. Table 28–1 lists several painful medical conditions that commonly occur in the geriatric population (Ferrell, 1991) and their signs and symptoms.

PAIN ASSESSMENT IN THE ELDERLY

The accurate initial and ongoing assessment of pain is the cornerstone of effective pain man-

Common Painful Conditions in the Elderly

Condition	Type of Pain	Signs and Symptoms
Musculoskeletal problems	Somatic	Tightness, stiffness, spasm, acute sharp pain
Rheumatoid arthritis	Somatic	Joint stiffness, joint swelling, tenderness, pain, malaise, fatigue
Osteoarthritis	Somatic	Deep aching pain in afflicted joints, morning stiffness, joint instability, preponderance of pain at rest
Cancer	Somatic, visceral, neuropathic	Variable, depending on the cause
Postherpetic neuralgia	Neuropathic	Burning, tingling, shocklike stabs
Temporal arteritis	Somatic	Headache, visual disturbances, intermittent claudication, polymyalgia rheumatica
Peripheral vascular disease	Somatic	Intermittent claudication, burning, stiffness
Traumatic injuries	Somatic, visceral, neuropathic	Variable, depending on the type of trauma and the tissues involved
Vertebral compression fracture	Somatic	Severe pain, localized tenderness, muscle spasm
Myocardial ischemia	Somatic	Tightness, squeezing, burning, pressing, choking, aching, feeling of indigestion, ill-characterized discomfort
Pleuritic pain	Somatic	Sharp, well-localized pain that worsens with coughing, sneezing, deep breathing, or movement
Gastroesophageal reflux	Somatic	Heartburn that occurs 30 to 60 minutes after meals; regurgitation (sour or bitter taste)

agement. The assessment of pain in an elderly patient requires (1) an understanding of the potential barriers to performing the assessment; (2) knowledge of the key components of the initial pain assessment; (3) knowledge of the critical questions related to the pain complaint; and (4) an understanding of the consequences of pain in the elderly that could potentially influence the patient's ability to describe his or her pain problem, affect the treatment regimen, or affect the patient's ability to recover.

Barriers to Pain Assessment with the Elderly

The major barriers to pain assessment in the elderly are listed in Table 28–2. Elderly patients may view pain as a normal part of the aging process and therefore ignore the problem or bear it as a part of life. Some patients may strive to play the role of the "good patient" and may therefore be reluctant to report pain problems for fear of being labeled a "complainer." Elderly patients may refrain from reporting pain complaints because they perceive that their healthcare professionals are too busy and should not be bothered. In addition, elderly patients may have multiple health problems of which pain is a low priority. Some patients may worry that reporting a pain problem will result in needless tests and additional expense. Others may worry about the meaning of the pain and fear that the pain is caused by a serious disease. Elderly patients may also fear being given pain medication that produces unwanted side effects or results in addiction (Dull & Stratton, 1991; Leech-Hofland, 1992).

TABLE 28-2

Barriers to Pain Assessment with the Elderly

Barrier	Corrective Strategy
1. Elderly perceive that pain is a normal part of the aging process	1. Inform the elderly that pain can occur with aging, that pain requires treatment, and that a health care professional needs to know about a pain problem to be able to effectively manage the pain.
2. Elderly want to be perceived as "good patients."	2. Give the elderly permission to tell their "pain story."
3. Elderly perceive that healthcare professionals are "too busy."	3. Provide an unhurried atmosphere and an attentive manner when conducting a history and physical examination. Do not use condescending language.
4. Elderly have multiple health problems, with pain low on the priority list.	4. Ask about pain as a routine part of every assessment.
5. Elderly worry about additional tests and expenses.	5. Reassure the patient that only necessary tests will be performed. Prepare the patient for the diagnostic test.
6. Elderly worry about what the pain may signify.	6. Provide patients with sufficient information about what might be causing the pain.
7. Elderly fear that pain medication may produce intolerable side effects and addiction.	7. Reassure patients that side effects will be managed. Educate patients about the difference among tolerance, dependence, and addiction.

Pain Assessment

The initial pain assessment includes a detailed history of the pain complaint, a past medical history, a psychosocial assessment, and a detailed physical examination.

DETAILED PAIN HISTORY

The specific components of a pain assessment and the appropriate questions to ask are outlined in Table 28–3 (Miaskowski, 1993). Patients may find it easier to describe their pain if they are provided a list of word descriptors such as those listed in the McGill Pain Questionnaire (Table 28–4; Melzack, 1975). The words patients use to describe their pain may provide clues to the cause of the pain. For example, an elderly patient with postherpetic neuralgia may describe his pain as sensations of burning, numbness, and tingling, with intermittent shocklike bolts of pain. In contrast, someone with a compression fracture of the lumbosacral spine may describe sharp, agonizing pain over the site of the compression frac-

ture. The location and pattern of radiation of the pain (if any) may provide clues to the cause of the pain and help focus the physical examination and diagnostic testing.

An evaluation of the severity or intensity of the pain in an elderly patient requires some

TABLE 28-3

Components of a Pain Assessment

1. *Description*—What does the pain feel like?
2. *Location*—Show me where it hurts (have patient point to anatomical site on themselves or on the clinician). Does the pain go anywhere else (i.e., is there radiation)?
3. *Severity or intensity*—On a scale of 0 to 10, with 0 being no pain and 10 being the worst pain you can imagine, how much does it hurt right now? at its worst? at its least?
4. *Aggravating or relieving factors*—What makes the pain better? What makes the pain worse?
5. *Previous treatments and effectiveness*—What drugs and treatments have you tried in the past to relieve your pain? How effective were these drugs and treatments in relieving your pain?

TABLE 28-4

Word Descriptions from the McGill Pain Questionnaire

Directions: Circle only one word in each of the 20 groups *if* the group contains a word that describes your pain. Leave out any group that is not suitable.

1	2	3	4	5
Flickering	Jumping	Pricking	Sharp	Pinching
Quivering	Flashing	Boring	Cutting	Pressing
Pulsing	Shooting	Drilling	Lacerating	Gnawing
Throbbing	Shocking	Stabbing		Cramping
Beating		Lancinating		Crushing

6	7	8	9	10
Tugging	Hot	Tingling	Dull	Tender
Pulling	Burning	Itchy	Sore	Taut
Wrenching	Scalding	Smarting	Hurting	Rasping
	Searing	Stinging	Aching	Splitting
			Heavy	

11	12	13	14	15
Tiring	Sickening	Fearful	Punishing	Wretched
Exhausting	Suffocating	Frightful	Grueling	Blinding
		Terrifying	Cruel	
			Vicious	
			Killing	

16	17	18	19	20
Annoying	Spreading	Tight	Cool	Nagging
Troublesome	Radiating	Numb	Cold	Nauseating
Miserable	Penetrating	Drawing	Freezing	Agonizing
Intense	Piercing	Squeezing	Icy	Torturing
Unbearable		Tearing		

Adapted from Melzack, R. (1975). The McGill Pain Questionnaire: Major properties and scoring methods. *Pain, 1,* 357–381.

judgment on the part of the healthcare professional. Recent clinical practice guidelines developed by expert panels for the Agency for Health Care Policy and Research recommend that simple, easy-to-use pain intensity measures be included as a routine part of pain assessment (Acute Pain Management Guideline Panel, 1992; Jacox et al., 1994). To date, however, no research has been done to determine what type of pain intensity measure is most appropriate for the elderly.

Several different pain intensity measures are illustrated in Figure 28–1. One of the easiest measures for the clinician to use is a verbal, numerical rating scale. Using this type of intensity scale, patients are asked to rate their pain on a scale from 0 (no pain) to 10 (the worst pain imaginable). Clinical experience, however, suggests that a 0 to 10 verbal numerical rating scale is sometimes difficult for an elderly person to understand. Clinicians have anecdotally reported having better success with scales from 0 to 5. One of the major advantages of a verbal numerical rating scale is that no additional equipment (e.g., visual analog scales, a list of word descriptors, or a faces scale) is required. Additional research is needed to determine what type of pain intensity measure is most appropriate for cognitively intact as well as cognitively impaired elderly patients (see the section on pain assessment in the cognitively impaired elderly).

The next section of the pain assessment focuses on evaluating aggravating and relieving

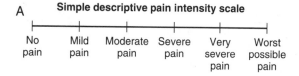

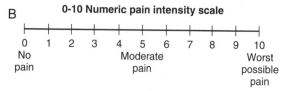

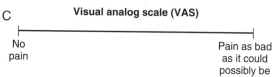

FIGURE 28–1. Pain intensity scales. *A,* Simple descriptive pain intensity scale. *B,* 0–10 numeric pain intensity scale. If either of these two is used as a graphic rating scale, a 10-cm baseline is recommended. *C,* Visual analog scale; a 10-cm baseline is recommend for this scale. (A to C redrawn from Jacox, A., Carr, D. B., Payne R., et al [1994]. *Management of cancer pain.* Clinical Practice Guideline No. 9. Agency for Health Care Policy and Research Publication No. 94-0592. Rockville, MD: U.S. Department of Health and Human Services, Public Health Service, Agency for Health Care Policy and Research.)

factors (i.e., what makes the pain better or worse). These factors often provide clues to the cause of the pain (e.g., a constricting garment that worsens the pain of postherpetic neuralgia). An analysis of the factors that worsen or relieve the pain can also help define specific nonpharmacological interventions that can be incorporated into the pain management plan.

A careful evaluation of previous treatment modalities and their effectiveness provides valuable information to guide the development of a treatment plan. The clinician should ask about specific pharmacological interventions (e.g., over-the-counter analgesics, opioid analgesics, and adjuvant analgesics) and nonpharmacological interventions (e.g., the use of heat or cold, massage, relaxation exercises, transelectrical nerve stimulation, and chiropractic therapy). A comprehensive evaluation of previous treatment modalities should help eliminate previously ineffective interventions. In addi-

tion, the opportunity may arise to clarify misconceptions about specific pain relief strategies (e.g., that the use of opioid analgesics results in addiction).

PAST MEDICAL HISTORY

The past medical history should include an evaluation of concurrent medical problems as well as a history of any other painful conditions (see Table 28–1). Obtaining information on how the patient coped with previous pain problems and the impact of the pain on the patient's functional status may help categorize the present pain as either acute or chronic.

As part of the past medical history, elderly patients should be asked to report any history of trauma (e.g., falls and fractures) and the extent of the injuries. A complete medication history also should be obtained at this time. Particular attention should be paid to obtaining an accurate estimate of the amount of over-the-counter medication the elderly person is taking (particularly acetaminophen, aspirin, and nonsteroidal antiinflammatory drugs).

PHYSICAL EXAMINATION

The physical examination should be used to confirm information obtained during the history. Careful attention should be paid to performing a detailed musculoskeletal and neurological examination. An important part of the physical examination is palpation for trigger points and sites of swelling and inflammation. Trigger points may result from tendonitis, muscle strain, or nerve irritation. Specific maneuvers that reproduce pain, such as straight leg raising and joint motion may provide diagnostic information as well as information about the extent of the individual's functional limitations. The neurological examination, including an evaluation of sensory and motor changes, may provide useful information for diagnosing neuropathic pain problems such as postherpetic neuralgia (Ferrell, 1991).

A functional assessment is critical in maximizing the elderly patient's mobility and independence. Information on functional status should be obtained from the patient history and physical examination. In addition, inquir-

TABLE 28-5
Components of a Psychosocial Assessment

1. The meaning of the pain to the patient or family.
2. Significant past instances of pain and their effects on the patient.
3. The patient's typical coping responses to stress or pain.
4. The patient's knowledge of, curiosity about, preferences for, and expectations of different pain management methods.
5. The patient's concerns about using controlled substances (e.g., opioids, anxiolytics).
6. The economic effect of the pain and its treatment.
7. Changes in mood that have occurred as a result of the pain (e.g., depression, anxiety).
8. Changes in social functioning that have occurred as a result of the pain.
9. Changes in sexual functioning that have occurred as a result of the pain.

Adapted from Jacox, A., Carr, D. B., Payne, R., et al. (1994). *Management of cancer pain.* Clinical Practice Guideline No. 9. Agency for Health Care Policy and Research Publication No. 94-0592. Rockville, MD: U.S. Department of Health and Human Services, Public Health Service, Agency for Health Care Policy and Research.

ies should be made about how pain interferes with ambulation or social activities. More detailed information may be obtained through the use of functional assessment scales such as the Tinetti gait evaluation scale (Tinetti, 1986) or the Lawton (Lawton & Brody, 1969) or Katz (Katz et al., 1963) activities of daily living scales, which may provide useful information on the magnitude of the pain problem.

PSYCHOSOCIAL ASSESSMENT

A comprehensive pain assessment should include a psychological evaluation. Questions that should be included in the psychosocial assessment of a pain problem are listed in Table 28–5. Specific attention should be placed on an evaluation of changes in the elderly person's mood, particularly the symptoms of anxiety and depression.

ONGOING PAIN ASSESSMENT

The clinical practice guidelines on acute pain (Acute Pain Management Guideline Panel, 1992) and cancer pain (Jacox et al., 1994) emphasize the importance of establishing a routine approach to pain assessment. This type of approach, which is used by all clinicians in a practice setting, is particularly important with an elderly population. Routine inquiries about pain problems should be perceived by elderly persons as a normal part of their care. By asking questions about pain problems, the clinician can provide patients an opportunity to report the symptom and, if necessary, to "tell their pain story."

Ongoing assessment is a critical part of the follow-up on a pain complaint and also a way to determine the efficacy of the treatment plan. Components of the ongoing assessment should include an evaluation of any changes in pain intensity, problems or side effects associated with the treatment plan, changes in the patient's functional status and mood, and consequences of the pain (Table 28–6).

A useful strategy, particularly for elderly individuals with short-term memory disturbances, is to have patients keep a *pain diary*, in which they record pain intensity scores, medi-

TABLE 28-6
Consequences of Pain in the Elderly

Depression
Decreased socialization
Sleep disturbances
Impaired ambulation
Deconditioning
Gait disturbances
Falls
Polypharmacy
Cognitive dysfunction
Malnutrition
Increased healthcare use and costs

cation intake, the use of nonpharmacological interventions, and activities of daily living. The patient can bring the pain diary to the clinician's office, or the clinician can review the information in the patient's home or in the nursing home. The clinician should make appropriate adjustments in the pain management plan based on the person's self-report.

Pain Assessment in the Cognitively Impaired Elderly

Because pain is a subjective experience, patient self-report has become the gold standard for evaluating pain complaints. In the United States, however, between 2 and 5 million people suffer from dementia, and by the year 2000 that number is likely to increase by 60% (Office of Technology Assessment, 1987). Dementia, caused by a variety of acute and chronic conditions, is defined as a decrease in mental functions in an otherwise awake and alert individual (Davitz & Davitz, 1980). Changes in mental functioning can markedly interfere with an individual's ability to report pain. A number of clinical issues need to be considered when attempting to assess pain in the cognitively impaired elderly; these include depression, sensory impairments (e.g., hearing, visual acuity), aphasia, and chemical and physical restraints (Parke, 1992).

Pain assessment in the cognitively impaired elderly must focus on creating a picture of the pain-free person. Data must be collected from all possible sources, including family members, nursing assistants, physicians, physical therapists, occupational therapists, and volunteers. Clinicians should focus on facial expressions, body movements, and changes in daily activities (Table 28–7). Normal patterns of behavior should be noted in the patient's record, as they can alert clinicians to changes in behavior that may be indicative of pain.

Clinicians must maintain a high index of suspicion that an elderly patient may be experiencing pain from one or more causes. Careful attention must be paid to the patient's medical history and physical examination. If a condition causes pain in an individual who can self-report pain, clinicians must assume that this

TABLE 28-7
Pain Assessment in the Cognitively Impaired Elderly

Facial expressions
  Wrinkling of forehead
  Tightly closed or widely opened eyes
  Grimacing or distorted expression
  Aggressive or withdrawn behavior
  Increase in hitting or biting
  Start of hitting or biting behavior
  Calling out or crying, or decrease in vocalizations
Body movements
  Moving head from side to side
  Rocking
  Pulling legs to abdomen
  Inability to keep hands still
  Changes in gait
  No movement or decreased movement
  Splinting or guarding
Changes in daily activities
  Sudden increase or decrease in activity
  Increase in periods of rest
  Irritability
  Decrease in social interaction
  Sudden stop in common routines
  Sudden onset of confusion

Adapted from Parke, B. (1992). Pain in the cognitively impaired elderly. *The Canadian Nurse, 88,* 17–20. Reproduced with permission from The Canadian Nurse/ L'infirmière canadienne, vol. 88, no. 7.

condition is painful in the cognitively impaired patient and must treat the pain empirically. Changes in facial expression, body movements, and daily activities should be evaluated to determine if the pain management program has been effective (Marzinski, 1991; Parke, 1992).

PRINCIPLES OF PAIN MANAGEMENT IN THE ELDERLY

To effectively manage pain in an elderly patient, clinicians should incorporate several fundamental principles into their routine practice (Table 28–8). Although assessment is the cornerstone of effective pain management, the implementation of a few specific measures should optimize an elderly patient's pain management plan. It is imperative that clinicians facilitate the diagnostic workup of the pain complaint by medicating patients during diagnostic pro-

TABLE 28-8
Principles of Pain Management in the Elderly

1. Always ask elderly patients about pain.
2. Accept the patient's word about pain and its intensity.
3. Never underestimate the potential effects of chronic pain on the patient's overall condition and quality of life.
4. Be compulsive about pain assessments. An accurate diagnosis will lead to more effective treatment.
5. Treat pain to facilitate diagnostic procedures. Don't wait for a diagnosis to relieve the pain and needless suffering.
6. Use a combination of pharmacological and nonpharmacological approaches whenever possible.
7. Mobilize patients physically and psychosocially. Involve patients in their own care.
8. Use analgesic drugs correctly. Start doses low and increase slowly. Titrate to desired effect or intolerable side effects.
9. Anticipate and attend to anxiety and depression.
10. Reassess responses to treatment at regular intervals. Alter therapy to maximize pain relief and improve functional status and quality of life.

Adapted from Ferrell, B. A. (1991). Pain management in elderly people. *Journal of the American Geriatrics Society, 39*, 64–73.

cedures that can cause or increase pain. This proactive approach should reduce needless pain, ensure a more accurate diagnostic test, and enable the development of a more effective treatment plan based on an accurate diagnosis.

The management of pain in the elderly should employ both pharmacological and nonpharmacological approaches. Patient preferences should play a major role in developing an effective pain management plan. The risks and benefits of the various treatment options should be explained so that the patient can make an informed decision. The costs of specific pain management options need to be considered when developing the treatment plan because many elderly patients live on a fixed income.

PHARMACOLOGICAL MANAGEMENT OF PAIN IN THE ELDERLY

The pharmacological management of pain in the elderly requires an in-depth understanding of the pharmacology of opioid, nonopioid, and adjuvant analgesics as well as an understanding of the physiological changes in renal and liver function that accompany aging and can influence analgesic drug metabolism and clearance (see Chapter 26). Several authors have provided detailed reviews on the pharmacological management of pain in the elderly (e.g., Enck, 1991; Ferrell, 1991; Kaiko et al., 1982; Portenoy, 1987; Reidenberg, 1982; Sager & Bennett, 1992; Wall, 1990). This section presents an overview of nonopioid, opioid, and adjuvant analgesics, including their mechanisms of action, indications for use, dosing and administration guidelines, and side effects. General principles governing the use of opioid analgesics are reviewed. The section concludes with a brief discussion of the changes in the pharmacokinetics of opioid analgesics (e.g., metabolism, clearance) that result from the physiological consequences of aging.

Nonopioid Analgesics

Nonopioid analgesics are the first-line pharmacological agents used to manage mild to moderate pain. The nonopioids include acetaminophen, aspirin, and the nonsteroidal anti-inflammatory drugs (NSAIDs). NSAIDs are used for a wide variety of pain complaints, including musculoskeletal aches and pains, headaches, toothaches, backaches, arthritis, gout, tendonitis, bursitis, and pain associated with bone metastasis. The use of NSAIDs has increased dramatically in the United States, with more than 100 million prescriptions written each year since 1986 (Brooks & Day, 1991). Over 40% of NSAIDs are prescribed for elderly patients, and many of the well-defined NSAID toxicities are associated with aging or age-related debility (Baum et al., 1985).

NSAIDs work by decreasing the levels of inflammatory mediators generated at sites of tissue injury by inhibiting the enzyme cyclooxygenase, which catalyzes the conversion of arachidonic acid to prostaglandins and leukotrienes (Sunshine & Olson, 1989). These mediators sensitize nerves to painful stimuli. NSAIDs work primarily in the peripheral ner-

TABLE 28-9
Commonly Used Nonopioid Analgesics

Drug	Usual Dose for Adults ≥50 Kg Body Weight
Acetaminophen (Tylenol)	650 mg every 4 hr 975 mg every 6 hr
Aspirin	650 mg every 4 hr 975 mg every 6 h
Choline magnesium trisalicylate (Trilisate)	1000–1500 mg 3 times/day
Diflunisal (Dolobid)	500 mg every 12 hr
Etodolac (Lodine)	200–400 mg every 6–8 hr
Fenoprofen calcium (Nalfon)	300–600 mg every 6 hr
Ibuprofen (Advil, Motrin, Nuprin)	400–600 mg every 6 hr
Ketoprofen (Orudis)	25–60 mg every 6–8 hr
Ketorolac (Toradol)	10 mg every 4–6 hr to a maximum of 40 mg/day—orally 60 mg initially, then 30 mg every 6 hr; intramuscular dose should not exceed 5 days
Naproxen (Naprosyn)	250–275 mg every 6–8 hr
Naproxen sodium (Anaprox)	275 mg every 6–8 hr

Adapted from Jacox, A., Carr, D. B., Payne, R, et al. (1994) *Management of cancer pain.* Clinical Practice Guideline No. 9. Agency for Health Care Policy and Research Publication No. 94-0592. Rockville, MD: U.S. Department of Health and Human Services, Public Health Service, Agency for Health Care Policy and Research.

vous system and are useful in the management of mild to moderate pain.

The most commonly used NSAIDs are listed in Table 28–9. These drugs are administered orally and do not produce tolerance or physical dependence. However, the analgesic effectiveness of the NSAIDs as well as aspirin and acetaminophen is limited by the pharmacological property known as the *ceiling effect*. A ceiling effect occurs when further escalation of the drug dose does not produce additional analgesia and, as is the case with this group of drugs, worsens drug-induced side effects and toxicities.

There is considerable individual variation in response to different classes of NSAIDs. Patients should be given a 2-week trial before switching to another drug. At low doses, the primary effect of the NSAIDs is analgesia; higher doses are needed to achieve an antiinflammatory effect. Elderly patients on chronic NSAID therapy must be monitored on an ongoing basis not only for the effectiveness of the therapeutic regimen but also for drug-induced side effects and toxicities.

The major side effects associated with NSAIDs are listed in Table 28–10. About 25% of patients on NSAIDs experience gastrointestinal complaints ranging from nausea and heartburn to abdominal pain (Sager & Bennett, 1992). Approximately 12.5% of patients on NSAIDs have

TABLE 28-10
Side Effects of Nonsteroidal Antiinflammatory Drugs

Gastrointestinal effects (e.g., nausea, heartburn, abdominal pain, bleeding, ulceration)
Nephrotoxicity
Bleeding
Bronchospasm
Hepatitis
Skin rash
Headache
Tinnitus
Hearing loss
Vertigo
Cognitive dysfunction
Psychosis
Central nervous system depression

gastric ulcers, and recent data suggest that the elderly are at the highest risk for developing NSAID-induced gastrointestinal complications (Carson et al., 1987; Griffin et al., 1988). Nephrotoxicity is another side effect associated with the administration of NSAIDs. The reversible renal insufficiency that can occur with these drugs (i.e., elevated blood urea nitrogen and creatinine) is caused by the inhibition of prostaglandins and occurs in approximately 20% of patients taking NSAIDs within the first several days of use (Sager & Bennett, 1992). Prostaglandin-mediated homeostasis of fluid and electrolyte excretion, renin release, and renal blood flow all are affected by NSAIDs. Disruption of these physiological processes results in sodium and water retention, hyperkalemia, and acute renal insufficiency.

Prostaglandin E_2 (PGE_2) inhibits the tubular reabsorption of sodium and chloride as well as the action of antidiuretic hormone (ADH), thereby promoting the excretion of sodium and water. The administration of NSAIDs inhibits the actions of PGE_2 and results in peripheral edema and weight gain in high-risk individuals. Inhibition of PGE_2 by NSAIDs also decreases the excretion of potassium, resulting in hyperkalemia. Finally, by inhibiting the action of prostacyclin (PGI_2), NSAIDs decrease glomerular filtration rates and predispose the patient to acute renal failure (Sager & Bennett, 1992).

In the elderly, significant risk factors for NSAID-induced renal toxicity include increased age, hemorrhage, the use of diuretics, congestive heart failure, cirrhosis, diabetes, hypertension, chronic pyelonephritis, and the use of antihypertensive drugs. Additional side effects of NSAIDs can include bleeding disorders, bronchospasm, hepatitis, skin rash, headache, tinnitus, hearing loss, vertigo, cognitive dysfunction, psychosis, and central nervous system depression.

Opioid Analgesics

Opioid analgesics work by binding to opioid receptors, largely within the central nervous system. These drugs are indicated for moderate to severe acute and chronic pain. Unlike NSAIDs, opioid analgesics produce tolerance and physical dependence; however, they do not exhibit a ceiling effect. The appropriate use of opioids is governed by an understanding of their relative analgesic potencies, oral to parenteral analgesic potencies, and pharmacokinetic properties.

Morphine is the prototypical opioid agonist against which all other opioids are compared. It has a short half-life (2–3 hours), a parenteral-to-oral ratio of 1:3, and an average duration of analgesia of 4 to 6 hours. In addition to the more common injectable form, morphine is available in sustained-release tablets; the two brands available are MS Contin and Oramorph SR. Sustained-release morphine preparations are an important innovation in pain management. The two formulations mentioned provide 8 to 12 hours of pain relief. One of the major advantages of sustained-release morphine is that it allows patients to sleep through the night. The most reliable way to design a sustained-release morphine regimen is to treat the patient with immediate-release morphine for at least 48 hours (or until adequate pain control is achieved) to learn the average daily dose requirement. Patients can then be converted to the sustained-release morphine preparation. Immediate release preparations should be available for breakthrough pain (American Pain Society, 1993). Table 28–11 lists the properties of the other commonly used opioids compared with morphine.

Hydromorphone (Dilaudid) is a potent opioid analgesic that is very similar to morphine. It is available in a highly concentrated form (10 mg/mL) that may be useful for parenteral administration in cachectic patients. In contrast to morphine and hydromorphone, which are short-acting opioids, levorphanol and methadone are potent analgesics with relatively long serum half-lives (i.e., 12–16 and 12–24 hours, respectively). These drugs require careful titration to achieve maximal analgesic effectiveness. Safe and effective use of opioids with long half-lives requires careful monitoring and dosage adjustments, especially in elderly patients or in patients with compromised hepatic or renal function (Wall, 1990).

The use of meperidine (Demerol) should be avoided in the management of acute and

TABLE 28-11

Dosing Chart for Common Opioid Analgesics

Opioid	Equianalgesic Doses		Duration of Analgesia (hr)	Plasma Half-Life (hr)	Usual Starting Dose for Moderate to Severe Pain	
	Oral (mg)	Parenteral (mg)			Oral	Parenteral
Morphine	30	10	4–6	2.5–3	30 mg every 3–4 hr	10 mg every 3–4 hr
Hydromorphone (Dilaudid)	7.5	1.5	4–6	2–3	6 mg every 3–4 hr	1.5 mg every 3–4 hr
Levorphanol (Levodromeran)	4	2	6–8	12–16	4 mg every 6–8 hr	2 mg every 6–8 hr
Methadone (Dolophine)	20	10	6–8	24	20 mg every 6–8 hr	10 mg every 6–8 hr
Meperidine (Demerol)	300	100	2–3	3–4	Not recommended	100 mg every 3 hr

Adapted from Jacox, A., Carr, D. B., Payne, R., et al. (1994) *Management of cancer pain.* Clinical Practice Guideline No. 9. Agency for Health Care Policy and Research Publication No. 94-0592. Rockville, MD: U.S. Department of Health and Human Services, Public Health Service, Agency for Health Care Policy and Research.

chronic pain, particularly in the elderly. Meperidine has a short duration of action (2.5–3.5 hours), and a poor oral potency (i.e., 50 mg meperidine administered orally is equivalent to 650 mg aspirin or acetaminophen). In addition, chronic administration of meperidine results in the accumulation of a toxic metabolite, normeperidine, which produces central nervous system hyperirritability ranging from changes in mood to tremors, multifocal myoclonus, and seizures. Normeperidine toxicity is increased in patients with impaired renal function (Kaiko et al., 1983).

Codeine is less potent than other opioid analgesics. Thirty mg of oral codeine produces analgesic effects equivalent to 650 mg of aspirin or acetaminophen. Two drugs that require special attention in the elderly are propoxyphene (Darvon) and pentazocine (Talwin) (Ferrell, 1991). Propoxyphene is a controversial drug that is probably overprescribed in the elderly. Reports suggest that its analgesic efficacy is equivalent to that of acetaminophen or aspirin; however, propoxyphene has a significant potential to produce psychological addiction and can precipitate renal failure (Beaver, 1988). Pentazocine is classified as a mixed agonist-antagonist. It should be avoided in the elderly because it has been associated with delirium and agitation.

Opioids can be administered through numerous routes. The oral route is preferred because of its convenience and the relatively predictable blood levels produced (Wall, 1990). Adjustments in doses must be made for parenteral administration owing to the first-pass effect in the liver. Equianalgesic dosing tables (see Table 28–11) must be used when converting from one route of administration to another. The intramuscular route of administration should be avoided because it is painful and absorption is inconsistent (Jacox et al., 1994).

A novel route of opioid administration is the transdermal drug delivery system. Currently, fentanyl (Duragesic) is the only opioid commercially available in a transdermal form. Transdermal delivery bypasses gastrointestinal absorption. Each patch contains a 72-hour supply of fentanyl, which is passively absorbed through the skin. Plasma levels of fentanyl rise slowly from 12 to 18 hours after patch placement, and the elimination half-life is approximately 21 hours. Patients who are receiving sustained-release morphine preparations (i.e., MS Contin, Oramorph SR) or transdermal fentanyl should have an immediate-release morphine preparation available for breakthrough pain.

Patients on opioid analgesics need to be monitored for side effects. The most common side effects associated with the *chronic* administration of opioids and selected management strategies are listed in Table 28–12.

Adjuvant Analgesics

Tricyclic antidepressants and anticonvulsants are two classes of adjuvant analgesics that may be particularly useful for pain problems seen in the elderly. The tricyclic antidepressants are helpful in controlling neuropathic pain (e.g., tic douloureux, postherpetic neuralgia, diabetic neuropathy, and poststroke thalamic pain syndrome). The tricyclic antidepressants act by blocking the reuptake of serotonin and norepinephrine at central nervous system synapses. These drugs are useful as analgesics at doses lower than those required to achieve an antidepressant effect. However, for patients experiencing chronic pain, the tricyclic antidepressants provide analgesia, improve sleep, and may alleviate depression.

In the elderly, the starting dose for the tricyclic antidepressants should be low (usually 10 mg), and the dose should be slowly increased in 10 to 25 mg increments every week until the desired effect is achieved. For most middle-aged individuals, a dose of 150 mg for amitriptyline (Elavil) or doxepin (Sinequan) is usually effective. The tricyclic antidepressants are usually administered 2 hours before bedtime. It may take 4 to 6 weeks for the patient to feel the therapeutic benefit of these drugs (Portenoy, 1992; Wall, 1990). Clinicians must be aware that the tricyclic antidepressants produce anticholinergic side effects, including dry mouth, blurred vision, tachycardia, urinary retention, constipation, confusion, delirium, and cognitive impairment.

The anticonvulsants—which include phenytoin (Dilantin), carbamazepine (Tegretol), sodium valproate (Depakene), and clonazepam (Klonopin)—are useful adjuvant analgesics for managing the lancinating pain of chronic neuralgias (e.g., trigeminal neuralgia, postherpetic neuralgia, glossopharyngeal neuralgia, and posttraumatic neuralgias). These drugs act by suppressing spontaneous neural firing through membrane stabilizing effects. The major dose-

TABLE 28-12
Management of Side Effects Associated with Chronic Opioid Administration

Constipation	1. Start patients on a bowel regimen containing docusate sodium (100–200 mg 2 or 3 times/day) and senna (1–2 tablets at bedtime). 2. Maintain adequate fluid intake. 3. Provide increased roughage if the patient can tolerate this in the diet.
Respiratory depression	1. Not a major problem in patients who are taking opioids chronically. 2. If respiratory depression occurs, withhold a dose of the opioid and stimulate the patient. 3. If an opioid antagonist is required, dilute 1 ampule (0.4 mg) of naloxone in 10 mL normal saline and administer *slowly*, titrating the drug to the patient's respiratory rate.
Sedation	1. Sometimes this side effect is difficult to avoid. 2. Dextroamphetamine in doses of 2.5–5 mg twice a day may be helpful.
Nausea and vomiting	1. Administer antiemetics as needed.

From Miaskowski, C. (1993). Current concepts in the assessment and management of cancer-related pain. *Med Surg Nursing, 2*(1), 113–118.

limiting toxicity for carbamazepine is bone marrow suppression (Wall, 1990).

Guidelines for Prescribing Opioids in the Elderly

Only a limited number of studies have evaluated changes in opioid metabolism or excretion as a result of aging. Early work suggested that elderly patients are more sensitive to the therapeutic effect of morphine than are younger patients (Belville, 1971). This age-related increase is primarily a function of an increased duration of action rather than a peak analgesic effect (Kaiko et al., 1982). Morphine's increased duration of action is most likely explained by the fact that the clearance of morphine is decreased in people older than 50 years. Additional research is needed to better understand age-induced changes in the pharmacokinetics of opioid and nonopioid analgesics.

Given these age-related changes in the pharmacokinetics of opioid analgesics, several principles are worth implementing when using opioid analgesics with the elderly. The old axiom "start low and go slow" is a basic principle to adhere to when initiating and titrating opioid analgesics. Elderly patients older than 70 years should be started on doses of opioids approximately 25 to 50% less than the recommended starting doses (American Pain Society, 1993). Opioids should be titrated slowly to the desired effect or side effects. In most instances, it is appropriate to administer opioid analgesics on a regular schedule—*not* on an as needed basis. The "around-the-clock" administration schedule maintains therapeutic blood levels of the drug. Side effects should be anticipated, and constipation, in particular, should be treated prophylactically. The use of these simple principles should result in optimal pain management for the elderly patient.

Tolerance, Dependence, and Addiction

One of the barriers to effective pain management is fear on the part of elderly patients of becoming addicted to opioid analgesics. This concern needs to be abated, and patients need to be educated about the differences among tolerance, physical dependence, and psychological addiction. Tolerance is a common physiological effect associated with chronic opioid administration. It means that, over time, a larger dose of opioid is required to maintain the same analgesic effect. One of the first signs of developing tolerance is a shortened duration of analgesia. Physical dependence represents a physiological adaptation of the body to an opioid such that abrupt cessation of the opioid produces an abstinence syndrome. Both tolerance and physical dependence are physiological effects associated with chronic opioid administration.

Psychological dependence or addiction is defined as a pattern of compulsive drug use characterized by a continued craving for an opioid and the need to use the opioid for effects other than pain relief (Jacox et al., 1994). Surveys suggest that the appropriate use of opioids rarely results in psychological addiction (Porter & Jick, 1980). Fears of psychological addiction are therefore unwarranted and should not impede appropriate pain management.

NONPHARMACOLOGICAL MANAGEMENT OF PAIN

Often elderly patients may benefit by combining pharmacological and nonpharmacological pain management strategies. Several types of nonpharmacological pain control strategies may be useful with the elderly; these include physical modalities, physical therapy, transelectrical nerve stimulation (TENS), biofeedback, hypnosis, relaxation therapy, and distraction techniques. Elderly patients should have these techniques described and patient preferences sought for use of the different options.

Physical Modalities

Superficial application of heat increases blood flow to the skin and produces vasodilation, which increases oxygen and nutrient delivery to damaged tissues. Heat also decreases joint stiffness by increasing the elastic properties of muscles. The superficial application of heat may be useful for the following conditions: muscle spasms, painful joint stiffness in arthritis, superficial thrombophlebitis, lower back pain, and anorectal pain. Superficial heat can be applied using a dry or moist electric heating pad; hot, moist compresses; or a chemical pack.

Superficial application of cold causes vasoconstriction and local hyperesthesia. This technique may be useful in reducing pain associated with the following conditions: muscle spasms, acute but not severe trauma (e.g., sprained ankle), bursitis, lower back pain, headache, and minor burns. Superficial cold can be applied using waterproof bags, frozen gel packs, or cold compresses.

Both heat and cold are usually applied to the site of pain for 20 to 30 minutes. They should be applied at a comfortable intensity (heat = 40 to 45°C; cold = 15°C). The elderly must be cautioned about the potential for thermal burns occurring with the prolonged use of heat or cold.

Physical therapy and regular exercise may serve as an adjunct to effective pain management and increase mobility and functional status. Elderly patients should be encouraged to exercise on a routine basis to maintain muscle strength, mobilize stiff joints, and maintain coordination, balance, and cardiovascular status.

TENS involves the application of low-voltage electrical stimulation to large, myelinated nerve fibers through skin electrodes to modify pain transmission. In this technique, the patient describes a sensation of tingling or vibration over the sites where the electrodes are applied. Transelectrical nerve stimulation has been used in patients with the following conditions: acute and chronic lower back pain, rheumatoid arthritis, sciatic pain, phantom limb pain, headache, and acute postoperative pain. The overall effectiveness of TENS is somewhat

---

TABLE 28-13
Simple Relaxation Exercises

Example: 1: Deep Breath/Tense, Exhale/Relax, Yawn for Quick Relaxation

1. Clench your fists; breathe in deeply and hold it a moment.
2. Breathe out slowly and go limp as a rag doll.
3. Start yawning.

Additional points: Yawning becomes spontaneous. It is also contagious, so others may begin yawning and relaxing too.

Example 2: Slow Rhythmic Breathing for Relaxation

1. Breathe in slowly and deeply.
2. As you breathe out slowly, feel yourself beginning to relax; feel the tension leaving your body.
3. Now breathe in and out slowly and regularly, at whatever rate is comfortable for you. You may wish to try abdominal breathing. If you do not know how to do abdominal breathing, ask your nurse for help.
4. To help you focus on your breathing and breathe slowly and rhythmically; breathe in as you say silently to yourself, "in, two, three"; breathe out as you say silently to yourself, "out, two, three"; *or* each time you breathe out, say silently to yourself a word such as peace or relax.
5. You may imagine that you are doing this in a place you have found very calming and relaxing for you, such as lying in the sun at the beach.
6. Do steps 1 through 4 only once or repeat steps 3 and 4 for up to 20 minutes.
7. End with a slow deep breath. As you breathe out say to yourself, "I feel alert and relaxed."

Additional points: If you intend to do this for more than a few seconds, try to get in a comfortable position in a quiet environment. You may close your eyes or focus on an object. This technique has the advantage of being very adaptable, in that it may be used for only a few seconds or for up to 20 minutes.

From McCaffery, M., & Beebe, A. (1989). *Pain: Clinical manual for nursing practice.* St. Louis, MO: Mosby-Year Book.

variable, although some patients have received excellent pain relief (Ferrell, 1991).

Cognitive-Behavioral Strategies

The use of cognitive-behavioral strategies such as relaxation, hypnosis, or biofeedback may provide patients with a sense of control over their pain. Although hypnosis and biofeedback require specialized training, clinicians can easily teach patients simple relaxation techniques to reduce pain and enhance their level of comfort. A simple relaxation technique is described in Table 28–13.

Relaxation exercises can be used to alleviate anxiety, reduce muscle tension, decrease pain, and enhance comfort and well-being. Relaxation exercises are easy to learn and require no specialized equipment or training. To facilitate elderly patients' use of this strategy, healthcare professionals can provide patients with relaxation tapes and headsets with recorders. The success of cognitive-behavioral techniques in the elderly has not been evaluated, however, and there may be some limitations in using these techniques with individuals who have cognitive impairments.

SUMMARY

The development of an effective pain management plan for elderly patients requires a coordinated and organized approach. A detailed assessment of the patient forms the cornerstone for the development of the plan. Knowledge of both pharmacological and non-pharmacological pain management strategies allows for the development of an individualized plan of care that includes patient preferences for specific treatment strategies. Plans must be made to ensure compliance with the treatment plan. For example, pain medications should be placed in non-childproof containers for easy access or counted out into a pill box if the patient has poor vision. The clinician must evaluate how much supervision the patient requires to carry out the therapeutic regimen. Only with careful planning and routine follow-up will optimal pain management for elderly patients become a reality.

REFERENCES

Acute Pain Management Guideline Panel (1992). *Acute pain management: Operative or medical procedures and trauma.* Clinical Practice Guideline. Agency for Health Care Policy and Research Publication No. 92-0032. Rockville, MD: U.S. Department of Health and Human Services, Public Health Service, Agency for Health Care Policy and Research.

American Pain Society (1993). *Principles of analgesic use in the treatment of acute pain and cancer pain* (3rd ed.). Skokie, IL: The American Pain Society.

Baum, C., Kennedy, D. L., & Forbes, M. B. (1985). Utilization of nonsteroidal anti-inflammatory drugs. *Arthritis and Rheumatism, 28,* 686–692.

Beaver, W. T. (1988). Impact of nonnarcotic oral analgesics on pain management. *American Journal of Medicine, 84*(5A), 3–15.

Belville, J. W. (1971). Influence of age on pain relief from analgesics: A study of postoperative patients. *Journal of the American Medical Association, 217,* 1835–1841.

Brattberg, G., Mats, T., & Anders, W. (1989). The prevalence of pain in a general population: The results of a postal survey in a county of Sweden. *Pain, 37,* 215–222.

Brooks, P. M., & Day, R. O. (1991). Nonsteroidal anti-inflammatory drugs: Differences and similarities. *New England Journal of Medicine, 324,* 1716–1725.

Carson, J. L., Strom, B. L., Soper, K. A., et al. (1987). The association of nonsteroidal anti-inflammatory drugs with upper gastrointestinal tract bleeding. *Archives of Internal Medicine, 147,* 85–88.

Crook, J., Rideout, E., & Browne, G. (1984). The prevalence of pain complaints among a general population. *Pain, 18,* 299–314.

Davitz, L. L., & Davitz, J. R. (1980). *Nurses' response to patients' suffering.* New York: Springer.

Dull, W. B., & Stratton, M. (1991). Current approaches to chronic pain in older patients. *Geriatrics, 46,* 47–52.

Enck, R. E. (1991). Pain control in ambulatory elderly. *Geriatrics, 46*(3), 49–60.

Ferrell, B. A. (1991). Pain management in elderly people. *Journal of the American Geriatrics Society, 39,* 64–73.

Ferrell, B. A., Ferrell, B. R., & Osterweil, D. (1990). Pain in the nursing home. *Journal of the American Geriatrics Society, 38,* 409–414.

Griffin, M. R., Ray, W. A., & Schaffner, W. (1988). Nonsteroidal anti-inflammatory drug use and death from peptic ulcer in elderly persons. *Annals of Internal Medicine, 109,* 359–363.

Harkins, S. W., Kwentus, J., & Price, D. D. (1984). Pain in the elderly. In C. Benedetti (Ed.), *Advances in pain research and therapy, vol. 7* (pp. 91–105). New York: Raven Press.

Jacox, A., Carr, D. B., Payne, R., et al. (1994). *Management of cancer pain.* Clinical Practice Guideline No. 9. Agency for Health Care Policy and Research Publication No. 94-0592. Rockville, MD: U.S. Department of Health and Human Services, Public Health Service, Agency for Health Care Policy and Research.

Kaiko, R. F., Foley, K. M., Grabinski, P. Y., et al. (1983). Central nervous system excitatory effects of meperidine in cancer patients. *Annals of Neurology, 13*(5), 180–185.

Kaiko, R. F., Wallenstein, S. L., Rogers, A., & Houde, R. W. (1982). Narcotics in the elderly. *Medical Clinics of North America, 66*(5), 1079–1089.

Katz, S., Ford, A. B., Moskowitz, R. W., et al. (1963). Studies in the aged: The index of ADL: A standardized measure of biological and psychosocial function. *Journal of the American Medical Association, 185,* 914–919.

Lau-Ting, C., & Phoon, W. O. (1988). Aches and pains among Singapore elderly. *Singapore Medical Journal, 29,* 164–167.

Lawton, M. P., & Brody, E. M. (1969). Assessment of older people: Self-maintaining and instrumental activities of daily living. *Gerontologist, 9,* 179–186.

Leech-Hofland, S. (1992). Elder beliefs: Blocks to pain management. *Journal of Gerontological Nursing, 18,* 19–24.

Marzinski, L. R. (1991). The tragedy of dementia: Clinically assessing pain in the confused, nonverbal elderly. *Journal of Gerontological Nursing, 17*(6), 25–28.

Melzack, R. (1975). The McGill pain questionnaire: Major properties and scoring methods. *Pain, 1,* 357–381.

Merskey, H. (1986). Classification of chronic pain: Descriptions of chronic pain syndromes and definitions of pain terms. *Pain, 12*(suppl. 3), 51–52.

Miaskowski, C. (1993). Current concepts in the assessment and management of cancer-related pain. *Med Surg Nursing, 2*(1), 113–118.

Office of Technology Assessment (1987). *Losing a million minds.* Washington, D.C.: U.S. Government Printing Office.

Parke, B. (1992). Pain in the cognitively impaired elderly. *The Canadian Nurse, 88,* 17–20.

Portenoy, R. K. (1987). Optimal pain control in elderly cancer patients. *Geriatrics, 42*(5), 33–44.

Portenoy, R. K. (1992). Pain management in the older cancer patient. *Oncology, 6*(2), 86–98.

Porter, J., & Jick, H. (1980). Addiction rare in patients treated with narcotics. *New England Journal of Medicine, 302,* 123.

Reidenberg, M. M. (1982). Drugs in the elderly. *Medical Clinics of North America, 66*(5), 1073–1078.

Roy, R., & Michael, T. (1986). A survey of chronic pain in an elderly population. *Canadian Family Physician, 32,* 513–516.

Sager, D. S., & Bennett, R. M. (1992). Individualizing the risk/benefit ratio of NSAIDs in older patients. *Geriatrics, 47*(8), 24–31.

Sunshine, A., & Olson, N. Z. (1989). Nonnarcotic analgesics. In P. D. Wall & R. Melzack (Eds.), *Textbook of pain* (2nd ed., pp. 670–685). New York: Churchill Livingstone.

Tinetti, M. E. (1986). Performance oriented assessment of mobility problems in elderly patients. *Journal of the American Geriatrics Society, 34,* 119–126.

Wall, R. T. (1990). Use of analgesics in the elderly. *Clinics in Geriatric Medicine, 6*(2), 345–364.

Elder Mistreatment

Terry T. Fulmer

Scope of the Problem	Nursing Management of Elder Mistreatment
Definitional Issues	Intervention
Assessment of Elder Mistreatment	Summary
Prevention of Elder Mistreatment	
Care Across Settings	

The 1990s are on their way to being known as one of the most violent decades in history. Rampant murders, muggings, and domestic violence plague our society. Although considerable attention has been placed on the assessment and management of abused children and battered women, in most healthcare settings it is not standard practice to detect and manage elder abuse. This chapter focuses on the nature of elder abuse, assessment strategies for the detection of mistreatment, and health promotion strategies for the prevention of elder abuse.

SCOPE OF THE PROBLEM

The exact prevalence and incidence of elder mistreatment is unknown. The prevalence of elder abuse is generally estimated at 750,000 to 1.2 million cases annually in the United States. In the most highly regarded epidemiological study, Pillemer and Finkelhor (1988) reported a 32 per 1000 prevalence rate from a randomized sample survey in the Boston area.

Research has been lacking on elder abuse. Clinicians need reliable data to be able to form responsible care plans that meet the needs of abused elders (Fulmer, 1994; Lachs & Fulmer, 1993). The absence of such data is largely because the National Center for Elder Abuse (NCEA; 810 First Avenue N.E., Suite 500, Washington, D.C., 20002-4267; 202-682-0100; fax, 202-289-6959) was not established until recently, nor were there any federal guidelines regarding mistreatment prior to its inception. Today, the NCEA has plans to conduct a national epidemiological survey on the prevalence of elder mistreatment.

Congressional testimony has documented that whereas 1 in 6 cases of child abuse come to public attention, only 1 in 10 cases of elder mistreatment do so (U.S. Select Committee on Aging, House of Representatives, 102nd Congress, 1991). The underreporting of elder mistreatment is related to health professionals' inability to appropriately conceptualize abuse and neglect; this inability stems largely from the fact that gerontology is a relatively young discipline and that clinicians have not been prepared to distinguish abuse from neglect, disease, and old age.

Fulmer and Ashley (1989) described how the cumulative effects of the normal aging process, when co-mingled with disease symptoms as well as any concurrent functional limitations, may mask the signs and symptoms of elder mistreatment. With normal aging, for example, older individuals develop lens opacities and a decreased ability of the lens to accommodate (presbyopia), both of which impair vision. If this visual impairment leads the elder to be poorly groomed or to make errors in self-medication, this might be viewed by some as self-neglect or, in cases where there is a caregiver, neglect. This example vividly illustrates the importance of context when reviewing a case. Clinicians should ask themselves several questions. What is the nature of the caregiving situation? Is there a paid provider or volunteer? Is the caregiver knowledgeable? If the elder has been removed from the situation, did he or she consent to this? Can a better situation be provided? If so, who will pay for it? Given these complex questions, it is not surprising that so many nurses, physicians, and social workers shy away from asking questions about elder abuse and neglect. Support and guidance in the process are essential.

Abuse and neglect have caused alarm in institutional settings such as nursing homes, adult homes, and adult daycare centers. Studies have suggested that vulnerable elderly individuals in these places are at risk for mistreatment (Pillemer & Bachman-Prehn, 1991; Pillemer & Hudson, 1993; Pillemer & Moore, 1989; Tellis-Nayak & Tellis-Nayak, 1989). In a randomized telephone survey of nursing homes in New Hampshire, staff members were asked to report any abuse by others that they had witnessed as well as any abuse that they had committed (Pillemer & Moore, 1989). Thirty-six percent of the 577 nursing personnel surveyed reported that they had seen at least one incident of physical abuse in the last year;

81% had observed psychological abuse; and 23% had witnessed the isolation of an elder. Ten percent of nursing home staff members reported having committed physical abuse, and 40% reported at least one psychologically abusive act. Staff members who reported that they had frequently thought about hitting a patient tended to believe that patients were like children. Nursing home staff members who scored poorly on the Maslach Burnout Inventory, indicating high conflict and a stressful personal life, were more likely to be abusive.

Several risk factors for elder mistreatment have been identified, although the research has been inconsistent, with conflicting information. One study (Lachs et al., 1997) found age, race, poverty, functional and cognitive impairments as risk factors; however, the influence of race and poverty were likely to have been overestimated owing to bias in reporting.

Little is known about the relationship between ethnicity and mistreatment. Generally, studies that have investigated elder abuse among minorities or included them as part of the sample have been inconclusive. In one study (Moon & Williams, 1993), 13 scenarios were used to measure and compare the perceptions of elder abuse and help-seeking behaviors of 90 African American, white, and Korean American older women. Significant group differences existed in the perceptions of elder abuse in six of the scenarios, with the Korean American women significantly less likely than the other groups to perceive a given situation as abusive. Differences were also observed in the intended use of formal and informal sources of help in the elder abuse scenarios, with African American women the least likely to rely on formal help. However, help-seeking patterns should not be overgeneralized because they seem to depend on the nature of the specific situation.

Internationally, even less is known about elder mistreatment. In Israel, Neikrug and Ronen (1993) conducted a survey of Israelis' attitudes regarding elder abuse, in which the severity of abuse was determined from short vignettes told by the subjects. The most severe ratings were given to those elders who resided in institutional settings for the aged. In this study, intrafamily abuse was rated as less severe, and physical abuse consistently more severe, than psychological abuse, neglect, or the abuse of rights and property. In Canada, Podnieks (1992) conducted a randomized telephone survey of 2008 community-dwelling elders. The findings indicated that approximately 40 people per 1000 experienced some form of maltreatment in their home from a relative, partner, or significant other. In Britain, Ogg (1993) conducted a representative survey of 2130 adults aged 65 years and older. Of the 593 individuals who reported mistreatment, 32% reported having been recently verbally abused by a close family member or relative, 2% reported physical abuse, and 2% reported financial abuse. This study suggested that there is currently less elder abuse in Great Britain than in the United States. Cross-national studies are needed for clinicians to learn from other societies about what seems to prevent abuse and neglect.

DEFINITIONAL ISSUES

Varying language is used to describe elder mistreatment. Each state that has a mandatory reporting law also has a set of definitions for operationalizing abuse and neglect. It is important to know which definitions are being used. For example, some definitions of abuse include neglect, whereas others do not. Similarly, neglect is sometimes divided into two subcategories: intentional versus unintentional and active versus passive. (There is, however, some question as to whether the terms *intentional* and *active* have the same meaning, and similarly, whether *unintentional* and *passive* are the same types of abuse.)

Johnson (1989) identified four main categories of elder mistreatment: physical, psychological, neglect, and legal; Table 29–1 identifies these categories along with indicators for each category. Nurses would benefit from a set of standard definitions that can be operationalized in the practice setting. For example, neglect should denote a set of circumscribed behaviors and outcomes that are considered institutional policy and should dovetail with state language.

ASSESSMENT OF ELDER MISTREATMENT

Problems in assessing elders for mistreatment abound. A significant problem is *ageism*, the prejudice that accompanies assessment of the elderly. With ageism, negative stereotypes are attributed to the elder simply because he or she is old. The term *ageism*, first coined by

TABLE 29–1
Indicators of Possible Elder Mistreatment

Physical	Psychological	Neglect-Related	Legal
Medication misuse	Humiliation	Isolation	Material misuse
Absence	Shame	Involuntary withdrawal	Property mismanagement
Improper use	Blame	Voluntary withdrawal	Contract mismanagement
Adverse interactions	Ridicule	Inadequate supervision	Blocked access to property
Unnecessary use	Rejection	Improper supervision	Blocked access to contract
Bodily impairment	Harassment	Role confusion	Theft
Unmet medical needs	Insults	Dependency on elder	Stealing property
Poor hygiene	Intimidation	Excessive expectations	Extorting property
Ingestion problems	Fearfulness	Misuse of living arrangements	Extorting contracts
Rest disturbance	Agitation	Household disorganized	Misuse of rights
Bodily assaults	Manipulation	Lack of privacy	Denied contracting
External injuries	Information withheld	Unfit environment	Involuntary servitude
Internal injuries	Information falsified	Abandonment	Unnecessary guardianship
Sexual assault	Unreasonable emotional dependence		Misuse of professional authority
Suicidal or homicidal act	Interference with decisions		

Adapted from Johnson, T. F. (1991). *Elder mistreatment: Deciding who is at risk* (pp. 19–20). Westport, CT: Greenwood Publishing Group, Inc. Copyright © 1991 by the Greenwood Publishing Group. Reproduced with permission of Greenwood Publishing Group, Inc., Westport, CT.

Robert Butler (1975) in the early 1970s, is illustrated clearly by the following example: If a child presents in an emergency department with multiple bruises in various stages of healing, most clinicians become concerned that child abuse is a possibility and will triage that child appropriately. These same bruises on an elderly person, however, may be overlooked because he or she is old and "all old people bruise easily," or "fall a lot." A major concern is that clinicians do not even ask questions about possible abuse. Advanced practice nurses need to become comfortable saying to

an older person, "You live with your daughter. Is she good to you? Are you happy in that setting? Is there anything that you'd like to say to me privately?"

During the 1990s, different groups and individuals have developed a number of assessment instruments, guidelines, and protocols to assist with the difficult task of assessing elder mistreatment. The Yale–New Haven Hospital in Connecticut uses an assessment form with a set of definitions and indicators to determine whether there is evidence of abuse, neglect, exploitation, or abandonment (Appendix 29–

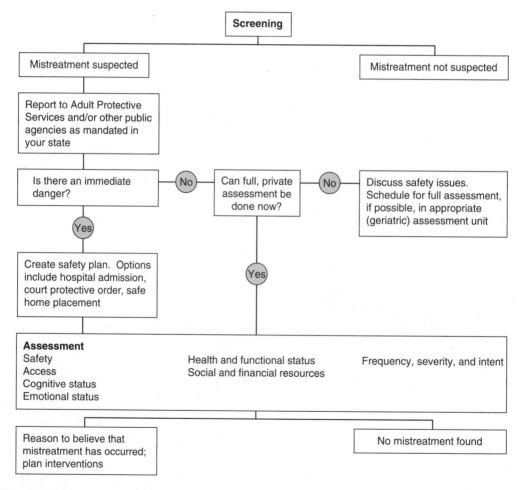

FIGURE 29–1. Screening and assessment for elder mistreatment. (Adapted from American Medical Association [1992]. *Diagnostic and treatment guidelines on elder abuse and neglect.* Chicago: American Medical Association. Copyright 1992 by the American Medical Association.)

1). In their book *Elder abuse and neglect: Causes, diagnosis, and intervention strategies*, Quinn and Tomita (1986) provide several forms and charts that can be easily adapted for use in other settings.

The American Medical Association (AMA; 1992) lists several protocols in addition to their own guidelines that can help assess and manage elder mistreatment (Figs. 29–1 and 29–2). The AMA guidelines provide examples of high-risk signs and symptoms useful in evaluating abuse, neglect, exploitation, and abandonment (Table 29–2) and suggest the key areas for assessment (Table 29–3). They also provide flow charts for the assessment and management of elder mistreatment (Figs. 29–1 and 29–2).

Although the AMA guidelines are excellent, many other helpful guidelines are available through protective service workers across the

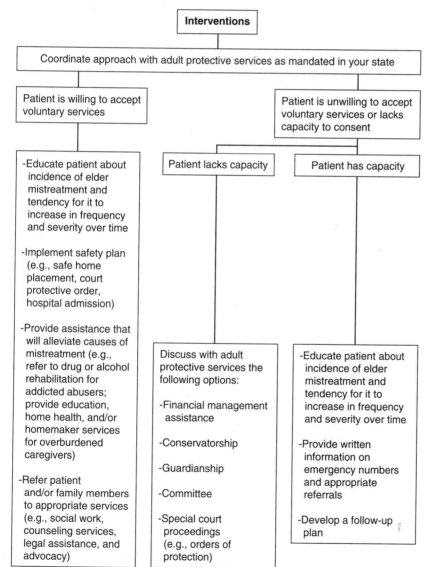

FIGURE 29–2. Interventions for elder mistreatment. (Adapted from American Medical Association [1992]. *Diagnostic and treatment guidelines on elder abuse and neglect.* Chicago: American Medical Association. Copyright 1992 by the American Medical Association.)

TABLE 29-2
High-Risk Signs and Symptoms of Elder Mistreatment

Abuse	Unexplained bruises Repeated falls Laboratory values inconsistent with history Fractures or bruises in various stages of healing *Any report by a patient of being physically abused should be followed up immediately.*
Neglect	Listlessness Poor hygiene Evidence of malnutrition Inappropriate dress Pressure ulcers or urine burns Reports of being left in an unsafe situation Reports of an inability to get needed medications
Exploitation	Unexplained loss of social security or pension checks Any evidence that material goods are being taken in exchange for care Any evidence that elder's personal belongings (e.g., house, jewelry, car) are being taken over without consent or approval of elder
Abandonment	Evidence that someone has "dropped off" elder at the emergency room or the family unit with no intention of coming back for him or her
Other High-Risk Situations	Drug or alcohol addiction in the family Isolation of the elder History of untreated psychiatric problems Evidence of unusual family stress Excessive dependence of elder on caretaker

country. Fulmer and Ashley (1986) provide a comprehensive review of assessment instruments that can help advanced practice nurses establish a procedure to detect and manage elder mistreatment. Open-ended formats and checklists are used as well as intensive interviews and structured protocols. The American Public Welfare Foundation in Washington, D.C., which houses the National Center for Abuse and Neglect, has a compendium of other screening instruments.

The choice of assessment format is based entirely on individual or agency preference, as there is no singularly correct way to assess for elder mistreatment. For some agencies, a narrative flow sheet detailing the patient's history works best. For other agencies, computerized Likert-type checklists are better. The assessment format selected will depend on the purpose of the assessment and how the data will be stored, compiled, and retrieved. The

key is to ensure that a process for evaluation is standardized before an elder abuse event is found.

At a minimum, every emergency department should have a protocol for detecting elder mistreatment. Just as clinicians ask questions about smoking and alcohol intake when taking a patient history, the assessment of every older individual should include an evaluation for possible mistreatment.

The creation of new forms and regulations for elder abuse and neglect assessment usually leads to a period of overreporting, as clinicians struggle to do the right thing by reporting, even when they would not previously have done so for a given symptom. This means that an elder who is not abused or neglected may be suspected and reviewed. Although some people may argue that a false positive is better than a false negative, such a review can be extremely disruptive to the caregiving system

<table>
<tr><td>

TABLE 29-3

Key Areas of Assessment for Elder Mistreatment

</td></tr>
</table>

Safety
Access
Cognitive status
Emotional status
Health and functional status
Social and financial status
Resources
Frequency, severity, and intent of abuse

Adapted from American Medical Association (1992). *Diagnostic and treatment guidelines on elder abuse and neglect.* Chicago: American Medical Association. Copyright 1992 by the American Medical Association.

and potentially harmful to someone trying his or her best to give good care. Most people, as in the case of child abuse, understand that such reporting is for the well-being of the elder and can justify the intrusion on that basis.

The best way to handle overreporting is to formulate an internal reporting mechanism. This can be an agency elder abuse team or one clinician who is willing to review all reports so that they can be considered carefully before a final report is made. False positive reporting has its hazards: Elders may lose their care provider if that care provider is insulted by the accusation, or they may be subjected to a police investigation. Conversely, a false negative case means that the abuse or neglect of an elder has gone undetected and unassessed and may be repeated. Therefore, it may be wise to set up a process that allows for overreporting to an internal screen before state offices are called.

In most states, after a report of elder abuse or neglect has been made, a protective services worker meets with the elder to verify the case. The elder is interviewed, and in some cases a medical agency becomes involved if the elder is in serious condition. Some states liberally provide protective services, whereas others have no such mechanism. The advanced practice nurse should become familiar with the process in his or her community and facility and should learn the appropriate channels for processing these concerns.

PREVENTION OF ELDER MISTREATMENT

Interventions that promote health and prevent elder mistreatment have two main facets: (1) actions that empower the elder and (2) actions on behalf of the nurse that ensure an adequate system of care. The American Association of Retired Persons has published a pamphlet entitled "Domestic Mistreatment of the Elderly: Toward Prevention/Some Dos and Don'ts" (1987). This pamphlet provides excellent health promotion suggestions directed toward the elderly individual, his or her family, and the community. To maintain autonomy and visibility, older people are encouraged to stay involved and participate socially to the greatest degree possible. They are advised to keep accurate records of financial accounts and property and to seek help when needed in maintaining such records. Elders are also strongly encouraged to leave abusive situations and seek the safety of friends and family who can help them when they are the victims of mistreatment. The pamphlet recommends that families discuss older relatives' wishes regarding healthcare and prepare for potential incapacitation by planning which family member will take responsibility when an elder needs help. Many agencies have similar pamphlets and brochures that are directed toward educating the elderly person and the public about the nature of elder mistreatment and actions that can be taken to stop it.

When an individual is being victimized, elder protective service workers are available to help in almost every community. Abuse is most frequently reported by a neighbor or friend who calls in to report a suspicion of elder mistreatment on behalf of an elderly individual. In some instances, the elder reports on his or her own behalf, but this is not common. Once the report has been made, an individual in the state department on aging or health and human services visits the elder and conducts an assessment to confirm whether elder mistreatment has occurred. If the abuse or neglect is confirmed, the case is opened, which leads to the provision of a large array and intensity of services (e.g., Meals on Wheels, home health aides, and case management) that ensure the safety and well-being of the elderly individual. If the caseworker does not concur that the elder has been mistreated or if the elderly individual refuses any services, the caseworker documents this information and the case is closed. It is not unusual for a particular older individual to be reported more than once in a given year or, in some cases, as many as four times within a year. In the absence of documentation that anything has been done, communities should be concerned about individuals who are being repeatedly reported. The consequences of omission—that is, of missing elder mistreatment—are very serious.

CARE ACROSS SETTINGS

Excellent communication across care systems is another way to stem the tide of elder mistreatment. As community health nurses, long-term care nurses, and acute care nurses become more comfortable with consulting each other to compare care plans, less of the rich clinical picture will be lost. This will become increasingly important, if not required, in a managed care healthcare system. Elder abuse and neglect victims will be less likely to fall between the cracks when improved methods of data transfer are developed.

NURSING MANAGEMENT OF ELDER MISTREATMENT

When nurses learn to ask the question "Is this elderly person a victim of mistreatment?," it will make a dramatic impact in stemming the violence against elders. With 2.2 million nurses in the United States, the health policy implications of revising practice to incorporate an elder abuse assessment are extraordinary. Clinical guidelines for elder mistreatment can be made readily available to nurses in all areas of practice and tailored to fit the practice environment. The most important and first step in detecting and assessing elder mistreatment is for acute care or community health nurses to be suspicious of any unusual signs or symptoms that do not fit logically with the patient, family, or caregiver's history (Table 29–4). The

documentation of potential abuse should include a careful record of the chief complaint along with the patient's history, detailed descriptions of any injuries, and abnormal laboratory values. In some instances, it may be important to take color photographs to document the elderly person's health status. The AMA guidelines (1992) provide useful documentation on how best to take such pictures:

1. Use color film
2. Photograph from different angles
3. Use a ruler to illustrate the size of an injury
4. Include the patient's face in at least one picture
5. Take at least two pictures of every trauma area
6. Mark the photographs with the patient's name and the date, time, and photographer; keep the materials in a confidential, safe location

In practice, nurses are concerned about the legal implications of becoming involved in a court case. The key issue is the absence of malicious intent and the documentation of elder mistreatment. When the nurse reports in "good faith," the law protects him or her even when elder mistreatment is not confirmed. The benefit of taking a stand may well be that of saving the elderly person's life. In summary, the key steps in approaching elder mistreatment are astute assessment, careful documentation (using pictures if necessary), and following through with the appropriate agencies.

Intervention

Once elder mistreatment is suspected, the most important action nurses can take is to work with the elder on a safety plan that he or she finds plausible and acceptable. As in other domestic violence situations, this may not be the first time that mistreatment has occurred. The nurse should ask the older person what he or she usually does when violence (or neglect or exploitation) occurs and how successful that plan has been in resolving the situation. Frequently, plans have been tried that do not use the full array of local and state agency

TABLE 29-4

Physical and Psychological Indicators of Elder Mistreatment

Type of Mistreatment	Possible Indicators

Abuse	Unexplained bruises and welts
	    on face, lips, or mouth
	    on torso, back, buttocks, or thighs
	    in various stages of healing
	    clustered, forming regular patterns
	    reflecting shape of article used to inflict the injury (e.g., electric cord, belt buckle)
	    that regularly appear after absence, weekend, or vacation
	Unexplained burns
	    from cigars or cigarettes, especially on soles, palms, or back of buttocks
	    from immersion (socklike, glovelike, and doughnut shaped on buttocks or genitalia)
	    patterned like electric burner or iron
	    from ropes on arms, legs, neck, or torso
	Unexplained fractures
	    to skull, nose, or facial structure
	    multiple or spiral, in various stages of healing
	Unexplained lacerations or abrasions
	    to mouth, lips, gums, or eyes
	    to external genitalia

Neglect	Consistent hunger, poor hygiene, or inappropriate dress Consistent lack of supervision, especially in dangerous activities or during long periods Constant fatigue or listlessness Unattended physical problems or medical needs Abandonment
Exploitation	Unexplained loss of social security or pension checks Evidence of materials being exchanged for services Threats of withdrawal of services if no exchange
Sexual Abuse	Difficulty in walking or sitting Torn, stained, or bloody underclothing Pain or itching in genital area Bruises or bleeding in external genitalia or vaginal or anal areas Venereal disease
Psychological Abuse	Behavior such as sucking, biting, or rocking Antisocial, destructive behavior Sleep disorders Speech disorders Hysteria Obsession Compulsion Phobias Hypochondriasis

Adapted from American Medical Association (1992). *Diagnostic and treatment guidelines on elder abuse and neglect.* Chicago: American Medical Association. Copyright 1992 by the American Medical Association.

services. Programs such as those run by State Offices for Aging can be very successful in changing elder mistreatment patterns; these programs can include Adult Protective Services, Meals on Wheels, Alzheimer's disease support groups, and victim services support groups. In some instances, direct communication and planning with local police may be essential. Alcohol counselors, drug counselors, clergy, social workers, and visiting nurses may already be known to the family and may have important insights into what has been tried in the past, what works best, and what triggers mistreatment events. The AMA flow chart on intervention strategies (1992; see Fig. 29–2) can serve as a useful guide for all clinicians as they cope with the difficult care planning required in these situations.

Nurses should be strongly encouraged to use an interdisciplinary team approach to solve problems in such cases. The nature of elder mistreatment events warrants a full array of professional perspectives to ensure the best possible outcome for the older adult.

SUMMARY

Advanced practice nurses have a key role in detecting and managing elder mistreatment. Thus, it is important for nurses to incorporate assessment strategies for elder abuse and neglect and to teach the requisite health promotion actions that can inform elders, their families, and communities about preventing elder mistreatment. Interdisciplinary collaboration is essential in managing elder mistreatment, as a full range of services may be required to achieve the best outcome for the mistreated individual.

REFERENCES

American Association of Retired Persons (1987). *Domestic mistreatment of the elderly: Toward prevention/Some dos and don'ts* [Pamphlet]. Washington, D.C.: American Association of Retired Persons.

American Medical Association (1992, November). *Diagnostic and treatment guidelines on elder abuse and neglect*, AA22: 92-698 20M. Chicago: American Medical Association.

Butler, R. (1975). *Why survive? Being old in America.* New York: Harper and Row.

Fulmer, T. T. (1994). Elder mistreatment. *Annual Review of Nursing Research, 12*, 51–64.

Fulmer, T. T., & Ashley, J. (1986). Neglect: What part of abuse? *Pride Institute Journal, 5*, 18–24.

Fulmer, T. T., & Ashley, J. (1989). Clinical indicators of elder abuse. *Applied Nursing Research, 2*(4), 161–167.

Johnson, T. F. (1989). Elder mistreatment identification instruments: Finding common ground. *Journal of Elder Abuse and Neglect, 1*(4), 15–36.

Lachs, M., & Fulmer, T. (1993). Recognizing elder abuse and neglect: *Clinics in Geriatric Medicine, 9*(3), 665–681.

Lachs, M. S., Williams, C., & O'Brien, S. (1997). Risk factors for reported elder abuse and neglect: A nine-year observational cohort study. *Gerontologist, 37*, 469–474.

Moon, A., & Williams, O. (1993). Perceptions of elder abuse and help-seeking patterns among African-American, Caucasian American, and Korean-American elderly women. *Gerontologist, 33*(3), 386–395.

Neikrug, S. M., & Ronen, M. (1993) Elder abuse in Israel. *Journal of Elder Abuse and Neglect, 5*(3), 1–19.

Ogg, J. (1993) Researching elder abuse in Britain. *Journal of Elder Abuse and Neglect, 5*(2), 37–54.

Pillemer, K., & Bachman-Prehn, R. (1991). Helping and hurting: Predictor of maltreatment of patients in nursing homes. *Research on Aging, 13*, 74–95.

Pillemer, K., & Finkelhor, D. (1988). The prevalence of elder abuse: A random sample survey. *Gerontologist, 28*, 51–57.

Pillemer, K., & Hudson, B. (1993). A model abuse prevention program for nursing assistants. *Gerontologist, 33*, 128–131.

Pillemer, K., & Moore, D. W. (1989). Abuse of patients in nursing homes: Findings from a survey of staff. *Gerontologist, 29*, 314–320.

Podnieks, E. (1992). National survey on abuse of the elderly in Canada. *Journal of Elder Abuse and Neglect, 4*, 5–58.

Quinn, M. J., & Tomita, S. K. (1986). *Elder abuse and neglect: Causes, diagnosis, and intervention strategies.* New York: Springer.

Tellis-Nayak, V., & Tellis-Nayak, M. (1989). Quality of care and the burden of two cultures: When the world of the nurse's aide enters the world of the nursing home. *Gerontologist, 29*, 307–313.

U.S. Select Committee on Aging, House of Representatives, 102nd Congress. *Elder abuse: What can be done?* Publication No. 1020808, May 15, 1991, 17–19.

U.S. Senate Select Committee on Aging (1991). *Aging America: Trends and projections.* Department of Health and Human Services Publication No. 91-28001, National Council on Aging.

Elder Abuse Assessment Form

PATIENT STAMP

Date: _____ Person completing form: _____

PATIENT INFORMATION

Name: _____ Age: _____ Unit #: _____

Street Address: _____

City, State, Zip: _____ Telephone #: _____

Residence: Home ☐   Nursing Home ☐

Accompanied to Emergency Department by: _____
Name

_____
Street Address   City, State, Zip

Telephone #: _____ Relationship to Patient: _____

Family Contact Person: _____
Name

_____
Street Address   City, State, Zip   Telephone #

Reason for visit (please check primary reason):

Cardiac ☐   Orthopedic ☐   Fall ☐   Gastrointestinal ☐   Psychiatric ☐

Changed mental status ☐   Other (describe) _____

Current mental status:

Oriented ☐   Confused ☐   Unresponsive ☐

Who provides home care? _____

1. **GENERAL ASSESSMENT**

	Good	Bad	Uncertain	Cannot Get Information
a. Clothing				
b. Hygiene				
c. Nutrition				
d. Skin integrity				

Additional Comments: _____

_____

_____

_____

_____

2. **POSSIBLE ABUSE INDICATORS**

	Yes	No	Uncertain	Cannot Get Information
a. Bruising				
b. Lacerations				
c. Fractures				
d. Various stages of healing of any bruises or fractures				
e. Evidence of sexual abuse				
f. Statement by elder regarding abuse				

3. POSSIBLE NEGLECT INDICATORS

	Yes	No	Uncertain	Cannot Get Information
a. Contractures				
b. Pressure ulcers				
c. Dehydration				
d. Diarrhea				
e. Depression				
f. Impaction				
g. Malnutrition				
h. Urine burns				
i. Poor hygiene				
j. Repetitive falls				
k. Failure to respond to warning of obvious disease				
l. Inappropriate medications (under or over)				
m. Repetitive hospital admissions owing to probable failure of healthcare surveillance				
n. Statement by elder regarding neglect				

4. POSSIBLE EXPLOITATION INDICATORS

	Yes	No	Uncertain	Cannot Get Information
a. Misuse of money				
b. Evidence				
c. Reports of demands for goods in exchange for services				
d. Inability to account for money or property				
e. Statement by elder regarding exploitation				

5. POSSIBLE ABANDONMENT INDICATORS

	Yes	No	Uncertain	Cannot Get Information
a. Evidence that a caretaker has withdrawn care precipitously without alternate arrangements				
b. Evidence that the elder is left alone in an unsafe environment for extended periods of time without adequate support				
c. Statement by elder regarding abandonment				

SUMMARY

	Yes	No	Uncertain	Cannot Get Information
a. Evidence of abuse				
b. Evidence of neglect				
c. Evidence of exploitation				
d. Evidence of abandonment				

COMMENTS

Copyright 1992 by Terry T. Fulmer.

Index